Advances in Controlled and Novel Drug Delivery

Advances in Controlled and Novel Drug Delivery

Edited by :

N.K. JAIN Ph.D.
Prof.,Deptt. of Pharmaceutical Sciences
Dr. H.S. Gour Vishwavidyalaya
Sagar(M.P.) 470003

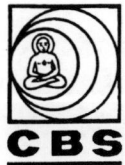

C B S

CBS Publishers & Distributors Pvt. Ltd.

New Delhi • Bengaluru • Chennai • Kochi • Kolkata • Mumbai
Hyderabad • Nagpur • Patna • Pune • Vijayawada

Advances in Control & Novel Drug Delivery

ISBN: 978-81-239-0727-7

First Edition: 2001

Reprint: 2003, 2006, 2008, 2010, 2011, 2013, 2017, 2023

Published by **Satish Kumar Jain** and produced by **Varun Jain** for
CBS Publishers & Distributors Pvt Ltd
4819/XI Prahlad Street, 24 Ansari Road, Daryaganj, New Delhi 110 002, India
Ph: 011-23289259, 23266861   Website: www.cbspd.com
                                    e-mail: delhi@cbspd.com

Corporate Office: 204 FIE, Industrial Area, Patparganj, Delhi 110 092, India
Ph: 011-4934 4934   Fax: 011-4934 4935   e-mail: publishing@cbspd.com;
                                    publicity@cbspd.com

Branches

- **Bengaluru:** Seema House 2975, 17th Cross, KR Road, Banasankari 2nd Stage, Bengaluru 560 070, Karnataka, India
  Ph: +91-80-26771678/79   Fax: +91-80-26771680   e-mail: bangalore@cbspd.com
- **Chennai:** 7, Subbaraya Street, Shenoy Nagar, Chennai 600 030, Tamil Nadu, India
  Ph: +91-44-26680620, 26681266   Fax: +91-44-42032115   e-mail: chennai@cbspd.com
- **Kochi:** 42/1325, 1326, Power House Road, Opp KSEB, Power House, Ernakulum Kochi 682 018, Kerala, India
  Ph: +91-484-4059061-65,67   Fax: +91-484-4059065   e-mail: kochi@cbspd.com
- **Kolkata:** 147, Hind Ceramics Compound, 1st Floor, Nilgunj Road, Belghoria, Kolkata-700056, West Bengal, India
  Ph: +033-25633055, 033-25633056   e-mail: kolkata@cbspd.com
- **Lucknow:** Basement, Khushnuma Complex, 7 Meerabai Marg (Behind Jawahar Bhawan),Lucknow-226001, UP, India
  Ph: +91-522-4000032   e-mail: tiwari.lucknow@cbspd.com
- **Mumbai:** PWD Shed, Gala no 25/26, Ramchandra Bhatt Marg, Next to JJ Hospital Gate no. 2, Opp. Union Bank of India Noorbaug, Mumbai-400009, Maharashtra, India
  Ph: 022-66661880/89   e-mail: mumbai@cbspd.com

Representatives

- Hyderabad   0-9885175004
- Patna   0-9334159340
- Jharkhand   0-9811541605
- Pune   0-9923910676
- Nagpur   0-9421945513
- Uttarakhand   0-9716462459

Printed at   Glorious Printers, Daryaganj, Delhi, India

Foreword

I have gone through the contents of the book "Advances in Controlled and Novel Drug Delivery" edited by Prof. N. K. Jain containing advanced information on various latest novel drug delivery systems. Prof. Jain has been working in this field for many years and has gained great insight in the subject of his specialization. All the chapters have been authored by dedicated academicians and scientists actively engaged in the field of design and development of advanced drug delivery systems. As a proven expert in this field for more than 30 years, I foresee that this book will be of great value not only to P.G. teachers and research scholars in the field of Pharmaceutics, but also to the industrial R&D scientists. The work contains substantial data for approving such new and novel drug delivery systems for the drug control administration. In the post-GATT era, a number of biotechnologically derived protein-rugs would have to be delivered for treatment of various diseases more effectively or in the case of gene therapy. The overall exposure of the subject by the various authors of different chapters of this book would go a long way in throwing new light in the area of advanced drug delivery.

I wish this endeavor great success which has culminated as a result of devotion, dedication and hard work of Prof. N. K. Jain, presently Professor of Pharmaceutics at Dr. H.S. Gour University, Sagar. I am confident the book will be very useful to pharmaceutical academics and scientists.

PROF. B. K. GUPTA
former Head of the Department,
Pharmaceutical Technology, Jadavpur University.
Hon'ble Chairman,
17 Sept., 2000
Calcutta
Gluconate Health Ltd.,
(A Govt. of West Bengal Undertaking)
President, Pharmacy Council, W.B.,
President, Indian Pharmaceutical Association, W.B. Branch,
Member, AICTE (ERC).

Preface

The optimum use of drugs for therapeutic purposes would be greatly improved by the possibili , of introducing them selectively into those cells where the pharmacological action is desired.

At the end of the nineteenth century, Paul Ehrlich suggested the use of "bodies which possess a particular affinity for a certain organ as carrier by which to bring therapeutically active groups to the organ in question". Unfortunately even today the concept is still at the experimental stage and has not been translated into practice.

Controlled and novel drug delivery envisage optimized drug delivery in the sense that the therapeutic efficacy of a drug is optimized which also implies nil or minimum side effects. It is expected that the twenty first century would witness sea changes in the area of drug delivery. The products may be more potent as well as safer. The conventional drug delivery systems and methods of administration may change drastically paving the way for more and more products based on genetic engineering, reflecting closer cooperation of scientists from different branches of science. Target specific drug delivery is likely to overcome much of the criticism of conventional dosage forms. The cumulative outcome could be summarized as 'optmized drug delivery' that encompasses greater potency and greater effectiveness, lesser side effects and toxicity, better stability, low cost hence greater accessibility, ease of administration, and best patient compliance. This is highly significant for the majority of world population particularly in underdeveloped and developing countries. The consumer awareness is likely to increase enormously so also the accountability of the manufacturer. Increasing competition amongst manufacturers may bring excellence and novelty in drug products.

The book entitled "Controlled and Novel Drug Delivery" edited by this author and published in 1997 comprised of seventeen exclusive chapters and its success, as a multi-author book of its own kind in India, is overwhelming. It has been widely accepted as a ready reference by scientists in academia and industry alike. Encouraged by such a response and the requests from colleagues and friends the editor is too pleased to accept the challenge and the present volume is the outcome. The book has 19 chapters and the greater emphasis is on the advances in Novel Drug Delivery. The subject matter encompasses topics from Ion-exchange resinates to Dendrimers, from Colon to Pulmonary drug delivery, from Implants to Nanoerythrosomes, Cancer chemotherapy, Protein and peptide drug delivery, Targeted drug delivery etc. Each chapter presents a review of the literature and conclusions include scope for further research. Thus an attempt has been made to provide most consolidated and uptodate information on different topics which is a time consuming and strenuous task otherwise.

The cooperation extended by the authors of different chapters is exemplary who have been kind enough to accommodate various types of editorial requests. My students Dr. Ajay Khopade, Dr. Sanjay Jain, Mr. Alok Namdeo and Mr. Prabhat Ranjan Mishra have been helpful in many ways. Mr. Satish Jain and Mr. Vinod Jain of CBS publishers and distributors have left no stone unturned in making this book a good presentation. Members of my family allowed me to encroach upon their time without making demands or complaints. I gratefully acknowledge all of them.

The learned readers and post-graduate students in India and abroad have been a constant source of encouragement and I request all of them to write to me about this book. The credit for any positive assessment goes to the authors of different chapter and shortcomings, if any, are attributable to me, as editor.

Sagar : 27 September, 2000

Professor N. K. Jain

List of Contributors

H. P. Bharadwaj, Ph.D.
Chief Research Scientist
Pharma Division
Wockhardt Research Centre
Aurangabad - 411 029 (M. S.)

N. S. Parmar, Ph.D.
Professor and Principal
K. B. Institute of Pharmaceutical Education &
Research
Gandhingar - 382 003 (Guj.)

S. K. Vyas, M. Pharm.
Torrent Research Centre
Gandhinagar - 382 428 (Guj.)

Navin Vaya, M. Pharm.
Torrent Research Centre
Gandhinagar - 382 428 (Guj.)

U. V. Singh, M. Pharm.
Department of Pharmaceutics
College of Pharmaceutical Sciences
Manipal - 576 119 (Karnataka)

B. Dinesh Shenoy, M. Pharm.
Department of Pharmaceutics
College of Pharmaceutical Sciences
Manipal - 576 119 (Karnataka)

N. Udupa, Ph.D.
Professor and Principal
College of Pharmaceutical Sciences
Manipal - 576 119 (Karnataka)

Padma V. Devarajan, Ph.D.
Reader in Pharmaceutics
University Department of Pharmaceutical
Technology
Mumbai - 400 019 (M.S.).

Y. S. R. Krishnaiah, M. Pharm.
Department of Pharmaceutical Sciences
Andhra University
Vishakhapatnam - 530 003 (A.P.)

S. Satyanarayan, Ph.D.
Professor of Pharmaceutis
Department of Pharmaceutical Sciences
Andhra University
Vishakhapatnam - 530 003 (A.P.)

A.N. Mishra, Ph.D.
Professor of Pharmaceutics
Pharmacy Department
Faculty of Technology and Engineering
M. S. University of Baroda
Vadodara - 390 001 (Guj.)

S. G. Deshpande, Ph.D.
C.U. Shah College of Pharmacy
S. N. D.T. Womens University
Mumbai - 400 049 (M.S.)

Amrita Bajaj, Ph.D.
C.U. Shah College of Pharmacy
S. N. D.T. Womens University
Mumbai - 400 049 (M.S.)

Sujata P. Sawarkar, M. Pharm.
C.U. Shah College of Pharmacy
S. N. D.T. Womens University
Mumbai - 400 049 (M.S.)

R. S. R. Murthy, Ph.D.
Professor of Pharmaceutics
Pharmacy Department
Faculty of Technology and Engineering
M. S. University of Baroda
Vadodara - 390 001 (Guj.)

Anilkumar S. Gandhi, M. Pharm.
University Department of Pharmaceutical
Technology
Mumbai - 400 019 (M.S.)

Alok Namdeo, M. Pharm.
Department of Pharmaceutical Sciences
Dr. H. S. Gour University
Sagar - 470 003 (M.P.)

N. K. Jain, Ph.D.
Professor of Pharmaceutics
Department of Pharmaceutical Sciences
Dr. H. S. Gour University
Sagar - 470 003 (M.P.)

M. Vimla Devi, Ph.D.
Professor of Pharmaceutics
Department of Pharmaceutical Sciences
Andhra University
Vishakhapatnam - 530 003 (A.P.)

P. S. S. Krishna Babu, M. Pharm.
Department of Pharmaceutical Sciences
Andhra University
Vishakhapatnam - 530 003 (A.P.)

J. K. Pandit, Ph.D.
Reader in Pharmaceutics
Department of Pharmaceutics
Banaras Hindu University
Varanasi - 221 005 (U.P.)

Romi Bharat, M. Pharm.
Department of Pharmaceutics
Banaras Hindu University
Varanasi - 221 005 (U.P.)

S. K Jain, Ph.D.
Reader in Pharmaceutics
Department of Pharmaceutical Sciences
Dr. H. S. Gour University
Sagar - 470 003 (M.P.)

Girish K. Jain, Ph.D.
Assistant Director
Division of Pharmaceutics
Central Drug Research Institute
Lucknow - 226 001 (U.P.)

Sanjay Jain, Ph.D.
Lecturer of Pharmaceutics
Department of Pharmaceutical Sciences
Dr. H. S. Gour University
Sagar - 470 003 (M.P.)

Ajay J. Khopde, Ph.D.
Research Scientist
Sun Pharmaceutical Advanced Research
Centre
Vadodora (Guj.)

Shelly Utreja, M. Pharm.
Department of Pharmaceutical Sciences
Dr. H. S. Gour University
Sagar (M.P.) - 470 003

Subheet Jain
Department of Pharmaceutical Sciences
Dr. H. S. Gour University
Sagar - 470 003 (M.P.)

Deepankar Bhadra
Department of Pharmaceutical Sciences
Dr. H. S. Gour University
Sagar - 470 003 (M.P.)

Roop K. Khar, Ph.D.
Professor of Pharmaceutics
Department of Pharmaceutics
Faculty of Pharmacy
Jamia Hamdard
New Delhi - 110 062.

Manish Diwan, Ph.D.
Reproductive Health and Vaccinology
International Centre for Genetic Engineering
& Biotechnology
New Delhi- 110 067.

Contents

Chapter 1

Biodegradable Microparticles of Peptide Drugs Using Polylactide Polymers

H. P. Bhagwatwar

1.1 ABSTRACT

Presently, peptides and proteins are available in plenty due to advances in synthetic chemistry, fermentation technology and recombinant technology. Most of these molecules have to be administered daily because of their short half-lives in-vivo, and parenterally because of their inherent chemical and physical instability, for extended periods of time causing discomfort to the patients and resulting in non-compliance. The challenge facing the pharmaceutical scientist lies in the development of controlled release formulations capable of reducing the frequency of dosing while providing reproducible, controlled plasma levels of the drug over extended periods of time. A few such products based on microencapsulation with biodegradable polymers are now available with quite a few more under development. Several researchers have reviewed the different methods of microencapsulation. But, a logical approach to the development of a process for the encapsulation of peptides for controlled release is missing. This chapter is an attempt to describe the logical development of the water-in-oil-in-water technique of microencapsulation for peptide drugs within biodegradable polymers.

1.2 INTRODUCTION

Peptides/polypeptides have gained considerable interest in the treatment of different disease conditions. Although various routes of administration (nasal, parenteral, vaginal, oral, transdermal, etc.) have been investigated for their delivery most products are administered parenterally because of their inherent physical and chemical instability and short biological half-lives (Lee, 1991). Usually a solution or a suspension formulation of the peptide (e.g. insulin, leuprolide, busereline, calcitonin, etc.) is administered intravenously, subcutaneously or intramuscularly. Repeated administration is essential to achieve prolonged effects over extended periods of time. Thus, controlled release parenteral dosage forms, which reduce the frequency of administration and minimize the fluctuations in plasma levels caused by repeated injections are essential.

Certain devices allow the continuous administration of a solution /suspension of the peptide at programmed rates over extended periods of time (external or implantable infusion pumps). These systems require implantation through surgery, causing discomfort to the patient and result in loss of patient compliance. Similarly, after the completion of drug release the systems may require surgical recovery. Alternatively, peptides could be entrapped in implants (gosereline acetate, Zoladex, ICI Pharmaceuticals) which has to be injected under the abdominal skin under local anesthesia. A drug delivery system which can be administered through a normal 22-23 gauge needle and which will not need surgical recovery after complete drug release is required. Biodegradable polymers are alternatives to these above-mentioned systems for the delivery of peptides.

A liquid injectable system capable of forming a biodegradable implant was developed (Dunn et al, 1994). The system comprises a biodegradable polymer dissolved in a biocompatible organic solvent such as N-methyl pyrrolidone, with a drug dissolved/dispersed in the polymer solution. The mixture upon being injected subcutaneously/intramuscularly through a conventional 22-23 gauge needle comes into contact with body fluids and causes the precipitation of the polymer forming an implant to entrap the drug substance for prolonged release through biodegradation. The system has the disadvantage that the implant formed varies in shape and size depending upon the site of injection.

Another viable alternative to this system is biodegradable drug delivery systems based on microencapsulation. Microencapsulation is a process by which a drug substance is entrapped within discrete free-flowing polymeric particle microencapsule products (Sanders et al, 1986; Mason-Garcia et al., 1988; Ogawa et al., 1988 a, b, c; Ruiz et al., 1989; Csernus et al., 1990; Cohen et al., 1991; Heya et al., 1991; Hermann & Bodmeier, 1995; Bittner et al., 1998).

Several methods of microencapsulation are known including solvent evaporation, phase separation, spray drying, supercritical fluid extraction, etc. Of these methods, the solvent evaporation method has attracted the most attention because of its ease of use and scale-up, lower residual solvent potential etc.

Table 1.1 : Commercially available controlled release peptide formulations

Drug substance	Brand name	Company
Leuprolide acetate	Lupron Depot	TAP Pharmaceuticals
Goserelin acetate	Zoladex	I.C.I.
Triptorelin	Decapeptyl	Debiopharma
Busereline acetate	Bigonist	Laboratoires Cassenne

A recent article which describes the United States Food and Drug Administration (USFDA) viewpoint on microencapsulated products for parenteral depot administration (Niu & Chiu, 1998) emphasizes the following : 1. polymer/copolymer, 2. organic solvents, 3. copolymer-peptide complexes, 4. sterilization, 5. in-vitro-in-vivo correlation's, 6. particle size, 7. diluent - suspending vehicle

The purpose of this chapter is to highlight the water-in-oil-in-water (w/o/w) emulsion solvent evaporation method for encapsulation of peptides within polylactide polymers and to serve as a guideline for the rational development of such a product. An attempt is made to bring out the interplay of the formulation and processing parameters affecting this process keeping the USFDA viewpoints in perspective.

1.3 DEVELOPMENT OF A MICROENCAPSULATION PROCEDURE

The oil-in-water (o/w) solvent evaporation method, also known as "in-water drying", originally developed for the encapsulation of water-insoluble drugs has been extensively used to date and its use with polylactide polymers was reviewed in detail (Jalil & Nixon, 1989, 1990 a &b). The method involves the preparation of a solution of a wall forming polymer in a water-immiscible organic solvent into which the drug is dissolved directly or with the aid of a cosolvent or dispersed in a fine state. This is then added in a controlled fashion into an aqueous solution of an emulsifying agent under intense agitation. This procedure usually yields a microsphere morphology and was applied to the encapsulation of a few water-insoluble peptides such as salmon calcitonin (Mehta et al, 1994, 1996, Li et al, 1995, Jeyanthi et al, 1996, 1997)) and cyclosporine (Chacon et al, 1999). It is generally not applicable to the encapsulation of highly water-soluble peptides within hydrophobic polymers because upon emulsification of the dispersion of the drug-organic polymer solution/dispersion into the external aqueous phase, most of the peptide partitions out into the external phase resulting into negligible entrapment in the microspheres.

In 1970 a multiple emulsion solvent evaporation microencapsulation procedure was patented by Vrancken and Claeys and further by DeJaeger and Tavernier in 1971. In brief, an aqueous solution of the drug substance was emulsified under high-speed homogenization or sonication into a solution of polymer in an organic solvent. This emulsion, known as the primary emulsion, was then poured under constant stirring into an external aqueous phase containing a suitable emulsifier. This procedure was further modified to enable the encapsulation of highly water-soluble peptides (Ogawa et al,1988a; Okada et al, 1995).

For the successful development of a microencapsulation procedure it is essential to have an excellent understanding and control on the polymer and its chemistry, the microencapsulation procedure in terms of its engineering and various parameters which affect the product and the stability of the peptide. Each of these are considered in detail in the forthcoming sections.

1.3.1 The Polymer

One of the preliminary requirements in the successful development of a microencapsulation procedure and in achieving a product of reproducible quality in terms of microencapsulation efficiency, yield, scale-up performance, and finally, drug release characteristics is the selection of a suitable polymer as the coating material and the complete characterization of the polymer.

The requirements for a parenterally acceptable biodegradable polymer for drug delivery include controlled biodegradation rate, production of nontoxic degradation products and metabolites, reproducible and economically viable manufacturing process for large scale manufacture, non-immunogenicity, absence of impurities such as residual solvents, catalysts, monomers, stabilizers, etc., and ease of processing.

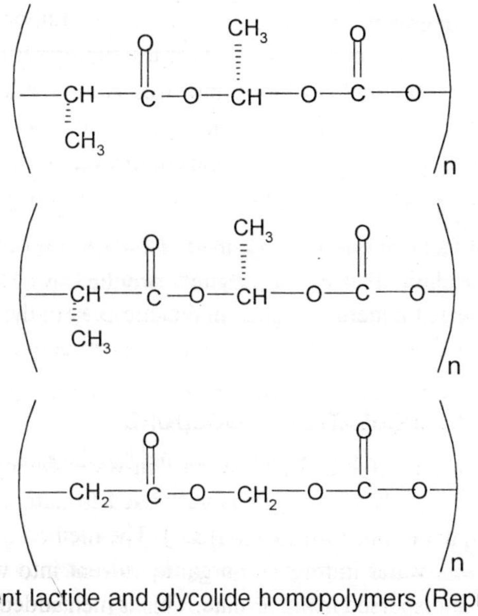

Fig 1.1: Structures of different lactide and glycolide homopolymers (Reproduced from DeLuca et al, 1993, with permission)

To meet these requirements it is important to understand the chemistry of the biodegradable polymers. The different classes of biodegradable polymers which have attracted attention for their use in drug delivery include natural polymers such as gelatin, albumin, caesin, etc. and synthetic polymers such as polyanhydrides, polyorthoesters, polyaminoacids, polyphosphazenes, polyhydroxy acids, etc. to name a few (Figure 1.1). The synthetic polymers are generally more accepted because of the reproducibility in their manufacture through

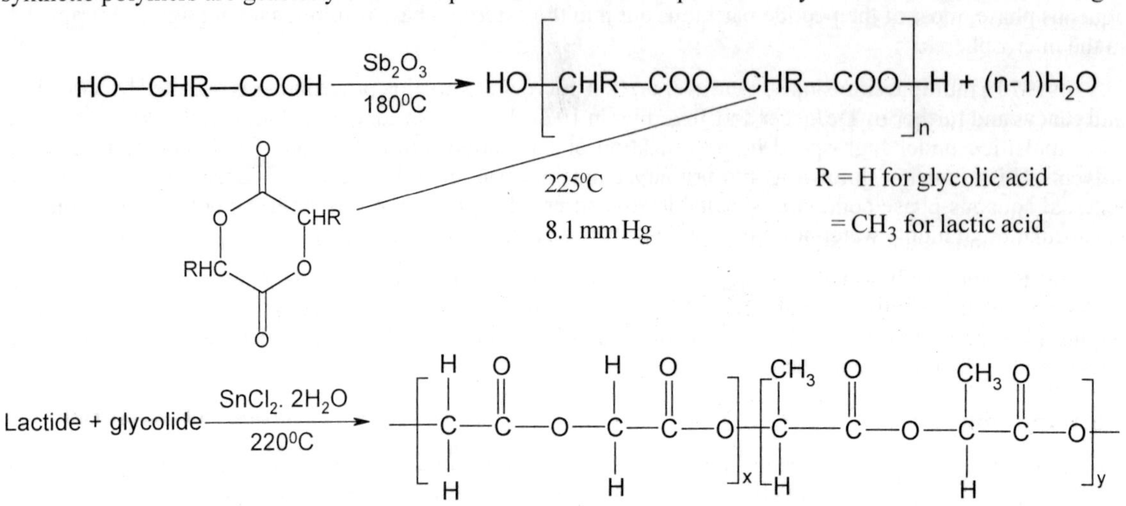

Fig 1.2: Methods of synthesis of the polylactide/polyglycolide polymer (Reproduced from DeLuca et al, 1993, with permission)

synthetic means, lack of immunogenicity, predictable biodegradation profiles, etc. Of these polylactic acid (PLA), polyglycolic acid (PGA) and their copolymers in different ratios of lactic to glycolic acid (PLGA) are the only classes of polymers currently approved for clinical use in drug delivery (Figure 1.1). These polymers have established use as sutures, drug carriers and prostheses (Jain et al, 1998). The biodegradation profile and safety of these polymers and their biodegradation products, lactic and glycolic acid, are well characterized. In addition, it is possible to achieve a wide variety of release profiles simply by blending different PLAs and PLGAs together and even more so by changing the co-monomer ratios. This will be discussed in a subsequent section.

It is essential to differentiate between the terms polylactic acid or polyglycolic acid and polylactide or polyglycolide. These polymers are synthesized mainly by two methods (Fig 1.2):

1. The direct polycondensation of lactic and/or glycolic acid in the presence of a catalyst such as antimony trioxide, ion exchange resins or clays. This method usually produces polymers in the molecular weight range of less than 10,000 D. These polymers are called polylactic or polyglycolic acid or their copolymers (Gilding & Reed, 1979; Ogawa et al, 1997).

2. The ring-opening melt-condensation of the cyclic dimers of lactic and/or glycolic acid (lactide/glycolide) in the presence of catalysts such as antimony, tin, zinc, titanium, etc. This method produces polymers with a molecular weight greater than 10,000 D, which are called polylactides or polyglycolides (Gilding & Reed, 1979; Lewis, 1990).

In order to get reproducible results in microencapsulation experiments using polylactide polymers it is essential to characterize the polymer completely in terms of the following parameters (methods of characterization): molecular weight and polydispersity (gel permeation chromatography), whether it has free carboxylic acid end groups or whether it is end-capped, acid number (percentage of free carboxylic acid end groups, acid number through non-aqueous titrimetry), content of low molecular weight oligomers (water extractable residue through gravimetry), residual monomers (HPLC, GC), residual catalyst (HPLC, GC), residual solvent (GC), thermal properties (differential scanning calorimetry), co-monomer ratio (nuclear magnetic resonance), solubility in organic solvents (cloud point titration), inherent viscosity (capillary viscometry), etc.

For a more detailed description of some of these characterizations the reader is directed to an excellent review by Hausberger & DeLuca (1995). A change in one or more of these properties could result in a drastic change in the microencapsulation efficiency, the yield, the porosity, the burst effect, etc. Several researchers have noted a difference in different lots of polymer supplied by the same manufacturer and between polymers supplied by different manufacturers but claiming the same molecular weight and co-monomer ratio (Mehta et al, 1996).

1.3.2 Biodegradation

Once a polymer has been identified it is important to know how the polymer behaves in-vitro and in-vivo. We thus have to understant the definitions of the different terms used to define these polymers. "Biomaterials", "biodegradation", "biocompatible", "bioerosion", etc. are terms which are used interchangeably to describe the polymers used for microencapsulation. Biomaterials is a broad term which encompasses all materials which are introduced into the body for therapeutic or diagnostic purposes. Biocompatibility pertains to the lack of adverse response, immunogenicity, histocompatibility of the material upon injection. Biodegradation on the other hand relates to the break down of the polymer into its component monomers or oligomers upon coming into contact with the bodily fluids, enzymes, microbial flora, etc (DeLuca et al, 1993). For the purposes of this chapter the discussion focuses on the biodegradation of the polymers. The reader is directed to several excellent articles about the biocompatibility and in-vivo behavior of these polymers (Zaikov, 1985; Visscher et al, 1985, 1988; Yamaguchi & Anderson, 1993; Tabata & Ikada, 1988; Williams & Mort, 1997; Salthouse & Matlaga, 1975).

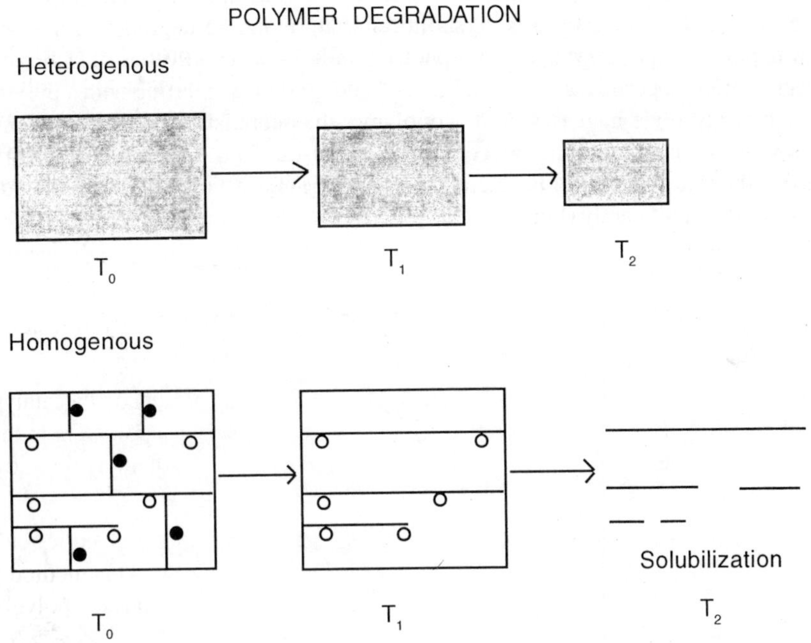

POLYMER DEGRADATION

Fig 1.3: The mechanism of degradation of biodegradable polymers (Reproduced from DeLuca et al, 1993, with permission)

Biodegradation of the polymer is of two kinds; homogeneous and heterogeneous (Fig 1.3). Heterogeneous biodegradation starts at the surface of the microparticle and proceeds to the layers beneath, with the drug being released as the polymer degrades (assuming that biodegradation is the major release rate controlling process). The degradation rate is constant in this case with the undegraded carrier retaining its integrity throughout the process. Homogeneous degradation involves a random cleavage throughout the bulk of the polymer matrix. In this case the molecular weight of the polymer steadily decreases until a critical value of the molecular weight is reached. Till this value is reached the carrier system retains its original shape, whereas beyond this value loss of mass and solubilization of the polymer commences.

The lactide-glycolide polymers degrade predominantly through a homogeneous degradation process. The different stages involved in the biodegradation of these polymers include:

1. Hydration of the polymer : There is initial uptake of the physiologic medium, swelling of the polymer and thus change in physical dimensions

2. Cleavage of covalent bonds throughout the matrix

3. Mass loss through step 2 and through solubilization of low molecular weight species

A critical molecular weight of approximately 1000 D is required to be reached before the polymer goes into solution. This process is thus associated with an uptake of the release medium and swelling of the polymer, a reduction in molecular weight, a decrease in the pH of the release medium as the low molecular weight species (lactic and glycolic acid) are released into the medium and finally complete disappearance of the pellet.

The rate of biodegradation of lactide/glycolide polymers depends strongly on the molecular weight, co-monomer ratio, the crystallinity of the polymer, porosity of the microsphere matrix, drug loading, additives, etc. A higher molecular weight of the polymer results in a significantly slower rate of degradation. The homopolymers poly(L-lactide) and polyglycolide are crystalline in nature and hence require longer degradation times when compared with their copolymers. In addition, lactic acid which has an asymmetric carbon gives rise to L and DL classes of polymers. Poly(L-lactide) is crystalline in nature and so degrades at a much slower rate when compared with poly-DL-lactide which is amorphous. Similarly, the copolymers of lactic and glycolic acid show different degradation properties as shown in Fig 1. 4 and Table 1.2. Starting with a polymer of DL-lactide, as the percentage of glycolide increases in the copolymer the degradation rate increases until a molar ratio of 50:50 %. Any further increase in the glycolide content results in a decrease in biodegradation rate. As the percentage of either the glycolide or the lactide increases the crystallinity of the polymer and hence its melting point also increases significantly (Fig 1.5). Table 1.2 demonstrates the properties of different polylactide and polyglycolide polymers.

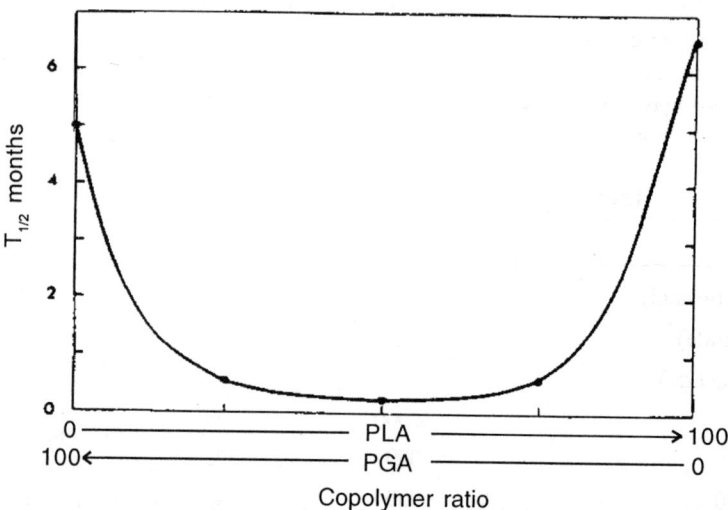

Fig. 1.4 : Schematic representation of the effect of the lactide and glycolide content on the biodegradation time of biodegradable polymers (reproduced from DeLuca et al, 1993, with permission)

The rate of biodegradation of the polymers is also affected by the nature of their endgroups. The original PLA/PGA polymers used as sutures, ligatures, etc. were endcapped polymers, where at the end of the polymerization reaction the terminal carboxylic group was blocked with some hydrophobic group. Many researchers observed that it would require months or years for these PLA/PGA polymers to disappear completely from the injection site because of their high hydrophobicity. To enhance the rate of biodegradation the hydrophilicity of the polymers was increased by having non-end-capped polymers with free terminal carboxylic groups.

The molecular weight of the polymer determines to a great extent the entrapment of the drug, the rate of biodegradation and so the rate and duration of drug release, and the final disappearance of the implanted pellet

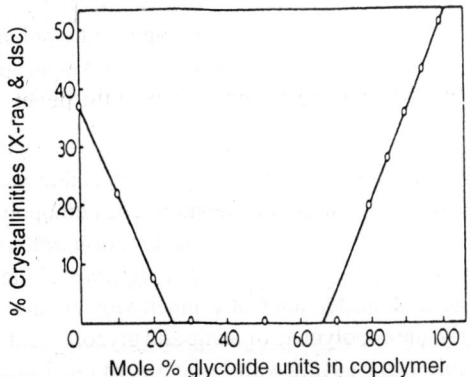 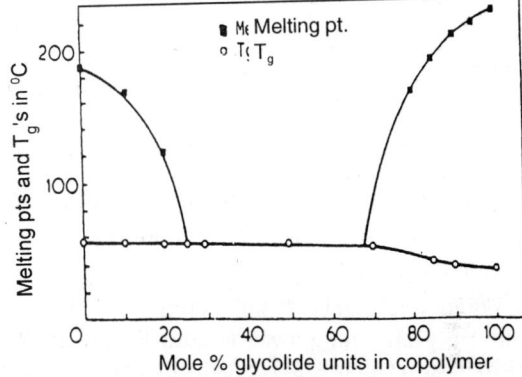

Fig 1.5 : The effect of the ration of the lactide/glycolide monomer content on the properties of biodegradabel polymers (reproduced from DeLuca et al, 1993 with permission)

from the site of injection. For development of products for parenteral controlled release it is essential to choose a polymer which will degrade slowly while providing release of the drug substance over the required time period. Subsequently, the implanted pellet should disappear completely from the site of injection. Generally, polymers with different molecular weights and comonomer ratios have to be tried before a suitable polymer is identified. Such a series of experiments demonstrated that a suitable polymer for a 1 month release formulation, for example, should have a molecular weight of 10,000-14,000 D and a lactide : glycolide comonomer ratio of 75 : 25 mole % (Ogawa et al, 1988a, b, c). This polymer provided a continuous release of leuprolide acetate over one month and the implanted pellet disappeared completely from the injection site after approximately 6 weeks.

Table 1.2 : Properties of some LA/GA homo and copolymers

Polymer	MW, D	Tg (°C)	Tm, (°C)
Poly (L-lactic acid)	2,000	40	140
Poly (L-lactide)	100,000	60	180
Poly (DL-lactide)	----	52	None
PLGA 85:15	232,000	49	None
PLGA 75:25	63,000	48	None
PLGA 50:50	12,000	40	None
PLGA 50:50	98,000	47	None
Poly (glycolide)	36,000	36	210-220

Adapted from DeLuca et al (1993) and modified

1.3.2. The Organic Solvent

In addition to the choice of the proper polymer for microencapsulation it is also essential to determine the appropriate solvent for the preparation of the primary emulsion. The selection of the solvent and the external continuous phase determine the microsphere formation and the entrapment efficiencies. A good solvent for microencapsulation should have the following properties:

1. Good solvency for the polymer: A highly concentrated polymer solution would precipitate rapidly on secondary emulsification with enhanced drug entrapment.

2. Poor solvency for the drug: A low drug solubility prohibits partitioning of the drug into the external aqueous phase during secondary emulsification with enhanced drug entrapment.

3. Low boiling point: A boiling point lower than that of water enables easier removal of the solvent without the use of harsh conditions such as high temperatures.

4. Should be immiscible with water yet should have a finite solubility in it : A high miscibility with water would result in the formation of a film or precipitation and not encapsulation, yet a minimum solubility is required for the solvent evaporation to occur.

5. Should not cause the degradation of the drug substance.

6. Should be acceptable for human use.

Methylene chloride is by far the most widely used solvent for microencapsulation using the solvent evaporation technique. It suffers from the drawback of being carcinogenic and has a low solubility in water. Other solvents with a lower toxicity than methylene chloride such as ethyl acetate have also been used in microencapsulation. Ethyl acetate suffers from the disadvantage of being a poor solubilizer for higher molecular weight polymers and those with a co-monomer ratio of 50: 50 mole % (lactide : glycolide) (Cleland, 1997).

1.3.3 The External Phase

The external phase in a solvent evaporation encapsulation method should be inexpensive, high boiling, non-toxic and immiscible with the organic solvent used. Water is the only medium, which fulfills all these requirements. Other external environments such as oils (cottonseed, mineral, olive, etc.), organic solvents, etc. have also been used to enhance entrapment efficiencies but they suffer from the disadvantage of residual levels in the finished product (Jain et al, 1998).

The external phase should also contain an emulsifier. As the solvent evaporation proceeds to a completion the droplets generated initially shrink in size as the organic solvent evaporates. During this early evaporation stage the droplets tend to coalesce and form agglomerates. A good emulsifier is required for the stabilization of the droplets to prevent coalescence by the formation of a thin film. As the evaporation proceeds, the emulsifier film helps to maintain the spherical shape of the droplets till such time as the droplets are hardened enough to be harvested. The emulsifier can then be washed off. Polyvinyl alcohol is by far the most commonly used emulsifier in solvent evaporation procedures. Other emulsifiers which have been used include poly(vinylpyrrolidone), gelatin, alginate, methylcellulose, polysorbates, hydroxypropylmethylcellulose, sodium lauryl sulfate, etc. (Jain et al, 1998).

1.3.4 The Process

Fig 1. 6 describes the different stages of the microencapsulation procedure and the different parameters, which need to be controlled to get a reproducible product.

1.3.4.1 Primary emulsification

The first step in the development of a successful microencapsulation procedure is the formation of a stable primary emulsion. Generally, during the preparation of the primary emulsion an aqueous solution of the peptide is emulsified under high shear into an oily phase consisting of a solution of the polymer in an organic solvent, with or without an emulsifier. The finer the internal droplet size the more stable is the primary emulsion. Peptides and proteins by their amphiphillic nature act to stabilise the primary emulsions (Hermann & Bodmeier, 1995). But, a higher drug loading is detrimental to the primary emulsion stability depending on the volume of internal water used for dissolving the drug.

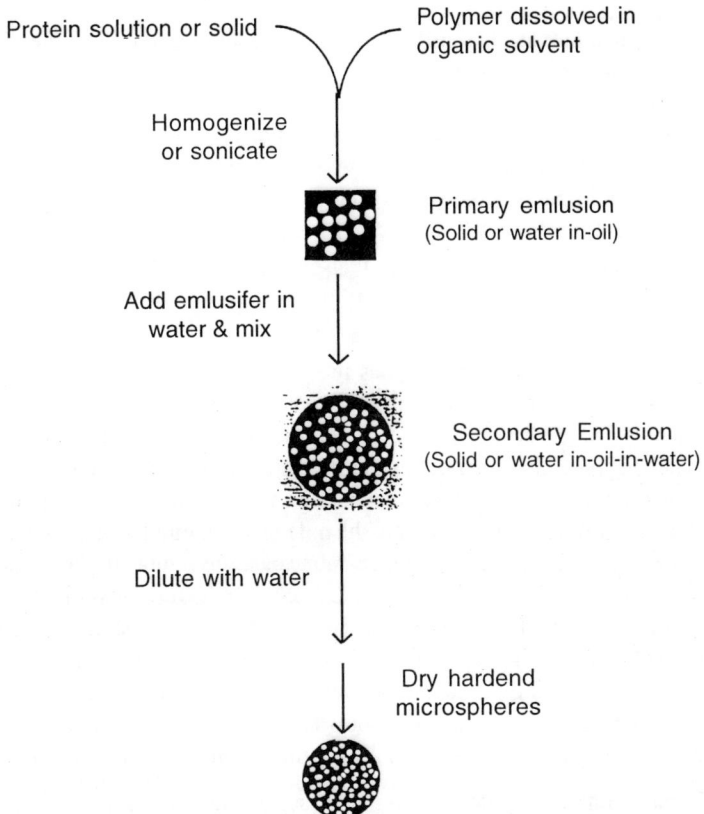

Fig 1.6 : Schematic representation of the water-in-oil-in-water microencapsulation procedure

Several modes of mixing have been used for primary emulsification including high speed homogenization, microfluidization, probe sonication, vortexing, static mixers, etc. A fine droplet size in the primary emulsion leads to a more dense structure of the final microsphere product. Vortex mixing generated larger droplet sizes and larger cavities in the microspheres than products using probe sonication (Hermann & Bodmeier, 1995). Probe sonication generates fine primary emulsions through the concept of cavitation but its use suffers from two major drawbacks. Degradation and reduction in molecular weights of PLGA polymers was observed during probe sonication probably due to the high localized increase in temperatures. Also, higher energy is required at the tip to sonicate solutions with a higher viscosity. In addition, it is difficult to use probe sonicators for higher volumes because of their localized action resulting in the inability to scale-up the product. High speed homogenization is by far the most popular method because of the different configurations of rotors, stators and their combinations available, the ease of scale-up when compared with other procedures, versatile application and their availability for use from volumes as low as 1 ml to production size batches. As the homogenization speed increases in rotor-stator homogenization the droplet size decreases until an equilibrium droplet size is achieved whereas the homogenization time does not have a major impact on the equilibrium droplet size (Maa & Hsu, 1996).

The stability of the primary emulsion has a profound impact on the surface and cross-sectional morphology, the entrapment and particle size of the final microsphere product ultimately also affecting the drug release characteristics (Nihant et al, 1994, Schugens et al., 1994, Maa & Hsu, 1997). Various formulation factors that affect the formation and stability of the primary emulsion include drug loading, polymer concentration, droplet size, viscosity, volume and pH of internal aqueous phase etc.

The volume of the internal aqueous phase affects the microsphere morphology, the drug entrapment and the rate of drug release. As the volume of the internal aqueous phase increases the phase volume ratio between the internal aqueous phase to the oil phase increases. This results in an insufficient volume of the oil phase and hence of the polymer being available for the entrapment of the internal aqueous droplets. Thus, upon secondary emulsification the internal aqueous phase is more prone to come in contact with the external aqueous phase thereby resulting in the loss of drug substance and hence a lower entrapment efficiency. Also, the internal water which gets entrapped in the microsphere matrix due to polymer precipitation diffuses out along with the solvent during solvent evaporation and creates pores and channels in the microsphere structure. The result is a microsphere system with a high porosity through which the drug substance is released at a faster rate (Hermann & Bodmeier, 1995).

The pH of the internal aqueous phase determines the state of ionization of the polymer and the drug substance which in turn determines the possible interactions between the polymer and the peptide. The dissociation constant of a poly(lactide-co-glycolide) was reported as approximately 4.0 (Makino et al, 1986). Thus, the polymer has a net negative charge at pH values above 4.0 as the carboxylic end groups are ionized. By adjusting the pH of the internal aqueous phase it should be possible to create an interaction between the negatively charged -COOH groups on the polymer and the positively charged groups on the amino acids from the peptide. Such an interaction is beneficial to enhance entrapment, to reduce the burst effect and to control the release rate of the drug as will be discussed in subsequent sections (Okada et al., 1995). This phenomenon was demonstrated for the encapsulation of somatostatin acetate within PLA microspheres (Hermann & Bodmeier, 1995) and for leuprolide acetate and thyrotropin within PLGA microspheres (Okada et al., 1995). This is the beneficial use of such a drug-polymer interaction. Other cases of drug-polymer interaction which result in the degradation of the drug or poor release profiles are also known (Cleland, 1997). It is thus essential to characterize such an interaction or the lack of it for microencapsulated formulations of peptide-protein drugs.

Generally, in the formulation of multiple emulsions w/o surfactants such as albumin or polyoxyethylene-polyoxypropylene block copolymers are needed to stabilize the primary emulsion. This may be detrimental to the final microsphere product as the primary surfactant could leach out into the external aqueous phase during secondary emulsification along with the diffusion of the internal water and organic solvent during solvent evaporation. This would probably generate a microsphere matrix which is more porous and would result in a large burst effect and a drug release which is governed more by diffusion through the movement of the dissolution medium into the pores and out rather than through the process of degradation of the polymer.

The overall viscosity of the primary emulsion influences the entrapment of the peptide, the particle size and the morphology. The viscosity can be increased through increasing the viscosity of the internal aqueous phase, adjusting the ratio of the internal aqueous phase to the polymer-organic solution phase, addition of a drug retaining substance, lowering of the temperature of the primary emulsion and increasing the concentration of the polymer in the organic solvent.

An increase in the concentration of the polymer in the organic solvent causes an increase in the viscosity of the polymer solution, the viscosity of the primary emulsion, the stability of the primary emulsion and also the rate at which the polymer precipitation occurs upon secondary emulsification. This results in a higher entrapment efficiency upon secondary emulsification. But, given the same processing conditions a much higher rate of shear is required to achieve the same particle size of the microparticulates.

The use of a drug retaining substance such as gelatin, albumin, pectin, etc., in the inner aqueous phase aids in achieving higher drug loading through an increased inner aqueous phase viscosity. Of course, the kind of drug retaining substance, its concentration, its molecular weight, etc. would also play a critical role. In addition, a reduction in the temperature of the primary emulsion aids in enhancing the entrapment ratio of the drug. But, as the overall viscosity of the primary emulsion increases the particle size also increases where above a certain viscosity the particles are actually deformed upon secondary emulsification (Okada et al., 1995).

1.3.4.2 Secondary emulsification

Once a stable primary emulsion is formulated the next step in the microencapsulation procedure is secondary emulsification (Fig 1. 6). In this step the primary emulsion is added into an external aqueous phase containing a suitable emulsifier, with intense agitation. The mode of addition of the primary emulsion during this step has an impact on the final particle size distribution. Several different modes of addition are practiced including direct pouring, slow addition with the use of a syringe or infusion pump, or through the use of a peristaltic pump, etc. Addition of the primary emulsion through a narrow bore tube or needle so that the emulsion is added at a slow controlled rate into the blades of the homogenizer/propeller usually provides the best results. A smaller droplet size to be subjected to secondary emulsification generates a finer final microparticulate product. A high speed of mixing during secondary emulsification usually leads to the formation of a smaller particle size. Also, the concentration of the emulsifier used helps to control the particle size of the final product.

It is essential at this point to understand the method of solvent evaporation. The solvent used in the procedure is usually immiscible with water. Upon secondary emulsification, the solvent from the surface of the droplet at the oil/water interface diffuses into the external aqueous phase, dissolves and then evaporates at the water to air interface (Fig 1. 7). The rate of evaporation is thus limited by the solubility of the solvent in the external aqueous phase. Methylene chloride has a solubility of approximately 1.32 %w/v in water at 25°C. This solubility may be further enhanced because of the presence of the surfactant. The rate can be modified by a rapid dilution of the external aqueous phase by gradual addition of a large excess of water. In addition, the temperature of the external aqueous phase could be raised suddenly or gradually in a programmed gradient to cause enhanced rates of solvent evaporation (Jeyanthi et al, 1996; Li et al, 1995). Another approach to enhance the rate of precipitation of the polymer is to add a water-miscible organic solvent such as isopropyl alcohol or acetone into the external aqueous phase. The presence of such a cosolvent results in the rapid extraction of the organic solvent from the droplets causing rapid hardening of the microspheres. It must be remembered that all of the techniques mentioned here for the enhancement of the rate of solvent evaporation also affect the microsphere morphology. It is important to characterize the effect that each such change has on the

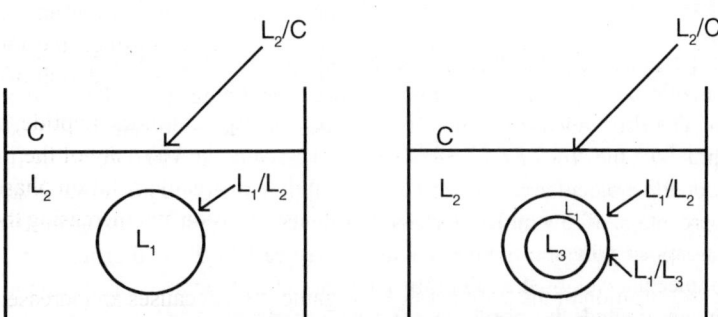

Fig 1.7: Schematic of the mode of solvent evaporation
(Reproduced from Benoit et al., 1996, with permission)

morphology of the final product. In addition, it is also essential to characterize the level of residual solvent in the microparticulates and the levels of residual emulsifier such as polyvinyl alcohol on their surface.

1.3.4.3 Hardening and Recovery

The microspheres in suspension have to be hardened by continuing the evaporation of the solvent. The hardened microspheres are recovered by filtration or centrifugation. The wet cake is then subjected to drying by one of various processes: heating, vacuum, lyophilization, etc. Lyophilization is the most preferred process because of the sensitivity of the peptide molecules. It must be remembered that raising the temperature of the product above the glass transition temperature of the polymer results in the agglomeration of the microspheres. So a careful control on the drying conditions is essential to achieve a product of reproducible quality.

1.3.4.5 Characterization of the microspheres

The microspheres formulated as described above have to be characterized thoroughly for the different properties. This is not the focus of the chapter and thus only a brief mention is made of the different properties and the methods by which this characterization should be carried out. The different properties include : peptide entrapment and entrapment efficiencies (HPLC), particle size (microscopy, sieve analysis, laser light scattering, coulter-counter, photon correlation spectroscopy), stability and activity of the peptide in the microspheres (HPLC and biological methods), yield of the process, bulk and tap density, porosity and specific surface area (mercury or helium intrusion porosimetry), drug release, thermal properties (differential scanning calorimetry, thermogravimetric analysis), moisture content (Karl Fischer titration, gravimetry, thermogravimetric analysis), surface and cross-sectional morphology (scanning electron microscopy, transmission electron microscopy, scanning probe microscopy, image analysis), biodegradation rate in-vitro (HPLC, GPC), residual organic solvent (GC, thermogravimetric analysis), surface and bulk sterility (microbiological methods), resuspendability, syringeability, etc.

Here a brief mention about the residual solvent levels has to be made. The residual organic solvent in the final microencapsulated product has to be characterized. The USFDA has allowed the product Lupron Depot to be marketed which has levels of less than 50 ppm residual methylene chloride. It is generally difficult to remove the organic solvents completely. Repeated lyophilization cycles or drying under vacuum at elevated temperatures may help reduce the residual levels. Temperatures in excess of 20°C may result in the agglomeration of the microspheres unless they are properly stabilized.

Mention of the use of alternate organic solvents such as ethyl acetate, methyl ethyl ketone, etc. for microencapsulation has been made earlier in this article. Approval for such use from the FDA for commercial manufacture would only be possible after establishing the residual solvent levels and the toxicity of such levels to human beings. Till then methylene chloride appears to be the solvent of choice for microencapsulation by solvent evaporation.

1.3.4.6 Drug release

One of the important aspects of the performance of the microencapsulated product is the drug release. The drug release profile from microencapsulated systems will differ depending upon whether it is a microsphere or a microcapsule system. The drug release profiles from biodegradable microspheres are governed by many properties, both of the polymer, the drug and the carrier system (Kissel et al, 1991; Washington, 1990). Polymer dependent factors include the molecular weight and its distribution, the comonomer ratio and the distribution of the monomers, the percentage of low molecular weight species, the crystallinity, whether the polymer is an end-capped or non-end-capped polymer, the percentage of free carboxylic end groups, etc. Drug dependent parameters include the molecular weight, the solubility in the dissolution medium and drug-polymer interactions. The carrier system parameters include the morphology, i.e. whether the product is a microcapsule or microsphere, the drug loading, the physical state of the drug in the polymer matrix, i.e. whether the drug is in the dispersed or dissolved state, the particle size and distribution, the porosity and the internal morphology of the microparticles depending upon the different parameters discussed above.

A general release profile from biodegradable microspheres is depicted in Fig 1.8. The drug release could be continuous acting through diffusion alone (as occurs for smaller molecules) or it could be triphasic (as occurs for most high molecular weight peptides and proteins). The triphasic profile also called the 'S' shaped profile is characterized by:

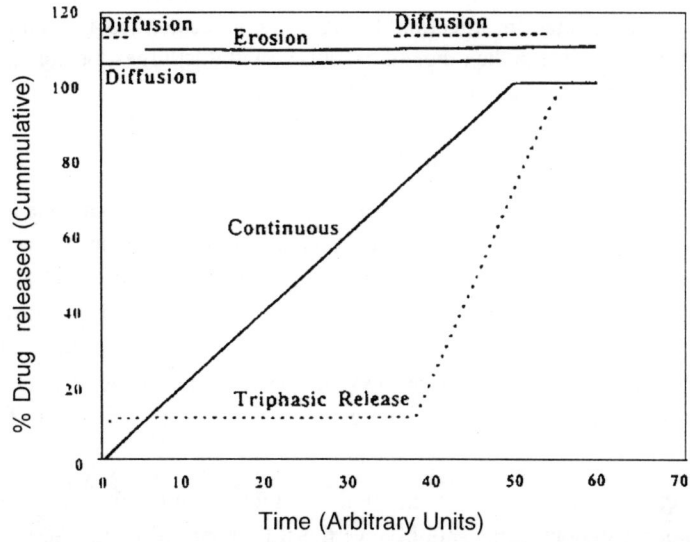

Fig 1.8 : A generalized release profile for drug substances from biodegradable microspheres (Reproduced from Cleland, 1997, with permission)

1. A burst effect which is a rapid initial release of the drug caused because of adsorbed or unentrapped drug
2. A lag time during which the polymer degrades and reaches the critical molecular weight where mass loss occurs
3. A controlled release of the drug substance through a combination of the degradation of the polymer and diffusion of the drug through newly generated pores and surfaces.

It is hoped to achieve a product with a minimum burst effect and which will release the drug in a zero order fashion. Several methods to control the burst effect have been used. The ionic interaction between the negatively charged polymer and the positively charged peptide was used to entrap leuprolide acetate within PLGA microspheres (Okada et al, 1995). The addition of a drug retaining substance into the internal aqueous phase helps to reduce the burst effect possibly through the formation of a barrier between the drug release medium and the drug substance (Okada et al, 1995). The presence of low molecular weight oligomeric species in the polymer also leads to an increased burst effect. Washing of polymer to reduce low molecular weight species helps to reduce this burst effect (Okada et al, 1995).

Additional medium related parameters which have to be controlled during drug release studies include volume, pH, osmolarity, buffer capacity, buffer species, ionic strength, additives, etc. Each of these has to be characterized in detail before a drug release method can be applied to a formulation. It is also essential to develop an accelerated dissolution method for the quick and reproducible characterization of the drug release from the product as an in-process test. This could be done through an increase in the temperature or a change in the medium or its pH, etc. For each such change it is essential to characterize the effect that the change has on the performance of the product.

1.3.4.7 Resuspendability and syringeability of the microspheres

The particle size of the microspheres is one of the important parameters which has to be finalized well in advance. The final particle size and the suspending vehicle for redispersion finally decide the syringeability of the suspension. The final pack for such a product would be either (a) a vial containing the microspheres, an ampoule with a diluent and a syringe needle assembly, or (b) a dual chambered prefilled syringe containing the microspheres in one chamber and the diluent in the other. In both cases the microsphere powder is to be resuspended in the diluent vehicle before injection. The microsphere suspension is injected subcutaneously or preferably intramuscularly through a 18 gauge needle, though needles as fine as 22-23 gauge have also been used. An 18 gauge needle has an internal diameter of 838µm (Lee et al, 1991). Thus, a maximum particle size of 100µm should be formulated for injection through such a needle. Most of the marketed microencapsulated products have a particle size in the range of 5-100µm, with the largest percentage of the particles in the less than 40µm range. A particle size larger than 100µm may lead to interparticulate interactions and a possible eventual clogging of the needle during injection though this problem could be prevented by the inclusion of suitable surfactants such as Tween 80 in the vehicle.

Another approach to improve the syringeability is the use of extremely fine particles. Such small particles have an extremely high surface area and hence pose problems for proper wetting and dispersion during resuspension. Secondly, small particles also show agglomeration and development of static charge, which are both potential problems when it comes to flow of material during vial filling. Thirdly, small particles sometimes demonstrate non-Newtonian flow properties. Thus, a perfectly fluid, well dispersed suspension of the microparticles suddenly stops flowing as excess shear is developed at the tip of the needle. On relaxation of the shear the suspension becomes fluid again. This cycle continues causing problems for the smooth administration of the product.

The microcapsules along with the suspending vehicle form the final injectable suspension. The vehicle for suspension and its components should have the following properties: easy and complete wetting of the product, rapid resuspension, stability of the suspension adequate for injection, uniform dispersion, adequate viscosity to prevent sedimentation and agglomeration but not so high as to prevent flow, should cause no local irritation, nontoxic, and isotonic.

It is also essential to determine the concentration of microparticles in the final suspension so that the final product has adequate syringeability. Generally, a mock trial is carried out where the microsphere suspension is injected through the final syringe and needle combination into a matrix, which exerts sufficient back pressure as in the case of the actual injection into human beings. A similar study should also be carried out using a needle with a smaller bore than that to be actually used, as a more stringent challenge to the formulation.

1.3.4.8 Sterilization

The microspheres described in this chapter are intended for intramuscular or subcutaneous administration. It is therefore essential to develop a product which will be sterile and pyrogen free. Several methods of sterilization known include: autoclaving, dry heat, ethylene oxide, irradiation, aseptic processing. Most peptides and polypeptides are known to be thermolabile. Similarly, the polylactides degrade through simple hydrolysis and show a higher rate of degradation at elevated temperatures. PLA/PGA polymers and their copolymers degrade rapidly when subjected to irradiation sterilization as a function of the irradiation dose. The degradation is seen through a decrease in the molecular weight, reduction in the viscosity and mechanical properties. This is more predominant in the PLA and PLGA polymers than for PGA polymers (Sintzel et al., 1997). Thus, for the preparation of the microspheres aseptic processing is the most acceptable method. The polymer solution in methylene chloride can be easily filtered through 0.22µm filters. Similarly, the internal aqueous phase, the external aqueous phase and the washing water can all be sterile filtered and the final compounding of the product can be carried out in a sterile environment. It is important to establish the sterility of the microspheres, not only on the surface but also internally by dissolving the microspheres in some mild nontoxic solvent such as DMA or DMSO and further subjecting it to sterility testing.

1.4 CONCLUSIONS AND SUGGESTIONS FOR FURTHER WORK

Microencapsulation of peptide or protein drugs is a challenging field for research. It can be seen from the above discussion that a variety of factors are responsible for achieving the correct microsphere characteristics of particle size, entrapment efficiency and drug release. In addition, other factors such as syringeability, sterility, residual solvent concerns, etc. have also been highlighted. The major challenges facing the pharmaceutical scientists include, scale-up problems, use of alternative solvents to replace methylene chloride, application of this and other techniques for the encapsulation of higher molecular weight proteins, to overcome the problems of peptide/protein degradation during microencapsulation and within the microspheres on stability and most important; the use of alternative biodegradable polymers to the polylactides/glycolides.

REFERENCES

Benoit J. P.; Herve M.; Rolland H. and Velde V.V. (1996) "Biodegradable microspheres : Advances in production technology", In : "Microencapsulation : Methods and industrial applications." Simon Benita (Eds), Marcel Dekker, New York, pg 35-72.

Bittner B.; Morlock M.; Koll H.; Winter G. and Kissel T. (1998) "Recombinant human erythropoietin (rhEPO loaded poly(lactide-co-glycolide) microspheres : influence of the encapsulation technique and polymer purity on microsphere characteristics." Eur. J. Pharm. Biopharm., 45(3) : 295-305

Chacon M.; Molpeceres J.; Berges L.; Guzman M. and Aberturas M.R. (1999) "Stability and freeze-drying of cyclosporine loaded poly(D,L lactide-glycolide) carriers." Eur. J. Pharm. Sci., 8(2) : 99-107

Cleland J. (1997) "Protein delivery from biodegradable microspheres" In : "Protein delivery : Physical systems." Pharmaceutical Biotechnology Series, Volume 10, Sanders L.M. and Hendren R. W. (Eds); Plenum Press, New York.

Cohen S.; Yoshioka T.; Lucarelli M.; Hwang L.H. and Langer R. (1991) "Controlled delivery systems for proteins based on poly(lactid-glycolic acid) microspheres." Pharm. Res., 8 : 713-720

Csernus V.J.; Szende B. and Schally, A.V. (1990) "Release of peptides from sustained delivery systems(microcapsules and microparticles) in vivo." Int. J. Peptide. Protein. Res., 35 : 557-565

Dejaeger N. C. and B. H. Tavernier (1971) British Patent, 1,405,108

DeLuca P.P.; Mehta R.C.; Hausberger A.G. and Thanoo B.C. (1993) "Biodegradable polyesters for drug and polypeptide delivery." In : Polymeric delivery systems, El-Nokaly,M.A., Piatt,D.M. and Charpentier, B.A. (eds.), pp. 53-79, American Chemical Society, Washington, DC.

Dunn R.L.; English J. P.; Cowsar D.R. and Vanderbilt D.P. (1994) "Biodegradable insitu forming implants and the method of producing the same." US Patent No. 5,278,201,

Gilding D.K. and Reed A.M. (1979) "Biodegradable polymers for use in surgery - polyglycolic / polylactic acid homo- and copolymers : I." Polymer, 20 : 1459-1464

Hausberger A.G. and DeLuca P.P. (1995) "Characterization of biodegradable poly(dl-lactide-co-glycolide) polymers and microspheres." Journal of Pharmaceutical and Biomedical Analysis, 13(6) : 747-760

Hermann J. and Bodmeier R. (1995) "Somatostatin containing biodegradable microspheres prepared by a modified solvent evaporation method based on w/o/w-multiple emulsions." Int. J. Pharm., 126 : 129-138

Heya T.; Okada H.; Tanigawara Y.; Ogawa Y. and Toguchi H. (1991) "Effect of counteranion of TRH and loading amount on control of TRH release from copoly(dl-lactic-glycolic acid) microspheres prepared by an in-water drying method." Int. J. Pharm., 69 : 69-75

Jain R.; Shah N.H.; Waseem Malick A. and Rhodes C.T. (1998) "Controlled drug delivery by biodegradable poly(ester) devices : Different preparative approaches." Drug Dev. Ind. Pharm., 24(8) : 703-727

Jalil R. and Nixon J.R. (1989) "Microencapsulation using poly(L-lactic acid). I : Microcapsule properties affected by the preparative technique." J. Microencapsul., 6(4) : 473-484

Jalil R. and Nixon J.R. (1990a) "Microencapsulation using poly(L-lactic acid). II : Preparative variables affecting microcapsule properties." J. Microencapsul., 7(1) : 25-39

Jalil R. and Nixon J.R. (1990b) "Microencapsulation using poly(L-lactic acid). III : Effect on polymer molecular weight on microcapsule properties." J. Microencapsul., 7(1) : 41-52

Jalil R. and Nixon J.R. (1990c) "Microencapsulation using poly(L-lactic acid). IV : Release properties of microcapsules containing phenobarbitone." J. Microencapsul., 7(1) : 53-66

Jalil R. and Nixon J.R. (1990d) "Microencapsulation using poly(DL-lactic acid). I: Effect of preparative variables on the microcapsule characteristics and release kinetics." J. Microencapsul., 7(2) : 229-44

Jalil R. and Nixon J.R. (1990e) "Microencapsulation using poly (DL-lactic acid). II : Effect of polymer molecular weight on the microcapsule properties." J. Microencapsul., 7(2) : 245-54

Jeyanthi R.; Thanoo B.C.; Mehta R.C. and DeLuca P.P. (1996) "Effect of solvent removal technique on the matrix characteristics of polylactide/glycolide microspheres for peptide delivery." J. Control. Rel., 38 : 235-244.

Jeyanthi R.; Mehta R.C.; Thanoo B.C. and DeLuca P.P. (1997) "Effect of processing parameters on the properties of peptide-containing PLGA microspheres." J. Microencapsul., 14(2) : 163-174

Kissel T.; Birch Z.; Bantle S.; Lancranjan I.; Nimmerfall F. and Vit F. (1991) "Parenteral depot systems on the basis of biodegradable polymers" J. Control. Rel., 16 : 27-42

Lee V. H. (1991) "Peptide and protein drug delivery." Marcel Dekker, New York

Lewis D.H. (1990) In : Biodegradable polymers as drug delivery systems. Chasin, M., Langer,R. (eds), Marcel Dekker Inc: New York, NY, pp. 1-41

Li W-I.; Anderson K.W.; Mehta R.C. and DeLuca P.P. (1995) "Prediction of solvent removal profile and effect on properties for peptide-loaded PLGA microspheres prepared by solvent extraction/evaporation method." J. Control. Rel., 37 : 199-214

Maa Y-F. and Hsu C. (1996) "Liquid-liquid emulsification by rotor / stator homogenization." J. Control. Rel., 38 : 219-228

Maa Y-F. and Hsu C. (1997) "Effect of primary emulsions on microsphere size and protein-loading in the double emulsion process." J. Microencapsulation, 14(2) : 225-241

Makino K.; Oshima H. and Kondo T. (1986) "Transfer of protons from bulk solution to the surface of poly(L-Lactide) microcapsules." J. Microencapsulation, 3 : 195-202

Mason-Garcia M.; Vaccarella M.; Horvath J.; Redding T.W.; Groot K.; Orsolini P. and Schally A.V. (1988) "Radioimmunoassay for octapeptide analogs of somatostatin : measurement of serum levels after administration of long-acting microcapsule formulations." Proc. Natl. Acad. Sci., USA, 85 : 5688-5692

Mehta R.C.; Jeyanthi R.; Calis S.; Thanoo B.C.; Burton K.W. and DeLuca P.P. (1994) "Biodegradable microspheres as depot system for parenteral delivery of peptide drugs." J. Control. Rel., 29 : 375-384

Mehta R.C.; Thanoo B.C. and DeLuca P.P. (1996) "Peptide containing microspheres from low molecular weight and hydrophilic poly(d,l-lactide-co-glycolide)." J. Control. Rel., 41 : 249-257

Nihant N.; Ch. Shugens, Ch. Grandfils, R. Jerome and Teyssie, Ph (1994) "Polylactide microparticles prepared by a double emulsion/evaporation technique. I. Effect of primary emulsion stability." Pharmaceutical Research 11(10) : 1479-1484

Niu C.H. and Chiu Y.Y. (1998) "FDA perspective on peptide formulation and stability issues." J. Pharm. Sci. 87(11): 1331-1334

Ogawa Y.; Yamamoto M.; Okada H.; Yashiki T. and Shimamoto T. (1988a) "A new technique to efficiently entrap leuprolide acetate into microcapsules of polylactic acid or copoly(lactic/glycolic) acids." Chem. Pharm. Bull. 36 : 1095-1103

Ogawa Y.; Yamamoto M.; Okada H.; Yashiki T. and Shimamoto T. (1988b) "Controlled release of leuprolide acetate from polylactic acid or copoly(lactic/glycolic) acid microcapsules : Influence of molecular weight and copolymer ratio of polymer." Chem. Pharm. Bull. 36 : 1502-1507

Ogawa Y.; Okada H.; Yamamoto M. and Shimamoto T. (1988c) "In-vivo release profiles of leuprolide acetate from microcapsules prepared with polylactic acids or copoly(lactic/glycolic acids) and in-vivo degradation of the polymers." Chem. Pharm. Bull., 36 : 2576-2581

Ogawa Y. (1997) "Injectable microcapsules prepared with biodegradable poly(alpha-hydroxy)acids for prolonged release of drugs." J. Biomater. Sci. Polym. Ed., 8(5) : 391-409

Okada H. and Toguchi H. (1995) "Biodegradable microspheres in drug delivery." Critical Reviews in Therapeutic Drug Carrier Systems, 12(1) : 1-99

Okada H.; Ogawa Y. and Yashiki T. (1987) "Prolonged release microcapsule and its production." US Patent 4,652,441

Ruiz J.M.; Tissier B. and Benoit J.P. (1989) "Microencapsulation of peptide : a study of the phase separation of poly(DL-lactic acid-co-glycolic acid) copolymers by silicone oil." Int. J. Pharm., 49 : 69-77

Salthouse T.N. and Matlaga B.F. (1975) "Approach to the numerical quantitation of actue tissue response to biomaterials." Biomater, Med. Devices Artif Organs, 3 47-56

Sanders L.M.; Kell B.A.; McRae G.I., and Whitehead G.W. (1986) "Prolonged controlled-release of nafarelin, a leutenizing hormone-releasing hormone analogue, from biodegradable polymeric implants : influence of composition and molecular weight of polymer." J. Pharm. Sci., 75 : 356-360

Shugens Ch.; Laruelle N.; Nihant N.; Grandfils Ch.; Jerome R. and Teyssie Ph. (1994) "Effect of emulsion stability on the morphology and porosity of semicrystalline poly l-lactide microparticles prepared by w/o/w double emulsion-evaporation." J. Control. Rel., 32 : 161-176

Sintzel M.B.; Merkli A.; Tabatabay C. and Gurny R. (1997) "Influence of irradiation sterilization on polymers used as drug carriers - A review." Drug Dev. Ind. Pharm. 23(9) : 857-878

Tabata Y. and Ikada Y. (1988) "Macrophage phagocytosis of biodegradable microspheres composed of L-lactic acid/glycolic acid homo- and copolymers." Journal of Biomedical Materials Research, 22 : 837-858

Visscher G.E.; Pearson J.E.; Fong J.W.; Argentieri G.J.; Robison R.L.; Maulding H.V., and (1988) "Effect of particle size on the in vitro and in vivo degradation rates of the poly(DL-lactide-co-glycolide) microcapsules." Journal of Biomedical Materials Research, 22 : 733-746

Visscher G.E.; Robison R.L.; Maulding H.V.; Fong J.W.; Pearson J.E. and Argentieri G.J. (1985) "Biodegradation of and tissue reaction to 50:50 poly(DL-lactide-co-glycolide) microcapsules." Journal of Biomedical Materials Research, 9 : 349-365

Vrancken M. N. and D. A. Claeys (1970) US Patent 3,526,906

Washington C. (1990) "Drug release from microdisperse systems : A critical review." Int. J. Pharm., 58 : 1-12

Williams D.F. and Mort E. (1997) "Enzyme-accelerated hydrolysis of poly glycolic acid." J. Bioeng, 1 : 231-238

Yamaguchi K. and Anderson J. (1993) "In vivo biocompatibility studies of medisorb 65/35 D,L-lactide/glycolide copolymer microspheres." J. Control. Rel., 24 : 81-93

Zaikov G.E. (1985) "Quantitative aspects of polymer degradation in the living body." J. Macromol. Sci. Rev. Macromol. Chem.Phys., C25 (4) : 551-597

Chapter 2

Osmotic Pump - A Novel Drug Delivery System

N. S. Parmar, S. K. Vyas, Navin Vaya

2.1 INTRODUCTION

During the past three decades significant advances have been made in the area of controlled drug delivery. This was, in part, due to the evolving disciplines of biopharmaceutics, pharmacokinetics and pharmacodynamics. In a typical therapeutic regimen, the drug dose and the dosing interval are optimized to maintain drug concentration within the therapeutic window, thus ensuring efficacy while minimizing toxic side effects. Surveys indicated that dosing more than once or twice daily greatly reduces patient compliance. Hence, the primary objective for controlled drug delivery is to maintain drug concentration within therapeutic window, improve patient compliance to the dosage regimen by decreasing dosing frequency, and improve drug efficacy while reducing toxic side effects. A diagrammatic illustration of controlled versus conventional dosage delivery is shown in Fig 2.1.

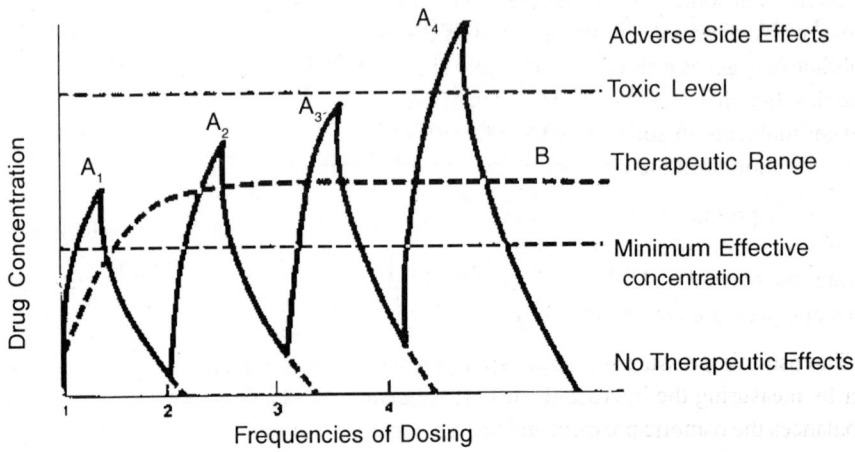

Fig 2.1 : Simulation of blood concentration profiles resulting from multiple doses of conventional dosage form (A$_1$, A$_2$, A$_3$ and A$_4$) as compared to a single dose of controlled release (Zero order) dosage Form (B).

Numerous technologies have been used to control the systemic delivery of drugs. One of the most interesting employs osmotic pressure as a source of energy. Osmotic pressure has been used extensively in the fabrication of drug delivery systems. This chapter describes controlled release devices based on the osmotic pressure concept. Main emphasis is given to oral osmotic pumps.

2.2 HISTORY

Since the beginning of antiquity, both pharmacy and medicine have sought effective delivery systems for administering beneficial drugs. The first written reference to a delivery system is to the Eber Papyrus, written about 1552 B.C., in 865-925 AD, Arab physician Rhazes invented coated pill. Primeval tablet was described in Arabian manuscripts written by al-Zahrawi, 936-1009 A.D. The earliest application of osmotic pressure to drug delivery was by Rose and Nelson (1955). The next quantum leap in osmotic dosage forms came in 1972 when Theeuwes invented elementary osmotic pump (Theeuwes, 1975). After that many modified osmotic pumps have been invented which enable controlled delivery of almost all drugs.

2.3. THEORY

Osmotic Pressure

Osmotic pressure, like vapour pressure and boiling point is a colligative property of a solution in which a nonvolatile solute is dissolved in a volatile solvent. If cobalt chloride is placed in a parchment sac and suspended in a beaker of water, the water gradually becomes red as the solute diffuses throughout the vessel. In this process of diffusion, both the solvent and solute molecules migrate freely. On the other hand, if the solution is confined in a membrane permeable only to solvent molecules, the phenomenon known as osmosis (Greek : a push or impulse) occurs, and the barrier that permits only the molecules of one of the components (usually water) to pass through is known as a semipermeable membrane. Osmosis is therefore defined as the passage of the solvent into a solution through a semipermeable membrane. This process tends to equalize the escaping tendency of the solvent on both sides of the membrane. It should be evident that osmosis can also take place when a concentrated solution is separated from a less concentrated solution by a semipermeable membrane.

Osmosis in some cases is believed to involve the passage of solvent through membrane by a distillation process, or by dissolving in the material of the membrane in which solute is insoluble. In other cases, the membrane may act as a sieve, having a pore size sufficiently large to allow passage of solvent but not of solute molecules. In either case the phenomenon of osmosis really depends on the fact that the chemical potential of a solvent molecule in solution is less than it exists in pure solvent. Solvent therefore passes spontaneously into the solution until the chemical potentials of solvent and solute are equal.

Osmotic pressure can be measured with the help of a simple experiment using an osmometer (Fig 2.2), one side of which contains a pure solvent, while the other contains a solution. A semipermeable membrane separates the two sides. The solvent will travel from the solvent side to the solution side until such time as the hydrostatic pressure created by the solvent flux is sufficiently high to stop further flux.

The osmotic pressure that is set up as a result of this passage of solvent molecules may be determined either by measuring the hydrostatic head (h) appearing in the solution or by applying a known pressure that just balances the osmotic pressure and prevents any net movement of solvent molecules into the solution. The latter is preferred technique. Osmotic pressure is defined as the excess pressure, or pressure greater than that above the pure solvent, which must be applied to the solution to prevent the passage of the solvent through a perfect semipermeable membrane.

Flow of solvent depends on following factors: semipermeable membrane characteristics, differential osmotic pressure between two sides of osmometer, differential hydrostatic pressure between two sides of osmometer, and the difference between osmotic pressure and hydrostatic pressure as the mass (volume) transfer process approaches equilibrium.

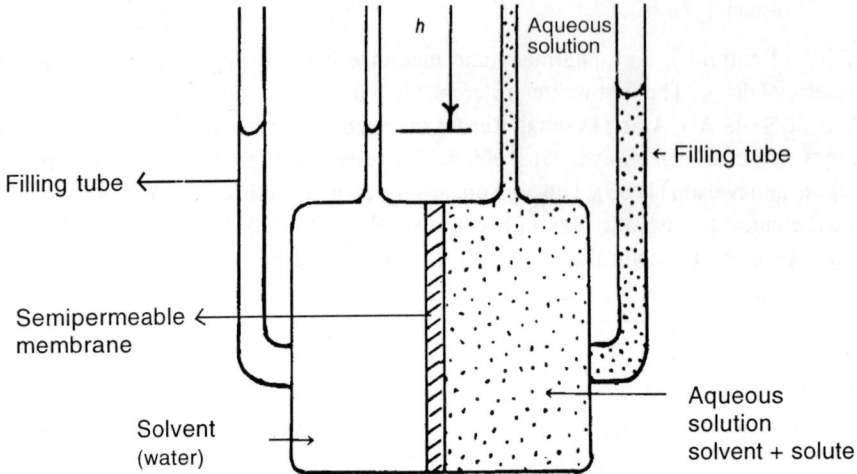

Fig 2.2 : Osmotic pressure osmometer

Osmotic pressure can also be calculated by using Van't Hoff and Morse equation:

$$\pi V = n RT \qquad ... (Eq.1)$$

in which π is osmotic pressure in atm, V is the volume of solution in liters, n is number of moles of solute, R is gas constant (0.082 liter atm/mole deg) and T is the absolute temperature (Martin, 1994).

Osmotic pressures for concentrated solutions of soluble solutes commonly used in controlled formulations are extremely high, ranging from 28 atm for sodium phosphate up to 500 atm for lactose : fructose mixture. Some commonly used osmotic agents are given in Table -2.1.

Table -2.1 : List of osmotic agents with their osmotic pressure (Theeuwes, 1981).

Compound or Mixture	Osmotic Pressure (atm)
Mannitol : Fructose	415
Sodium chloride	356
Fructose	355
Lactose : Sucrose	250
Potassium chloride	245
Lactose : Dextrose	225
Mannitol : Dextrose	225
Dextrose : Sucrose	190
Mannitol : Sucrose	170
Dextrose	82
Potassium sulfate	39
Mannitol	38
Sodium phosphate tribasic. 12 H_2O	36
Sodium phosphate dibasic. 7 H_2O	34
Sodium phosphate dibasic. 12 H_2O	31
Sodium phosphate dibasic anhydrous	29
Sodium phosphate monobasic. H_2O	28

These osmotic pressures can produce high water flows across semipermeable membranes. The osmotic water flow across a membrane is given by this equation:

$$\frac{dv}{dt} = \frac{A}{h} Lp \left(\sigma\Delta\pi - \Delta P \right) \qquad\qquad \text{(Eq. 2)}$$

Where dv/dt is the water flow across the membrane of area A, thickness h; $\Delta\pi$ & ΔP are the osmotic and hydrostatic pressure differences, respectively, on either side of the membrane; Lp is the mechanical permeability; σ is the reflection coefficient (leakage of solute through membrane). In terms of membrane performance and predictability, it is important to select a material whose reflection coefficient is close to 1. Water permeabilities of membranes can vary over a wide range, but most osmotic devices generally use relatively water permeable materials. Cellulosic materials, particularly cellulose acetate, are widely used. Table-2.2 gives list of various polymers for semipermeable membranes. Semipermeable membrane has important role in controlling drug release. Hence, the membrane must meet several performance criteria. First, the material must possess sufficient wet strength ($\sim 10^5$ psi) and wet modulus ($\sim 10^5$ psi) so as to retain its dimensional integrity during the operational lifetime of the device. Second, the polymer membrane must exhibit sufficient water permeability so as to attain water flux rate (dv/dt) in the desired range. Third, the reflection coefficient (σ), "leakiness" of the membrane to the osmotic agent, should approach the limiting value of 1. Finally, the membrane should be biocompatible.

Table-2.2 : List of semi permeable polymers with their water vapour transmission rates (WVTR) (Johnson, 1980).

Polymers Membrane	WVTR(g/100m²/24hr/mm thick)
Polyvinyl alcohol	100
Polyurethane	30-150
Methyl cellulose	70
Cellulose acetate	40-75
Ethyl cellulose	75
Cellulose acetate butyrate	50
Polyvinyl chloride (cast)	10-20
Polyvinyl chloride (extruded)	6-15
Polycarbonate	8
Polyvinyl fluoride	3
Ethylene vinyl acetate	1-3
Polyesters	2
Cellophane (polyethylene coated)	> 1.2
Polyvinyledine fluoride	1.0
Ethylene propylene copolymer	0.8
Polypropylene	0.7
Polyvinyl chloride (rigid)	0.7

2.4 CLASSIFICATION

2.4.1 Implantable Osmotic Pumps (Santus & Baker, 1995)

2.4.1.1 The Rose Nelson Pump

In 1955, two Australian physiologists reported the first osmotic pump. They were interested in delivery of drugs to the gut of sheep & cattle. The pump consisted of three chambers (Fig 2..3): a drug chamber with an orifice, a salt chamber with elastic diaphragm containing excess solid salt, and a water chamber. A semipermeable membrane separates the drug and water chamber. The difference in osmotic pressure across the membrane moves water from the water chamber into the salt chamber. The volume of the salt chamber increases because of this water flow, which distends the latex diaphragm separating the salt and drug chambers, thereby pumping drug out of the device.

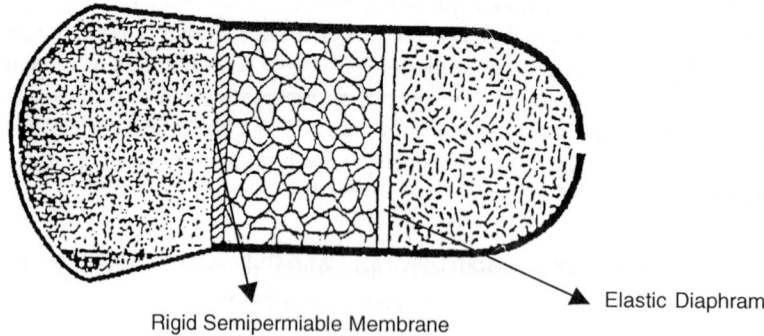

Rigid Semipermiable Membrane · · · · · · · · · · · Elastic Diaphram

Fig 2.3 : Rose - Nelson osmotic pump

The pumping rate of Rose-Nelson pump is given by the equation.

$$\frac{dm}{dt} = \frac{dv}{dt} C \qquad (Eq.3)$$

Where dm/dt is the drug release rate, dv/dt is the volume flow of water into the salt chamber, and C is concentration of drug into the drug chamber. Substituting eq.2 in eq.3 gives

$$\frac{dm}{dt} = \frac{A}{h} Lp (\sigma\Delta\pi - \Delta P)C \qquad (Eq.4)$$

These basic equations can be used to describe the behaviour of all the devices described in this chapter.

The osmotic pressure of saturated salt solution is high, on the order of tens of atmosphere, and the small pressure required to pump the suspension of active agent is insignificant in comparison. Therefore, the rate of water permeation across the semipermeable membrane remains constant as long as sufficient salt is present in the salt chamber to maintain a saturated solution and hence a constant osmotic pressure driving force.

2.4.1.2 Higuchi - Leeper Pump

Design of Higuchi - Leeper pump described in Fig 2.4, represents the first simplified version of Rose-Nelson pump. It contains a rigid housing and the semipermeable membrane, which is supported on a perforated frame. Rigid housing is divided in two chambers by a movable separator. The benefit over Rose-Nelson pump is that it does not have water chamber, and the device is activated by water imbibed from the surrounding environment. This means the pump can be prepared loaded with drug and then stored for weeks or months prior to use.

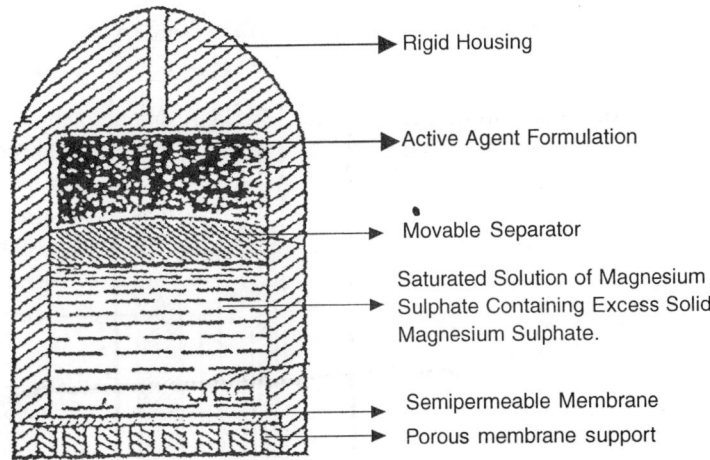

Fig 2.4 : Higuchi - Leeper pump

2.4.1.3 Higuchi - Theeuwes Pump

In early 1970s, Higuchi and Theeuwes developed a simpler form of Rose-Nelson Pump. As shown in Fig 2..5, semipermeable wall itself acts as a rigid outer casing of the pump. The device is loaded with drug prior to use. When the device is placed in aqueous environment, release of the drug follows a time course set by the salt used in the salt chamber and the permeability of the outer membrane casing.

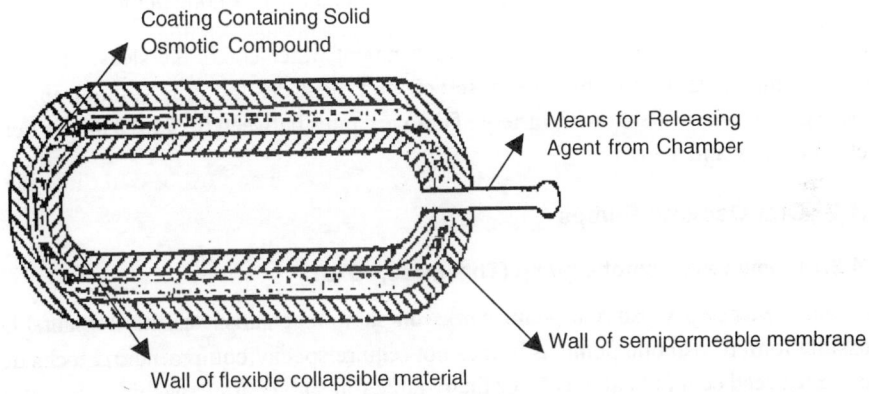

Fig 2.5 : Higuchi - Theeuwes pump.

4.1.4 Implantable Mini Osomotic Pump

This is most advanced version in the category of implantable pumps developed by Alza Corporation. As shown in Fig 2..6, it is composed of three concentric layers - the drug reservoir, the osmotic sleeve and the rate controlling semipermeable membrane. The additional component called flow moderator is inserted into the body of the osmotic pump after filling.

The inner most compartment is drug reservoir which is surrounded by a osmotic sleeve, a cylinder containing high concentration of osmotic agent. The osmotic sleeve is covered by a semi permeable membrane

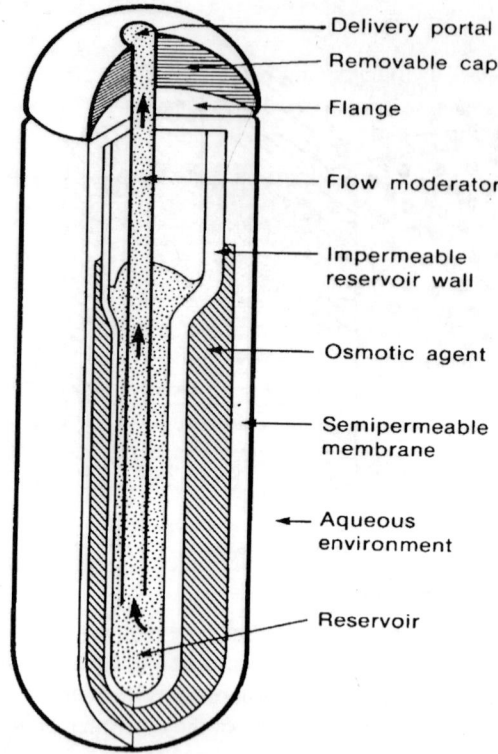

Delivery portal
Removable cap
Flange
Flow moderator
Impermeable reservoir wall
Osmotic agent
Semipermeable membrane
Aqueous environment
Reservoir

Fig 2.6 : Implantable mini osmotic pump

When the system is placed in aqueous environment water enters the sleeve through semipermeable membrane, compresses the flexible drug reservoir and displaces the drug solution through the flow moderator. These pumps are available with variety of delivery rates between 0.25 to10 ml per hour and delivery duration between 1 day and 4 weeks.

2.4.2 Oral Osmotic Pumps

2.4.2.1 Elementary osmotic pump (Theeuwes, 1975)

Although elementary osmotic pump works on same mechanism as the implantable pumps, it is simplest possible form of osmotic pump as it does not require special equipment and technology (Fig 2.7). It can be mass-produced economically using ordinary tabletting and coating machine and a facility to drill an orifice.

The elementary osmotic pump consists of an osmotic core containing drug, which is coated with a semipermeable membrane, usually cellulose acetate, with a delivery orifice. The core may or may not contain an osmotic agent depending on the osmotic activity of the drug. When exposed to aqueous environment, the core imbibes water osmotically at a controlled rate through the semipermeable membrane, forming a saturated drug solution inside the system. The membrane being non-extensible, internal volume of the pump remains constant. The system delivers, via the orifice, in any time interval, a volume of saturated solution of drug equal to volume of water uptake. This process continues at a constant rate until all solid drug inside the tablet has been dissolved and only a solution filled shell remains. The residual dissolved drug continues to be delivered, but at a declining rate, until the osmotic pressure inside and outside the pump is equal. The typical release rate

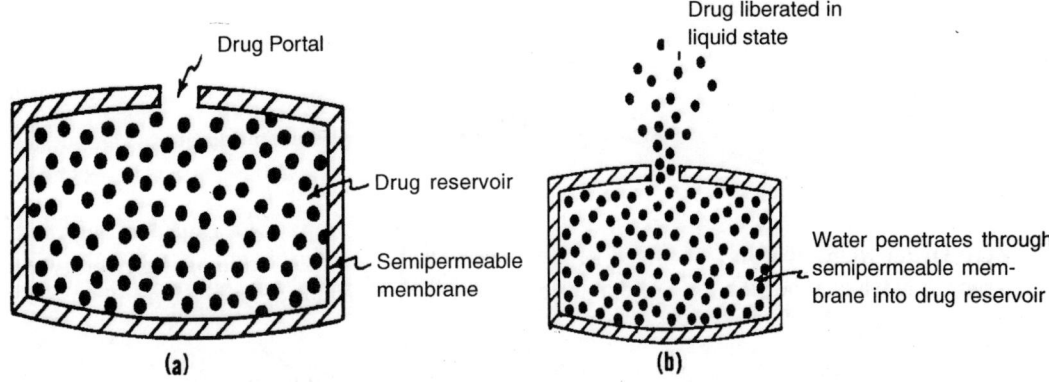

Fig 2.7 : The elementry osmotic pump (a) Before operation (b) After operation

obtained from this system is illustrated in Fig 2.8. Elementary osmotic pump is most appropriate for delivery of drugs having moderate solubility (50 to 500 mg/ml) in water. It typically delivers 60-80% of its contents at constant rate.

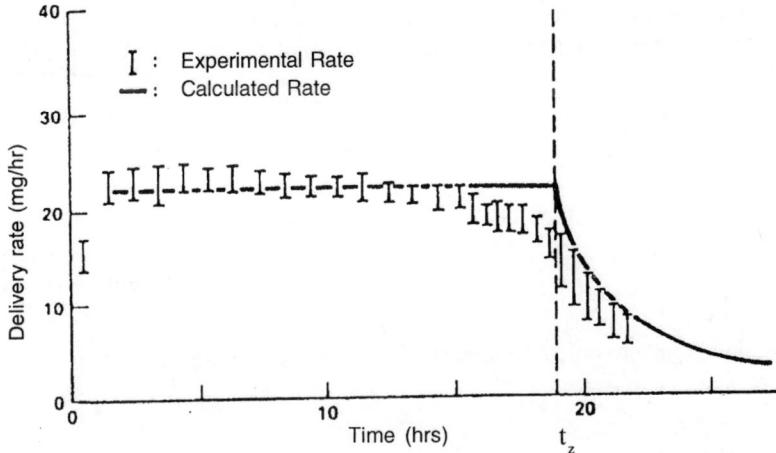

Fig 2.8 :In vitro delivery rate profile of potassium chloride elementry osmotic pumps in water at 37°C.

Delivery rate of the drug is dependent on membrane permeability, the osmotic pressure of the core formulation, and the solubility of the drug in question. The delivery rate is independent of the release orifice size as long as the cross sectional area (A_o) is within two critical limits; $A_{min} \leq A_o \leq A_{max}$. The size of the orifice must be larger than a minimum size, A_{min}, to minimize hydrostatic pressure within the device. This is a necessary step in achieving zero order drug release. The presence of any significant hydrostatic pressure would decrease the delivery force for drug delivery. In addition, larger hydrostatic pressure could deform the device. The size of orifice must be smaller than a maximum size, A_{max}, to minimize diffusional contribution to the delivery rate.

The general expression for the solute delivery rate, dm/dt, obtained by pumping through the orifice is described by Rose-Nelson equation is given below:

$$\frac{dm}{dt} = \frac{A}{h} Lp \, (\sigma \Delta \pi - \Delta P) \, C \qquad (Eq.4)$$

As the delivery orifice increases, hydrostatic pressure inside the system is minimized as expressed by the condition $\Delta\pi \gg \Delta P$.

When the osmotic pressure of the formulation (π) is large compared to the osmotic pressure of the environment, π can be substituted for $\Delta\pi$. Eq. 4 then reduces to a much simpler expression in which the constant k replaces the product $L_p\sigma$:

$$\frac{dm}{dt} = \frac{A}{h} k\pi C \qquad \text{(Eq.5)}$$

Zero-Order Delivery Rate - The release rate from the elementary osmotic pump is zero order from $t = 0$ until a time t_z, at which time all of the solid in the core has dissolved and is described by:

$$\left(\frac{dm}{dt}\right)_z = \frac{A}{H} k\pi_s S \qquad \text{(Eq. 6)}$$

where S is the solubility, and ps is the osmotic pressure at saturation.

The rate of dissolution of a single compound within the system is much larger than the rate of pumping as given in Eq.6. For this reason, the concentration, C, can be replaced by the component solubility, S, from time $t = 0$ to $t = t_z$.

Nonzero-Order Release Rate - The nonzero-order release rate from the system (Eq 5) is obtained by describing the concentration, C, as a function of time. For simplicity, the volume flux into the system is replaced by the symbol F:

$$F = \frac{A}{h} k\pi \qquad \text{(Eq.7)}$$

and F_s represents the flux during the zero-order time and is related to F by:

$$\frac{F_s}{F} = \frac{\pi_s}{p} = \frac{S}{C} \qquad \text{(Eq.8)}$$

By substituting Eq. 8 into Eq. 5, the nonzero-order release rate as a function of concentration is given by:

$$\frac{dm}{dt} = \frac{F_s}{S} C^2 \qquad \text{(Eq.9)}$$

Beyond t_z the mass m, of component dissolved into the elementary pump volume, V, is given by:

$$m = CV \qquad \text{(Eq.10)}$$

The change in mass at constant volume V, causes a concentration change, dC/dt, given by:

$$\frac{dm}{dt} = -V \frac{dC}{dt} \qquad \text{(Eq.11)}$$

The delivery rate, dm/dt, can be eliminated between Eqs.9 and 11 as shown by:

$$-\frac{dC}{dt} = \frac{Fs}{VS} C^2 \qquad \text{(Eq.12)}$$

The concentration, C, inside the system is obtained by integrating Eq.12 from time tz to t, when the concentration changes from S to C:

$$-\int_{s}^{c} \frac{dC}{C^2} = \frac{Fs}{V_s} \int_{z}^{t} dt \qquad \text{(Eq 13)}$$

Solving Eq.13 and rearranging terms result in an expression for the concentration as a function of time:

$$C = \frac{VS}{V + F_s(t-t_z)} \qquad \text{(Eq.14)}$$

Substituting Eq. 13 into Eq. 8 gives the release rate as a function of time, indicating the parabolic decline.

$$\frac{dm}{dt} = \frac{F_s S}{\left[1 + \dfrac{F_s}{V}\left(t - t_z\right)\right]^2} \qquad \text{(Eq 15)}$$

The nonzero - order release rate can also be expressed as a fraction of the zero order rate.

$$\frac{dm}{dt} = \frac{\left(dm/dt\right)_z}{\left[1 + \dfrac{1}{SV}\left(\dfrac{dm}{dt}\right)_z (t - t_z)\right]^2} \qquad \text{(Eq 16)}$$

The delivery rate discussed in this section is the rate from the elementary osmotic pump when most of the contents are delivered by pumping. When the membrane is not ideally semipermeable, a fraction of the agent is delivered by diffusion through the membrane.

Mass Delivered at Zero Order, mz, and Zero-Order Delivery Time, t_z - For a total mass, m_t, contained in the core of the elementary osmotic pump, only an amount mz is delivered at zero order, and an amount m_{NZ} is delivered at a parabolically declining rate given by Eq.15. The amount m_{NZ} is the mass that just fills the internal volume of the system with a saturated solution, as shown by:

$$m_{NZ} = SV \qquad \text{(Eq.17)}$$

The internal volume, V, of the system containing a pure component is related to the total mass mt, by the density, r, of the core by:

$$m_t = \rho V \qquad \text{(Eq.18)}$$

The fraction not delivered at zero order is obtained from Eqs.17 and 18 and given by:

$$\frac{m_{NZ}}{m_t} = \frac{S}{\rho} \qquad \text{(Eq.19)}$$

Since the sum of mNZ and mz is equal to mt, the fraction of the total mass delivered at zero order can be given by:

$$\frac{m_z}{m_t} = 1 - \frac{S}{\rho} \qquad \text{(Eq.20)}$$

The time tz at which the mass mz is delivered for an ideal system, with zero start up time, is obtained from:

$$\frac{m_z}{m_t} = \left[\frac{dm}{dt}\right]_z \qquad \text{(Eq.21)}$$

Combining Eqs.20 and 21 gives:

$$t_z = m_t \left[1 - \frac{S}{\rho} \frac{1}{(dm/dt)_z} \right] \qquad \text{(Eq.22)}$$

The membrane being semipermeable in nature, does not allow any ion to pass through, it allows only the passage of water, which makes the delivery rate of drug from the system independent of the pH of the environment (Fig 2.9). Since there is no requirement for the system to disintegrate for release of drug to occur and there is no influence of stirring rate (Fig 2.10) or surfactants on in vitro release rates, the in vivo delivery rate of drug is expected to be the same as that in vitro.

2.4.2.2 Push-pull Osmotic pump (Wong et al, 1992)

Push pull osmotic pump is a modified elementary osmotic pump through which it is possible to deliver both poorly water-soluble and highly water-soluble drugs at constant rate. The system resembles a standard bilayer coated tablet (Fig 2.11). One layer (depicted as the upper layer) contains drug (accounts for 60-80% of tablet weight) in a formulation of polymeric, osmotic agent, and other tablet excipients. This polymeric osmotic agent has the ability to form a suspension of drug in situ when this tablet layer imbibes water. The other layer (accounts for 20-40% of tablet weight) (depicted as the lower layer), contains osmotic and coloring agents, polymers and tablet excipients. These layers are formed and bonded together by tablet compression to form a single bilayer core.

The tablet core is then coated, using standard film coating equipment and techniques, with a semipermeable membrane. After the coating has been applied, a small hole (orifice) is drilled through the membrane by a laser or mechanical drill on the drug layer side of the tablet. The drug layer can be detected by light sensors (for mass

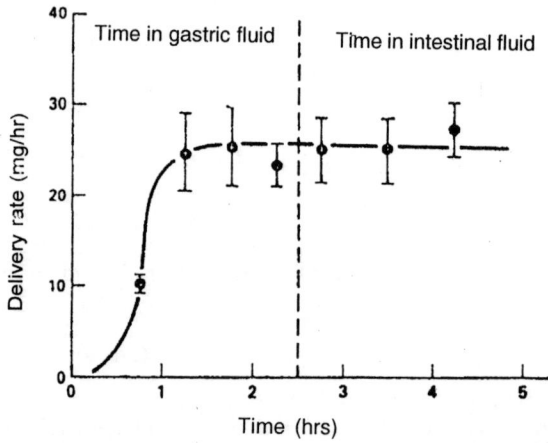

Fig 2.9 : Effect of pH conditions on in-vitro delivery rate profile of sodium phenobarbitone from elementry osmotic pump system in gastric and intestinal fluid USP (without enzymes).

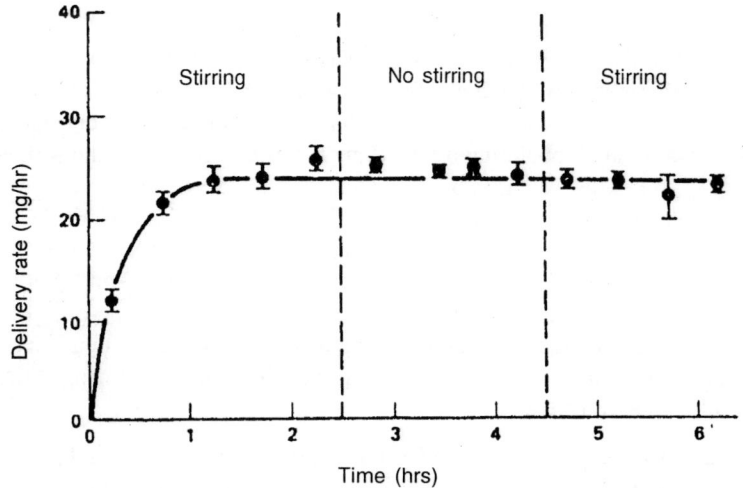

Fig 2.10 : Effect of hydrodynamic conditions on in-vitro delivery rate profile of potassium chloride elementry osmotic pump in water at 37°C.

production) or by an eye, which differentiates between the drug and the non-drug layers of the tablet based on colour (from the colourant added to the non-drug layer). A film coat can be applied (for cosmetic purpose or to protect light sensitive drugs) over the cellulose membrane to complete the fabrication.

When the system is placed in an aqueous environment, water is attracted into the tablet by an osmotic pressure gradient across the membrane. The gradient develops because of high affinity of the osmotic agents for water and the low water activity in the dry tablet core. The osmotic attractant in the drug layer pulls water into that compartment to form in situ a suspension of drug. The osmotic agent in the non-drug layer simultaneously attracts water into that compartment, causing it to expand volumetrically as shown in Fig 2.10. Since the membrane is insoluble and rigid in nature, it maintains constant shape and volume of the system and the expansion of non-drug layer pushes the drug suspension out of the delivery orifice. The delivery orifice is

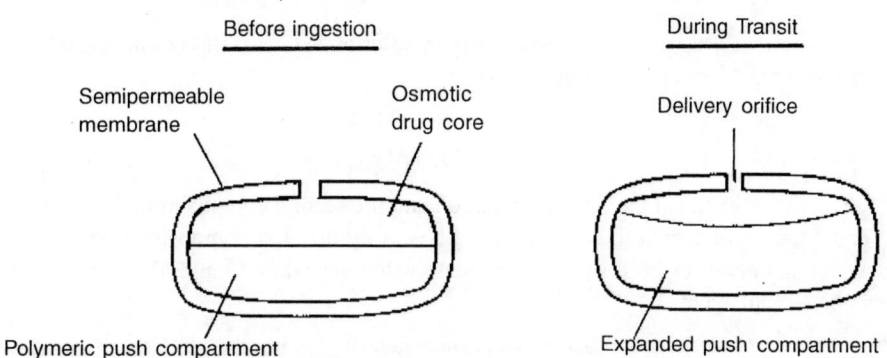

Fig 2.11 : The Push - Pull osmotic pump

large enough to eliminate the build up pressure within the system and yet not large enough to permit uncontrolled leaching of drug from the orifice.

The operation of the system can be compared to a piston within a cylinder. The non drug layer acts like a piston, pushing almost all the drug suspension out of the orifice as it expands. At the completion of delivery cycle, the membrane shell contains only the expanded non-drug layer.

The drug layer and the non-drug layer act together to substantially ensure that the delivery of drug from the compartment is controlled and constant over a prolonged period of time by two methods. First, the drug layer imbibes external fluid across the wall, thereby forming a dispensable composition, which is substantially delivered at non-zero order rate, without the record composition present, since the driving force decays with the time. Second, the non-drug layer operating by imbibing external fluid across the wall continuously and consequently, increases in volume as well as imbibition area, thereby exerting a force which can be constant, increasing or decreasing with time (depending on the osmotic formulation) against the drug layer and diminishing its volume, thus directing drug to the passage way at a controlled rate from the compartment. Additionally, as the drug layer is squeezed out, which is delivered from the device, the osmotic composition closely contacts the internal wall and generation constant delivery rate in conjunction with the non-drug layer. The swelling and expansion of the non-drug layer, with its accompanying increase in volume, along with the simultaneous corresponding reduction in volume of the drug layer, assures the delivery of drug through the osmotic passageway at a controlled rate over time.

In case of push-pull osmotic pump, the volume rate delivered by the device F_t is composed of two sources; the water imbibition rate by the first composition Ft and the water imbibition rate of the second composition Q wherein:

$$F_t = F + Q \qquad\qquad\qquad \text{(Eq.23)}$$

Since the boundary between the first composition and the second composition hydrates very little during the functioning of the device, there is insignificant water migration between the compositions. Thus, the water imbibition rate of the second composition, Q, equals the expansion of its volume:

$$\frac{dv_p}{dt} = Q \qquad\qquad\qquad \text{(Eq.24)}$$

The total delivery rate from the osmotic device is then,

$$\frac{dm}{dt} = F_t \cdot C = (F + Q)C \qquad\qquad\qquad \text{(Eq.25)}$$

wherein C is the concentration of drug in the delivered slurry or solution. Conservation of the osmotic device volume, V, and the surface area A, gives equations 26 and 27.

$$V = V_d + V_p \qquad\qquad\qquad \text{(Eq.26)}$$
$$A = A_d + A_p \qquad\qquad\qquad \text{(Eq.27)}$$

Wherein V_d and V_p equal the volumes of the first composition and the second composition, respectively, and wherein A_d and A_p equal the surface area in contact with the wall by the first composition and the second composition, respectively. In operation, both V_p and A_p increase with time, while V_d and A_d decrease with time as the device delivers beneficial agent.

The volume of the second composition that expands with time when fluid is imbibed into the compartment is given by eq.28:

$$V_p = f \frac{W_H}{W_p} \qquad\qquad\qquad \text{(Eq.28)}$$

wherein W_H is the weight of the fluid imbibed by the second composition, W_p is the weight of the second composition initially present in the device, W_H/W_p is the ratio of fluid to initial solid of the second composition, and

$$V_p = \left[1 + \frac{W_H}{W_p}\right] \frac{W_p}{\rho} \qquad (Eq.29)$$

wherein ρ is the density of the second composition corresponding to W_H/W_p. Thus, based on the geometry of a cylinder, where r is the radius of the cylinder, the area of imbibition is related to the volume of the swollen second composition as follows:

$$A_p = \pi r^2 + \frac{2}{\rho} \frac{W_p}{p} (1 + W_H/W_p) \qquad (Eq.30)$$

The fluid imbibition rates into each composition are:

$$A_d = A - A_p \qquad (Eq.31)$$

The fluid imbibition rates into each composition are:

$$F = \frac{k}{h} (A_d - \Delta\pi_d) \qquad (Eq.32)$$

$$Q = \frac{k}{h} (A_p - \Delta\pi_p) \qquad (Eq.33)$$

wherein k equals the osmotic permeability of the wall, h equals the wall thickness, $\Delta\pi_p$ and $\Delta\pi_d$ are the osmotic gradients for the first composition and the second composition respectively. The total delivery rate, therefore, is equation:

$$\frac{dm}{dt} = \frac{k}{h} C \left[A - \pi r^2 - \frac{2}{r} \frac{Wp}{\rho} (1 + W_H/W_p)\right] \Delta\pi_d + \left[\pi r^2 + \frac{2}{r} \frac{W_p}{\rho} (1 + W_H/W_p)\right] \Delta\pi_d \qquad (Eq.34)$$

The system typically delivers more than 80% of their contents at a constant rate.

2.4.2.3 Controlled Porosity Osmotic Pumps

As discussed earlier permeability of semipermeable membrane plays important role in rate of release of drugs from the osmotic pumps. To increase the permeability of membrane and maintaining its semipermeable nature two layers of membrane are applied on pumps. The inner membrane is micro-porous membrane, which is made up of cellulosic materials containing some water- soluble pore forming agents. A semipermeable membrane covers this layer. When the system is placed is an aqueous environment the soluble components of first layer of coating dissolve, resulting in a micro-porous membrane, which provides greater flux of water into the system.

2.4.2.4 Osmotic Bursting Osmotic Pumps

This system is similar to an elementary osmotic pump except delivery orifice is absent and size may be small. When it is placed in an aqueous environment, water is imbibed and hydraulic pressure is built up inside until the wall ruptures and the contents are released to the environment. Varying the thickness as well as the area of the semipermeable membrane can control release of drug. This system is useful to provide pulsated release of drug.

2.4.2.5 Combination of Effervescent Agents with the Drug (Rastogi et al, 1995)

This is a commercially important variation of elementary osmotic pump. Drugs, which are poorly soluble at low pH, may precipitate at the pH of gastric fluid, when such drug (indomethacin) is delivered through osmotic pump it may precipitate on the orifice affecting its functioning. An effervescent compound such as potassium bicarbonate can be incorporated to overcome this problem. When delivered from the pump with the drug solution, the bicarbonate reacts with acid in the exterior environment generating carbon dioxide. The expansion of gas dispenses the precipitated drug, allowing for rapid absorption of the drug and preventing blockage of the orifice.

2.4.2.6 Pump for Insoluble Drugs

In this system for delivering insoluble drugs, particles of osmotic agents are coated with an elastic semi-permeable membrane. These coated particles are then mixed with the relatively insoluble drug and tableted and coated with the rigid semipermeable membrane in usual way. When this system is placed in an aqueous environment, water is drawn through the two-membranes in-turn into the osmotic agent particles, which swell and hydrostatic force delivers the insoluble drug out of the orifice.

2.5 ADVANTAGES (Rastogi et al, 1995)

Apart from reduced dosing frequency, reduced systemic side effects and improved patient compliance, other unique advantages of osmotic pump are as follows:

1. It delivers drugs at zero-order release kinetics. Constant delivery rate is an important specification for chronic treatment.

2. The attainable delivery rate is significantly greater than the rate that can be attained with diffusion based systems with comparable size. This is especially important for cases where large dosage of drugs must be administered.

3. Delivery rate is independent of pH and outside agitation. This therefore suggests that the delivery rate is independent of the variation in pH throughout the GIT (advantage over normal enteric coated tablet) and GI motility.

4. Delivery of drugs takes place in solution form, which is ready for absorption. Thus it is an in situ prepared liquid dosage form.

5. In vitro delivery rate can be accurately predicted since the system is well described by relevant equation and the delivery rate in GI tract is equal to in vitro delivery rate.

6. It is possible to design an osmotic pump for drugs with wide range of water solubilities.

7. Due to its zero order release profile it is used in very early stages of drug research, such as drug screening, animal toxicology and pharmacology and initial clinical testing.

Limitations

Special equipment is required for making an orifice in the system.

1. Residence time of the system in the body varies with the gastric motility and food intake.

2. It may cause irritation or ulcer due to release of saturated solution of drug.

2.6 APPLICATIONS

In his pioneering work, Theeuwes (1975) developed the elementary osmotic pump of potassium chloride and phenobarbital sodium and demonstrated the effect of hydrodyanamic conditions, pH of media and pore size on the rate of release. The release rate from the systems was obtained by transferring each pump at regular intervals from one test tube to the other, each tube containing fixed volume of dissolution medium and measuring the amount released in each test tube. The potassium chloride elementary osmotic pump were agitated with a stroke of 2-5 cm at a frequency of 0.5 stroke/sec. For in vivo experiments the elementary osmotic pump were administered to three dogs at recorded time intervals. The dogs were sacrificed, the devices were retrieved, and the in vivo release rates were determined gravimetrically.

The results of his studies exhibited a constant release rate under stirred and stagnant conditions. Also the release rate was independent of the pH of environment. He inferred that the delivery rate of KCl and phenobarbital sodium from elementary osmotic pump is governed by the osmotic pressure within the formulation and the water permeability of the membrane. He also studied the effect of pore size on release rate but found no systematic trend in delivery rate within the pore size range from 75 to 274 μm. He also observed good correlation between in vivo and in vitro release rates.

Theeuwes and co-workers (Theeuwes et al, 1983) fabricated elementary osmotic pump of sodium indomethacin trihydrate with release rate of 7, 8 and 12 mg/hr. They used potassium bicarbonate as osmotic agent due to its high osmotic pressure and buffer capacity and coated the systems using an air suspension coater. In vitro release rates were determined by differential release apparatus and USP dissolution apparatus and were found to be independent of pH of environment and stirring conditions. In vitro release rates were similar to in vivo studies conducted on dogs.

Liu and co-workers (Liu et al, 1984) conducted in vitro studies to compare the release of phenylpropanolamine hydrochloride from the oral osmotic pump and one marketed long-acting appetite-suppressant product (Spansules). It was found that osmotic pump delivered phenylpropanolamine hydrochloride at a rate, which was independent of hydrodynamic conditions in a well-controlled, validated dissolution apparatus and no significant difference in drug release profiles were observed at pH 1.2 or 7.4. The effect of environmental osmotic pressure on the delivery rate was studied and a linear decrease in delivery rate of phenylpropanolamine hydrochloride from osmotic pump was observed with increase in the osmotic pressure. The marketed product however, gave zero-order release up to 7 hours as compared to 18 hours from osmotic pump. The results led the authors to conclude that osmotic pressure controlled drug delivery system provides better control over drug release than the sustained release Spansule system.

Ramadan and Tawashi (Ramadan & Tawashi, 1987) investigated the effect of hydrodynamic conditions and orifice size on drug release rate from elementary osmotic pump systems. In this study, neat potassium chloride tablets were prepared, coated in accordance with patent literature, and orifices of various sizes were mechanically created. Release characteristics were examined using the USP basket method at different rotation speeds, and a Turbula mixer, using equivalent volume of distilled water (200 mL) at 37°C. The drug release was found to be dependent on rotational speed of particular apparatus. Moreover release rate was considerably higher under turbulent conditions operating in Turbula mixer. Using USP rotating basket at low stirring rates and at static condition the drug release followed zero-order kinetics but at 100 and 250 rpm, the release rate deviated from zero-order. The authors explained that the increase in drug delivery as a function of fluid velocity could be due to agitation increased water influx into the core of elementary osmotic pump by forcing water through the pores of the membrane and/or through the delivery orifice.

The study of release profile of potassium chloride from elementary osmotic pump, over a range of 70-500 μm orifice reflected the role of hydrodynamic conditions. In static condition and at low agitational speed there was no significant difference in average release rates but in turbulent conditions and under high rotating speeds, the difference was found to be significant. This may further be attributed to the increase of water influx through the delivery orifice.

Bindschaedler et al (1986) reported their study on elementary osmotic pump of potassium chloride with cellulose acetate coatings prepared from organic solutions or aqueous dispersions. A release orifice of 250μm was created using a microdrill and release experiments were conducted in 500 mL distilled water. Based on their observation, the authors concluded that aqueous-based latex films exhibit a shorter lag time to constant release with a higher release rate, in comparison to organic-based coatings of the same film weight.

Theeuwes et al (1985) developed elementary osmotic pump for metoprolol and oxprenolol for once daily administration. For the desired solubility succinate salt of oxprenolol and fumarate salt of metoprolol were used along with sodium bicarbonate as osmotic agent. Highly efficient method of laser drilling was used with rate of failure less than one in million. The systems were found to be stable after storage period of 2, 1, and 1 years at 23°, 37° and 51°C, respectively. In vitro release study was conducted using differential method apparatus, which indicated substantial drug delivery (60%) at zero-order rates. Vyas et al (1995) designed elementary osmotic pump, push-pull osmotic pump and diffusion pump of ciprofloxacin HCl using empty gelatin capsule shell. Elementary osmotic pump and push-pull osmotic pumps were coated with solution of cellulose acetate and diffusion pump was coated with emulsion of cellulose acetate solution and dextran solution (99:1). In case of push-pull osmotic pump, a swellable polymer was added in 1/3 part of capsule and separated drug and polymer layers with a septum. The extent of drug release was found in the decreasing order of push-pull osmotic pump (80%), elementary osmotic pump (60%) and diffusion pump (45%). This was explained on the basis of extra mechanical forces that developed inside the push-pull osmotic pump and elementary osmotic pump.

Mc Clelland et al (1991) developed solubility-modulated osmotic pump of diltiazem hydrochloride. The solubility of drug was determined in various concentrations of sodium chloride solution and the solubility of drug in presence of 1 M sodium chloride solution was reduced to 155 mg/mL from >590 mg/mL (37°C), the normal solubility of drug in distilled water. The devices were prepared with core that contained diltiazem hydrochloride and sufficient sodium chloride granules coated with a microporous cellulose acetate butyrate 381-20 film to maintain a 1M sodium chloride concentration within the drug compartment over a 16-hr period. Core was coated with a microporous membrane of cellulose acetate, sorbital and PEG-400. The device resulted in releasing 75% of the initial diltiazem hydrochloride load with zero-order kinetics over a period of 14 to 16 hours.

In another study (Zentner, 1989), diltiazem hydrochloride was granulated with a water insoluble non-diffusible resin (Dowex-1), bearing the same charge as drug, and other optional ingredients and then tableted. The tablets were coated with a semipermeable membrane made of cellulose acetate, PEG-400 and sorbitol. In vitro results showed a constant sustained release pattern of the drug after a brief lag period irrespective of the pH of dissolution media (pH 1.2 or 8.0) over 12 hours. In the absence of the charged resin, the drug release was found to be pH dependent (Jain et al, 1986).

An osmotic controlled release bilayer tablet for water soluble drugs was described by Wright et al (1992). In their device, the drug compartment containing the drug and an osmopolymer, a low molecular weight CMC (as thixotropic transport means), was placed together side by side with the osmotic compartment which had a higher molecular weight CMC as osmotic agent preferably with another osmotically active compound. The contracting drug compartment and the pushing compartmnet were coated with semipermeable membrane (made of cellulose ester and flux enhancer) which had an exit pore for the drug to be pushed out. Both low and high molecular weight CMC in the device cooperated to exhibit a high level of hydrodynamic and osmotic activity adequate for controlled delivery of the drug over the time with minimum (as little as 3.7%) residual drug left in the device.

For controlled delivery of a calcium antagonist, Wong et al (1992) prepared granules separately both from the drug, poly(ethylene oxide) (Molecular wt., 200,000), HPMC and KC1, and from poly(ethylene oxide) (Molecular wt., 5,000,000) and sodium chloride, and made two layered cores from the granules. The core was coated with semipermeable membrane made from cellulose acetate (95%) and HPMC (5%). The device showed controlled release of drug over 24-30 hours when studied both in vitro and in vivo in dogs. In another report, Wong et al (1992) described a similar system proclaimed to give time varied pattern delivery of drug. The device gave a drug free interval after administration prior to delivery of the drug. In this case, they used poly (ethylene oxide) only in one compartment in combination with HPMC, Fe_2O_3 and magnesium stearate. The other compartment contained polyvinyl pyrolidone, noncrosslinked polyvinyl pyrolidone and magnesium stearate.

Wenzel et al. (1990) described a system in which core contained diltiazem hydrochloride, polyvinyl alcohol, potassium sulphate and magnesium stearate, and was coated with a semipermeable membrane made from cellulose-2, 5-acetate and PEG-600. They found this system to give a controlled release pattern of drug (in vitro and in humans) which was adequate for single daily dose treatment. A similar pump device (Haslam & Rork, 1989), where the drug core containing diltiazem L-malate, sodium bitartrate and povidone coated with cellulose acetate, sorbitol and PEG-400, released 50% of drug in 6-7.5 hours when tested in vitro in different dissolution media having pH 1.2 to 7.5.

Theeuwes et al (1985) developed several osmotic pumps for metoprolol, which gave zero order drug release up to 10-15 hrs. In a subsequent study in humans, Godbillon et al (1985) examined the in vivo performance of OROS systems with different duration of drug release. In another study with six subjects, metoprolol OROS was dosed in a crossover fashion and using the Nelson-Wagner method (Wagner & Nelson, 1964), the in vivo delivery rate was determined. The in vivo release was found to correlate well with the in vitro release, but the lag time was found to differ by one hr. The authors concluded that the blood level curves substantiate the claim of extended drug release from the devices, with subsequent absorption from the gastrointestinal(GI) tract.

Swanson et al (1987) detailed the development of push-pull osmotic pump for 24 hrs oral controlled delivery of nifedipine. Zero-order release rates for the systems were 1.7, 3.4, and 5.1 mg/hr and total amount of drug released was 30, 60 and 90 mg, respectively. Chung et al (1987) conducted in vivo investigations to compare the osmotic pump system with conventional capsules by controlled delivery. Nifedipine administered by controlled oral delivery system was found to be well absorbed from GI tract. The oral osmotic pump system was observed to achieve a sustained plasma level of nifedipine with minimal fluctuation, while conventional dosing showed substantial seesaw-shaped fluctuation. Vetrovec et al (1987) evaluated the clinical efficacy of nifedipine releasing oral osmotic pump in the treatment of angina pectoris. Results from the trial indicated that the nifedipine osmotic pump is more effective in reducing angina attacks than conventional dosage forms. This may result from the controlled delivery of nifedipine from osmotic pump, which achieves a more consistent blood level within the therapeutic effective range for prolonged duration.

Soons et al (1989) compared the pharmacokinetics and pharmacodynamic data after administration of tablet and osmotic pump of nitrendipine in healthy subjects. Administration of osmotic pump of nitrendipine resulted in a relatively smooth plasma concentration-time profile in comparison with tablet. The mean bioavailability of nitrendipine from osmotic pump (8.2 ± 1.6%) was found lower than from the tablet (11.1 ± 4.5%), which is probably due to release of nitrendipine in lower parts of GI tract where absorption is not or less possible. The osmotic pump produced less side effects (as headache) than the tablet.

Kendall et al (1982) conducted a crossover double blind study on conventional sustained release formulation and osmotic pump of metoprolol. The pharmacokinetic behavior of the osmotic pump system was found to be consistent with its in vitro release profile, in that the formulation produced constant plasma levels over longer

Table 2.3 : Patents on osmotic pumps

Year of Patent	US Patent number	Details of Patent
1974	3,845,770	First general patent describing osmotic pump and list of polymers for semi permeable membrane along with their WVTR
1975	3,916,899	Continuation of patent number 3,845,770 gives calculation of the optimum diameter of the passage way including Amax and Amin
1977	4,008,719	Use of two adjacent semipermeable coatings of different composition in osmotic pumps.
1977	4,036,227	Delaying drug release by using bioerodible outer coating
1978	4,088,864	Details of laser drilling in osmotic pumps.
1978	4,111,201	Osmotic pump containing expandable mini pumps which control release of drug.
1981	4,256,108	Use of two adjacent membranes (semipermeable and microporous), a list of dispersants is given
1981	4,271,113	Automatic orifice formation during coating due to recess in core tablet
1982	4,326,525	Improved drug delivery properties by use of buffer compounds to moderate drug solubility
1982	4,344,929	Use of effervescent activity to prevent blocking of orifice due to preciptation of drug in acidic environment.
1982	4,309,996	Bicompartment osmotic pump contains a swellable osmopolymer forming expandable chamber.
1982	4,327,725	Bilayered osmotic device with hydrogel as driving member
1985	4,522,625	Semipermeable membrane blended with enteric coatings.
1986	4,612,008	Osmotic pump of diclofenac sodium with dual thermodynamic activity.
1988	4,751,071	Zero order delivery of drugs joined with pulsed release of drugs.
1991	4,992,278	Delivery of poorly water soluble drug in the suspension form (using a swelling agent) from single layer osmotic pump.
1992	5,082,668	Calculation for bilayered osmotic devices.
1993	5,208,037	Use of different molecular weight sodium carboxymethylecellulose in different compartment
1993	5,232,705	Device for time varying patterns of drug delivery like providing drug free interval, pulsated drug delivery
1993	5,221,536	Bilayered osmotic pump for antiparkinsonism drugs.
1993	5,252,338	Push pull osmotic pump for delayed drug release (after adminis tration initially a drug free period).

periods compared with the commercial slow-release formulation. Osmotic pump formulation elicited a more uniform haemodynamic response and a greater pre-dosing effect when administered once daily.

Bayne et al (1982) evaluated two osmotically driven controlled release dosage forms of indomethacin in a multiple dose crossover study in 12 healthy subjects. Following equivalent daily doses, less frequent dosing of both controlled release forms resulted in plasma concentration profiles that were more uniform than those following capsule regimen.

Based on principle of osmoregulation, Jain et al (1984, 1986) prepared GI tract resistant hard-gelatin capsule of tetracycline hydrochloride and a zero order release was attained through laser drilled pores. The concept was successfully employed in case of propranolol hydrochloride (Jain & Naik, 1989) and theophylline (jain et al, 1992).

2.7 BRIEF DETAILS ON PATENTS OF OSMOTIC PUMPS

A number of papers have described controlled release devices that are based on osmotic pressure concept, but a great deal of information is found only in the patent literature, which is not available to researchers. Up to December 1993, 240 US patents were issued on various types of osmotic pumps and most of them are assigned to Alza Corporation, California, US. Some information about US patents on important oral osmotic pumps is given in Table 2.3.

2.8 CONCLUSION

In this chapter we have tied to provide a guide to the fundamental principles underlying the application of osmotic pressure in controlled delivery of drugs. Therapeutic value of a controlled release pharmaceutical product largely depends on dosage form technology.

Osmotic system technology has been extended to allow rate-controlled, constant drug delivery over a wide range of water solubility. Delivery rates and duration can be designed to limits imposed by GI transit time and absorption capacity. In general these systems made 4- and 3- times-a-day regimens obsolete. Instead they made once-a-day dosing practical for many agents, including some with short half-lives. For these and the other reasons, the future of osmotic technology in drug delivery is bright.

2.9 ACKNOWLEDGEMENTS

The authors thank Sajeev N.D for his assistance in the preparation of this manuscript. The authors also thank M.I.Bhatt for graphical assistance and V.K.Gupta for his constructive comments.

REFERENCES

Bayne, W.; Place, V.; Theeuwes, F.; Rogers, J.D.; Lee, R.B.; Davies, R.O. and Kwan, K.C. (1982) "Kinetics of osmotically controlled indomethomethacin delivery systems after repeated dosing." Clin. Pharmacol. Ther., 32(2) : 270-276.

Bindschaedler, C.; Gurny, R. and Doelker, E. (1986) "Osmotically controlled drug delivery systems produced from organic solutions and aqueous dispersions of cellulose acetate." J. Control. Rel., 4: 203-212.

Chung, M.; Reitberg, D.; Gaffney, M. and Singleton, W. (1987) "Clinical pharmacokinetics of nifedipine gastrointestinal therapeutic system: controlled release formulation of nifedipine." Am. J.Med., 83(Suppl. 6B) : 10-14.

Godbillion, J.; Gerardin, A.; Richard, J.; Leroy, D. and Moppert, J. (1985) "Osmotically controlled delivery of metoprolol in man: in vivo performance of Oros system with different durations of drug release." Br. J Clin. Pharmac., 19 : 213S-218S.

Haslam, J.L. and Rork, G.S. (1989) European Patent, EP 309051 A1.

Jain, N.K and Jain, R.K. (1992) Controlled release of theophylline from capsule exploring laser drilling. Ind. J.Hosp. Pharm., XXIX (3) : 107-111.

Jain, N.K. and Jain, R.K. (1989) "In vitro and in vivo performance of a slow release capsule - compared with a conventional capsule." Drug Dev. Ind. Pharm., 15(1) : 117-132

Jain, N.K. and Naik, S.U. (1984) "Design of a slow-release capsule using laser drilling." J. Pharm. Sci., 73(12) : 1806 - 1811.

Jain, N.K.; Naik, S.U.; Sainath, B.R. and Dab, S.K. (1986) "Design and performance evaluation of a novel sustained release capsule." J. Control. Rel., 3 : 177-183.

Johnson, J. (1980) "Sustained Release Medications, Noyes Data Corporation." N.J.

Kendall, M.J.; Jack, D.B.; Woods, K.L.; Laugher, S.J.; Quarterman, C.P. and John, V.A. (1982) "Comparison of pharmacodynamic and pharmacokinetic profiles of single and multiple doses of a commercial slow-release metoprolol formulation with a new Oros® delivery system." Br. J. Clin. Pharmac., 13 : 393-398.

Liu, F.; Farber, M. and Chien, Y. (1984) "Comparative release of phenylpropanotamine HCl from long active appetite supressant products." Drug Dev. Ind. Pharm., 10: 1639-1661.

Martin, A. (1994) "Physical Pharmacy." 4th edition, B.I. Wavery Pvt. Ltd., New Delhi.

McClelland, G.A.; Sutton, S.C.; Engle, K. and Zentner, G.M. (1991) "The solubility-modulated osmotic pump: In vitro/in vivo release of diltiazem hydrochloride." Pharm. Res., 9(1) : 88-92.

Ramadan, M.A. and Tawashi, R. (1987) "The effects of hydrodynamic conditions and delivery orifice size on the rate of drug release from elementary osmotic pump system (EOP)." Drug Dev. Ind. Pharm., 13(2) : 235-248.

Rastogi, S.K.; Vaya. N., and Mishra, B. (1995) "Osmotic pump: A novel concept in rate controlled oral drug delivery." Eastern Pharmacist, 38(452): 79-82.

Rose, S. and Nelson, J.F. (1955) "A continuos long-term injector." Aust. J. Exp. Biol., 33:415

Santus, G. and Baker, R.W. (1995) "Osmotic drug delivery: a review of patent literature." J. Control Rel., 35 : 1 - 21.

Soons, P.A.; Boer, A.G.D.; Brummelen, P.A. and Breimer, D.D. (1989) "Oral absorption profile of nitrendipine in healthy subjects: a kinetic and dynamic study." Br. J. Clin. Pharmac., 27: 179-189.

Swanson, D.; Barclay, B.; Wong, P. and Theeuwes, F. (1987) "Nifedipine gastrointestinal therapeutic system." Am. J.Med., 83 (Suppl.6B) : 3-10.

Theeuwes, F. (1975) "Elementary osmotic pump." J.Pharm. Sci., 64(12) : 1987- 1991.

Theeuwes, F. (1981) "Microporous - Semipermiable Laminated Osmotic Systems." U.S. Patent 4,256,108.

Theeuwes, F.; Swanson D.; Wong, P.; Bonsen, P.; Place, V.; Heimrich, K. and Kwan, K.C. (1983) "Elementary osmotic pump for indomethacin." J. Pharm. Sci., 72(3), 253-258.

Theeuwes, F.; Swanson, D.R.; Guittard, G.; Ayer, A. and Khanna, S. (1985) "Osmotic delivery systems for the B-adrenoceptor antagonists metaprolol and oxprenalol: design and evaluation of systems for once daily administration." Br. J. Clin. Pharmac., 19: 69S-76S.

Vetrovec, G.; Parker, V.; Cole, S.; Procacci, P.; Tabatznik, B. and Terry R. (1987) "Nifedipine gastrointestinal therapeutic system in stable angina pectoris: Results of a multicenter open label crossover comparison with standard nifedipine." Am. J.Med., 83(Supl. 6B) : 24-29.

Vyas, S.P.; Guleria, R. and Singh, R. (1995) "Development and in vitro characterization of elementary osmotic pump bearing ciprofloxacin HCl." Eastern Pharmacist, 38(447) : 133-135.

Wagner, J. and Nelson, E. (1964) "Kinetic analysis of blood levels and urinary excretions in the absorptive phase after single dosage of drug." J.Pharm. Sci.; 53 : 1392.

Wenzel, U.; Metzner, J.; Rosin, T.; Jaeger, H. and Salama, Z.B. (1990) European Patent, EP 381181 A2.

Wong, P.S.L.; Barclay, B.L.; Deters, J.C. and Theeuwes, F. (1992) "Controlled release system with constant pushing force." U.S. Patent 5,082,668.

Wong, P.S.L.; Jao, F.; Theeuwes, F. and Lam, A. (1992) International Patent, WO 92/00729.

Wright, J.D.; Barclay, B.L. and Swanson, D.R. (1992) International Patent, WO 92/18102.

Zentner, G.M. (1989) European Patent. EP 302693 A2.

Chapter 3

Novel Carriers in Cancer Chemotherapy

U.V. Singh, B. Dinesh Shenoy, N. Udupa

3.1 INTRODUCTION

New drugs are being developed and made available for clinical use at an amazing pace and as a result of this, there has been considerable increase in both number and classes of anticancer agents. However, most of the drugs developed have narrow therapeutic index with greater potential for causing side effects. Drugs being mainly palliative, the life expectancy has increased negligibly. Simply making available new compounds that have therapeutic potential does not provide benefit to the patient unless an effective means of drug administration exists. The amount of intact drug that ultimately reaches the site of activity must be adequately large to achieve the desired therapeutic effect, but, insufficient to cause untoward side effects. The primary objective of novel drug delivery systems is to ensure safety and to improve efficacy of drugs as well as patient compliance.

3.1.1 Cancer - an enigma

Cancer is a disease of cells characterized by reduction or loss of normal cellular control and maturation mechanisms. Cancer is a leading cause of death in the world today. There are varieties of malignancies, each one possibly due to many causes. Strictly speaking, one should use the term 'neoplasm' (meaning a 'new growth') rather than the term 'cancer'. Neoplasms that have only the characteristics of localized growth are classified as benign. Neoplasms with additional characteristics of invasiveness and/or capacity to metastasize are classified as malignant. The most deleterious effects of cancer on the host are because of this ability to metastasize and invade into other tissues/organs. The etiology of every class of tumors (often used interchangeably with cancer) and among the same class of tumors occurring at different sites is a complex problem. Neoplasms are not always fatal and are considered to be amenable to treatment. The therapy is determined on the basis of stage of diagnosis, treatment(s) available, and patients compliance towards these treatments. The oncological characteristics of most tumors require one of the following treatments: total excision of tumor tissue, combination chemotherapy, immunotherapy, radiation therapy and a combination of the above.

3.2 THERAPEUTIC MODALITIES AND THEIR LIMITATIONS

The war against cancer has been launched in four segments namely, (1) prevention of cancer, (2) early detection of cancer, (3) regional cancer cure, and (4) systemic cancer control. The most commonly employed modalities for the treatment of established cancer are surgery, radiotherapy and chemotherapy. Immunotherapy and gene therapy are the other two therapeutic tools that are gaining importance in recent years.

3.2.1 Surgery

Surgery, a locoregional therapy, is the oldest treatment for cancer. Even today, it continues to be the most important aspect in the treatment of patients presenting with solid tumors. But the use of surgery has been limited to those cases in which the tumor has not yet spread beyond the limits of surgical excision. Unfortunately, more than 70% of patients with solid tumors are reported to have developed secondary tumors when they are first diagnosed. This is due to the spread of micrometastasis beyond the primary site. Hence, the advances in modern clinical research in oncology have combined surgery with other adjuvant therapies.

3.2.2 Radiotherapy

In 1895, Roentgen discovered X-rays and their biological effects, cell-killing effect in particular, became apparent. Soon then, radiotherapy established a major role in the radical and palliative treatment for locally advanced malignant disease. Despite the advancement in the field of radiotherapy, its success in clinics is hampered by the inherent factors such as tumor hypoxia, tumor size, normal tissue sensitivity and distant metastasis. Hence, radiotherapy is usually combined with surgery and/or chemotherapy.

3.2.3 Hyperthermia

The use of hyperthermia in treatment of cancers has a long tradition. Heat has been used for centuries as a therapeutic agent.

Hippocrates (470-377 BC) stated "those illnesses which are not cured by drugs will be cured by knife, those which are not cured by knife will be cured by fire, those which are even not cured by fire will be incurable" (Streffer, 1990).

Many of the difficulties in the field of hyperthermia in cancer therapy have concerned, and still do concern, the method of applying heat to tumors. Numerous techniques of heating have been tried, ranging from microwaves to regional perfusion (Selawry et at., 1958; Crile, 1961; Suzuki, 1967). Each method has its own inherent difficulties.

With microwaves, the heating effect is governed by the wave length used; different degrees of transmission and absorption of the waves by various tissues (fat, muscles, bone, tumor etc.) and reflection of the waves at tissue boundaries render this form of heating difficult to control. The use of ultra sound for hyperthermia has been hampered by the need to maintain some form of physical continuity between the probe and the tissue during treatment. The simplest method of heating tumor is by water bath immersion. Foot tumors, leg tumors and subcutaneous tumors on the abdomen can be readily treated in this way.

Heat directly kills cells, especially at higher temperatures (>43°C). It seems that, in principle, this effect does not differ qualitatively between a malignant and a normal cell. However, therapeutic benefit can be obtained from certain special factors which exist, such as low blood flow (Vaupel, 1979), low pH (Wike-Hooley et al., 1984; Thistlethwaite et al., 1985), hypoxia (Gerweck et al., 1974; Kim et al., 1975; Overgaard & Bichel, 1977) and low nutrient supply, which favor hyperthermic cell killing (Laval & Mitchell, 1982., Gerweck et al., 1984; Hahn et al., 1993). Hyperthermia is at present receiving widespread interest as a potential method of treating cancer. High temperature has been shown to selectively destroy several types of cancer cells in vitro and in vivo (Overgaard & Overgaard, 1972 a, 1972b; Kase & Hahn, 1975; Hahn, 1982; Giovanella, 1983; Streffer, 1985a, 1985b, 1990).

3.2.4 Chemotherapy

Chemotherapy of cancer has survived several years of criticism and is now an established means of cancer treatment. It was almost many decades before firm evidence was obtained that chemotherapy could actually cure cancer. Today, with cures documented in some proportions over a dozen different malignancies, it can be said that chemotherapy has joined surgery and radiotherapy as a significant treatment modality.

Two basic types of agents are recognized - cell cycle (phase) specific agents (CCS) and cell cycle (phase) - nonspecific agents (CCNS) (DeVita, 1971; Chabner, 1993).

3.2.4.1 Cell cycle (phase) - specific agents

The major cytotoxic activities of anticancer drugs in this class are seen in a particular phase of the cell cycle. These agents are technically phase-specific drugs rather than cycle-specific agents. It was noted in animal species that these particular agents produced a greater cell kill if an amount of drug was divided and given in multiple, repeated fractions rather than as a single large dose. These agents are then also termed "schedule dependent" (Skipper et al., 1967; Jones et al., 1977; Lippman et al., 1978). Examples of S-phase (DNA synthesis) dependent drugs are antimetabolites like Methotrexate, 5-Fluorouracil (Moran & Stranus, 1975; Martin et al., 1978); M-phase (mitosis) dependents are Vinca alkaloids (Vincristine/Vinblastine), Colchicine and Podophyllotoxin (Fries et al., 1964); G2-phase (premitotic interval) dependent is Bleomycin (Tobey, 1972; Rao, 1993), and G1-phase (synthesis of components for DNA synthesis) dependents are L-Asparaginase and Corticosteroids (Miller et al., 1969; Capizzi et al., 1971; Lippman et al., 1978).

3.2.4.2 Cell cycle (phase) - Non specific agents

In contrast, the cell cycle (phase)-nonspecific agents are equally effective in large tumor in which the growth fraction, labeling index and mitotic index are low. Moreover, drugs in this group are not schedule dependent but are dose dependent. In other words, the degree of cell kill is directly proportional to the absolute dose given, a single bolus injection generally kills the same number of cells as repeated fractions totaling the same amount (Salmon & Apple, 1972; Tobey & Crissman, 1975). Examples include alkylating agents like Cyclophosphamide (Proceedings, 1976); antitumor antibiotics like Doxorubicin; nitrosoureas like Bis-2-chloroethyl-1-nitrosourea (BCNU) (Tobey & Crissman, 1975); Cisplatin (Roberts & Pascoe, 1972).

The utilization of cancer chemotherapy breaks down into three major categories:

(a) Curative to some degree in clinically evident disseminated malignancy. e.g.: childhood leukemia, Hodgkin's disease.

(b) Curative to some degree in clinically evident localized and regional malignancy in combination with surgery and/or irradiation. e.g.: breast cancer, osteogenic sarcoma.

(c) Palliative in clinically evident disseminated malignancy (prolongation of survival). e.g.: ovarian cancer, multiple myeloma, breast cancer.

In the past two decades, considerable progress has been made in the understanding of some important factors that influence the effectiveness of chemotherapy. They include:

(a) The log-kill hypothesis (Salmon & Apple, 1973; Tobey & Crissman, 1975)

(b) Cell kinetics of both normal and malignant cells (Chabner, 1993).

(c) The mechanism of action of different cytotoxic drugs and their effect on the cell cycle (Jones et al., 1977; Lippman et al., 1978).

(d) The influence of drug scheduling (pharmacokinetics) (DeVita et al., 1970; DeVita, 1985).

(e) Drug toxicity, especially the effects on the haematopoietic and immune systems.

(f) Selectivity of cytotoxic drugs for certain histological cell types.

(g) Drug resistance.

The ability to cure cancer with local means - surgery or radiotherapy - is hindered by the presence of viable metastasis outside the treatment field. Malignant tumors, as they grow, may invade their surrounding stroma and will pass through the basement membrane. During this process it would constantly shed cells. Some of these cells are able to establish metastatic clones even before the primary mass reaches a clinically detectable level. In such instances, systemic therapy of cancer using chemical agents has been proved useful. Drugs can in some instances cure by themselves or help to cure when combined with surgery and radiotherapy.

For a wide range of disseminated cancers, drugs can achieve clinical remissions and regressions, which have a favorable impact on quality of life as well as survival.

Vexing problems with current chemotherapeutic approaches:

Compared with chemotherapy of bacterial diseases, it has proved difficult to find general, exploitable, biochemical differences between cancer cells and normal body cells. Major obstacles to the cure of neoplastic diseases using chemotherapeutic agents are:

1. Development of multidrug resistance.
2. Tumor heterogeneity.
3. Dose dependent host tissue toxicity.

Tumor heterogenecity and development of multidrug resistance are the two unresolved problems in cancer research and no clear cut understanding in this regard has been achieved till date. Besides the above two, the inherent problem of non-specificity of chemotherapeutic agents is a major area of research interest. This non-specificity is due to very subtle metabolic differences that exist between a cancerous and a normal cell. So, unlike in a bacterial infection, a cancer chemotherapeutic agent cannot exclusively act on the metabolic pathways of cancerous cells while leaving the rapidly dividing normal cells unaffected.

3.2.5 Strategies to optimize cancer chemotherapy

As the fundamental advances continue in the chemotherapy of neoplastic disorders, the greatest progress in the recent past is in the conceptual therapeutic developments. These include:

(a) The design of more effective regimens for concurrent administration of drugs, including combinations of neoplastic agents with 'biologic response modifiers.'

(b) The increased use of adjuvant and neoadjuvant chemotherapy.

(c) The greater insight into mechanisms of resistance to antineoplastic agents.

(d) The acquisition of knowledge of mechanism of action of many antitumor agents, which facilitates the design of new methods to prevent or minimize drug toxicity.

(e) Increased knowledge about such vital processes as tumor initiation and the dissemination, implantation and development of metastasis.

3.3 METHODS DEVELOPED TO ENHANCE SPECIFICITY OF CHEMOTHERAPEUTIC AGENTS

Antineoplastic agents are, therefore, neither specific nor targeted to cancer cells. Improved delivery of anticancer drugs to tumor tissues, thus, appears to be a challenging and achievable effort. Significant efforts have been directed towards the improvement of anticancer drug delivery in the recent years. At present, the specificity of antineoplastic agents is achieved by one of the three approaches, namely,

(a) Chemical conversion of a drug to an inactive pro-drug form. Conversion to an active drug is control led by intrinsic physiological process, and thus inappropriate drug activity is theoretically reduced.

(b) Utilization of simple soluble macromolecules to which a drug is immobilized. The macromolecular carriers exhibit intrinsic targeting properties and delivery of an active drug bound to the macromolecular carriers is controlled by processes intrinsic to the carrier and endogenous ligands.

(c) Utilization of more complex particulate multicomponent carriers within which the drug is shielded from degradative processes during transit. Delivery of an active drug is controlled by enhanced drug survival and may be targeted by the addition of specific ligands to the carrier.

3.3.1 Drug targeting - A "state-of-the-art" technique

For antineoplastic agents that have narrow therapeutic window and require localization to a particular site in the body, it is essential that they be delivered to their target sites intact, in adequate concentration and in an efficient, safe, convenient and cost effective manner. The behavior of drug in vivo can often be changed in dramatic fashion by coupling the drug to a carrier moiety. The plasma clearance kinetics, tissue distribution, metabolism and cellular interaction of the drug will be dictated, or atleast strongly influenced, by the behavior of the carrier. In some cases, manipulation of these changes in pharmacodynamic behavior can lead to a higher therapeutic index of the drug. As antitumor agents have a high potential to induce side effects and toxicity, localization of the drugs to tumor sites would certainly optimize therapy. There are different types of targeting, namely,

1. First order targeting (delivery to a discrete organ).

2. Second order targeting (targeting to a specific cell type within a tissue or organ. For example, tumor cells Vs normal cells).

3. Third order targeting (delivery to a specific intracellular compartment in the cells. For example, lysosomes).

Further, targeting may belong to one of the following classes:

A. Passive targeting: This relies on the natural distribution pattern of the drug carrier system. For example, particles of 5mm or smaller are readily removed from the circulation by macrophages of the RES when administered systematically.

B. Active targeting: This employs a deliberately modified drug-drug carrier molecule capable of recognizing and interacting with a specific cell, tissue or organ. Modification may include a change in the molecular size, alteration of the surface properties, incorporation of antigen-specific antibodies, or attachment of cell receptor-specific ligands.

C. Physical targeting: This refers to a delivery system that releases a drug only when exposed to a specific microenvironment, such as a change in pH or temperature, or the use of an external magnetic field.

3.3.2 Pro-drugs

A pro-drug is a compound resulting from chemical modification of a biologically active compound that will liberate the active form in vivo by enzymatic or hydrolytic cleavage. The primary purpose in forming a pro-drug is to modify the physico-chemical properties of the drug, usually to alter the membrane permeability of the parent compound. The change influences the ultimate localization of the drug itself. The derivative or pro-drugs are comparable to the zymogenic forms of enzymes. They exist in inactive altered forms until activated by other specific enzymes or biochemicals. Pro-drug systems have been taken even further by including as polymeric pro-drugs, in which a drug is covalently linked to a polymer backbone. This type of system could encompass a staggering number of possibilities. Encouraging results have been shown with Mitomycin (Kojima et al., 1980).

There are two major challenges to pro-drug constructs that limit the technology to specific applications. First, the technology requires that an activatable version of the drug can be manufactured in a zymogen-like form, and thus research into pro-drug development is comparable in cost to drug development. Second, the technology does not necessarily place the drug where it is most needed. Although activation of pro-drug forms is controlled anatomically by the site of its activating enzyme, its delivery is generalized. The drug, regardless of how it is administered, arrives at the diseased tissues or cells "by chance" in a fraction of the original concentration. The pro-drug may be activated only by involved cells, but its uptake may occur in many of the surrounding cells and tissues where adverse effects may occur. The pro-drug approach may be improved by a targeting carrier system. Work to ensure that pro-drug methods of delivery are more specific is being done with notable success (Kumar et al., 1993a; Kumar et al., 1993b; Brown & Anderson, 1993).

3.3.3 Simple soluble macromolecular systems

3.3.3.1 Glycoproteins

The family of glycoproteins includes many enzymes, acute phase reactant proteins and plasma proteins. Albumin and lysozyme, although common plasma proteins, are not glycoproteins. Mannose, galactose and sialic acid are the principal sugars that form the carbohydrate components of these simple macromolecules and tend to confer receptor specificity. They are not, however, exquisitely selective and glycoproteins that have larger sugar components may interact with more than one receptor. If enzymes are used in the chemical derivatization process to reproduce specific sugar residues on the carriers, a mixture of terminal sugars is usually produced thereby further reducing targeting specificity. To counter this problem, some carrier systems use neoglycoproteins that are synthesized under very controlled conditions.

In addition to targeting problems, the integrity and biological effectiveness of a drug may be compromised when the drug is bound to the glycoprotein. Gross conformational changes and loss of flexibility in the protein molecule due to drug binding or sugar manipulation may produce an inactivated or ineffective drug carrier complex. First, the drug may no longer exhibit pharmacological activity. Second, the carrier may lose cell specificity and may even become immunogenic.

Overall, the use of glycoprotein as a delivery system for antineoplastic agents is attractive conceptually because of the targeting specificity afforded by the ligand-receptor interaction principle and the relatively low cost of production. On the down side, glycoproteins can carry only a small drug load. Moreover, direct linking of the drug to the ligand by covalent bonding may induce conformational changes and charge changes that could simultaneously inactivate the drug and degrade the specificity of the targeting.

3.3.3.2 Recombinant technology as a carrier system

Recombinant proteins, largely devoid of carbohydrate moieties, are appealing drug delivery vehicles because they are not plagued by the technical challenges of carbohydrate chemistry. Many recombinant ligands and receptors are under investigation. While the specificity of recombinant proteins may exceed that of glycoproteins, there are several pitfalls. First, most of the recombinant technology is very expensive and to produce a drug delivery system on a commercial scale using this method may not be cost effective. Second, the concerns raised previously on the matter of conformational integrity and the consequences of covalent bonding on both the pharmacologic activity of the drug and the binding specificity of the carrier apply here as well.

3.3.3.3 Monoclonal antibodies

An alternative drug delivery system makes use of macromolecular attachment for delivery using monoclonal antibodies as the macromolecules. By definition, the monoclonal antibodies are very specific to their immuno-logical ligand and are thus very appealing drug carriers (Vitetta & Uhr, 1985). Although this usually does not provide much of a sustaining mechanism, the problem of spatial placement is addressed. The advantage in this is that far less drug is used, and side effects can be reduced substantially (Lee et al., 1990). Monoclonal antibodies have been coupled to cytotoxic anticancer agents such as Doxorubicin and the carrier substrate dextran. The monoclonal antibodies used in these formulations were directed, in theory, against epitopes found only on cancer cells. Unfortunately, in vivo trials have shown little improvement in the efficacy of the drug as compared to conventional administration (Brich et al., 1992). There are many other anticancer drugs that have been conjugated to monoclonal antibodies or their fragments, a few are Daunomycin, Chlorambucil and Vindesine. When choosing a drug for this type of delivery, one must consider many things such as, whether the drug is active extra- or intra-cellularly, if it must be cleaved from the antibody to be active, and the strength and method of coupling.

There are a few potential problems with monoclonal antibody based-delivery system. While antibodies are highly specific in their binding of ligands, the ligands may be present on many tissues. Non-affected cells that have targeted epitopes on their surface will receive the drug and may be damaged or killed in a process of selective toxicity. Another problem is that, because the antibody-drug construct does not always stimulate internalization of the carrier system, the drug may remain ineffective and bound to the antibody on the cell surface. A third concern is that, diseased cells may alter their expression of ligand thereby rendering targeting more difficult. Fourth, the antibody-drug conjugate may induce its own immunogenicity and be removed from the system before interacting with the target (Shea et al., 1989). Moreover, if an immune response towards the complex is delayed, the reaction may be directed ultimately against those cells that have bound to the complex. Fifth, conformational changes consequent to covalent bonding are also of concern. However, unlike recombinant protein and glycoproteins, antibodies tend to be very conformationally stable and usually retain their binding specificity when combined with other molecules. The same can not be said for most pharmacological agents.

3.3.3.4. Soluble synthetic polymers

Rather than targeting receptors or ligands, the backbone of a polymeric carrier molecule provides both control-led, sustained release pattern and a means of protecting the drug from the physiological environment until it is needed. The synthetic polymeric carriers are large enough to avoid filtration and removal by the kidneys but small enough to avoid trapping by the liver and spleen (Duncan & Lloyd, 1991; Lloyd, 1991). Many natural and synthetic biodegradable polymers have been investigated as implants, microcapsules, microparticles and nanocapsules in order to achieve prolonged release and targeting of a variety of drugs (Jalil, 1990; Venkatesan et al., 1995). In vivo a pharmacologic agent is progressively released from the carrier by diffusion. If the complex is phagocytosed, the pharmacologic agent is released following polymer degradation. Two soluble polymers, dextran and N-2-hydroxypropyl methacrylamide have been combined with both a drug and a target-ing agent with limited success. Otherwise, intravascular applications of these systems have been overshad-owed by extravascular uses. As with all of the other soluble systems described above, targeting specificity and molecular conformation are critical concerns. Especially in view of some of the apparent success, the use of soluble polymers as a drug delivery system may be better applied as sustained release vehicles rather than as targeting carriers.

3.3.3.5 A few examples for soluble macromolecular systems in cancer chemotherapy

Song et al.,(1993), prepared macromolecular conjugates between N-succinyl-chitosan and Mitomycin C. Acute toxicity was studied in normal mice and antitumor activity in mice bearing P388 leukemia. The LD50 of the conjugate and the life span were about 3 times that of Mitomycin.

Hashida et al., (1978a), synthesized a prolonged release derivative of Cytosine arabinoside (Ara-C), Cytosine arabinoside-agarose bead conjugate (Ara-C-AB). Following intraperitoneal administration of the conjugate the radioactivity could be detected in plasma and urine of mouse for four days compared to only 24 hours for plain drug.

Hashida et al., (1977a, 1978b), synthesized a derivative of Mitomycin C, Mitomycin D-agarose-bead conjugate by using cyanogen bromide method. Biologically active Mitomycin-C was released successively from the conjugate with a half-life of about 6 days in vitro, and also in vivo following subcutaneous injection of conjugate. The conjugate exhibited identical inhibitory effect against Ehrlich ascites carcinoma cells to free Mitomycin-C and less toxicity to mouse than free Mitomycin-C. The therapeutic index of the conjugate was two times greater compared to free Mitomycin-C.

Hashida et al., (1980a, 81, 82, 83, 84a,b, 85, & 1986) synthesized high molecular weight derivatives of Mitomycin-C (MMC) using dextrans of various molecular weights (MMC-D), polyglutamic acid (MMC-PGA) and bovine serum albumin (MMC-BSA) as carrier moieties. After intraperitoneal administration of MMC-D, free MMC could be detected in plasma and urine for 5 to 8 hours while MMC administered as a free form was eliminated rapidly. MMC-D showed reduced toxicity and increased life span in mice bearing Ehrlich ascites carinoma or B16 melanoma. MMC was liberated from MMC-D in vitro with a half-life of 24 hours regardless the size of dextran, while the liberation half-lives of MMC-PGA and MMC-BSA were 35.5 and 20.2 hours respectively. The regeneration characteristics and biological activities of MMC-D were also investigated in comparison to MMC. MMC-D showed about one tenth of the antitumor activity of MMC in vitro in contact with L1210 leukemia cells, but showed almost equal efficiency in vivo after intraperitoneal injection suggesting that MMC-D exhibited activity after being regenerated to the parent drug in the body. The factors dominating the antitumor effects of MMC-D, plasma disposition and in vitro and in vivo antitumor activities of MMC-D were studied in comparison to free MMC. The molecular weight of dextran or route of administration had no effect as far as sustained action was concerned, since the action was similar. The results suggested that MMC-D had some direct interaction with tumor cells and this interaction played an important role in manifestation of antitumor activity in vivo, as well as modified pharmacokinetic behavior in the body. A single intraperitoneal injection of MMC-D exhibited higher antitumor activity against intraperitoneally inoculated B16 melanoma, Ehrlich ascites carcinoma, and P388 leukemia than MMC, but lower activity against BDF mouse transplanted L1210 leukemia. Intratumoral injection of MMC-D showed a superior effect on subcutaneously implanted B16 melanoma, while intravenous injection of MMC-D exhibited reduced activity against P388 and L1210 leukemia compared with MMC. The disposition of MMC-D after intravenous bolus injection revealed that radioactivity was accumulated in liver, spleen and lymph nodes. The usefulness of MMC-D as a lymphotropic delivery system for preventing lymphatic metastasis of cancer was also suggested. Cellular interaction played an important role in the manifestation of the antitumor effect of MMC-D and these phenomenon resulted from physicochemical properties of macromolecular pro-drugs such as electric charge and molecular weight.

Table 3.1:Macromolecule-drug conjugates and properties of their linkage (Sezaki & Hashida, 1984)

Method and position of conjugation	Macromolecule	Property of linkage
Nitrogen mustard derivatives		
Mixed anhydride, carbodiimide	Polypeptide	
Chlorambucil		
Carbodiimide	Lectin	
Cyclophosphamide derivatives		
Reaction with acid anhydride	Pyran copolymer	Slowly hydrolyzed *in vitro*
Trenimon		
Reaction between free SH group and unsubstituted carbon of quinone nucleus	γ-globulin; antibody	
p-Phenylene diamine mustard		
Carbodiimide (via polyglutamic acid intermediary)	Antibody	
Methotrexate		
Carbodiimide (amide linkage at α and γ-carboxyl groups of glutamic acid moiety	Albumin Aminoethyldextran Immunoglobulin	Hydrolyzed in cells

Contd...

Method and position of conjugation	Macromolecule	Property of linkage
	Poly-L-lysine	Intracellular breakdown of
	Poly-D-lysine	L-isomers
	Poly-L-lysine	Breakdown of lysosomal protease
	Albumin	
	Concanavalin A	
	Lectin	
	Antibody	
	Poly (iminoethylene)	
Carbodiimide (via albumin intermediary)	Antibody	
Transesterification (O-ester at glutamic acid moiety)	Poly (vinyl alcohol) Carboxymethylcellulose	Breakdown by enzyme
Mixed anhydride; N-hydroxy-succinimide	Antibody	
Reaction with acid anhydride (pteridinyl amino group)	Pyran copolymer	Chemically hydrolyzed
Cytosine arabinoside		
Coupling to BrCN activated agarose	Agarose bead	Chemical prolonged release
Carbodiimide	Albumin	Estimated to be hydrolyzed in lysosome
Mitomycin C		
Carbodiimide (amide at lα-N position)	Dextran	Prolonged release by base-catalyzed hydrolysis
Coupling to BrCN activated agarose	Agarose bead	Chemical prolonged release
Adriamycin		
Periodate oxidation of intermediary dextran		
Schiff base condensation at amino group of sugar moiety	Polyglutaraldehyde microspheres	Stable in vitro
N-hydroxysuccinamide	Agarose bead	Stable in vitro
Daunomycin		
Reaction with hydrazide at keto group (formation of hydrazones)	Carboxymethyldextran; polyglutamate; alginic acid; carboxymethyl cellulose	Hydrolyzable

Contd. . .

Method and position of conjugation	Macromolecule	Property of linkage
Periodate oxidation of amino-sugár moiety of the drug (Schiff-base condensation)	Antibody Concanavalin A Melanotropin	Estimated to be hydro-lyzed in lysosome
Carbodiimide; gluteraldehyde	Antibody	
Periodate oxidation of dextran (Schiff-base condensation at amino group of drug)	Dextran Antibody-dextran	
Amide at amino-sugar moiety (via oligopeptide spacer)	Albumin enzyme	Breakdown by lysosomal
Amido at amino-sugar moiety (via cis-aconityl spacer)	Poly-D-lysine at low pH	Chemically hydrolyzed
N-hydroxysuccinimide (via spacer arm containing L-arginyl-L-leucine)	Wheat germ agglutinin	Hydrolyzed in the cell
Ester linkage (via methyl-ketone side chain)	Poly-L-aspartic acid	Hydrolyzable
Vindesine		
Acid hydrazide	Antibody	
Neocarzinostatin		
N-hydroxysuccinimide	Agarose	Stable in storage
Carbodiimide	Antibody	
Amide linkage at α-amino group in Ala-1 and ε-aminogroup in Lys-20	Poly (maleic acid)-styrene oligomer	Degraded in vivo to parent drug
L-asparaginase		
gluteraldehyde	Albumin Concanavalin A	
Fragment A of diphtheria toxin		
Disulfide linkage	Antibody	
Disulfide linkage (sulfonated fragment A)	F ab fraction of antibody	
Disulfide linkage (cystamine derivatized concanavalin A)	Concanavalin A	
Toluene diisocyanate	Antibody	
Chlorambucil: mixed anhydride	Antibody	
Fragment A of ricin		
Disulfide linkage	Antibody Epidermal growth factor	

3.3.3 Complex particulate multicomponent systems

3.3.3.1 Liposomes

The specific association of drugs with their targets could be achieved by means of a versatile carrier capable of transporting drug molecules from the site of application directly to the site of action (Gregoriadis, 1977) and this concept has been utilized to modify drug disposition. The liposomes are phospholipid vesicles or microscopic particles composed of lipid bilayer membrane which can carry water-soluble drugs in their aqueous compartments and lipid-soluble drugs in the lipid bilayers. This makes the liposomal carrier a versatile drug delivery system for both hydrophilic and lipophilic drugs (Grubber, 1987). Liposomes are chiefly composed of natural or synthetic phospholipids especially lecithins hence can be metabolized in vivo and are generally nontoxic and nonantigenic. The chemical composition of the phospholipid membrane controls membrane fluidity, permeability and surface properties. Agents can be entrapped without chemical bond to offer a controllable time dependent release due to restricted permeability. Entrapment of drug leads to different pharmacokinetics hence can result in better therapeutic index and enhanced cellular uptake. The importance of liposomes as drug delivery vehicle is now becoming well established (Roerdnik et al., 1987; Gregoriadis et al., 1984; Lopez-Berestein et al., 1985). This applies particularly to the ability of liposomes to buffer the toxicity of entrapped drugs while maintaining efficacy. Some areas in which liposomes display therapeutic promises are as carriers for anticancer agents, antifungal drugs, antibacterials, antivirals and antiparasites (Lopez-Beres & Juliano, 1987; Kim et al., 1994).

The behaviour of liposomes in vivo is strongly dependent upon vesicle size, lipid composition and lipid dose. Smaller vesicles are cleared more slowly than their larger counterparts (for the same lipid dose) and are less avidly sequestered by the liver. The circulation times are also sensitive to the lipid dose, higher doses lead to longer circulation time.

The most promising applications of liposomes rely either on the spontaneous uptake of liposomes by the RES (for example, in intracellular microbial infections and vaccination), or on the extended retention of small liposomes in the circulatory system for intravascular or extravascular access to cells, such as cancer or infected cells. Over the past 10-15 years, there has been a substantial investment in the research and development of liposome (or lipid-based) formulations destined for such applications and some of the resulting formulations are largely licensed for use in certain European countries and elsewhere, including USA; some are awaiting approval, and others are in phase I-III clinical trials. Annamycin, Daunorubicin (DaunoXome - Aronex Pharmaceuticals, USA), Vincristine (VincaXome - NeXstar Pharmaceuticals, USA) are some anticancer agents/ liposome based anticancer formulations which are undergoing clinical trials. Doxorubicin (Doxil - SEQUUS Pharmaceuticals, USA; D99 - The Liposome Company, USA) is being developed as liposomal formulation.

3.3.3.2 Niosomes

The vesicles, formed when a mixture of cholesterol and a single alkyl chain, non-ionic surfactant is hydrated, are termed as "niosomes". They can entrap solutes and drugs and are osmotically active and stable. In addition, handling and storage of the surfactant requires no special conditions. Niosomes behave in vivo like liposomes, prolonging the circulation of entrapped drug and altering its organ distribution and metabolic stability (Baillie et al., 1985).

Non-ionic surfactant vesicles (niosomes) prepared from a non-ionic surfactant (hexadecyl triglyceryl ether), cholesterol and dicetyl phosphate by Azmin et al. (1985) was used as a carrier for Methotrexate and was shown to modify tissue distribution of entrapped Methotrexate. Rogerson et al. (1988) Baillie et al. (1986) and Hunter et al. (1988) have used niosomes as drug carriers for Doxorubicin and Sodium stibogluconate, with and without cholesterol. The methods of preparation of niosomes have been described by Baillie et al. (1985). Niosomes may be regarded either as inexpensive alternatives, of non biological origin to liposomes or perhaps in vivo as carrier systems physically similar to the liposomes, but with its own peculiar properties which can be exploited to attain different drug distribution and release characters (Baillie et al., 1986).

Niosomes and liposomes of Methotrexate have extensively been studied by many researchers (Chandraprakash et al., 1993; Colley & Ryman, 1975; Kimelberg, 1976; Kosloski et al., 1978; Kimelberg & Atchison, 1978; Fry et al., 1979; Freise et al., 1979, 1981; Macy & Leserman, 1980; Magin & Weinstein, 1980; Todd et al., 1980,1982; Fry & Goldman, 1982; Patel et al., 1982; Woo et al., 1983; Claassen & Van-Rooijen, 1984; Patel & Baldeschweiler., 1984; Basset et al., 1986; Machy et al., 1986; Shek et al., 1986). Also, niosome encapsulated Bleomycin (Raja Naresh & Udupa, 1996), Plumbagin (Raja Naresh et al., 1996), Vincristine (Parthasarathi et al., 1994) etc. have been evaluated for anticancer activity.

3.3.3.3 Ultrafine colloidal capsules (Nanoparticles)

The loading of drugs into ultrafine colloidal capsule in the nanometer size range (10 to 1000 nm) is another technique used for the optimization of drug delivery to the desired site with the drug encapsulated, dissolved, adsorbed, or covalently attached. These colloidal capsules are termed as nanoparticles or nanocapsules and some of these carriers may assist cellular uptake via endocytosis (Couvreur et al., 1977,1993).

Nanoparticles can be prepared using alkylcyanoacrylates and due to their polymeric nature, these nanoparticles appear to be more stable than liposomes in biological fluids and during storage. They can entrap various agents in a stable and reproducible fashion. Stabilizers such as dextran and it's derivatives can be incorporated into the nanoparticle surface by a process of polymer grafting to modify the characteristics of the nanoparticle surface charges and surface behavior. The drug thus can either be directly incorporated during the polymerization process or by adsorption onto preformed nanoparticles. Selectivity in drug targeting can be achieved by the attachment of certain form of "homing devices" such as monoclonal antibody or lecithin. The binding capacity of these nanoparticles to Dactinomycin (90%), Vinblastine (36-85%) and Methotrexate (15-40%) exceeds that of these drugs incorporated into liposomes (Couvreur et al., 1979a, 1980).

Polyalkylcyanoacrylate nanoparticles appear to be new drug delivery devices for cells generally exhibiting endocytic uptake, since they are ultrafine, degradable units that are able to associate with various drugs in a non-specific manner. However, adsorption of certain anticancer drugs to polyalkylcyanoacrylate nanoparticles can modify drug distribution in tissue. Differential and selective increase in tissue uptake of anticancer agents would be of interest in cancer chemotherapy and polyalkylcyanoacrylate nanoparticles could be useful in this area (Couvreur et al., 1979b; Florence et al., 1979; Gipps et al., 1986; Kreuter et al., 1983; Manil et al., 1995).

Nanoparticles show great promise as devises for the controlled release of drugs, provided that the choice of material for nanoparticle formation is made with the appropriated considerations of the drug cargo, administration route, and the desired site of action.

3.3.3.4 Cells as carriers

Red blood cells, leukocytes, lymphocytes and fibroblasts have all been used as potential delivery vehicles for drugs (Jain & Jain,, 1997). They have an advantage of inherent biocompatibility, but they can not cross barriers and can not easily fuse with other cells. Erythrocytes have been explored as possible carriers for Methotrexate and Adriamycin (Kato, 1983). These carriers have relatively few practical applications and are not cost effective.

3.3.3.5 Microspheres/Microcapsules

Many of the more biocompatible polymers can be used as small soluble molecular drug carriers or they can be assembled as both soluble and particulate drug vehicles. Large amounts of drugs or agents can be incorporated through non-covalent forces into these assembled polymers. These particulate systems are best utilized as sustained release vehicles (Jayakrishnan & Latha, 1997). The use of albumin microspheres in drug delivery was first suggested by Kramer (1974). Several methods have been reported in the literature for the preparation of albumin microspheres (Gallo et al, 1984; Burgess & Davis, 1986; Gupta et al., 1986). Most of the methods involve application of suspension and emulsion technology. Factors involved in the formation of beads in the emulsification process are discussed in these reports. A wide range of therapeutic agents with different physical and chemical properties can be entrapped in the albumin matrix. Bovine albumin or Bovine Serum Albumin (BSA) and Human Serum Albumin have been extensively investigated for target-specific and sustained delivery of cancer chemotherapeutic agents (Lewis et al., 1992; Gizurarson & Bechgaard, 1991; Goldberg et al., 1982, 1990; McArdle et al., 1988; Willmot & Cummings, 1987; Willmot et al., 1985a,b; Fujimoto et al., 1985a,b; Morimoto & Fujimoto, 1985; Sugibayashi et al., 1979; Goosen et al., 1983; Verrijk et al., 1991; Truter, 1995). Gupta & Hung, (1989a,b) have reviewed the experimental and chemical applications of albumin microspheres in drug delivery along with an account of the toxicological properties of these particles.

Nishioka et al. (1990) and Wang et al. (1996a) prepared Cisplatin chitosan microspheres incorporating chitin to suppress the burst effect during initial phase of drug release. The microspheres showed enzymatic degradation by lysozyme. Microsphere properties were affected by the type and concentration of chitosan, drug concentration, cross-linking process (Akbuga & Durmaz, 1994; Murata et al., 1993; Thanoo et al., 1992; Li et al., 1991; Nishioka et al, 1989, 1990). Chitosan has also been utilized as a polymer for microparticulate carrier system for Mitoxantrone (Jameela et al. 1996), 5-Fluorouracil (Akbuga and Bergisadi, 1996) and Methotrexate (Singh & Udupa, 1998).

Recent advances on the use of PLGA microparticles and nanoparticles in controlled drug delivery have been extensively reviewed by Brannon-Peppas (1995). Biodegradable microspheres of PLGA have been prepared for sustained delivery of bioactive agents such as cardiovascular drugs (Labhasetwar et al., 1994; Sansdrap & Moes, 1993; Bodmeier & McGinity, 1988), anticancer agents (Yoshida et al., 1995; Niwa et al., 1993; Spenlehauer et al., 1988; Juni et al., 1985), peptides and hormones (Heya et al., 1994a,b; Niwa et al., 1994; Jeffrey et al., 1993; Ruiz & Benoit, 1991; Ruiz et al., 1990; Sanders et al., 1984), immunogenic agents (Alonso et al., 1994, 1993) etc. Apart from microspheres, other dosage forms have also been tried with PLGA for long-term drug delivery through subdermal implantation. The biocompatibility of PLGA implants of Carboplatin and Etoposide with the rat brain tissue has been demonstrated by (Fallon et al., 1996). Wang et al., (1996b) and Boisdron-Cell et al., (1995) have reported that PLGA microspheres could be used as efficient carriers for Taxol and 5-Fluorouracil. Methotrexate and Plumbagin also have been encapsulated into PLGA microspheres with enhanced antitumor activity and reduced toxicity (Singh et al., 1996, 1997e).

Yoshikawa et al. (1989) prepared Aclarubicin encapsulated polylactic acid microsphere for targeting. The intraperitoneal administration of microspheres sustained the drug release over a period of time. Kumanohoso et al., (1995) have reported incorporation of Bleomycin into poly-d,l-lactic acid microspheres and the in vivo activity of the same in dogs.

There are also reports about using haemoglobin (Yapel, 1985; Willmot et al., 1985a), gelatin (Oner & Groves, 1993b; Tabata & Ikada, 1987; Yoshioka et al., 1981; Narayani & Rao, 1996), collagen (Rubin et al., 1973), gelatin ((Narayani & Rao, 1993) and casein (Latha & Jayakrishnan, 1994; Jayakrishnan et al., 1994; Willmot et al., 1992) as natural biodegradable carriers of drugs for microparticulate administration.

3.3.3.6 Magnetic microcapsules/microspheres

These were developed to minimize the reticuloendothelial clearance and to increase target site specificity. The magnetic microcapsules/microspheres can be used to entrap a variety of drugs and this system has great potential in the treatment of localized tumors in the regions of well defined blood supply. They are composed of denatured human serum albumin matrix that serves as the vesicle in which an anticancer agent and ultrafine particles of magnetite (Fe_3O_4) are entrapped. They are susceptible to the effects of a magnetic field, hence with the aid of external magnetic field, these systems are aimed at concentrating drugs at a defined target site. This technique has been developed specifically for directing drugs away from the reticuloendothelial system. These delivery systems are capable of altering the distribution of chemotherapeutic agents in the body and hence they offer the possibility of improving the therapeutic efficacy of the entrapped drugs (Kramer, 1974; Widder et al., 1979; Gupta & Hung, 1989a).

The tumoricidal activity of magnetically responsive albumin microspheres tagged with either Doxorubicin or Staphylococcal protein A was tested against an induced mammary adenocarcinoma 13762, implanted subcutaneously in the tail of female Fischer - 344 rats (Rettenmaier et al., 1987). Tumor growth rate was significantly suppressed in intra-arterially magnetically localized treatment group when compared with intravenously administered non-localized treatment group. The results suggest that magnetically responsive albumin microspheres can be an effective delivery system for cytotoxic agents and biological response modifiers. From the experimental evidence, with some limitations, magnetic microcapsules have demonstrated dramatic effects in directing anticancer drugs to a target site.

Table 3.2: List of complex particulate multicomponent systems reported with anticancer drugs (Kato, 1983)

Carriers	Drugs
Erythrocytes	Methotrexate, Adriamycin
Synthetic systems	
Liposomes / Niosomes	Actinomycin D, 5-Fluorouracil
	Neuraminidase, Methotrexate
	Bleomycin, Cytosine arabinoside
	Colchicine, L-Asparaginase, Plumbagin
	Bis-2-chloroethyl-1- nitrosourea, Vinblastine
Fat emulsion	5-Fluorouracil, Bleomycin, Mitomycin C
Albumin microspheres	6-Mercaptopurine, 5-Fluorouracil, Adriamycin
Poly (glutamic acid)	Phenylalanine mustard, Cyclophosphamide
Agarose beads	Mitomycin C, Cytosine arabinoside
Ethylcellulose microcapsules	Mitomycin C, Adriamycin, 5-Fluorouracil,
	Bleomycin, Carboquone, Peplomycin
Ferromagnetic ethylcellulose microcapsule	Mitomycin C
Magnetic albumin microspheres	Adriamycin
Poly (alkyl 2-cyanoacrylate)	Dactinomycin, Vinblastine, Methotrexate
Poly (L-lysine)	Methotrexate
Dextran	Mitomycin C
Gelatin microspheres	Mitomycin C
PLA & PLGA microspheres	Cisplatin, Bleomycin, Doxorubicin, Cyclosporin

3.3.3.6 Emulsions

Hydrophilic and lipophilic drugs can be administered as w/o or o/w emulsion respectively and can sustain the release of the drug. One of the major limitations of cancer chemotherapy is systemic drug toxicity on normal replicating cells. To reduce drug toxicity, low density lipoproteins (LDL) have been studies as novel carrier system for antineoplastic agents (Counsell & Pohland, 1982; Halbert et al., 1984). This is because of the greater uptake (Welsh et al., 1982) and metabolism (Gal et al., 1981) of LDL by tumors than normal cells. **Lipid-soluble** antineoplastic agents such as Methotrexate diester were incorporated into microemulsions which act as readily obtainable synthetic, protein free analogues of LDL. However, in vitro activity of the microemulsion against L1210 murine leukemia cells was found to be low (Halbert et al., 1984).

The efficiency of water-in-oil (w/o) and gelatin-microsphere-in-oil (w/o-G) emulsions as drug delivery systems for achieving specificity into lymphatics was evaluated in rat stomach by Hashida et al. (1977b,c). Improved bioavailability was achieved since increased transfer of Tripalmitin indicated the facilitation of lymphatic transport of Iodohippuric acid following injection of w/o and w/o-G emulsion.

Sezaki et al. (1982), demonstrated some pharmaceutical clinical characteristics of gelatin spheres in oil as a lymphotropic carrier as well as the potential application of isolated gelatin spheres independently or in combination with pro-drug modification. The efficiency of water-in-oil and gelatin microspheres-in-oil emulsion as a delivery system for delivering 5-Fluorouracil specifically into lymphatics was evaluated in rats (Hashida et al., 1977d). Increased bioavailability, pronounced retardation of release of 5-Fluorouracil and decreased peak plasma concentrations were obtained.

Hashida et al. (1980b,c) studied the stability, release characteristics and factors affecting lymphotropicity of water-in-oil and spheres-in-oil emulsion and suggested the superiority of sphere-in-oil emulsion compared to water-in-oil emulsion.

Delivery of Bleomycin in lymph as w/o emulsion and o/w emulsion by intraperitoneal and intramuscular injection was studied by Nakamoto et al. (1975). A comparison of concentration of Bleomycin in thoracic duct lymph showed that w/o emulsion was the most effective.

3.3.3.7 Implantable drug delivery systems

Polymeric implants follow the concept of controlled release systems that deliver a drug at a predetermined rate for a definite time period. In general, release rates are determined by the design of the system and are nearly independent of environmental conditions, such as pH. Implantable controlled release systems provide several advantages over conventional drug therapies (Danckwerts & Fassihi, 1991) viz.,

1. Improved control of drug levels at the specific site of action is possible due to the elimination of "peaks and troughs" resulting from periodic and uneven dosing intervals. In addition, less total drug is required to elicit the same therapeutic effect.

2. Preservation of medications that are rapidly destroyed by the body (this is particularly important for biologically sensitive molecules such as proteins).

3. Immediate removal of implants is possible in contrast to conventional drug delivery systems, in case of extreme allergies or side effects due to the drug already administered.

4. Reduced need for follow-up care and improved patient compliance.

However, there are few disadvantages of implantable controlled release drug delivery systems and these must be weighed against the advantages while developing one such system. Disadvantages include:

1. Toxicity or lack of biocompatibility of the materials used for the implant.

2. Harmful by-products may be formed from the systems, particularly for biodegradable types.

3. Most implantable controlled release drug delivery systems require minor surgery to implant and to remove from the administered site, if it is not a biodegradable type.

4. Dose dumping and variable imprecise drug release may occur if not formulated properly.

5. Pain and discomfort may be caused by the presence of the implant.

6. These systems can be more expensive than the conventional dosage forms.

However, proper formulation, extensive preclinical and clinical studies, strict quality control procedures etc, can take care of the above shortcomings of the implantable controlled release systems and hence, they may not be considered as inherent disadvantages.

Fabricating drugs in a polymeric device is a common technique, where drug release is regulated either by diffusion through the polymer barrier or by erosion of the polymer matrix. The non-biodegradable polymeric systems necessitate surgical removal of the implant after complete drug depletion. To overcome these problems, the concepts of biodegradable polymers for sustained release parenteral drug delivery began to be developed in the early 1970s. Ever since then, there has been considerable volume of research carried out in this particular area (Murthy, 1997). A number of implantable drug delivery systems have been developed for antineoplastic agents like Cisplatin (Fallon et al., 1996), Methotrexate (Singh et al., 1997a,b)etc.

The implantable pumps and reservoirs are being developed for the treatment of selected organs or for regional perfusions. This method provides an external control of delivery rate and delivers an amount of drug larger than the capabilities of conventional controlled release formulations. Regional artery drug infusion pump is promising with reports of prolonged survival compared with previously used methods of treatment (Vitale et al., 1986). Several recent studies comparing the performance of continuous hepatic arterial infusion using totally implantable pumps with conventional access systems for regional arterial chemotherapy of liver tumors have been described (Kemeny et al., 1986). Though the results of the studies were overwhelmingly positive, significant rehospitalization rate for complications and marginal increases in survival indicates that further improvements for this treatment are required.

Another major development in the recent years is the formulation of biodegradable "in situ gel-forming" drug delivery systems. Dunn et al. (1991), Tipton et al.(1992), Shah et al. (1993) have used PLGA copolymers in a formulation which forms a gel-matrix immediately on contact with aqueous fluids. This property of formulation can circumvent the need for making a surgical incision to implant the matrix. The gel-matrix thus formed will release the incorporated drug slowly, over a period of weeks to months, and ultimately biodegrade depending on the composition of the polymer used. This novel formulation design for a biodegradable injectable implant can provide prolonged release while avoiding the necessity for any surgical procedures. This particular carrier has been employed for Methotrexate (Singh et al., 1997c,d) with encouraging results.

3.4 INTRA-TUMORAL DRUG DELIVERY (Gupta et al, 1993)

The concept of administration of drug directly into the tumor arose from the non-uniform and inadequate accumulation of drug or drug carrier in the tumor. In intra-tumoral (i.t.) drug delivery novel strategies were employed due to non-maintenance of effective drug level in the tumor tissue for sufficiently longer time. Prodrug approach has been successfully utilized for i.t. chemotherapy for a variety of drugs. Mitomycin C was conjugated with dextran and subcutaneously implanted in B16 melanoma followed by i.t. delivery of free and conjugated MMC which resulted in considerable reduction in tumor growth. Melphalan was conjugated to 60 and 14K poly (1-glutamic acid) and subcutaneously implanted in Yoshida sarcoma rat. This was followed by i.t. delivery of free and conjugated drug. Significant reduction in tumor growth was observed in case of conjugated drug. Methotrexate was conjugated with human serum albumin and it was found that i.t. delivery was more effective than i.p.

Intra-tumoral delivery can also be optimized using polymeric implants. Cisplatin-Collagen matrix, Vinblastine-Collagen matrix, BCNU (bis-2-chloroethyl-1-nitrosourea)-Polyanhydride implant, Methotrexate-Polylactide implant, all have resulted in considerable suppression of tumor. However, the i.t. implantation chemotherapy requires surgical manipulation and only tumor cells which come in direct contact with the drug are the ones which are largely affected.

3.5 CHEMOEMBOLIZATION

Embolization is widely acknowledged form of endovascular therapy. It consists of delivering an embolic material locally through a catheter that has been previously inserted in the vessels supplying the pathological area. Embolization has proved to be effective in the treatment of diseases such as hemorrhage, blockade (gastrointestinal, pulmonary), vascular malformations (aneurysm, arteriovenous fistula and arteriovenous malformation). Chemoembolization involves the selective arterial embolization of a tumor together with a simultaneous or subsequent local delivery of chemotherapeutic agents. Comparative studies (Fujimoto et al., 1985a; Morimoto et al., 1989) have shown that intra-arterial hepatic chemoembolization of the albumin microspheres containing Mitomycin C (MMC) is preferred to the conventional intra-arterial hepatic continuous infusion of 5-Fluorouracil (5-FU) and MMC in achieving a higher survival in inoperable hepatic cancer

Table 3.3: Characteristics of the microspheres adopted in chemoembolization (Flandroy et al., 1993)

Polymer	Mean size (μm)	Shape	Degradation pattern	Drug	Kinetics of drug release
Ethyl cellulose	200-300	Irregular	Non-biodegradable	Cisplatin	Burst effect
PLGA	100-200	Spherical	Biodegradable: few days to months	Cisplatin, Adriamycin, Aclarubicin	Sustained release
Albumin	7-80	Spherical	Degradable, few days	Adriamycin, Mitomycin C	Burst effect
Wax	125-800	Spherical	Non-biodegradable	5 Fluorouracil	Ist order release
Chitosan	150-200	Spherical	Biodegradable	Cisplatin	Sustained release

patients. Adriamycin entrapped in microspheres can localize in lung tissue and release the drug in such a way as to both obviate the high serum peak levels associated with bolus injection and maintain serum levels longer (Willmot et al., 1985b). Intra-arterial administration of heated albumin microspheres containing MMC to rabbits with VX-2 tumor resulted in conspicuous antitumor efficacy compared to conventional MMC. Albumin microspheres containing MMC was better than free drug when administered through hepatic artery to 22 patients with hepatic malignancies, consisting of 8 primary and 14 metastatic tumor. Effective tumor regression was observed in 14 patients (64%) and no serious side effect was seen. Antitumor activity and fate of Adriamycin incorporated into biodegradable albumin microspheres was examined in vivo, after direct intra tumor injection. Goldberg et al., (1992) have reported that the drug loaded albumin microspheres containing Adriamycin are more potent in their antitumor effect than the drug in solution. Their demonstration of intracellular drug in target tissue 4 days after microsphere infusion suggested that Adriamycin loaded albumin microspheres have "slow-release" properties in vivo which sustain high target tissue drug levels for much longer than those achieved with regional administration of the drug in solution. Studies conducted by Mizushima et al., (1986) suggested that lipid microspheres can be used as drug delivery carriers for lipid soluble antitumor agents. Starch microspheres have also been evaluated for intra-arterial chemotherapeutic drug delivery. This aspect of microcapsule bound regional chemotherapy has the greatest potential because it is possible that the potency of existing cytotoxic drugs may be increased. In addition, improved response rates at lower dosage and hence increase in therapeutic potential which may allow dose escalation, can be achieved with a microcapsule bound formulation.

3.6 CONCLUSIONS

Incidence of cancer is increasing consequent to dramatic changes in the demographic profile of an aging society. This is true especially in developing countries like India. A multitude of antineoplastic agents have been discovered and synthesized in the past three decades. Unfortunately, majority of conventional cancer chemotherapies have relied on episodic or bolus administration of antineoplastic agents and the patients are frequently exposed to peak drug concentrations, which are well above the toxic levels. On the other hand, critical therapeutic levels are not always maintained for sufficiently long for effective treatment of neoplasms.

In the last few years we have witnessed an explosion in research aimed at creating new drug delivery systems. A variety of novel carriers differing in the degree of sophistication are available to control, sustain and target the drugs via parenteral route. Although delivery systems that could target drugs to specific body sites or precisely control drug release rates for prolonged times have long been dreamed of, only in recent years has the development of such systems become practical. Yet, in a short time, new drug delivery systems have had an impact on nearly every branch of medicine including cardiology, ophthalmology, endocrinology, pulmonology, immunology, pain management and oncology. Annual sales of advanced drug delivery systems in United States exceed $10 million and are rising rapidly.

Drug delivery is a remarkable interdiciplinary field. Important contributions have come from material scientists, engineers, biologists, pharmaceutical scientists and others who have developed important concepts and brought them to clinical applications. Certainly one activity that will take place in the next 10 to 20 years is the clinical introduction and evaluation of many of the new delivery systems.

Progress in immunology and human genomics should lead to a greater insight into the type of targeting molecules that can be used to achieve site-specific drug delivery. Advances in comibinatorial chemistry are already been used to create new biomaterials and may enable large numbers of new biomaterials to be screened more rapidly. Progress in microelectronics and nanotechnology may some day lead to tiny robots that may be able to travel through the blood stream and perform both physical and chemical functions. The understanding of transport phenomena through various portals in the body such as the intestine, lung and skin may lead to new drug delivery strategies. In addition, the development of mathematical model that can predict delivery performance will facilitate the design of various delivery systems.

Gene therapy is a powerful new technology that still requires several years before it will make a noticeable impact on the treatment of cancer. Several major deficiencies still exist including poor delivery systems, both viral and non-viral, and poor gene expression after genes are delivered. The reason for the low efficiency of gene transfer and expression in human patients is that we still lack the basic understanding of how vector should be constructed, what regulatory sequences are appropriate for which cell types, how in vivo immune defenses can be overcome, and how to manufacture efficiently the vectors we do make. It is not surprising that we have not yet had notable clinical successes. Nonetheless, the lessons we are learning in the clinic are invaluable in illuminating the problems that future research must solve. Despite our present lack of knowledge, gene therapy will almost certainly revolutionize the practice of medicine over the next 25 years. In every field of medicine, the ability to give the patient the therapeutic genes offers extraordinary opportunities to treat, cure and ultimately prevent a vast range of diseases that now plague mankind. The design of ideal carrier for applications such as gene therapy will be extremely important. The possibility of designing materials that can simultaneously avoid the RES, target specific cell types, be taken by those cell types in such a way as not to destroy their DNA, and made to release the DNA unharmed so that the DNA can travel to the nucleus will be an important challenge. Nonetheless, with the progress being made in biology, chemistry, biomaterials, engineering and pharmaceutical sciences, this field should have a bright and rapidly evolving future.

Use of polymeric materials particularly of biodegradable type has gained lot of importance during the last two decades in drug delivery research. In spite of the advent of many synthetic biodegradable polymers, the use of natural polymers to deliver drugs looks to be an active area of research due to obvious reasons of compatibility, economy and ready availability. Out of many natural polymers investigated collagen, gelatin, albumin, polysaccharides like dextran, starch show promising potentialities. As our understanding of the drug action and pathogenesis of different types of neoplasms becomes clearer, more rational approaches to the design of therapeutic systems with functions that selectively target the tumors, or deliver the drug cargo to it's intended site of action, with no or reduced side effects, will emerge. Current research in this area involves various novel systems, many of which have strong therapeutic potential. The future of this area is limited only by the imagination of those who choose to become involved in this field.

REFERENCES

Akbuga, J. and Bergisadi, N. (1996) "5-Fluorouracil-loaded chitosan microspheres: preparation and release characteristics." J. Microencapsul., 13(2) : 161-168.

Akbuga, J. and Durmaz, G. (1994), "Preparation and evaluation of cross-linked chitosan microspheres containing furosemide." Int. J. Pharm., 111: 217-222.

Alonso, M.J.; Cohen, S.; Park, T.G.; Gupta, R.K.; Siber, G.R. and Langer, R. (1993) "Determinants of release rates of tetanus vaccine from polyester microcapsules." Pharm. Res., 10 : 945-953.

Alonso, M.J.; Gupta, R.K.; Min, C.; Siber, G.R. and Langer, R. (1994) "Biodegradable microspheres as controlled release tetanus toxoid delivery systems." Vaccine, 12: 299-306.

Azmin, M.N.; Florence, A.T.; Handjani-Vila, R.M.; Stuart, J.F.B.; Vanlerberghe, G. and Whittaker, J.S. (1985) "The effect of non-ionic surfactant vesicle (Niosome) entrapment on the absorption and distribution of methotrexate in mice." J. Pharm. Pharmacol., 37: 237-242.

Baillie, A.J.; Coombs, G.H.; Dolon, T.F. and Laurie, J. (1986) "Non-ionic surfactant vesicles, Niosomes, as a delivery system for the antileishmanial drug Sodium stilbogluconate." J. Pharm. Pharmacol., 38: 502-505.

Baillie, A.J.; Florence, A.; Hume, L.R.; Muirhead, G.T. and Rogerson, A. (1985) "The preparation and properties of niosomes - non-ionic surfactant vesicles." J. Pharm. Pharmacol., 38: 863-865.

Basset, J.B.; Anderson, R.U. and Tacker, J.R. (1986) "Use of temperature-sensitive liposomes in the selective delivery of methotrex-ate and cisplatinum analogues to murine bladder tumor." J. Urol., 135: 612-615.

Bodmeier, R. and McGinity, J.W. (1988) "Solvent selection in the preparation of poly (dL-lactide) microspheres prepared by solvent preparation method." Int. J. Pharm., 43 : 179-186.

Boisdron-Cell, M.; Menei, P.; and Benoit, J.P. (1995) "Preparation and characterization of 5-fluorouracil-loaded microparticles as biodegradable anticancer drug carriers." J. Pharm. Pharmacol., 47(2) : 108-114.

Brannon-Peppas, L. (1995) "Recent advances on the use of biodegradable microparticles and nanoparticles in controlled drug delivery." Int. J. Pharm., 116 : 116-119.

Brich, Z.; Ravel, S.; Kissel, T.; Fritsch, J. and Schoffmann, A. (1992) "Preparation and characterization of a water soluble dextran immunoconjugate of Doxorubicin and the monoclonal antibody (ABL 364)." J. Control. Rel., 19 : 245-258.

Brown, M.R., and Anderson, B.E. (1993) "Receptor-ligand interactions between serum amyloid P component and model soluble immune complexes." J. Immunol., 151(4) : 2087-2095.

Burgess, D.J. and Davis, S.S. (1986) "Prednisolone release from albumin microspheres In vitro and in vivo studies by intra-articular injection into rabbits." J. Pharm. Pharmacol., 38(suppl) : 23.

Capizzi, R.L.; Bertino, J.R. and Steel, R.T. (1971) "L-asparaginase: clinical, biochemical, pharmacological and immunological studies." Ann. Intern. Med., 24 : 893-901.

Chabner, B.A. (1993) "Anticancer drugs." In: DeVita, V.T.; Hellman, S. and Rosenberg, S.A., (eds.), "Cancer. Principles and Practice of Oncology", 4th edition, JB Lippincott, Philadelphia: 325.

Chandraprakash, K.S.; Udupa, N.; Uma Devi, P. and Pillai, G.K. (1993) "Effect of niosome encapsulation of methotrexate, macrophage activation on tissue distribution of methotrexate and tumor size." Drug Delivery, 1: 133-137.

Claassen, E. and Van Rooijen, N. (1984) "The effect of elimination of macrophages on the tissue distribution of liposomes containing [3H] methotrexate." Biochem. Biophys. Acta., 802: 428-434.

Colley, C.M. and Ryman, B.E. (1975) "Liposomes as carriers in vivo for methotrexate." Biochem. Soc. Trans., 3 : 157-159.

Counsell, R.E. and Pohland, R.C. (1982) "Lipoproteins as potential site-specific delivery systems for diagnostic and therapeutic agents." J. Med. Chem., 25 : 1115-1120

Couvreur, P.; Kaute, B.; Roland, M. and Speiser, P. (1979a) "Absorption of antineoplastic drugs to polyalkyl cyanoacrylate nanoparticles and their release in calf serum." J. Pharm. Sci., 68: 1521 -1524.

Couvreur, P.; Tulkens, P.; Roland, M.; Trouet, A. and Speiser, P. (1977) "Nanocapsules: a new lysosomotropic carrier." FEBS Lett., 84 : 323-326.

Couvreur, P.; Rajaonarivony, M.; Vantheir, C.; Couarraze, G. and Puieseux, F. (1993) "Development of a new drug carrier made from alginate." J. Pharm. Sci., 82 : 912-917.

Couvreur, P.; Kaute, B.; Roland, M.; Guiot, P.; Bandin, P. and Speiser, P. (1979b) "Polycyanoacrylate nanocapsules as potential lysosomotropic carriers: Preparation, morphological and sorptive proper-ties." J. Pharm. Pharmacol., 31: 331-332.

Couvreur, P.; Kaute, B.; Lenaerts, V.; Scaitteur, V.; Roland, M. and Speiser, P. (1980) "Tissue distribution of antitumor drugs associated with polyalkyl cyanoacrylate nanoparticles." J. Pharm. Sci., 69 : 199-202.

Crile, G. (1961) "Heat as an adjunct to the treatment of cancer, experimental studies." Cleveland. Clin. Quart., 28 : 75-78.

Dankwerts, M. and Fassihi, A. (1991) "Implantable controlled release drug delivery system: A review." Drug Dev. Ind. Pharm., 17 : 1465-1502.

DeVita, V.T. (1971) "Cell kinetics and the chemotherapy of cancer." Cancer. Chemother. Rep., 3 : 23-25.

DeVita, V.T.(1985) "Principles of chemotherapy". In: "Cancer. Principles and practice of oncology.," DeVita, V.T.; Hellman, S. and Rosenberg, S.A., (eds..), Vol. 2, Lippincott Co., London : 257-285.

DeVita, V.T.; Serpick, A.A. and Carbone, P.P. (1970) "Combination chemotherapy in the treatment of advanced Hodgkin's disease." Ann. Intern. Med., 73 : 891-895.

Duncan, R., and Lloyd, J.B. (1991) "Biological evaluation of soluble synthetic polymers as drug carriers." In: "Recent Advancers in Drug Delivery Systems." Anderson, J..M. and Kim, S.W., (eds.), Plenum Press, New York: 1-22.

Dunn, R.L.; Tipton, A.J. and Menardi, E.M. (1991) "A biodegradable in situ forming drug delivery system." In Proceed 19th Inter. Symp. Control. Rel. Bioact. Mater. : 465.

Fallon, P.A.; Whateley, T.L.; Robertson, L. and Rampling, R. (1996) "Poly (lactide-co-glycolide) implants for in vivo sustained delivery of carboplatin and etoposide to the brain." J. Pharm. Pharmacol.., 47 : 1123-1127.

Flandroy, P.M.J.; Grandfils, C. and Jerome, R.J. (1993) "Clinical application of microspheres in embolization and chemoembolization : A comprehensive review and perspectives." In: Pharmaceutical particulate carrier.", Allain Roland (ed.), Marcel Dekker, New York, 321-365.

Florence, A.T.; Whateley, T.L. and Wood, D.A. (1979) "Potentially biodegradable microcapsules with poly (alkyl 2-cyanoacrylate) membranes." J. Pharm. Pharmacol., 31 : 422-424.

Freise, J.; Muller, W.; Broelsch, C. and Magerstedt, P. (1981) "Influence of a portacaval shunt on the distribution of 14C-chol-PC-DCP-liposomes and liposome entrapped 3H-methotrexate in the organs of rats." Hepatogastroenterology. 28 : 90-92.

Freise, J.; Schmidt, F.W. and Magerstedt, P. (1979) "Effect of liposome entrapped methotrexate on Ehrlich ascites tumor cells and uptake in primary liver cell tumor." J. Cancer. Res. Clin. Oncol., 94 : 21-27.

Fries, E.; Whang, J. and Scoggins, R.B. (1964) "The stathmokinetic effect of vincristine." Cancer Res. 24 : 1918-1920.

Fry, D.W. and Goldman, I.D. (1982) "Further studies on the charge-related alterations of methotrexate transport in Ehrlich ascites tumor cells by ionic liposomes: Correlation with liposome-cell associa-tion." J. Membr. Biol., 66 : 87-95.

Fry, D.W.; White, J.C. and Goldman, I.D. (1979) "Alterations of the carrier-mediated transport of an anionic solute, methotrexate, by charged liposomes in Ehrlich ascites tumor cells." J. Membr. Biol., 50 : 123-140.

Fujimoto, S.; Miyasaki, M.; Endoh, F.; Takahashi, O.; Okari K.; Okai, K. and Morimoto, Y. (1985a) "Effect of intra-arterial infused biodegradable microspheres containing Mitomycin-C." Cancer., 56 : 2404-2410.

Fujimoto, S.; Miyazaki, M.; Endoh, F.; Takahashi, O.; Okui, K.; Sugibayashi, K. and Morimoto, Y. (1985b) "Mitomycin-C carrying microspheres as a novel method of drug delivery." Cancer. Drug. Deliv., 2 : 173-181.

Gal, D.; MacDonald, P.E.; Porter, J.E., and Simpson, E.R. (1981) "Cholesterol metabolism in cancer cells in monolayer culture. IV. LDL metabolism." Int. J. Cancer., 28 : 315-319.

Gallo, J.M.; Hung, C.T. and Perrier, D.G. (1984) "Analysis of albumin microsphere preparation." Int. J. Pharm., 22 : 63-74.

Gerweck, L.E.; Dahlberg, W.K.; Epstein, L.F. and Shimm, D.S. (1984) "Influence of nutrient and energy deprivation on cellular response to single and fractionated heat treatments." Radiat. Res., 99: 573-581.

Gerweck, L.E.; Gillete, E.L. and Dewey, W.C. (1974) "Killing of Chinese hamster cells in vitro by heating under hypoxic or aerobic conditions." Eur. J. Cancer. 10: 691-693.

Giovanella, B.C. (1983) "Thermosensitivity of neoplastic cells in vitro. In: Hyperthermia and cancer therapy." Strom FK ed., Hall, Boston: 55.

Gipps, E.M.; Arshady, R.; Kreuter, J.; Groscurth, P. and Speiser, P.P. (1986) "Distribution of Polyhexyl cyanoacrylate nanoparticles in nude mice bearing human osteosarcoma." J. Pharm. Sci., 75: 256-258.

Gizurarson , S. and Bechgaard, E. (1991) "Insulin-carrying microspheres: In vitro studies." Chem. Pharm. Bull., 39: 1892-1893.

Goldberg, V.A.; Kerr, D.J.; Willmot, N.; McKillop, J.H. and McArdle, C.S. (1990) "Regional chemotherapy for colorectal liver metastases: a phase II evaluation of targeted hepatic arterial 5-fluorouracil for colorectal liver metastases." Br. J. Surg., 77: 1238-1240.

Goldberg, V.A.; Willmot, N.; Kerr, D.J.; Sutherland, C. and McArdle, C.S. (1982) "An in vivo assessment of adriamycin-loaded albumin microspheres." Br. J. Cancer., 65: 393-395.

Goldberg, J. A.; Willmot, N.; Kerr, D.I.; Sutherland, C. and McArdle, C. S. (1992) "An in vivo assessment of adriamycin loaded albumin microspheres." Br. J .Cancer., 65: 393-395.

Goosen, M.F.A.; Leung, Y.F.; O'Shea, G.M.; Chou, S., Sun, A.M. (1983) "Slow release of insulin from a biodegradable matrix implanted in diabetic rats." Diabetes., 32: 478-481.

Gregoriadis, G. (1977) "Targeting of drugs." Nature., 265: 407-411.

Gregoriadis, G.; Senior, J.; Wolff, B.; and Kirby, C. (1984) "Fate of liposomes in vivo : Control leading to targeting." In: "Receptor-mediated Targeting of drugs." Gregoriadis, G.; Poste, G.; Senior J. and Trouet, A. (eds.), Plenum Press, New York: 243.

Gruner, S.M. (1987) "Materials properties of liposomal bilayers" In: "Liposomes - From biophysics to therapeutics.", Ostro, M.J., ed., Marcel Dekker: 1-39.

Gupta, P.K. and Hung, C.T. (1989a) "Effect of carrier dose on the multiple tissue disposition of doxorubicin hydrochloride administered via magnetic microspheres in rats." J. Pharm. Sci., 78: 745-748.

Gupta, P.K. and Hung, C.T. (1989b) "Albumin microspheres II: Applications in drug delivery." J. Microencapsul., 6: 463-472.

Gupta, P.K.; Hung, C.T. and Lam, F.C. (1993) "Application of particulate carriers in intratumoral drug delivery" In: "Pharmaceutical Particulate Carriers.", Allain Rolland (ed.), Marcel Dekker, New York, 135-164.

Gupta, P.K.; Hung, C.T. and Perrier, D.G. (1986) "Albumin microspheres. I: Release characteristics of adriamycin." Int. J. Pharm., 33: 137-146.

Hahn, G.M. (1982) ed., "Mechanisms of heat action." In: "Hyperthermia and Cancer.", New York and London, Plenum Press: 87.

Hahn, G.M.; Kapp, D.S. and Carlson, R.W. (eds) (1993) "Principles of hyperthermia. In: Cancer Medicine." 3rd edn., Holland, Lea and Febiger, Philadelphia, London: 566.

Halbert, G.W.; Stuart, J.F.B., and Florence, A.T. (1984) "The incorporation of lipid soluble antineoplastic agents into microemulsions-protein-free analogues of low density lipoprotein." Int. J. Pharm., 21: 219-226

Hashida, M.; Kojima, T.; Takahashi, Y.; Muranishi, S. and Sezaki, H. (1977a) "Timed-release of mitomycin-C from its agarose bead conjugate." Communication to the editor. Chem. Pharm. Bull., 25: 2456-2458.

Hashida, M.; Sigawa, M.; Muranishi, S. and Sezaki, H. (1977b) "Role of intramuscular administration of water-in-oil emulsion as a method for increasing the delivery of anticancer agents to regional lymphatics." J. Pharmacokinet. Biopharm., 5: 225-239.

Hashida, M.; Takahashi, Y.; Muranishi, S. and Sezaki, H. (1977c) "An application of water-in-oil and gelatin microsphere-in-oil emulsion to specific delivery of anticancer agent into stomach lym-phatics." J. Pharmacokinet. Biopharm., 5: 241-255.

Hashida, M.; Muranishi, S. and Sezaki, H. (1977d) "Evaluation of water-in-oil and microsphere in oil emulsions as a specific delivery system of 5-fluorouracil into lymphatics." Chem. Pharm. Bull., 25: 2410-2418.

Hashida, M.; Kojima, T.; Muranishi, S. and Sezaki, H. (1978a) "Antitumor activity of prolonged release derivative of cytosine arabinoside, cytosine arabinoside-agarose conjugate." Gann., 69: 839-843.

Hashida, M.; Kojima, T.; Muranishi, S. and Sezaki, H. (1978b) "Antitumor activity of timed-release derivative of mitomycin-C, agarose bead conjugate." Chem. Pharm. Bull., 26: 1818-1824.

Hashida, M.; Kojima, T.; Muranishi, S. and Sezaki, H. (1980a) "Mitomycin-C-dextran conjugate. a novel high molecular weight prodrug of mitomycin-C." J. Pharm. Pharmacol., 32: 30-34.

Hashida, M.; Yoshioka, T.; Muranishi, S. and Sezaki, H. (1980b) "Dosage form characteristics of microsphere-in-oil emulsion-I. Stability and drug release." Chem. Pharm. Bull., 28: 1009-1015.

Hashida, M.; Liao, M.H.; Muranishi, S. and Sezaki, H. (1980c) "Dosage form characteristics of microsphere-in-oil emulsion-II. Examination of some factors affecting lymphotropicity." Chem. Pharm. Bull., 28: 1659-1666.

Hashida, M.; Kato, A.; Kojima, T.; Muranishi, S.; Sezaki, H.; Tanigawa, N.; Satomura, K. and Hikasa, Y. (1981) "Antitumor activity of mitomycin-C-dextran conjugate against various murine tumors." Gann., 72: 226-234.

Hashida, M.; Takakura, Y.; Kato, A.; Kimura, T. and Sezaki, H. (1982) "Physicochemical and antitumor characteristics of high molecular weight prodrugs of mitomycin-C." Chem. Pharm. Bull., 30: 2951-2957.

Hashida, M.; Takakura, Y.; Matsumoto, S.; Sasaki, H.; Kato, A.; Kojima, T.; Muranishi, S. and Sezaki, H. (1983) "Regeneration characteristics of mitomycin-C-dextran conjugate in relation to its activ-ity." Chem. Pharm. Bull., 31: 2055-2063.

Hashida, M.; Kato, A.; Takakura, Y. and Sezaki, H. (1984a) "Disposition and pharmacokinetics of a polymeric prodrug of mitomycin-C, mitomycin-C-dextran conjugate, in the rat." Drug Metabol. Disposition., 12: 492-498.

Hashida, M.; Takakura, Y.; Matsumoto, S. and Sezaki, H. (1984b) "Enhanced lymphatic delivery of mitomycin-C conjugated with dextran." Cancer Res., 44 : 2505-2510.

Hashida, M.; Matsumoto, S.; Arase, Y.; Takakura, Y. and Sezaki, H. (1985) "Plasma disposition and in vivo and in vitro antitumor activities of mitomycin-C-dextran conjugate in relation to the mode of action." Chem. Pharm. Bull., 33: 2941-2947.

Hashida, M.; Matsumoto, S.; Yamamoto, A.; Takakwa, Y.; Tanigawa, N. and Sezaki, H. (1986) "Cellular interaction and in vitro antitumor activity of mitomycin-C-dextran conjugate." Cancer Res., 46: 4463-4468.

Heya, T.; Mikura, Y.; Nagai, A.; Miura, Y.; Futo, T.; Tomida, Y.; Shimizu, H. and Toguchi, H. (1994b) "Controlled release of thyrotropin releasing hormone from microspheres. Evaluation of release profiles and pharmacokinetics after subcutaneous administration." J. Pharm. Sci., 83: 798-801.

Heya, T.; Okada, H.; Ogawa, Y. and Toguchi, H. (1994a) "In vitro and in vivo evaluation of thyrotropin releasing hormone release from copoly (DL-lactic/glycolic acid) microspheres." J. Pharm. Sci., 83: 636-640.

Hunter, A.; Dolon, T.F.; Coombs, G.H. and Baillie, A.J. (1988) "Vesicular systems (Niosomes and Liposomes) for delivery of sodium stilbogluconate in experimental murine visceral leishmaniasis." J. Pharm. Pharmacol., 40: 161-165.

Jain, S. and Jain, N.K. (1997) "Resealed erythrocytes as drug carriers." In: "Controlled and Novel Drug Delivery", Jain, N.K., (ed.), CBS Publishers and Distributors, New Delhi, pp. 256-291.

Jalil, R. (1990) "Biodegradable poly(lactic acid) and poly(lactide-co-glycolide) polymers in sustained drug delivery." Drug. Dev. Ind. Pharm., 16: 2353-2367.

Jameela, S.R.; Latha, P.G.; Subramonium, A. and Jayakrishnan, A. (1996) "Antitumor activity of mitoxantrone-loaded chitosan microspheres against Ehrlich ascites carcinoma." J. Pharm. Pharmacol., 48: 685-688.

Jayakrishnan A. and Latha M.S. (1997) "Biodegradable polymeric microspheres as drug carriers." In: "Controlled and Novel Drug Delivery", Jain, N.K., (ed.), CBS Publishers and Distributors, New Delhi, pp. 236-255.

Jayakrishnan, A.; Knepp, W.A. and Goldberg, E.P. (1994) "Casein microspheres. Preparation and evaluation as a carrier for controlled drug delivery." Int. J. Pharm., 106: 221-228.

Jeffery, H.; Davis, S.S. and O'Hagan, D.T. (1993) "Preparation and characterization of poly(lactide-co-glycolide) microparticles. Part 2. entrapment of a model protein using a (water-in-oil) in-water emulsion solvent evaporation technique." Pharm. Res., 10: 362-368.

Jones, B.; Holland, J.F. and Glidewell, O. (1977) "Optimal use of L-asparaginase (NSC-109229) in acute lymphocytic leukemia." Med. Pediatr. Oncol., 3: 387-390.

Juni, K.; Ogata, J.; Nakano, M.; Ichihara, T.; Mori, K. and Akagi, M. (1985) "Acid microspheres containing doxorubicin." Chem. Pharm .Bull., 33: 313-318.

Kase, K. and Hahn, G.M. (1975) "Differential heat response of normal and transformed human cells in tissue culture." Nature., 255: 228-230.

Kato, T. (1983) "Encapsulated drug in targeted cancer therapy." In: "Controlled drug delivery.", Stephen Bruck, ed., CRC press, 190 -234.

Kemeny, H.M.; Hogan, J.M.; Goldberg, D.A.; Lien, C.; Beaty, J.D.; Kokal, W.A.; Riihimaki, D.U. and Terz, J.J. (1986) "Continuous hepatic artery infusion with and implantable pump : problems and hepatic artery anomalies." Surgery., 99: 501-504.

Kim, C.K.; Lee, M.K.; Han, J.H. and Lee, B.J. (1994) "Pharmacokinetics and tissue distribution of methotrexate after intravenous injection of differently charged liposome entrapped methotrexate to rats." Int. J. Pharm. 108:21-29.

Kim, S.H.; Kim, J.H. and Hahn, E.W. (1975) "The radiosensitization of hypoxic tumor cells by hyperthermia." Radiology., 114: 727-728.

Kimelberg, H.K. and Atchison, M.L. (1978) "Effects of entrapment in liposomes on the distribution, degradation and effectiveness of methotrexate in vivo." Ann. New York Acad. Sci., 308: 395-410.

Kimelberg, H.K. (1976) "Differential distribution of liposome-entrapped [3H] methotrexate and labeled lipids after intravenous injection in a primate." Biochem. Biophys. Acta. 44: 531-550.

Kojima, T.; Hashida, M.; Muranishi, S.; and Sezaki, H. (1980) "Mitomycin C-dextran conjugate: A novel high molecular weight pro-drug of Mitomycin C." J. Pharm. Pharmacol., 32: 30-34.

Kosloski, M.J.; Rosen, F.; Milholland, R.J. and Papahadjopoulos, D. (1978) "Effect of lipid vesicle (liposome encapsulation of methotrexate on its chemotherapeutic efficacy in solid rodent tumors." Cancer Res. 38: 2848-2853.

Kramer, P.A. (1974) "Albumin microspheres as vehicles for achieving specificity in Drug delivery." J. Pharm. Sci., 63: 1646-1647.

Kreuter, J.; Nefzger, M.; Liehl, E.; Czok, E. and Vogesh. (1983) "Distribution and elimination of poly methyl methacrylate nanoparti-cles after subcutaneous administration to rats." J. Pharm. Sci., 72: 1146-1150.

Kumanohoso, T.; Natsogoe, S.; Shimada, M.; Aikou, T.; Nakamura, K.; Yamada, K., and Fukuzaki, H. (1995) "In vivo activity of bleomycin incorporated with biodegradable poly-d,l-lactic acid and implanted in the mediastinum of dogs." J. Surg. Oncol., 57(3): 178-182.

Kumar, G.N.; Hammer, R.H. and Bodor, N.S. (1993b) "Soft drugs 13: Design and evaluation of phenylsuccinic analogues of scopolamine as soft anticholinergics. Drug Design and Discovery" 10(1): 1-9.

Kumar, G.N.; Hammer, R.H.; Wu, W.M., and Bodor, N.S. (1993a) "Soft drugs 15: mydriatic activity and ranscorneal penetration of phenyl succinic soft analogues of methscopolamine as short acting mydriatics." Curr. Eye Res., 12(6): 501-506.

Labhasetwar, V.; Underwood, T.; Gallagher, M.; Murphy, G.; Langberg, J. and Levy, R.J. (1994) "Satolol controlled release systems for arrhythmias: In vitro characterization, in vivo drug disposition and electrophysiologic effects." J. Pharm. Sci., 83: 156-164.

Latha, M.S. and Jayakrishnan, A. (1994) "Gluteraldehyde cross linked bovine casein microspheres as a matrix for the controlled release of theophylline : In vitro studies." J. Pharm. Pharmacol., 46: 8 -13.

Laval, F. and Michel, S. (1982) "Enhancement of hyperthermia-induced cytotoxicity upon ATP deprivation." Cancer Lett., 15: 61-65.

Lee, K.C.; Lee, Y.J.; Kim, W.B. and Cha, C.Y. (1990) "Monoclonal anti-body based targeting of MTX loaded microspheres." Int. J. Pharm., 59: 27-33.

Lewis, D.A.; Field, W.N.; Hayes, K. and Alpar, H.O. (1992) "The use of albumin microspheres in the treatment of carrageenan-induced inflammation in the rat." J. Pharm. Pharmacol., 44: 271-74.

Li, Y.P.; Machida, T.Y.; Sannan, T. and Nagai, T. (1991) "Preparation of Chitosan microspheres containing fluorouracil using `drug-in-oil' method and its release characteristics." STP. Pharm. Sci., 1: 363- 368.

Lippman, M.E.; Yarbro, G.K. and Leventhal, B.G. (1978) "Clinical implications of glucocorticoid receptors in human leukemia." Cancer Res., 38: 4251-4254.

Lloyd, J.B. (1991) "Soluble polymers as targetable drug carriers." In: "Drug Delivery Systems: Fundamentals and techniques." Johnson, P. and Lloyd-Jones, J.G. (eds.), Ellis Horwood, New York, 95-105.

Lopez-Berestein, G. and Juliano, R.L. (1987) "Application of liposomes to the delivery of antifungal agents." In: "Liposomes - From biophysics to therapeutics.", Ostro, M.J., (ed.), Marcel Dekker, New York: 253-276.

Lopez-Berestein, G.; Juliano, R.L.; Mehta, K.; Mehta, R.; McQueen, T., and Hopfer, R.L. (1985) "Liposomes in antimicrobial therapy." In: "Targeting of drugs with synthetic systems" (NATO ASI - Series. Series A, Life Sciences; V. 113) Gregoriadis, G.; Senior, J. and Post, G., (eds.), Plenum Press, New York: 193.

Machy, P.; Arnold, B.; Alino, S. and Leserman, L.D. (1986) "Interferon sensitive and insensitive MHC variants of a murine thymoma differentially resistant to methotrexate-containing antibody-direct-ed liposomes and immunotoxin." J. Immunol., 136: 3110-3115.

Macy, P. and Leserman, L.D. (1980) "Elimination or rescue of cells in culture by specifically targeted liposomes containing methotrexate or formyl-tetrahydrofolate." Embo. J., 3: 971-977.

Magin, R.L. and Weinstein, J.N. (1980) "Selective delivery of drugs in "temperature-sensitive" liposomes." In: "Liposomes and Immunobiology", Tom, B.H. and Six, H.P. (eds.), Elsevier/North-Holland, Amsterdam, pp. 315-325.

Manil, L.; Couvruer, P. and Mahieu, P. (1995) "Acute renal toxicity of doxorubicin (adriamycin)-loaded cyanoacrylate nanoparticles." Pharm. Res., 12(1): 85-87.

Martin, D.S.; Stolfi, R.L. and Spiegelman, S. (1978) "Striking augumentation of the in vivo anticancer activity of 5-flurouracil (FU)by combination with pyrimidine nucleosides. An RNA effect." Proc. Am. Assoc. Cancer Res., 19: 221-222.

McArdle, C.S.; Lewis. H.; Hansell, D.; Kerr, D.J.; McKillop, J. and Willmot, N. (1988) "Cytotoxic - loaded albumin microspheres; a novel approach to regional chemotherapy." Br. J. Surg., 75: 132-134.

Miller, H.K.; Slaser, J.S. and Balis, M.E. (1969) "Amino acid levels following L-asparagin amino hydrolase therapy." Cancer Res., 29: 183-187.

Mizushima, Y.; Shoji, Y.; Kato, T.; Fukushima, M. and Kurozumi, S. (1986) "Use of lipid microspheres as drug carriers for antitumor drugs." J. Pharm. Pharmacol., 38: 132 -134.

Moran, R.E. and Straus, M.J. (1975) "Cell cycle synchronization prior to phase-specific therapy with increased survival." Proc. Am. Assoc. Cancer Res., 20: 123-126.

Morimoto, Y. and Fujimoto, S. (1985) "Albumin microspheres as drug carriers." Crit. Rev. Ther. Drug Carrier Syst. 2: 19-63.

Morimoto, Y.; Natsume, H.; Sugibayashi, K. and Fujimoto, S. (1989) "Effect of chemoembolization of albumin microspheres containing Mitomycin-C on AH272 liver metastasis in rats." Int. J. Pharm., 54: 27-32.

Murata, Y.; Maeda, T.; Miyamoto, E. and Kawashima, S. (1993) "Preparation of chitosan - reinforced alginate gel beads- effects of chitosan on gel matrix erosion." Int. J. Pharm., 96: 139-145.

Murthy, R.S.R. (1997) "Biodegradable Polymers." In: "Controlled and Novel Drug Delivery", Jain, N.K. (ed.), CBS Publishers and Distributors, New Delhi: 27-51

Nakamoto, Y.; Hashida, M.; Muranishi, S. and Sezaki, H. (1975) "Studies on pharmaceutical modification of anticancer agents-II. Enhanced delivery o bleomycin into lymph by emulsions and drying emulsions." Chem. Pharm. Bull. 23: 3125-3131.

Narayani, R. and Rao, K.P. (1993) "Preparation, characterization and in vitro stability of hydrophilic gelatin microspheres using a gelatin-methotrexate conjugate." Int. J. Pharm., 95: 85-91.

Narayani, R. and Rao, K.P. (1996) "Biodegradable microspheres using two different gelatin drug conjugates for the controlled delivery of methotrexate." Int. J. Pharm. 128: 261-268.

Nishioka, Y.; Kyotani, S.; Masui, H.; Okamura, M.; Miyazaki, M.; Okazaki, K.; Ohnishi, S., Yamamoto, Y. and Ito, K. (1989) "Preparation and release characteristics of cisplatin albumin microspheres containing chitin and treated with chitosan." Chem. Pharm. Bull. 37: 3074-3077.

Nishioka, Y.; Kyotani, S.; Okamura, M.; Miyazaki, M.; Okazaki, K.; Ohnishi, K.; Yamamoto, Y. and Ito, K. (1990) "Release characteristics of cisplatin chitosan microspheres and effect of containing chitin." Chem. Pharm. Bull., 38: 2871-2873.

Niwa, T.; Takeuchi, T.; Hino, T. and Kawashuma, Y. (1994) "In vitro drug release behaviour of D,L-lactide/ glycolide co-polymer (PLGA) nanospheres with narfarelin acetate prepared by a novel spontaneous emulsification solvent diffusion method." J. Pharm. Sci., 83: 727-732.

Oner, L. and Groves, M.J. (1993) "Optimization of conditions for preparing 2-5 micron range gelatin microparticles by using chilled dehydration agents." Pharm. Res., 10: 621-626.

Overgaard, J. and Bichel, P. (1977) "The influence of hypoxia and acidity on the hyperthermic response of malignant cells in vitro", Radiology., 123: 511-514.

Overgaard, K. and Overgaard, J. (1972a) "Investigations on the possibility of a thermic tumor therapy. I. Short-wave treatment of a transplanted isologous mouse carcinoma." Eur. J. Cancer., 8: 65-78.

Overgaard, K. and Overgaard, J. (1972b) "Investigations on the possibility of a thermic tumor therapy: II. Action of combined heat and roentgen treatment on a transplanted mouse mammary carcinoma." Eur. J. Cancer., 8: 573-575.

Parthasarathi G.; Udupa, N.; Uma Devi, P. and Pillai, G.K. (1994) "Niosome encapsulated of Vincristine sulfate: Improved anticancer activity with reduced toxicity in mice." J. Drug Targeting., 2: 173-182

Patel, K.R. and Baldeschwieler, J.D. (1984) "Mouse Lewis lung carcinoma and hepatoma ascites treatment by combination of liposome chemotherapy and non-specific immunotherapy." Int. J. Cancer., 34: 717-723.

Patel, K.R.; Jonah, M.M. and Rahman, Y.E. (1982) "In vitro uptake and therapeutic application of liposome-encapsulated methotrexate in mouse hepatoma 129." Eur. J. Cancer. Clin. Oncol., 18: 833-843.

Proceedings of the symposium on the metabolism and mechanism of action of cyclophosphamide. (1976) Cancer Treat. Rep., 60: 299-301.

Raja Naresh R.A., and Udupa, N. (1996) "Niosome encapsulated bleomycin." S.T.P. Pharma. Sciences., 6(1): 61-71

Raja Naresh R.A.; Udupa, N. and Uma Devi, P. (1996) "Niosomal Plumbagin with reduced toxicity and improved anticancer activity in Balb/C mice." J. Pharm. Pharmacol., 48: 1128-1132.

Rao, B.S.S. (1993) "Response of transplanted mouse tumor to radiation, chemicals and hyperthermia." Ph.D. thesis, University of Mangalore, India..

Rettenmaier, M. A.; Stratton, J. A.; Berman, M.L.; Senyei, A.; Widder, K.; White, D.B. and Disaia. P.J. (1987) "Treatment of a synergic rat tumor with magnetically responsive albumin microspheres labelled with doxurubicin or protein A." Gynecol. Oncol., 27: 34-43.

Roberts, J.J. and Pascoe, J.M. (1972) "Cross-linking of complementary strands of DNA in mammalian cells by antitumor platinum compounds." Nature., 235: 282-284.

Roerdnik, F.H.; Daemen, T.; Bakker-Woundenberg, I.A.J.M.; Storm, G.; Crommelin, D.J.A. and Scherphof, G.L. (1987) "Therapeutic utility of liposomes", In: "Drug Delivery Systems, Fundamentals and Techniques", Johnson, P. and Jones J.G.L., (eds.), Ellis Horward, Chichester: 67.

Rogerson, A.; Cummings, J.; Willmott, N. and Florence, A.T. (1988) "The distribution of doxorubicin in mice following administration in niosomes." J. Pharm. Pharmacol., 40: 337-342.

Rubin, A.L.; Stenzel, K.H.; Miyata, T.; White, M.J. and Dunn, M. (1973) "Collagen as a vehicle for drug delivery." J. Clin. Pharmacol., 14: 309-312.

Ruiz, J.M. and Benoit, J.P. (1991) "In vivo peptide release from poly (dl-lactic acid co-glycolic acid) polymers 50/50 microspheres." J. Control. Rel., 16: 177-186.

Ruiz, J.M.; Burnel, J.P. and Benoit, J.P. (1990) "Influence of average molecular weights of poly (DL-lactic acid-co-glycolic acid) copolymers 50/50 in vitro drug release from microspheres." Pharm. Res., 7: 928-935.

Salmon, S.E. and Apple, M. (1972) "Cancer chemotherapy." In Meyer, F.H.; Jawetz, E. and Goldfien, A. (eds.), "Review of Medical Pharmacology", CA, Lange Medical Publications, Los Atlos, pp. 448.

Sanders, L.M.; Kent, J.S.; McRae, G.I.; Vickery, B.H.; Tice, T.R. and Lewis DH. (1984) "Controlled release of a luteinizing hormone-releasing hormone analogue from poly (dl lactide-glycolide) microspheres." J. Pharm. Sci. 73: 1294-1297.

Sansdrop, P. and Moes, A.J. (1993) "Influence of manufacturing parameters on the size characteristics and the release profiles of nifedipine from poly (DL-lactide-co-glycolide) microspheres." Int. J. Pharm., 98: 157-164.

Selawry, O.S.; Carlson, J.C. and Moore, G.E. (1958) "Tumor response to ionizing rays at elevated temperatures. A review and discussion." Am. J. Roentgenol., 80: 833-839.

Sezaki, H. and Hashida, M. (1984) "Macromolecular-drug conjugates in targeted cancer chemotherapy." Crit. Rev .Ther. Drug. Carrier. Syst., 1: 1-388.

Sezaki, H.; Hashida, M. and Muranishi, S. (1982) "Gelatin microspheres as carriers for antineoplastic agents." In: "Optimization of drug delivery.", Bundgaard, H.; Hansen, A.B.; Kofod, H. and Munksgaard., (eds.), Alfered Benzon symposium 17, Copenhagen.

Shah, N.H.; Railkar, A.S.; Chan, F.C.; Tarantino, R.; Kumar, S.; Murjani, M.; Palmer, D.; Infeld, M.H. and Malick, A.W. (1993) "A biodegradable injectable implant for delivering micro and macro mole-cules using poly(Lactic-co-glycolic) acid PLGA co-polymers." J. Control. Rel., 27: 139-147.

Shea, C.R.; Chen, N.; Wimberly, J. and Hasan, T. (1989) "Rhodamine dyes as potential agents for photochemotherapy of cancer in human bladder carcinoma cells." Cancer Res., 49: 3961-3965.

Shek, P.N.; Lopez, N.G. and Heath, T.D. (1986) "Immune response mediated by liposome-associated protein antigens. IV. Modulation of anti-body formation by vesicle-encapsulated methotrexate." Immunology., 57: 153-157.

Singh, U.V.; Bisht, K.S.; Rao, S.; Uma Devi, P. and Udupa, N. (1996) "Plumbagin loaded PLGA microspheres with reduced toxicity and enhanced antitumor efficacy in mice." Pharm. Sciences., 2: 407-409.

Singh, U.V.; Pandey, S.; Udupa, N. and Uma Devi, P. (1997a) "Preparation, characterization and antitumor efficacy of biodegradable poly (lactic acid) methotrexate implantable films." Drug Delivery., 4: 101 - 106.

Singh, U.V. and Udupa, N. (1997b) "Implantable methotrexate films using polycaprolactone as biodegradable carriers." Indian J. Pharm. Sci., 59: 55-56.

Singh, U.V.; Bisht, K.S.; Rao, S.; Uma Devi, P. and Udupa, N. (1997c) "Reduced toxicity and enhanced antitumor efficacy of plumbagin using poly(lactic-co-glycolic) acid biodegradable injectable implant." Indian J. Pharmacol., 29: 168-172.

Singh, U.V.; Udupa, N.; Kamath, R. and Uma Devi, P. (1997d) "Enhanced antitumor efficacy of methotrexate gel implants in mice bearing Sarcoma-180. Pharm." Sciences., 3: 133-136.

Singh, U.V. and Udupa, N. (1997e) "In vitro characterization of methotrexate loaded poly(lactic-co-glycolic) acid microspheres and antitumor efficacy in Sarcoma-180 mice bearing tumor." Pharm. Acta. Helv., 72: 165-173.

Singh, U.V. and Udupa, N. (1998) "Methotrexate loaded chitosan and chitin microspheres - in vitro characterization and pharmacokinetics in mice bearing Ehrlich ascites carcinoma." J. Microencapsul. 15: 581-594.

Skipper, H.E.; Schabel, F.M. and Wilcox, W.S. (1967) "Experimental evaluation of potential anticancer agents. XXI scheduling arabinozyl cytosine to take advantage of its S-phase specificity against leukemic cells." Cancer Chemother. Rep., 51: 125-128.

Song, Y.; Onishi, H. and Nagai, T. (1993) "Conjugate of mitomycin-C with N-succinyl-chitosan. In vitro drug release properties, toxicity and antitumor activity." Int. J. Pharm., 98: 121-130.

Spenlehauer, G.; Vert, M.; Benoit, J.P.; Chabot, F. and Veillard. M. (1988) "Biodegradable cisplatin microspheres prepared by the solvent evaporation method. Morphology and release characteristics." J. Control. Rel., 7: 217-229.

Streffer, C. (1985a) "Mechanism of heat injury." In: "Hyperthermia oncology.", Overgaard, J., (ed.), Taylor and Francis, London: 213-222.

Streffer, C. (1985b) "Metabolic changes during and after hyperthermia." Int. J. Hyperthermia., 1: 305-319.

Streffer, C. (1990) "Biological basis of thermotherapy." In: "Biological basis of oncologic thermotherapy.", Gutherie, M., (ed.), Springer Verlag, Berlin, Heidelberg: 1-71.

Sugibayashi, K.; Morimoto, Y.; Nadai, T.; Kato, Y.; Hasegawa, A. and Arita, T. (1979) "Drug-carrier property of albumin microspheres in chemotherapy II. Preparation and tissue distribution in mice of microsphere entrapped 5-fluoroucacil." Chem. Pharm. Bull., 27: 204-209.

Suzuki, K. (1967) "Application of heat to cancer chemotherapy." J. Med. Sci., 30: 1-21.

Tabata, Y. and Ikada, Y. (1987) "Macrophage activation through phagocytosis of muramyl dipeptide encapsulated in gelatin microspheres." J. Pharm. Pharmacol. 39: 698-704.

Thanoo, B.C.; Sunny, M.C. and Jayakrishnan. (1992) "Crosslinked chitosan microspheres : Preparation and evaluation as a matrix for the controlled release of pharmaceuticals." J. Pharm. Pharmacol., 44: 283-286.

Thistlethwaite, A.J.; Leeper, D.B.; Moylan, D.J. and Nerlinger, R.E. (1985) "pH distribution in human tumors." Int. J. Radiat. Oncol. Biol. Phys., 11: 1647-1652.

Tipton, A.J.; Fujita, S.M.; Frank, K.R. and Dunn, R.L. (1992) "Release of naproxen from a biodegradable injectable delivery system." Proc. 19th Int. Symp. Control. Rel. Bioact. Mater. : 314.

Tobey, R.A. (1972) "Arrest of Chinese hamster cells in G2 following treatment with the antitumor drug bleomycin." J. Cell. Physiol., 79: 259-263.

Tobey, R.A. and Crissman, H.A. (1975) "Comparative effects of three nitrosourea derivatives on mammalian cell cycle progression." Cancer Res., 35: 460-465.

Todd, J.A.; Levine, A.M. and Tokes, Z.A. (1980) "Liposome-encapsulated methotrexate interactins with human chronic lymphocytic leukemia cells." J. Natl. Cancer Inst., 64: 715-719.

Todd, J.A.; Modest, E.J.; Rossow, P.W. and Tokes, Z.A. (1982) "Liposome encapsulation enhancement of methotrexate sensitivity in a transport resistant human leukemic cell line." Biochem. Pharmacol., 31: 541-46.

Truter, E.J. (1995) "Heat stabilized albumin microspheres as a sustained drug delivery system for the antimetabolite, 5-fluorouracil." Artif. Cells Blood Substit. Immobil. Biotechnol., 23(5):579-586.

Vaupel, P. (1979) "Oxygen supply to malignant tumors." In: "Tumor blood circulation: Angiogenesis, vascular morphology and blood flow of experimental and human tumors.", Peterson, H.I., (ed.), CRC, Boca Ration: 143-168.

Venkatesan, N.; Sood, A.; Singh, R. and Vyas, S.P. (1995) "Biodegradable polymers as microparticulate drug carriers." Indian Drugs., 32: 520-529.

Verrijk, R.; Smolders, I.J.H.; VcVie, J.G. and Begg, A.C. (1991) "Polymer coated albumin microspheres as carriers for intravascular tumor targeting of cisplatin." Cancer Chemother. Pharmacol., 29: 117-121.

Vitale, G.C.; Henser, L.S. and Polk, H.C. (1986) "Malignant tumors of the liver." Surg. Clin. North America., 66: 723-741.

Vitetta, E.S. and Uhr, J.W. (1985) "Immunotoxins." Annual Rev. Immunol., 3: 197-212.

Wang, Y.M.; Sato, H.; Adachi, I. and Horikoshi, I. (1996a) "Optimization of the formulation design of chitosan microspheres containing cisplatin." J. Pharm. Sci., 85(11): 1204-1210.

Wang, Y.M.; Sato, H.; Adachi, I. and Horikoshi, I. (1996b) "Preparation and characterization of poly(lactic-co-glycolic acid) microspheres for targeted delivery of a novel anticancer agent", taxol. Chem. Pharm. Bull., 44(10): 1935-1940.

Welsh, J.; Calman, K.C.; Stuart, J.F.B.; Clegg, J.; Stewart, J.M.; Packard, C.J.; Morgan, H.G.; and Shepard, J. (1982) "Low density lipoprotein uptake by tumors", Clin. Sci., 63: 44-50.

Widder, K.; Flouret, G. and Senyie, A. (1979) "Magnetic microspheres : synthesis of novel parenteral drug carrier." J. Pharm. Sci., 68: 79-82.

Wike-Hooley, J.L.; Van der Zee, J.; Van, Rhoon., G.C.; Van Den Berg, A.P. and Reinhold, H.S. (1984) "Human tumor pH changes following hyperthermia and radiation therapy." Eur. J. Cancer. Clin. Oncol., 20: 619-623.

Willmot, N. and Cummings, J. (1987) "Increased antitumor effect of adriamycin-loaded albumin microspheres is associated with anaerobic bioreduction of drug in tumor tissue." Biochem. Pharmacol. 36: 521-526.

Willmot, N.; Cummings, J. and Florence, A.T. (1985a) "In vitro release of adriamycin-loaded albumin and haemoglobin microspheres." J. Microencapsul., 2: 293-304.

Willmot, N.; Cummings, J.; Stuart, J.P. and Florence, A.T. (1985b) "Adriamycin loaded albumin microspheres preparation, in vivo distribution and release in rats." Biopharm. Drug Disp., 6: 91-104.

Willmot, N.; Magee, G.A.; Cummings, J.; Halbert, G.W. and Smyth, J.F. (1992) "Doxorubicin-loaded casein microspheres: protein nature of drug incorporation." J. Pharm. Pharmacol., 44: 472-475.

Woo, S.Y.; Dilliplane, P.; Rahman, A. and Sinks, L.F. (1983) "Liposomal methotrexate in the treatment of murine L1210 leukemia." Cancer Drug Deliv., 1: 59-62.

Yapel, A.F. (1985) "Heat and chemical stabilization." In: "Drug and enzyme targeting: Part A. Methods in enzymology.", Widder, K.J. and Green, R., (eds.), Vol 112, Academic Press Inc, New York: 3-18.

Yoshida, M.; Asano, M.; Omichi, H.; Hayashi, Y.; Yamaguchi, I. and Matsuda, K. (1995) "Study of biodegradable co-poly (L-lactic acid/glycolic acid) formulation with controlled release of Z-100 for application in radiation therapy." Int. J. Pharm., 115: 61-67.

Yoshikawa, H.; Nakao, Y.; Takada, K.; Muranishi, S.; Wada, R.; Tabata, Y,; Hyon, S.H. and Ikada, Y. (1989) "Targeted and sustained delivery of aclarubicin to lymphatics by lactic acid-oligomer microspheres in rats." Chem. Pharm. Bull., 37: 802-804.

Yoshioka, T.; Hashida, M.; Muranishi, S. and Sezaki, H. (1981) "Specific delivery of mitomycin C to the liver, spleen and lung: nano and microspherical carriers of gelatin." Int. J. Pharm., 8: 131-141.

Chapter 4

In Vitro and In Vivo Models for Oral Transmucosal Drug Delivery

Padma V. Devarajan, Anilkumar S. Gandhi

4.1 INTRODUCTION

The discovery and development of new drugs that are orally bioavailable continues to be a tremendous challenge in the pharmaceutical industry. In the discovery setting, increased reliance on genomics and high throughput screening to identify pharmacologically active lead compounds, as well as reliance on combinatorial chemistry to increase molecular diversity and achieve desired activity through structural optimisation can result in drug candidate having pharmaceutical properties that are not conducive to oral bioavailability. (Stratford et al, 1999; Irache et al, 1994). Recent years have seen enormous advances in the field of protein and peptide engineering by means of biotechnology and recombinant DNA techniques and today possibilities are to produce significant quantities of a wide variety of biologically active peptides and proteins that are therapeutically applicable. In most of the cases such compounds are indicated for chronic therapy where they will need to be administered by an appropriate delivery system. (LueBen et al, 1994; Senel et al, 1994). Hence, increasing efficiency and specificity of drugs by suitable delivery system is a major objective in pharmaceutical technology.

Recently, there has been a growing interest in exploring the buccal delivery route especially for metabolically unstable drugs such as peptides, as the absorption of therapeutic compounds from the oral mucosa provides a direct entry of the drug into the systemic circulation. (Bodde et al., 1990; Lopez et al, 1998). The mucosa is well supplied with both vascular and lymphatic drainage and gives rapid onset of action, high blood levels, avoids first pass metabolism of drugs and has excellent accessibility. (Garren & Repta, 1988; Rathbone & Hadgraft, 1991; Cassidy et al 1993; Lopez et al, 1998). Because of its natural function, the buccal mucosa is less sensitive to irritation and damage with added advantage of better patient compliance than other mucosae. (Senel et. al 1994; Aungst & Rogers, 1989; Ishida et al 1981). Buccal administration thus provides an alternative to insufficient oral delivery and inconvenient parenteral delivery of hydrophilic macromolecular drugs such as peptides and proteins. (Nagai, 1985; De Vries et al, 1991a; Hoogstraate et al, 1996c; Quadros et al 1991). A number of small molecular weight drugs including the nitrates, morphine, fentanyl and buprenorphine have been found to permeate through oral mucosa tissue at sufficient rates to achieve effective plasma concentrations within clinically reasonable times. Even peptide drugs were found to pass the oral mucosae (Ishida et al, 1981; Anders & Markle, 1983; Schurer & Ziegler 1983; Zhang et al, 1994; Bell et al, 1985). However, the major limitation to buccal delivery is low flux through the tissue resulting in a low bioavailability due to a relatively small surface area and low tissue permeability. Unlike surface area which is unchangeable, permeability of the oral mucosa can be temporarily altered to allow greater amounts of drug to be delivered to the systemic circulation.

The rational design of drug delivery system for use on oral cavity membranes requires amongst other things information on and an understanding of, the incorporated drug's ability to permeate the oral cavity membrane that it must cross to reach the systemic circulation. Such information might also provide the investigator with an insight into those factors which influence, control and govern the permeability of drug across biological membranes. Consequently in the development of an oral mucosal drug delivery system there is a need for experimental methods which allow the release characteristics and permeability of a drug through membrane to be determined. A number of in vitro, ex vivo, in vivo and cell culture techniques have been reported for this purpose. Each method is associated with its own advantages and limitations and yet there is no ideal methodology currently available. The purpose of this chapter is to review the reported methods.

4.2 METHODS FOR IN VITRO RELEASE STUDIES

Over the years, in vitro drug release studies have been employed as a quality control procedure in pharmaceutical production, in product development etc. Sensitive and reproducible release data derived from physicochemically and hydrodynamically defined conditions are necessary. The influence of technologically defined conditions and difficulty in simulating in vivo conditions has led to development of a number of in vitro release methods for buccal formulations, however no standard in vitro method has yet been developed. Different workers have used apparatus of varying designs and under varying conditions, depending on the shape and application of the dosage form developed.

4.2.1 Beaker Method

The dosage form in this method is made to adhere at the bottom of the beaker containing the medium and stirred uniformly using overhead stirrer. Volume of the medium used in the literature for the study varies from 50-500 ml and the stirrer speed from 60-300 rpm. (Venkatesh, 1989; Badrinarayan, 1991; Tanaka et al, 1977; Ishida et al, 1983a; Collins & Deasy, 1990).

4.2.2 Interface Diffusion System

In this method developed by Dearden & Tomlinson (1971a) compartment A (995 ml) (Fig 4.1) represents the

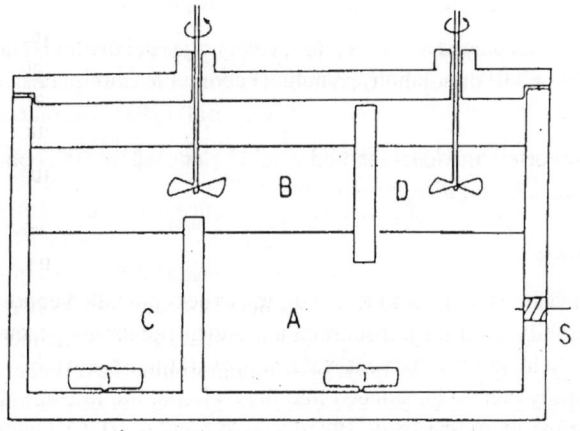

A : Appropriate concentration of drug in buffer (995 ml).

B : 1- Octanol (475 ml).

C : 0.2 M Hydrochloric acid (480 ml).

D : 1 Octanol (100 ml)

S : Sampling port.

Fig 4.1 : Interface diffusion system

oral cavity, and initially contained an appropriate concentration of drug in a buffer. Compartment B (475 ml) representing the buccal membrane, contained 1-octanol, and compartment C (480 ml), representing body fluids, contained 0.2M hydrochloric acid. Compartment D (100 ml) which may be taken as representing protein binding also contained 1-octanol. Before use the aqueous phase and 1-octanol were saturated with each other. Samples were withdrawn and returned to compartment A with a syringe.

4.2.3 Modified Keshary Chien Cell

A specialised apparatus was designed in the laboratory. It comprised of a Keshary Chien cell containing

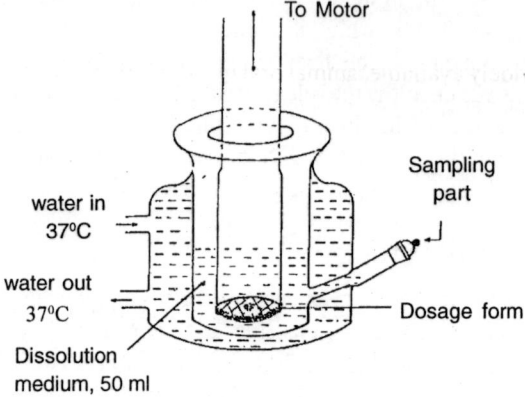

Fig. 4.2 : Modified Keshary Chien cell for in vitro release studies

distilled water (50 ml) at 37°C as dissolution medium (Fig 4.2) . TMDDS was placed in a glass tube fitted with a 10# sieve at the bottom which reciprocated in the medium at 30 strokes per minute (Save & Venkitachalam, 1994; Devarajan et al, 1999).

4.2.4 Dissolution apparatus

Standard USP or BP dissolution apparatus have been used to study in vitro release profiles using both rotating elements paddle (Lopez et al 1998; Parodi et al 1996; Smart, 1992; Chien et al, 1991) and basket (Cassidy et al 1993; Dortune et al, 1998). Dissolution medium used for the study varied from 100-500 ml and speed of rotation from 50-100 rpm.

4.2.5 Other methods

Few other methods involving plexiglass sample blocks placed in flasks (Guo, 1994), agar gel method (Nagai et al, 1980), Valia-Chein cell (Chein & Nair,1996) USP n2 III dissolution apparatus (Fabregas & Garcia, 1995a), etc. have also been reported.

Although a number of methods have been reported, the ideal method would be one where sink condition is maintained and dissolution time in vitro simulates dissolution time in vivo.

4.3 METHODS FOR EX VIVO RELEASE STUDIES

Ex vivo\methods enable anatomically well defined areas of mucosa to be studied under controlled conditions, usually by clamping between diffusion cells (usually used for transdermal and other membrane permeation studies). Provided that the specimen is securely held so as to prevent leakage around the edge of the tissue, a known concentration of the penetrant under study can be introduced into one cell and the rate at which it appears in the second cell is determined (Chidambaram & Srivastav, 1995; Tolo & Jonson, 1975). Compared with in vivo assessment, ex vivo permeability measurements offer a number of advantages and have been a useful tool to study the mechanism of oral mucosal drug absorption. Experimental set up is simple and experimental conditions can be easily manipulated. Data correlates well with in vivo studies with an added advantage of minimal or no sample pretreatment (Zhang & Robinson, 1996). The great disadvantage of the diffusion chambers is that considerable mechanical manifestation of the tissue is required and as the tissue is removed from systemic influences and placed in a highly artificial environment, the extrapolation of results obtained under these circumstances at the in vivo situation requires caution (Chidamabarm & Srivastav, 1995). A number of animal models have been suggested for this purpose.

4.3.1 Animal Models

Since human oral mucosa is not widely available, animal oral mucosa is routinely used for in vitro studies. The main criteria of choosing a particular animal model is resemblance of the animal mucosa to the oral mucosa of human beings in both ultrastructure and enzyme activity which represents the physical and metabolic barrier of the oral mucosa.

Many laboratory animals have been tested for ex vivo permeability studies. The most commonly used animals are dogs (Squier & Hall, 1984; Tobey et al, 1988; Siegal et al, 1981), rabbits (Cassidy et al, 1993; Chien et al, 1991) Rhesus monkeys (Squier et al, 1984; Mehta et al, 1991), guinea pigs (Alfano et al, 1975; Tolo, 1971), rats (Hussain et al, 1987) and hamsters (Tsutsumi et al, 1998; Egros et al, 1992). The oral mucosa of dogs, pigs, rabbits and Rhesus monkeys are believed to be similar to the oral mucosa of humans primarily because the epithelia are nonkeratinised. In vivo buccal absorption studies of flurbiprofen in humans and dogs revealed that permeabilities are approximately equal (Barsuhn et al, 1988). Ex vivo permeability coefficient of tritiated water in humans and pig oral mucosa are also similar (Lesch et al, 1989). Rats and hamsters however have heavily keratinised oral mucosa which differ from the buccal mucosa of humans. Such keratinised mucosa might be expected to represent a more formidable physical barrier and thus exhibit lower permeability than the corresponding human tissue (Garren & Repta, 1989).

Dogs, rabbits, pigs and hamsters are the most commonly used animals. The choice of a particular animal is commonly controlled by cost and availability apart from its similarity with human tissue. The physiology of the oral mucosa of dog closely resembles that of man and is accepted to be a good model for oral mucosal research. Both dogs and pigs have a large mucosal area that permits multiple simultaneous experiments using same animal which will minimise the individual biological variations. Rabbits are relatively cheap compared to dogs and pigs and also easy to handle so are hamsters. However the surface area of rabbit buccal mucosa is very small. Though it has keratinised mucosa, the hamster cheek pouch model for oral mucosal research is appealing due to economy and convenience (Veillard et al, 1987).

4.3.2 Tissue Preparation

Animals are sacrificed before the start of an experiment. Oral mucosa with a fair amount of underlying connective tissue is surgically removed from the oral cavity. In case of hamsters, the cheek pouch is carefully removed from the mouth and placed in ice-cold buffer solution (Veillard et al, 1987; Garren & Repta, 1989). The tissue is then pinned epithelial side down onto a dissecting dish and the connective tissue is carefully removed as thoroughly as possible with the help of a dissecting microscope (Siegel et al, 1981; Senel et al, 1994; Quadros et al, 1991). Tissue is then mounted in a thermostated diffusion chamber with blank buffer on both the sides. After an equilibration period of approximately 30 min., the buffer in donor chamber (representing mucosal side) is filled with solution of permeant in buffer whereas the acceptor chamber (representing serosal side) is filled with a fresh medium. Carbogen (a mixture of 95% oxygen and 5% carbon dioxide) is bubbled through both compartments to maintain tissue viability and to provide mixing or stirred mechanically. Samples are collected from the donor/acceptor chamber or both and analysed .

4.3.3 Methods of Tissue clean up

Although the functional permeability barrier of the oral mucosa, like that of skin is located in the epithelium and occupies the superficial layers (Squier & Hall, 1985; Squier, 1973) the connective tissue like a stagnant layer may significantly affect permeability. Since the surgical removal procedures are time consuming and require skill and patience, chemical (De Vries, et al, 1991b; Le Brun et al, 1989), thermal (De Vries, et al, 1991b) and enzymatic (Garren & Repta, 1989) methods of splitting have been developed. In chemical splitting intact tissue is incubated with EDTA solution in buffer at different temperature conditions for different periods of time. However these chemical and thermal splitting methods substantially affect the barrier properties of the oral mucosa. In case of enzymatic method, the intact hamster cheek pouch was treated with 0.5% collagenase solution on the endothelial side at 37°C for 20 min (Garren & Repta, 1989). Mechanical methods involving use of electro-dermatome have also been employed which allow the epithelium to be sliced to various thickness and structures (De Vries, et al, 1991b; Senel et al, 1998).

4.3.4 Permeability Measurement Studies

Studies of the permeability of mucosal tissue provide unique challenges. Specimens of mucosa from animal or human biopsies are rarely as large as skin samples. It is also necessary to have a donor chamber sufficiently large to provide adequate loading of the penetrant. Finally, it is also desirable to agitate or oxygenate the surface of the mucosa. Two compartment diffusion cells, with buccal mucosa clamped inside are widely used for the permeation studies. The advantage of such cells is that the amount of drug actually transported through the tissue can be determined. Various types of diffusion cells have been employed for this purpose: Modified Ussing Chamber (Quadros et al, 1991; Hoogstraate, et al, 1996a), Franz diffusion cells (Egros et al, 1992; Senel et al, 1998; Ferreira et al, 1995), Valia Chien cell (Nair et al, 1997) etc. Among these the Modified Ussing Chamber (Fig 4.3) and Franz cell (Fig 4.4) are most commonly used. Apart from these, few other modified diffusion cells (Squier & Hall, 1984; Veillard, et al, 1987; Lee & Chien, 1995) and continuous flow cells (Squier et al, 1997) have also been reported.

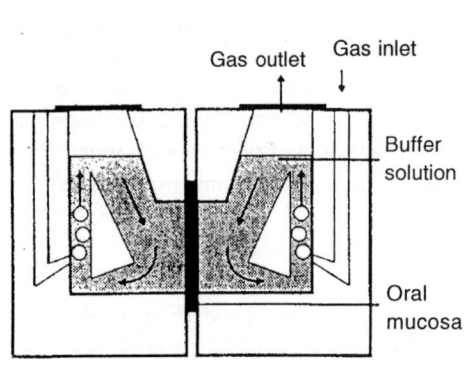

Fig 4.3: Modified Ussing chamber

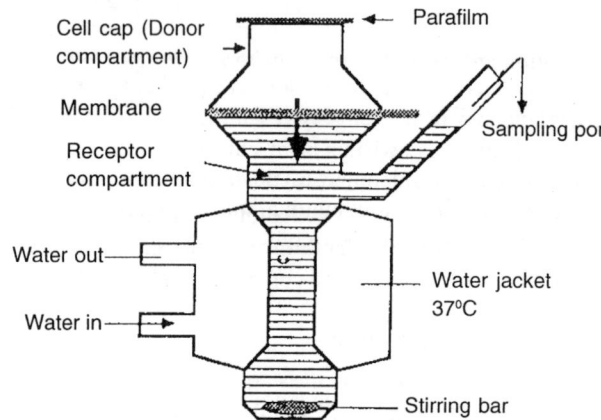

Fig 4.4 : Franz cell

Ex vivo methods measure the rate at which a compound permeates from one side of a membrane to the other and can be used to explore the mechanism of oral mucosal drug permeation and to obtain a first approximation of the expected in vivo absorption rate. Considerable information regarding the permeability behaviour of the oral mucosa to a variety of variables, such as partition coefficient dependency, pH dependency, effect of penetration enhancer etc., can be determined and may be useful in subsequent formulation work. However, since the tests are conducted outside the complex and dynamic physiological environment, results obtained cannot be extrapolated directly to in vivo conditions.

4.4 IN VIVO METHODS

Methods for studying the permeability of intact mucosa comprise of techniques that exploit the biological response of the organism locally or systemically and those that involve direct local measurement of uptake or accumulation of penetrants at the surface. Some of the earliest and simple studies of mucosal permeability utilised the systemic pharmacological effects produced by drugs after application to the oral mucosa. However the most widely used methods include in vivo studies using animal models, buccal absorption tests and perfusion chambers for studying drug permeability (Rathbone et al, 1996).

4.4.1 Animal Models

Animal models are used mainly for the screening of a series of compounds, investigating the mechanisms and usefulness of permeation enhancers or evaluating a set of formulations. A number of animal models have been reported in the literature, however, very few in vivo (animal): in vivo (human) correlation have been reported in the literature. Hence selection of a animal model is very important. Animal models such as the dog (Lu & Hui, 1996; Hosny & Al-Meshal, 1994; Yukimatsu, et al, 1994; Nozaki, et al, 1993; Heiber, et al, 1994; Ebert et al, 1994, Zhang, et al, 1994), rats (Hussain et al, 1986,1987; Hansen et al, 1992; Aungst & Rogers, 1989; Bland, et al 1991; Siegel, 1984; Siegel & Gordan, 1985), rabbits (Oh & Ritshel, 1988a; Oh & Ritshel 1988b; Bergman et al, 1968), cat (Kellaway & Warren, 1991), hamster (Ishida et al, 1983a; Ishida et al, 1983b, Tananka et al, 1980, Kurosaki et al, 1989, Kurosaki et al, 1988; Kurosaki et al, 1991), pigs (Hoogstraate et al, 1996b) and sheep (Burnside et al, 1989; Maddox et al, 1990) have been reported. In general, the procedure involves anesthetising the animal followed by administration of the dosage form. In case of rats, the oesophagus is ligated to prevent absorption pathways other than oral mucosa. At different time intervals, the blood is withdrawn and analyzed.

4.4.2 Buccal Absorption Test

The buccal absorption test developed by Beckett & Triggs (1967) is a simple and reliable method for measuring the extent of drug loss from the human oral cavity for single and multicomponent mixtures of drugs. The test has been successfully used to investigate the relative importance of drug structure, contact time, initial drug concentration and pH of the solution while the drug is held in the oral cavity (Rathbone , 1991a).

4.4.2.1 General method

The method involves swirling of a buffered drug solution of known concentration around the mouth by movement of cheeks and tongue 60 times per minute. After a known period of time the solution is expelled and the subjects rinse their mouth with aliquots of buffer. The drug solution and rinse are combined, adjusted to volume and analysed for drug content. The difference between the amount of drug contained in original buffered drug solution and the amount recovered was assumed to be the amount of drug lost into the oral cavity mucosa (Beckket & Moffat, 1968, 1969a, 1969b, 1970, 1971; Dearden & Tomlinson, 1971b; Hicks, 1973; Chan, 1979).

However, the method does not take into account the amount of drug that may be swallowed and moreover method is unsuitable for kinetic studies (Beckett & Moffat, 1968; Beckett, et al, 1971). Hence a number of modifications have been suggested.

4.4.2.2 Non absorbable marker compound

To account for non absorbable losses that might occur due to swallowing of drug during buccal absorption test, use of non absorbable markers have been suggested. Inulin (Manning & Evered , 1976), ^{125}I-labelled polyvinylpyrrolidone (Past et al, 1979), polyethylene glycol (Meyer et al, 1974) and phenol red (Schurmann & Turner, 1978) have been used to assess the extent of drug loss arising from non-absorbable sources during a 5 min buccal absorption test.

4.4.2.3 Pre-test wash out

In order to cleanse mouth and adjust pH prior to a buccal absorption test, mouth was rinsed by subjects for 10-30s, prior to a test with 20 ml of the buffer used in the test. (Tucker, 1988; Randhawa, et al, 1986).

4.4.2.4 Post-test rinsing

Immediately after a buccal absorption test, subjects rinsed their mouth with an aliquot of fresh drug-free buffer or distilled water for a short period of time. Beckett & Triggs (1967) employed a 10 ml, 10s rinse, whereas others have used a 10 ml, 5s rinse (Manning & Evered, 1976), 20 ml, 30s rinse, (Randhawa et al, 1986) and 5 ml, 3s rinse (Beckett & Pickup, 1975). It is clear that the post-test swirling period, although required, should involve small volumes and be restricted to short periods of time. This is particularly important with drugs that can readily return to the oral cavity from the membranes.

4.4.2.5 Kinetics of drug absorption

In order to estimate the transfer kinetics of a given drug the buccal absorption test requires repeated swirling over different time periods upto a maximum of 15 minutes, a process which can take days for the mapping of a drug's kinetic profile (Tucker, 1988). In this respect, Tucker, (1988) reported a technique which enables kinetic data to be collected in a single 15 min trial. The method validated using verapamil involved multiple samples being withdrawn from the mouth throughout the duration of test.

4.4.2.6 Monitoring of drug appearance in blood

Drug loss from the oral cavity during buccal absorption test may lead to entry of drug in systemic circulation. Studies measuring drug loss from the oral cavity and appearance in the blood are sparse in literature. Younes et al (1991) used a 5 min buccal absorption test to investigate the absorption of flurbiprofen. Blood samples were collected upto 48 hr post dosing.

Although the buccal absorption test is simple to perform, non invasive and both the rate and extent of drug loss from the oral cavity from aqueous solution can be measured, the test does suffer from some disadvantages. The amount of intact drug that reaches the systemic circulation remains unknown as only loss from the oral cavity is monitored whereas differences in the absorption characteristics of different membranes that line the oral cavity cannot be determined as absorption simultaneously takes place all over the mucosa. Furthermore, the determination of the kinetics of absorption is time consuming.

4.4.3 Disc Methods

These methods have advantage that the absorption across a defined oral cavity mucosa can be studied. A polytef disc with a diameter of approximately 3.5 cm and height of 1 cm was used in a study (Schurr & Ziegler, 1983). The disc had a central circular depression depth of 4 mm. A water soaked filter paper disc was placed in the depression and known amount of drug spread onto it. Once the drug had dissolved the device was placed onto a defined oral mucosal surface and maintained in place for 5 min. After removal, a non impregnated disc was used to wipe the oral mucosa, the discs combined and analysed.

Disc techniques allow investigators to study drug loss across a fixed area of defined oral cavity membrane. Major limitation of the technique include adherence of the disc to the membrane, leakage of drug from the disc and interference from salivary secretions.

4.4.4 Absorption cells

Absorption cells involve techniques which restrict known volume of an aqueous test solution to a defined area of the oral mucosa. The cell can be open or closed to the oral environment, but in either case, the test solution within the cell is protected from salivary secretions and therefore does not change in volume and also the test solution is not stirred.

The simplest reported absorption cell is a rubber O ring (Siegel 1984; Siegel & Gorden, 1985). A rubber O ring with an internal diameter of 2.64 mm was fixed to the ventral surface of the tongue of adult male Sprague-Dawley rats using a cyanoacrylate adhesive. Ten mL of radiolabelled substance dissolved in suitable buffer was placed into the ring and absorption characteristics determined by blood levels and test solution in the O ring. A cup with an area of 2.2 cm² was used to study the absorption characteristics of novel angiotensin converting enzyme across the buccal mucosa of anesthetised dogs (Quadros et al, 1988).

Kellawey & Warren (1991) developed a small cell comprising two concentric sealed chambers made of perspex. The inner chamber (0.6cm. diameter, 0.483 cm³ volume) contained the drug solution while the outer chamber was used to apply vacuum which maintained the cell in position on the buccal mucosa of anesthetised cat. The inner chamber was equipped with two pipes to allow solution to be introduced by injecting through the inlet pipe, excess of drug solution until it drained from outlet tube (Fig. 4.5a,b). The absorption characteristics of the drug under test were determined by blood sampling.

Zhang & co-workers (1989) described a cell (Fig. 4.6 a,b) which allowed a drug solution to remain in direct contact with a defined area of the inner side of the cheek of anesthetised dogs. To determine the transbuccal permeation rate of fentanyl, the authors introduced a known volume of solution containing a known amount of drug into the cell. After particular time intervals the samples were withdrawn from the cell and analysed. A stainless steel diffusion cell was also developed by Zhang & co-workers (1994). The cell has four completely segregated compartments, each acting as an independent cell and allowing the solution to directly contact the mucosa through an area of 2.0cm².

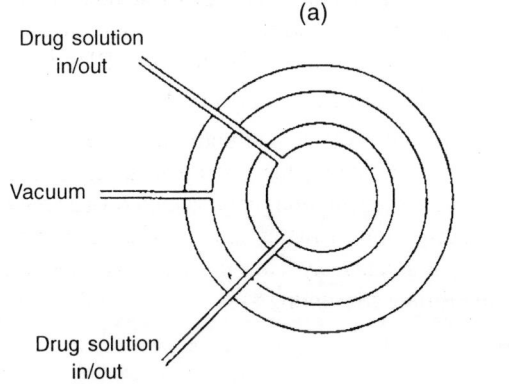

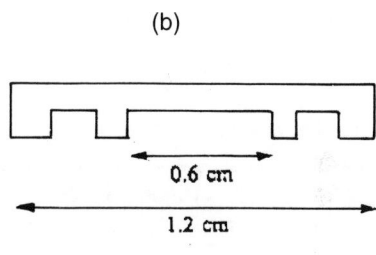

Fig. 4.5 : a) Diagrammatic representation of the b) Section through the cell showing dimensions.
absorption cell used by Kellaway et al (1991).

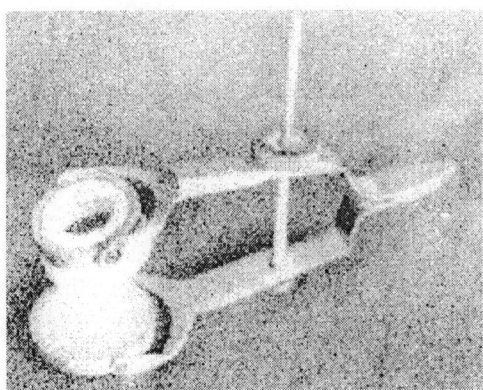

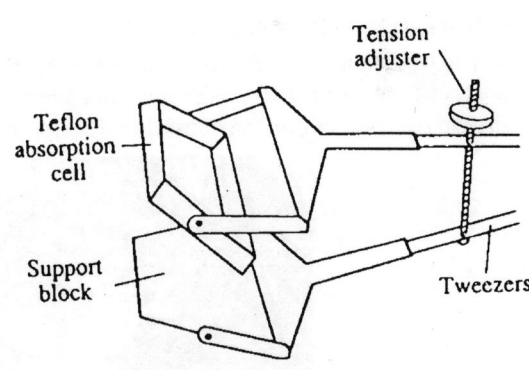

Fig. 4.6 (a) Absorption cell used by Zhang et al (1994) b) Diagrammatic representation of the absorption cell

4.4.5 Perfusion cells

Perfusion cell techniques are characterised by the restriction of known volumes of an aqueous solution to a defined area of oral mucosa using cells that are closed to the oral environment. In contrast to absorption cells, the test solution is well stirred and continuously perfused across the mucosal surface throughout the duration of an experiment. The absorption characteristics of the drug can be determined either by monitoring drug loss from the perfusing solution or by measurement of blood levels.

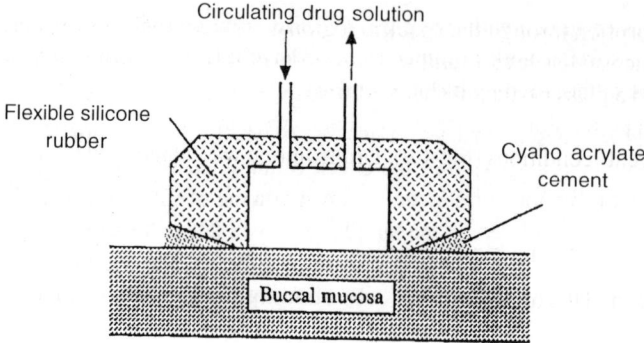

Fig 4.7: Diagrammatic representation of perfusion cell used by Veillard et al (1987).

4.4.5.1 Perfusion cells for Animal studies

A small perfusion chamber (0.07 cm^3 and 0.25cm^2) made from medical grade silicone polymer as shown in Fig 4.7.

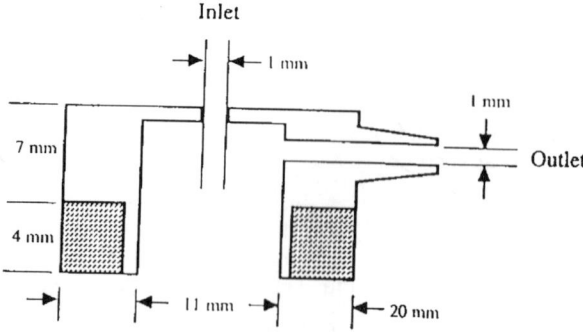

Fig 4.8 Dimensions of perfusion cell designed by Yamahara et al (1990)

was developed by Veillard et al (1987). Polyethylene tubing (0.75 mm I.D.) was used as the input and output lines. The perfusion chamber was attached to the buccal mucosa of the upper lip of an anesthetised dog using cyanoacrylate adhesive. Drug in the aqueous solution was circulated through the device for 30 min. (1 mg/ ml/ 5 min) and collected in 1 ml fractions. Blood samples were withdrawn and analysed. This method is very useful

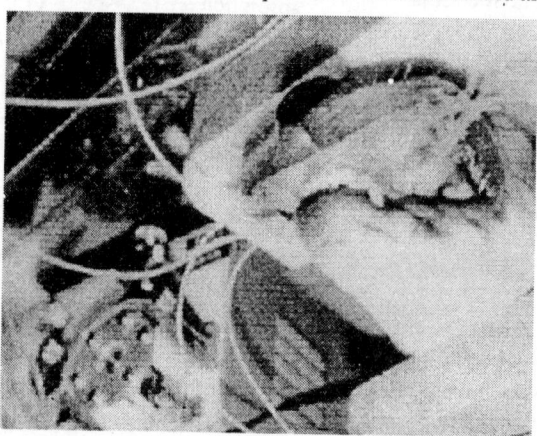

Fig. 4.9 Photograph of four perfusion cell designed by Yamahara et al (1990) simultaneously attached to the buccal mucosa of a dog

in determining the drug absorption through the specific region of oral mucosa, however cyanoacrylate adhesive used can damage the mucosal tissue resulting in poor reproducibility.An in situ perfusion device consisting of a circulating pump and a glass perfusion chamber with a harmless bioadhesive polymer was developed by Yamahara et al (1990) (Fig 4.8). Four of the perfusion cells were adhered to the buccal membrane and each cell was studied under different conditions (Fig 4.9). Drugsolution was maintained in a reservoir thermostated to 37°C and recirculated at a rate of 2 ml/min. by a peristaltic pump. The surface area of membrane exposed to perfusion solution was 0.95 cm². Drug loss was monitored by either taking samples from the reservoir and replacing with fresh solvent or by taking blood samples.

Weaver et al (1992) reported the use of a Teflon cell in anesthesized dogs which was held in place against

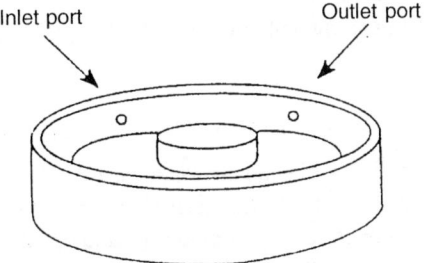

Fig. 4.10 : Diagram of the perfusion cell used by perfusion Weaver et al (1992)

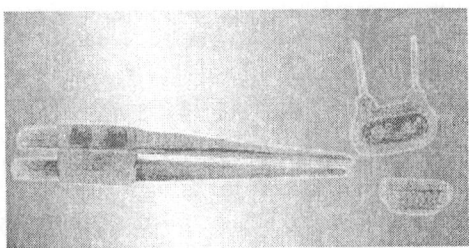

Fig. 4.11: Photograph of the buccal of Barsuhn et al (1988)

the surface of the buccal mucosa by the use of forceps and a rigid backing held against the cheek. The cell (Fig. 4.10) has an area of 2.8 cm² and two 19 gauge needles provide inlet and outlet ports which allows the aqueous drug solution to be flushed across the mucosa.

4.4.5.2 Perfusion cells for human studies

Barsuhn et al (1988) constructed a pliable cell made of a hydrophilic vinyl polysiloxane polymer which had an internal volume of 1 ml and allowed a 1.8 cm² area of buccal membrane to be perfused (Fig. 4.11). The design also incorporated a sealing lip to prevent leaks. Before placement of the perfusion cell the membrane of each subject was rinsed with sterile saline solution applied with a cotton gauze. Cells were placed visually and maintained in position by the natural suction created by the perfusion circuit and the extended clamp. Perfusing drug solution was maintained at 37°C and recirculated at 10 ml/min using a reciprocating piston pump. Samples were removed from the stirred reservoir and analysed. The closed perfusion cell apparatus is a significant improvement over both the buccal absorption test and disc methods for estimating kinetic rate constants for disappearance across a specified oral cavity membrane.

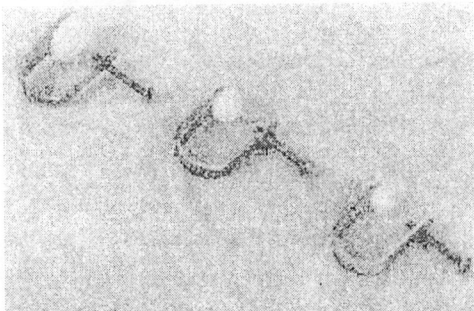

Fig. 4.12 : Buccal perfusion cells used by Rathbone et al (1991a)

Rathbone (1991a,b) reported a buccal perfusion cell design constructed from inflexible material such as nylon or teflon (Fig 4.12). The buccal perfusion cell was circular with an internal diameter of 1 cm and depth of 0.5 cm and allowed 3.14 cm^2 area of buccal membrane to be perfused. Buffered aqueous solution of model drug maintained at 37°C was continuously circulated across buccal membrane at 10 ml/min for the duration of the experiment. Drug concentrations were continuously monitored as a function of time by pumping the drug solution through a flow cell in a spectrophotometer.

Buccal perfusion cells of the types mentioned above offer fixed (known) interfacial areas over which transfer can take place into a defined oral cavity membrane. The isolation of the area over which transfer occurs prevents interference from salivary secretions; thus aqueous phase volume, pH and temperature of the perfusant remain constant throughout the duration of experiment. Buccal perfusion cells may provide an investigator with a technique suitable to quantify those factors which influence, control and govern drug permeability across oral cavity membranes.

4.5 CELL CULTURE METHODS

In vitro cell culture models involving monolayers of cells of epithelial origin and grown on permeable support membranes have been increasingly used to study transepithelial drug transport and metabolism (Imanidis et al, 1996). In vitro cultures of the cells have many advantages over conventional techniques (Audus et al, 1990; Borchardt, 1990; Audus, 1996) including, a) rapid assessment of the potential permeability, b) the opportunity to elucidate the molecular mechanisms of drug transport, c) expanding limited human or animal tissue samples, d) the possibility of establishing a cell line which would provide a consistent, continuous supply of tissue, e) the ability to readily manipulate experimental conditions, f) the accessibility of both mucosal and serosal surfaces of tissue, and g) the opportunity to minimise time consuming, expensive and sometimes controversial animal studies.

There remains, however, a formidable challenge to the establishment and development of an appropriate stratified squamous epithelial cell culture systems. Challenge is the defining of conditions for the establishment of a culture system that completely mimics the complex in vivo tissue with respect to cell growth and differentiation, permeability and metabolism.

4.5.1 General factors to be considered in developing a cell culture model system.

4.5.1.1 Cell line

In order to successfully mimic biological barriers with an in vitro cell culture system, the selection of cell line becomes particularly important. The cell line can offer convenient, consistent and unlimited sources of buccal epithelium. The transport and metabolic properties of cultured cells can vary depending on whether the cells are primary cultured, passaged lines or transformed lines.

4.5.1.2 Microporous membrane

A microporous membrane by itself or after treatment with an appropriate matrix material (e.g. collagen) will support cell attachment and cell growth. Many microporous membranes for cell culture (e.g. polycarbonate, nitrocellulose) are commercially available. Careful selection of the microporous membrane including the physico-chemical properties of the membrane, its pore size, surface area, nature and thickness of the support matrix (e.g. collagen), is critical so as to avoid generating artifactual data in transport experiments (Shah et al, 1989)

4.5.1.3 Diffusion apparatus

Another critical factor particularly in the study of the transport of lipophilic molecules is the selection of diffusion apparatus. Whether the apparatus is stagnant or stirred can influence the thickness of the aqueous boundary layer on the surface of the cell monolayer and thus, the permeability of lipophilic solutes. (Hidalgo et al, 1989). The types of diffusion apparatus currently employed for studying transport across monolayers include, a) the unstirred cell insert system, b) side by side diffusion system stirred mechanically, and c) the side by side diffusion system stirred by gas lift.

4.5.1.4 Buccal cell cultures

The use of a particular cell or tissue culture system to mimic a biological barrier in drug delivery studies requires that it fulfills certain criteria with respect to basic anatomy. Although not technically possible for most cell and tissue culture systems in general, ideally the first requirement would be that the in vitro biological barrier precisely reflect the in vivo biological barrier. Successful development of an appropriate in vitro cell culture model for drug delivery studies depends on generating not only a system that retains the restrictive intercellular epithelial barrier but one that also retains similar expression of enzyme systems and other morphological and biochemical properties typical of oral cavity epithelia. The development of cell cultures has been aided by the establishment of several specific differentiation parameters and biochemical markers, cytokines 4, 5, 6, 13, 14, 17 and 19 (Shaban , et al, 1989), involucrin expression (Banks-Schlegel & Green, 1981), lipids (Squier et al, 1991), Phemigus antigen (Acosta & Ivanyl, 1985), cell surface glycoconjugate or mucin receptor and blood group markers (Audus, 1996) for buccal epithelium have been documented.

In first type of tissue culture system, oral keratinocytes derived from human buccal explants have been grown in primary culture. Epithelial cells migrate out from explants placed on suitable growth surfaces divide and form a stratified tissue system. The tissue grown in this system is similar but not identical to the parent tissue. This system is relatively easy to establish but may retain non epithelial cells that may or may not be significant in drug studies (Audus et al, 1990).

In second type of buccal tissue culture system, hamster pouch buccal cells have been enzymatically dissociated and grown in primary culture (Tavakoli-Saberi, & Audus, 1989a). In this method hamster cheek pouch was excised and washed. One longitudinal incision was made in pouch and incubated in a medium. After incubation the cells were further seeded in plastic culture dishes containing polycarbonate discs coated with cross-linked rat tail collagen and fibronectin and incubated. (Tavakoli-Saberi & Audus , 1989b). The major difference between the hamster derived primary culture system and parent tissue is the absence of a completely keratinised epithelium typical of the hamster cheek pouch in vivo. In this respect, the cultured tissue more closely resembles the less differentiated or non keratinised buccal epithelium of man.

More recently, Nielson et al (1999) established the human cell line, TR146 as an in vitro model for studying transport pathways or mechanisms. TR146 cells are squamous carcinogenic cells derived from a neck node metastasis of a human buccal carcinoma. When cultured on filters it shows some morphological similarities to the human buccal epithelium (Jacobson et al, 1995).

The cell culture systems offer dynamic, living systems with the added flexibility of permitting manipulation of several experimental variables. They appear useful for screening substances for metabolic, pharmacological and toxicological factors associated with drug delivery. The tissue culture models require additional refinements to duplicate fully the absolute permeability barrier exhibited in vivo. However, the tissue culture models do have the potential as useful models for studying the role of physicochemical factors in determining the relative buccal permeability characteristics of a substance.

4.6 CONCLUSION

Numerous in vitro and in vivo studies of oral mucosal drug absorption have been reported in the literature utilising a wide range of animal tissues, experimental designs and probe molecules. In vitro methods employing USP dissolution apparatus can be useful for routine analytical purposes. As against in vitro methods, ex vivo methods employing animal tissues provide information about amount of drug that is actually permeated through the tissue. Most widely used tissues are rabbit, dog and pig oral mucosa and hamster cheek pouch. Animal models play an important role in the development of oral mucosal formulations, in particular when there is relatively limited toxicological data available. However, the limitation of animal models is their unsuitability for predicting human oral mucosal drug absorption. Buccal absorption test is the most widely used human model for passive transfer of drug through lipid membranes and provides a simple and reliable method for estimating drug loss from oral cavity. Perfusion cells have been reported to study drug transfer kinetics. Recently developed hamster cheek pouch and TR143 cell lines also provide an effective way of determining drug permeation across oral mucosa. Thus, although a number of methods have been reported, each has its own advantages and disadvantages, and the choice of a particular method depends on number of factors like purpose of the study, formulation factors, and the availability of the instrument or tissue samples.

4.7 SUGGESTIONS FOR FURTHER WORK

As indicated earlier, research in oral mucosal delivery systems is lacking in developing a standard method that can be universally accepted for in vitro release. Evaluation of membranes as alternative to tissues is another area where the need for extensive studies is indicated. The development of cell culture techniques is an important step towards harmonizing drug permeation methods, however there is a need to establish the crucial in vivo-in vitro correlation to validate these methods.

REFERENCES

Acosta, E. and Ivanyi, L. (1985) "Oral epithelial cells as the origin of phemigus antigen in human saliva." Arch. Oral Biol., 30: 23.

Alfano, M. C.; Drummond, J. F. and Miller, S. A. (1975) "Localisation of rate limiting barrier to penetration of endotoxin through nonkeratinised oral mucosa in vitro." J. Dent. Res., 54: 1143.

Anders, R. and Merkle, H. P. (1989) "Evaluation of laminated mucoadhesive patches for buccal drug delivery." Int. J. Pharm., 49: 231-240.

Audus, K. L. (1996) "Buccal epithelial cell cultures as a model to study oral mucosal drug transport and metabolism." In : Rathbone, M. J. (ed.), Oral mucosal drug delivery, Marcel Dekker Inc., New York, pp 101-119.

Audus, K. L.; Bartel R. L.; Hidalgo, I. G. and Borchardt R. T. (1990) "The use of cultured epithelial and endothelial cells for drug transport and metabolism studies." Pharm. Res., 7(5): 435-450.

Aungst, B. J. and Rogers, N. J. (1989) "Comparison of the effects of various transmucosal absorption promoters on buccal insulin delivery." Int. J. Pharm., 53: 227-235.

Badrinarayan, N. (1991) "Utilisation and evaluation of plant products in pharmaceutical formulations." M. Pharm. thesis submitted to SNDT Woman's University.

Banks-Schlegel and Green H. (1981) "Involucrin synthesis and tissue assembly by keratinocytes in natural and cultured human epithelia." J. Cell Biol., 90: 732.

Barsuhn, C. L.; Olanoff, L. S.; Gleason, D. D.; Adkins, E. L. and Ho, N. F. H. (1988) "Human buccal absorption of flurbiprofen." Clin. Pharmacol. Ther., 44: 225.

Beckett, A. H. and Moffat, A. C. (1970) "Kinetics of buccal absorption of some carboxylic acids and the correlation of the rate constants and n-heptane: aqueous phase partition coefficients." J. Pharm. Pharmacol., 22: 15-19.

Beckett, A. H. and Moffat A. C. (1968) "The influence of alkyl substitution in acids of their performance in the buccal absorption test." J. Pharm. Pharmacol., 20: 239S-247S.

Beckett, A. H. and Moffat, A. C. (1969b) "Correlation of partition coefficients in n-heptane aqueous systems with buccal absorption data for a series of amines and acids." J. Pharm. Pharmacol., 21: 144S-150S.

Beckett, A. H.; Grech., O. and Mihailova, D. (1971) "The influence of nitrogen, chain and ring substitution on some physico-organic properties and on buccal absorption of amphetamines." J. Pharm. Pharmacol., 27: 67P.

Beckett, A. H. and Moffat, A. C. (1969a) "The influence of substitution in phenylacetic acids on their performance in the buccal absorption test." J. Pharm. Pharmacol., 21: 139S-143S.

Beckett, A. H. and Moffat, A. C. (1971) "The buccal absorption of some barbiturates." J. Pharm. Pharmacol., 23: 15-18.

Beckett, A. H. and Pickup, M. E. (1975) "A model for steroid transport across "biological membranes." J. Pharm. Pharmacol., 27: 226-234.

Beckett, A. H. and Triggs, E. J. (1967) "Buccal absorption of basic drugs and its application as an in vivo model of passive drug transfer through lipid membranes." J. Pharm. Pharmaco., 19: 31S-41S.

Bell, M.D. D.; Mishra, P.; Weldon, B. D.; Murrey, G. R.; Calvey, T. N. and Williams, N. E. (1985) "Buccal morphine - a new route for analgesia?" Lancet, 1: 71-73.

Bergman, S.; Siegel I, A. and Ciancio, S. (1968) "Absorption of carbon 14 labelled lidocaine through oral mucosa." J. Dent. Res., 47: 1184.

Bland, C. R.; Davis, S. S. and Rawlins, D. A. (1991) "Buccal absorption of b-blockers in the rat." J. Pharm. Pharmacol., 43 (Suppl.): 116P.

Bodde, H. E.; De Vries, M. E. and Junginger, H. E. (1990) "Mucoadhesive polymers for the buccal delivery of peptides, structure - adhesiveness relationships." J. Control. Rel., 13: 225-231

Borchardt, R. T. (1990) "Assessment of transport barriers using cell and tissue culture systems." Drug Dev. Ind. Pharm., 16(18): 2595-2612.

Burnside, B. A.; Keith, A. D. and Snipes, W. (1989) "Microporous hollow fibers as a peptide delivery system via the buccal cavity." Proceed. Intern. Symp. Control. Rel. Bioact. Mater., 16: 94.

Cassidy, J. P.; Landcert, N. M. and Quardos, E. (1993) "Controlled buccal delivery of buprenorphine." J. Control. Rel., 25: 21-29.

Chan, K. (1979) "The effect of physicochemical properties of pethidine and its basic metabolites on their buccal absorption and renal elimination." J. Pharm. Pharmacol., 21: 160-168.

Chidambaram, N. and Srivatsav, A. K. (1995) "Buccal drug delivery systems." Drug Dev. Ind. Pharm., 21(9): 1009-1036.

Chien, Y. W. and Nair, M. (1996) "Mucosal adhesive device for long acting delivery of pharmaceutical combinations in oral cavity." US Patent No. 5578315.

Chien, Y. W.; Corbo, D. C. and Liu, J. C. (1991) "Mucosal delivery of progestational steroids from a controlled release device: in vitro/ in vivo relationship, Drug Dev. Ind. Pharm., 17(17): 2269-2290.

Collins, A. E. and Deasy, P. B. (1990) "Bioadhesive lozenge for the improved delivery of cetypyridinium chloride." J. Pharm. Sci., 79(2): 116-120.

De Vries M. E.; Bodde H. E.; Verhoef, J. C. and Junginger, H. E. (1991a) Developments in buccal drug delivery." Crit. Rev. Ther. Drug Carrier Syst., 8: 271-303.

De Vries, M. E.; Bodde, H. E.; Verhoef, J. C.; Ponec, M.; Craane, W. I. H. M. and Junginger, H. E. (1991b) "Localisation of the permeability barrier inside porcine buccal mucosa : a combination in vitro study of drug permeability, electrical resistance and tissue morphology." Int. J. Pharm, 76: 25.

Dearden, J. C. and Tomlinson, E. (1971a) "A new buccal absorption model." J. Pharm. Pharmacol., 23: 68S-72S.

Dearden, J. C. and Tomlinson, E. (1971b) "Buccal absorption as a parameter of analgesic activity of some p-substituted acetanilides." J. Pharm. Pharmacol., 23: 73S-76S.

Devarajan, P. V.; Gupta S.; Gandhi A. S.; Niphadkar, P. V. and Shah, M. (1999) "Transmucosal drug delivery systems of salbutamol sulfate." 26th Int. Symp. Control. Rel. Bioact. Mater., 6501

Dortune, B.; Ozer, L. and Uyanik, N. (1998) "Development and in vitro evaluation of buccoadhesive pindodlo tablet formulation." Drug Dev. Ind. Pharm., 24(3): 281-288.

Ebert, C. D.; Heiber, S. J.; Dave, S. C.; Kim, S. W. and Mix, D. (1994) "Mucosal delivery of macromolecules." J. Control. Rel., 28: 37-44.

Egros, A. C.; Maitani, Y.; Veillard, M.; Machida, Y. and Nagai, T. (1992) "Combined effects of pH, cosolvent and penetration enhancer on the in vitro buccal absorption of propranolol through excised hamster cheek pouch." Int. J. Pharm., 84: 117-128.

Fabregas, J. L. and Garcia, N. (1995) "In vitro studies on buccoadhesive tablet formulations of hydrocortisone hemisuccinate." Drug Dev. Ind. Pharm., 21(14): 1689-1696.

Ferreira, L. A. M.; Seiller, M.; Grossiard, J. L.; Marty, J. P. and Wepierre, J. (1995) "Vehicle influence on in vitro release of glucose: w/o, w/o/w and o/w systems compared." J. Control. Rel. ,33: 849-856.

Garren, K. W. and Repta, A. J. (1988) "Buccal drug absorption 1. Comparative levels of esterase and peptidase activities in rat and hamster buccal and intestinal homogenates." Int. J. Pharm., 48: 189-194.

Garren, K. W. and Repta, A. J. (1989) "Buccal drug absorption II : In vitro diffusion across the hamster cheek pouch." J. Pharm. Sci., 78(2): 160.

Guo, J. H. (1994) "Bioadhesive polymer buccal patches for buprenorphine controlled delivery: formulation, in vitro adhesion and release properties." Drug Dev. Ind. Pharm., 20(3): 315-325.

Hansen, H. B.; Jorgesen, A.; Rasmussen, S. N.; Louring, L. and Bundgaard, H. (1992) "Buccal absorption of ketobemidone and various ester prodrugs in the rat." Int. J. Pharm., 88: 243-250.

Heiber, S. J.; Ebert, C. D.; Dave, S. C. and Smith, K. (1994) "In vitro buccal delivery of calcitonin." J. Control. Rel., 28: 269-271.

Hicks, D. C. (1973) "The buccal absorption of some b-adrenoceptor blocking drugs." Br. J. Pharmacol, 47: 680P-681P.

Hidalgo, I.J.; Hillgren, K.M.; Grass, G.M. and Borchardt, R.T. (1989) "Characterization of the aqueous boundary layer in Caco-2 cells using a novel diffusion cell." Pharm. Res., 6: S-114 (abstr. PD950).

Hoogstraate, A. J.; Senel, S.; Cullander, C.; Verhoef, J.; Junginger, H.E. and Bodde, H. E. (1996a) "Effects of bile salts on transport rates and routes of FITC-labelled compounds across porcine buccal epithelium in vitro." J. Control. Rel, 40: 211-221.

Hoogstraate, A. J.; Verhoef, J. C.; Tuk, B.; Pijpers, A.; Verheijden, J. H. M.; Jungiger, H. E. and Bodde, H. E. (1996b) "In vivo buccal delivery of fluorescein isothiocyanate-dextran 4400 with glycodeoxycholate as an absorption enhancer in pigs." J. Pharm. Sci., 85(5): 457-460.

Hoogstraate, A. J.; Verhoef, J. C.; Tuk, B.; Pijpers, A.; Verheijden, J. H. M.; Leengoed, L. A. M. G.; Jungiger, H. E. and Bodde, H. E. (1996c) "Buccal delivery of fluorescein isothiocyanate-dextran 4400 and peptide drug buserelin with glycodeoxycholate as an absorption enhancer in pigs." J. Control. Rel., 41: 77-84.

Hosny, E. A. and Al-Meshal, M. A. (1994) "In vivo evaluation of a bioadhesive containing indomethacin tablets." Drug Dev. Ind. Pharm., 20(17): 2715-2720.

Hussain, M. A.; Aungst, B. J.; Kearney A. and Shefter, E. (1987) "Buccal and oral bioavailability of naloxone and naltreoxone in rats." Int. J. Pharm., 36: 127.

Hussain, M. A.; Aungst, B. J. and Shefter, E. (1986) "Buccal and oral bioavailability of nalbupine in rats." J. Pharm. Sci., 75(2): 218-219.

Imanidis G.; Waldner C.; Mettler C. and Leu enberger H. (1996) "An improved diffusion cell design for determining drug transport parameters across cultured cell monolayers." J. Pharm. Sci., 85(11): 1196-1203.

Irache, J.M.; Durrer, C.; Duchene, D. and Ponchel G. (1994) "In vitro study of lectin-latex conjugates for specific bioadhesion." J. Control. Rel., 31: 181-188.

Ishida, M.; Machida, Y.; Nambu, N. and Nagai T. (1981) "New mucosal dosage form of insulin." Chem. Pharm. Bull., 209: 810-816.

Ishida, M.; Nambu, N. and Nagai, T. (1983a) "Highly viscous gel ointment containing carbopol for application to the oral mucosa." Chem. Pharm. Bull., 31: 4561.

Ishida, M.; Nambu, N. and Nagai, T. (1983b) "Ointment type oral mucosal dosage form of carbopol containing prednisolone for the treatment of aphtha." Chem. Pharm. Bull., 31: 1010.

Jacobsen, J.: Deurs B. V.: Pedersen M. and Rassing M. R. (1995) "TR146 cells grown on filters as a model for human buccal epithelium. I : Morphology, growth, barrier properties and permeability." Int. J. Pharm., 125: 165.

Kellaway, I. W. and Warren, S. J. (1991) "Mucoadhesive hydrogels." Proc. Intern. Symp. Control. Rel. Bioact. Mater., 18: 73.

Kurosaki, Y.; Hisaichi, S.; Hamada, C.; Nakayama, T. and Kimura, T (1988) "Effects of surfactants on the absorption of salicylic acid from hamster cheek pouch as a model of keratinised oral mucosa." Int. J. Pharm., 47: 13.

Kurosaki, Y.; Hisaichi, S.; Nakayama, T. and Kimura, T. (1989) "Enhancing effect of 1-dodecylazacycloheptan-2-one (Azone) on the absorption of salicylic acid from keratinised oral mucosa and the duration of enhancement in vivo." Int. J. Pharm., 51: 47.

Kurosaki, Y.; Takatori, T.; Nishimura, H.; Nakayama, T. and Kimura, T. (1991) "Regional variation in oral mucosal drug absorption : Permeability and degree of keratinisation in hamster cheek oral cavity." Pharm. Res., 8: 1297.

Le Brun, P. P. H.; Fox, P. L. A.; De Vries, M. E. and Bodde, H. E. (1989) "In vitro penetration of some b-adrenoreceptor blocking drugs through porcine buccal mucosa." Int. J. Pharm., 49: 141-145.

Lee, Y. and Chien, Y. W. (1995) "Oral mucosa controlled delivery of LHRH by bilayer mucoadhesive polymer systems." J. Control. Rel., 37: 251-261.

Lesch, C. A.; Squier, C. A.; Cruchley, A.; Williams D. M. and Speight, P. (1989) "The permeability of human oral mucosa and skin to water." J. Dent. Res., 68: 1345.

Lopez, C. R.; Portero, A.; Vila-Jato, J. C. and Alonso, M. J. (1998) "Design and evaluation of chitosan/ethylcellulose mucoadhesive bilayered devices for buccal drug delivery." J. Control. Rel., 55: 143-152.

Lu, M. F. and Hui, H. W. (1996) "Delivery of renin inhibitor through mouth mucosa." Drug Dev. Ind. Pharm., 22(11): 1167-1171.

LueBen, H. L.; Lehr, C. M.; Rentel, C. O.; Noach, A. B. J.; De Boer, A. G.; Verhoef, J. C. and Junginger H. E. (1994) "Bioadhesive polymers for the peroral delivery of peptide drugs." J. Control. Rel., 29: 329-338.

Maddox, D. H.; Burnside, B. A. and Keith A. D. (1990) "Buccal delivery of progesterone." Proc., Intern. Symp. Control. Rel. Bioact. Mater., 17: 291.

Manning, A. S. and Evered, D. F. (1976) "The absorption of sugars from the human buccal cavity." Clin. Sci. Mol. Med., 51: 127-132.

Mehta, M.; Kemppainen, B. W. and Stafford R. G. (1991) "In vitro penetration of tritium labeled water and [3H]PbTx-3 (a red tide toxin) through monkey buccal mucosa and skin." Toxicology letters, 55: 185.

Meyer, W.; Kaye, C. M. and Turner, P. (1974) "A study of the influence of pH on the buccal absorption and renal excretion of procainamide." Eur. J. Clin. Pharmacol. 7: 287-289.

Nagai T. (1985) "Adhesive topical drug delivery systems." J. Control. Rel., 2: 121-134.

Nagai, T.; Machida, Y.; Suzuki Y. and Ikura, H. (1980) "Method and preparation for administration to the mucosa of the oral or nasal cavity" US Patent No. 4226848

Nair, K.; Chetty, D. J.; Ho, H. and Chien, Y. W. (1997) "Membrane permeation of nicotine: Mechanistic studies with porcine mucosa and skin." J. Pharm. Sci., 86(2): 257-262.

Nielsen H. M.; Verhoff J. C.; Ponec M. and Rassing M. R. (1999) "TR146 cells grown on filters as a model for human buccal epithelium : permeabiilty of fluoresein isothiocyanate labelled dextrans in the presence of sodium glycocholate." J. Control. Rel., 60: 223-233.

Nozaki, Y.; Kakumoto, M.; Ohta, M. and Yukimatsu, K. (1993) "A new transmucosal therapuetic system : overview of formulation development and in vitro / in vivo clinical performance." Drug Dev. Ind. Pharm., 19(1 & 2): 221-275.

Oh, C. K. and Ritschel, W. A. (1988a) "Biopharmaceutical aspects of buccal absorption of insulin in rabbits I. Effect of dose, size, pH and sorption enhancers : in vivo in vitro correlation." Pharm. Res., 5: S-100.

Oh, C. K. and Ritschel, W. A. (1988b) "Biopharmaceutical aspects of buccal absorption of insulin in rabbits II. Absorption characteristics of insulin through the buccal mucosa" Pharm. Res., 5- S-100.

Parodi, B.; Russo, E.; Caviglioli, G.; Cafaggi, S. and Binardi, G. (1996) "Development and characterisation of a buccoadhesive dosage form of oxycodone hydrochloride." Drug Dev. Ind. Pharm., 22(5): 445-450.

Past, T.; Tapsonyi, Z. S. and Hortobagyi, I. (1979) "Relationship between the dipole moment and rate of absorption of drugs." Acta Med. Acad. Sci. Hun, 36: 137-147.

Quadros C.; Cassidy J.; Gniecko K. and LeRoy S. (1991) "Buccal and colonic absorption of CGS16617, a novel ACE inhibitor." J. Control. Rel., 19: 77-86

Quadros, E.; Cassidy, J. P.; Rosenzweig, K. A. and Berner, B. (1988) "Permeation of a novel angiotensin converting enzyme inhibitor in vivo and in vitro." Proceed. Intern. Symp. Control. Rel. Bioact. Mater., 15:325.

Randhawa, M. A.; Blackett, A. N. and Turner, P. (1986) "Spectrofluorimetric analysis and buccal absorption of medifoxamine." J. Pharm. Pharmacol., 38: 629-630

Rathbone, M. J. (1991a) "Human buccal absorption I. A method for estimating the transfer kinetics of drugs across the human buccal membrane." Int. J. Pharm., 69: 103.

Rathbone, M. J. (1991b) "Human buccal absorption II. A comparative study of the buccal absorption of some paracetamol hydroxybenzoic acid derivatives using the buccal absorption test and a buccal perfusion cell." Int. J. Pharm., 74: 189.

Rathbone, M. J. and Hadgraft, J. (1991) "Absorption of drugs from the human oral cavity." Int. J. Pharm., 74: 1924.

Rathbone, M. J.; Purve, R.; Ghazati, F. A. and Ho, P. C. (1996) "In vivo techniques for studying the oral mucosal absorption characteristics of drugs in animals and humans." In Rathbone, M. J. (ed.), Oral Mucosal Delivery Systems, Marcel Dekker Inc. New York, 121-156.

Save T. and Venkitachalam P. (1994) "Bioadhesive tablets of Nifedipine: Standardisation of a novel buccoadhesive erodible carrier." Drug Dev. Ind. Pharm., 20(19): 3005-3014.

Schurmann, W. and Turner, P. (1978) "A membrane model of the human oral mucosa as derived from buccal absorption performance and physicochemical properties of the b-blocking drugs atenolol and propranolol." J. Pharm. Pharmacol., 30: 137-147.

Schure, W. and Ziegler, R. (1983) "Buccal absorption of protirelin : an effective way to stimulate thryrotropin and prolactin." J. Pharm. Sci., 72: 1481-1483.

Senel, S.; Duchene D.; Hincal, A. A.; Capan, Y. and Ponchel G. (1998) "In vitro studies on enhancing effect of sodium glycocholate on transbuccal permeation of morphine hydrochloride." J. Control, Rel., 51: 107-113.

Senel, S.; Hoogstraate, A. J.; Spies, F.; Verhoef, J. C.; Geest, A. B.; Junginger, H. E. and Bodde, H. E. (1994) "Enhancement of in vitro permeability of porcine buccal mucosa by bile salts : kinetic and histological studies." J. Control. Rel., 32: 45-56.

Shaban A. H. M.; Ouhayoun J. P.; Sawaf, M. H. N. and Forest (1989) "A biochemical and immunological analysis of cytokeratin patterns in the oral epithelium of miniature pig and man." Arch. Oral Biol., 34: 249.

Shah M. V.; Audus K. L. and Borchardt R. T. (1989) Pharm. Res., 6: 624-627,.

Siegel, I. A. (1984) "Permeability of the rat oral mucosa to organic solutes measured in vivo." Arch. Oral Biol., 29(1): 13-16.

Siegel, I. A. and Gordan, H. P. (1985) "Surfactant induced increases of permeability of rat oral mucosa to non electrolytes in vivo." Arch. Oral Biol., 30(1): 43-47.

Siegel, I. A.; Izutsu, K. T. and Watson, E. (1981) "Mechanism of non electrolyte penetration across dog and rabbit oral mucosa in vitro." Arch. Oral Biol., 26: 357-361.

Smart, J. D. (1992) "Some formulation factors influencing the rate of drug release from bioadhesive matrices." Drug Dev. Ind. Pharm., 18(2): 223-232.

Squier C. A.; Cox P. and Wertz P. W. (1991) "Lipid content and water permeability of skin and oral mucosa." J. Invest. Dermatol., 96: 123.

Squier, C. A. (1973) "The permeabilty of keratinised and nonkeratinised oral epithelium to horseradish peroxidase." J. Ultrastruct. Res., 43: 160.

Squier, C. A. and Hall, B. K. (1984) "The permeability of mammalian nonkeratinised oral epithelia to horseradish peroxidase applied in vivo and in vitro, Arch. Oral Biol., 29: 45-49.

Squier, C. A. and Hall, B. K. (1985) "In vitro permeability of porcine oral mucosa after epithelial separation, stripping and hydration." Arch. Oral Biol., 30(6): 485-491.

Squier, C. A.; Kremer, M. and Wertz, P. W. (1997) "Continuous flow mucosal cells for measuring in vitro permeability of small tissue samples." J. Pharm. Sci., 86(1): 82-84.

Stratford, R. E. Jr.; Clay, M. P.; Heinz, B. A.; Kuhfeld, M. T.; Osborne, S. J.; Phillips, D. L.; Sweetana, S. A.; Tebbe, M. J.; Vasudevan, V.; Zornes L.L. and Lindstrom, T. D. (1999) "Application of oral bioavailability surrogates in the design of orally active inhibitors of rhinovirus replication." J. Pharm. Sci., 88 (8) : 747

Tanaka, M.; Yanagibashi, N.; Fukuda, H. and Nagai T. (1980) "Absorption of salicylic acid through the oral mucous membrane of hamster cheek pouch." Chem. Pharm. Bull., 28: 1056-1061.

Tanaka, W.; Akito, E.; Yoshida, K.; Terada, T. and Ninomiya, H. (1977) "Pharmaceutical preparations for oral cavity administration" US Patent No. 4059686.

Tavakoli-Saberi, M. R. and Audus K. L. (1989a) "Physicochemical factors affecting b-adrenergic antagonists permeation across cultured hamster pouch buccal epithelium." Int. J. Pharm., 56: 135-142.

Tavakoli-Saberi, M. R. and Audus K. L. (1989b) "Cultured buccal epithelium: an in vitro model derived from hamster pouch for studying transport and metabolism" Pharm. Res., 6: 160-166,.

Tobey, N. A.; Schreiner, V. J.; Readling, R. D. and Orlando, R. C. (1988) "The acute effects of smokeless tobacco on transport and barrier function of buccal mucosa." J. Dent. Res., 67: 1414.

Tolo, K. J. and Jonson, B. J. (1975) "In vitro penetration of tritiated dextrans through rabbit oral mucosa." Arch. Oral Biol., 20: 419-422.

Tolo, K. (1971) "A study of permeability of gingival pocket epithelium to albumin in guinea pigs and Norwegian pigs." Arch. Oral Biol., 16: 881.

Tsutsumi, K.; Obata, Y.; Takayama, K.; loftsson, T. and Nagai T. (1998) "Effect of cod liver oil extract on the buccal permeation of ergotamine tartrate." Drug Dev. Ind. Pharm., 24(8): 757-762.

Tucker, I. G. (1988) "A method to study the kinetics of oral mucosal drug absorption from solutions." J. Pharm. Pharmacol., 40: 679-683.

Veillard, M. M.; Longer, M. A.; Martens, T. W. and Robinson, J. R. (1987) "Preliminary studies of oral mucosal delivery of peptide drugs." J. Control. Rel., 6: 123-131.

Venkatesh H. (1989) "A buccal delivery system of salbutamol sulphate." M. Pharm. Thesis submitted to University of Mumbai.

Weaver, M. L.; Tanzer, J. M. and Kramer, P. A. (1992) "Salivary flow induction by buccal premucosal pilocarpine in anesthetised beagle dogs." J. Dent. Res., 71: 1762.

Yamahara, H.; Suzuki, T.; Mizobe, M.; Noda, K. and Samejima, M. (1990) "In situ perfusion system for oral mucosal absorption in dogs." J. Pharm. Sci., 79(11): 963.

Younes, I. G.; Wagner, J. G.; Gaines, D. A.; Ferry, J. J. and Hageman, J. M. (1991) "Absorption of flurbiprofen through human buccal mucosa." J. Pharm. Sci., 80(9): 820-823.

Yukimatsu, K.; Nozaki, Y.; Kakumoto, M. and Ohta, M. (1994) "Development of a transmucosal controlled release device for systemic delivery of antianginal drugs pharmacokinetics and pharmacodynamics." Drug Dev. Ind. Pharm, 20(4): 503-534.

Zhang H. and Robinson J. R. (1996) "In vitro methods for measuring permeability of the oral mucosa" In : Rathbone, M. J. (ed.), Oral mucosal drug delivery, Marcel Dekker Inc., New York, 85-100.

Zhang J., Niu, S.; Ebert, C. and Stanley, T. H. (1994) "An in vivo dog model for studying recovery kinetics of the buccal mucosa permeation barrier after exposure to permeation enhancers : apparent evidence of effective enhancement without tissue damage." Int. J. Pharm., 101: 15-22.

Zhang, J.; Niu, S.; Ebert, C.; McJames, S.; Gijsman, H. J. and Stanley T. H. (1989) "Transbuccal permeability of isoproterenol - a dog model." Pharm. Res., 6: S-135.

Chapter 5 _____

Colon-specific
Drug Delivery Systems

Y.S.R. Krishnaiah, S. Satyanarayana

5.1 INTRODUCTION

Inflammatory bowel diseases including irritable bowl syndrome, ulcerative colitis and Crohn's disease are considered serious colonic disorders. Ulcerative colitis, if not treated, leads to colon cancer. More than 66,000 cases of colon cancer are reported to occur every year in India. Cancer of the large intestine accounts for about 15% of cancer deaths in India. The incidence is still high in western countries. The mainstay of treatment for colon cancer is still surgery. In most cases, partial colectomy (removal of the part of the colon) is performed followed by chemotherapy.

Most of the conventional drug delivery systems for treating the colon disorders such as inflammatory bowel diseases (e.g. irritable bowel syndrome, ulcerative colitis, Crohn's disease etc.), infectious diseases (e.g. amoebiasis) and colon cancer are failing as the drugs do not reach the site of action in appropriate concentrations. Thus, an effective and safe therapy of these colonic disorders, using site-specific drug delivery systems is a challenging task to the pharmaceutical technologists. The therapeutic advantages of targeting drug to the diseased organ include:

(a) delivery of drug in its intact form as close as possible to the target site,

(b) the ability to cut down the conventional dose, and

(c) reduced incidence of adverse side effects.

In the recent times, the colon-specific delivery systems are also gaining importance for the systemic delivery of protein and peptide drugs. This is because of the unprecedented rapid development of biotechnology and genetic engineering resulting in the availability of peptide and protein drugs at a reasonable cost. The peptide and protein drugs are destroyed and inactivated in acidic environment of the stomach and/or by pancreatic enzymes in the small intestine. These drugs are usually administered by parenteral route, which is inconvenient and expensive. Due to negligible activity of brush-border membrane peptidase activity and less activity of pancreatic enzymes, the colon is considered to be more suitable for delivery of peptides and protein in comparison to small intestine (Lee, 1991; Ikesue et al, 1991). Besides this low hostile environment, the colonic transit time is long (20-30 hours) and the colonic tissue is highly responsive to the action of absorption enhancers (Digenis & Sandefer, 1991; Taniguchi et al, 1980). The longer residence time, less peptidase activity, natural absorptive characteristics and high response to absorption enhancers make the colon a promising site for the delivery of protein and peptide drugs for systemic absorption. Thus, colonic delivery of analgesic peptides, contraceptive peptides, oral vaccines, insulin, growth hormone, erythropoietin, interferons and interleukins was attempted for systemic absorption (Saffran et al, 1988 & 1988a; Mackay & Tomilinson, 1993). Further, drug targeting to colon would prove useful where intentional delayed drug absorption is desired from therapeutic point of view in the treatment of diseases that have peak symptoms in the early morning such as nocturnal asthma (Quadros et al, 1995) angina or arthritis. Colonic drug delivery is also found useful for improving systemic absorption of drugs like nitrendipine, metoprolol, theophylline, isosorbide mononitrate etc. However, a substantial amount of research is needed in order to find out to what extent these molecules can be absorbed after oral administration.

Colonic delivery can be accomplished by oral or rectal administration. Rectal dosage forms such as suppositories and enemas are not always effective since a high variability in the distribution of these forms is observed (Wood et al, 1985). Suppositories are only effective in the rectum because of the confined spread (Jay et al, 1985), and enema solutions can only offer topical treatment to the sigmoid and descending colon (Hardy, 1989). Therefore, oral administration is preferred, but for this purpose, many physiological barriers have to be overcome. Absorption or degradation of the active ingredient in the upper part of the GI tract is the major obstacle and must be circumvented for successful colonic drug delivery.

There are several ways in which colon-specific drug delivery has been attempted (Van den Mooter & Kinget, 1995; Rama Prasad et al, 1996). Prodrugs, coating with pH dependent polymers, design of timed-release dosage forms and the use of carriers that are degraded exclusively by colonic bacteria are an array of such attempts. This chapter provides a review of colon function, physiology, and drug absorption characteristics relevant to pharmaceutical scientists and of the technologies available for colon-specific drug delivery.

5.2 FACTORS TO BE CONSIDERED IN THE DESIGN OF COLON-SPECIFIC DRUG DELIVERY SYSTEMS

5.2.1 Anatomy and physiology of colon

The GI tract is divided into stomach, small intestine and large intestine. The large intestine extending from the ileocaecal junction to the anus is divided into three main parts. These are the colon, the rectum and the anal canal The colon itself is made up of the caecum, the ascending colon, the hepatic flexure, the transverse colon, the splenic flexure, the descending colon and the sigmoid colon. It is about 1.5 m long, the transverse colon being the longest and most mobile part (Meschan, 1975), and has an average diameter of about 6.5 cm, although it varies in diameter from approximately 9 cm in the caecum to 2 cm in the sigmoid colon (Mrsny, 1992).

The wall of the colon is composed of four layers: the serosa, the muscularis externa, the submucosa and the mucosa. The serosa is the exterior coat of the large intestine and consists of areolar tissue that is covered by a single layer of squamous mesothelial cells. The major muscular coat of the large intestine is the muscularis externa. This is composed of an inner circular layer of fibers that surrounds the bowel and of an outer longitudinal layer. The submucosa is the layer of connective tissue that lies immediately beneath the mucosa. Lining the lumen of the colon, the mucosa is divided into epithelium, lamina propria and muscularis mucosae. Closely spaced crypts extend down into the surface of the mucosa. The muscularis mucosa consists of a layer of smooth muscle and separates the submucosa from the lamina propria. The lamina propria supports the epithelium, and occupies space between the crypts and beneath the crypts. Within the lamina propria are located blood capillaries and lymphatic lacteals. The space also acts as a reservoir for macrophages, neutrophils, eosinophils, lymphocytes and plasma cells, which locally produce IgA antibodies.

The epithelium consists of a single layer of cells, which lines the crypts and covers the surface of the mucosa. Three major cell types found in the epithelium are the columnar absorptive cells, goblet (mucous) cells and enteroendocrine cells. Adjacent columnar absorptive cells are attached to one another near their apical margins by a junctional complex. Mucus production in the colon is a function of goblet cells and the proportion of goblet cells increases in the elderly.

The arterial blood supply to the proximal colon is from the superior mesenteric artery and the inferior mesenteric artery supplies the distal colon. The venous drainage is via the superior (proximal colon) and inferior (distal colon) veins. The arterioles and capillary branches pass to the epithelial surfaces between the crypts and form an extensive network of capillary plexi.

The colon serves four major functions; (i) creation of suitable environment for the growth of colonic microorganisms; (ii) storage reservoir of faecal contents   (iii) expulsion of the contents of the colon at an appropriate time and (iv) absorption of potassium and water from the lumen, concentrating the faecal content, and secretion and excretion of potassium and bicarbonate. In vitro and in vivo electrophysiological studies have demonstrated that the mechanism of sodium absorption is an active transport (Binder et al, 1987; Hawker et al 1978). Furthermore, it is influenced by mucosal cyclic adenosine monophosphate level, pH, osmolarity and compounds such as fatty acids, and bile acids. Water is absorbed passively, while potassium and bicarbonate are actively secreted by colonic epithelium. The active secretion of potassium is stimulated by mineral corticoids (Gingell et al, 1968).

5.2.2   pH in the colon

The pH of the GI tract is subjected to both inter- and intra-subject variations. Table 5.1 gives an overview of the pH of the GI tract (Wilson & Washington, 1989).

Table 5.1 Average pH in the GI tract

Location	pH
Oral cavity	6.2 - 7.4
Oesophagus	5.0 - 6.0
Stomach	Fasted condition: 1.5 - 2.0
	Fed condition: 3.0 - 5.0
Small intestine	Jejunum: 5.0 - 6.5
	Ileum: 6.0 - 7.5
Large intestine	Right colon: 6.4
	Mild colon and left colon: 6.0 -7.6

Radiotelemetry has been used to measure the gastrointestinal pH in healthy human subjects. The highest pH levels (7.5 ± 0.5) were found to be in the terminal ileum. On entry into the colon, the pH dropped to 6.4 ± 0.6. The pH in the mid-colon was found to be 6.6 ± 0.8 and in the left colon, 7.0 ± 0.7 (Evans et al, 1988). The presence or absence of food in the stomach determines the gastric pH range, which varies from 1.5 to 3 in the fasted state and rises to approximately 4 or 5 in the fed (Wilson & Washington, 1989; Friend, 1991). In duodenum, the pH ranges from 1.7 to 4.3 in the fed state and from 3 to approximately 6 in fasted state (Ovesen et al, 1986). Passing from the jejunum through the mid small bowel and ileum, the pH rises slightly from approximately 6.6 to 7.5 and this falls to about 6.4 in the right colon. The mid and left colon have pH values of about 6.6 and about 7.0 respectively (Meldrum et al, 1972; Brown et al, 1974; Evans et al, 1988). Interspecies variability in pH is a major concern when developing and testing colon-specific delivery systems in animals and applying the information to humans. Colonic pH has been shown reduced in disease. The mean pH in a group of 7 patients with untreated ulcerative colitis was 4.7 ± 0.7 whereas in 5 patients receiving treatment it was 5.5 ± 0.4 (Raimundo et al, 1992). The in vitro fermentation of the pharmaceutical polysaccharides such as ispaghula and guar gum resulted in the reduction of pH in the presence of faecal bacteria (Tomlin & Read 1988).

5.2.3 Gastrointestinal transit

Gastric emptying of dosage forms is highly variable and depends primarily on whether the subject is fed or fasted and on the properties of the dosage form such as size and density. The arrival of an oral dosage form at the colon is determined by the rate of gastric emptying and the small intestinal transit time. The transit times of small dosage forms in GI tract are given in Table 5.2.

The presence of food generally increases gastric residence and, in some cases, with regular feeding, dosage forms have been shown to reside in the stomach for periods in excess of 12 hours (Davis et al, 1984). Small intestinal transit is surprisingly constant at 3-4 hours and appears to be independent of the dosage form and the subject's fasted or fed state (Davis et al, 1986). Therefore, a dosage form could take from as little as 4 hours to longer than 12 hours to arrive at the colon following oral administration. However, the movement of materials through the colon is slow and tends to be highly variable and influenced by a number of factors such as diet, dietary fiber content, mobility, stress, disease and drugs (Bararow et al, 1991). In healthy young and adult males, dosage forms such as capsules and tablets pass through the colon in approximately 20-30 hours,

Table 5.2 The transit time of dosage forms in GI tract

Organ	Transit time (hr)
Stomach	<1 (Fasting)
	>3 (Fed)
Small intestine	3 - 4
Large intestine	20 - 30

although the transit time of a few hours to more than 2 days can occur (Hardy, 1989). Diseases affecting colonic transit have important implications for drug delivery: diarrhoea increases colonic transit and constipation decreases it. However, in most disease conditions, transit time appears to remain reasonably constant (Hardy et al, 1988; Cann et al, 1983).

5.2.4 Colonic microflora

A large number of anaerobic and aerobic bacteria are present throughout the entire length of the human GI tract. The microflora found in the GI tract of man is given in Table 5.3 (Simon & Gorbach, 1984).

The upper region of the GIT has a very small number of bacteria and predominantly consists of Gram-positive facultative bacteria. The concentration of bacteria in the stomach is usually less than 10^3 colony-forming units/ml (CFU/ml) and the most commonly isolated species are *Streptococci, Staphylococci, Lactobacilli*, and various fungi (Simon & Gorbach, 1984). Under normal conditions, the microflora of the proximal small bowel are similar to those of the stomach, the bacterial concentration being 10^3-10^4 CFU/ml (Simon & Gorbach, 1986). In the distal part of the small intestine, a higher concentration of anaerobic bacteria is found. The lower ileum has a bacterial concentration of 10^7-10^8 CFU/ml and the distal ileum usually contains bacteria similar to those found in the colon (Gustafsson, 1982). In the ileocaecal sphincter, the bacterial concentration increases dramatically. The concentration of bacteria in the human colon is 10^{11}-10^{12} CFU/ml. The bacterial flora of the colon is predominantly anaerobic and composed of more than 400 strains. The anaerobic bacteria outnumber the aerobic by a factor of 10^3 to 10^4. The most important anaerobic bacteria are *Bacteroides, Bifidobacterium, Eubacterium, Peptococcus, Peptostreptococcus, Ruminococcus, Propionibacterium and Clostridium*. Important facultative bacteria in the large intestine are Escherichia coli and Lactobacillus (Drasar & Hill, 1974; Simon & Gorbach, 1983). The faecal flora are representative of the flora of the large bowel. Approximately 30% of the dry weight of faeces consist of bacteria. The influence of dietary factors appears to be of little importance in terms of the composition of the microflora (Hill, 1981). Orally administered antibiotics, however, can cause serious alterations in colonic flora (Nord & Heimdahl, 1986; Smith et al, 1990).

Table 5.3 The microflora found in the GIT of man

Bacterial counts (CFU/ml)	Stomach	Jejunum	Ileum	Faeces
Total bacterial count	$0\text{-}10^3$	$0\text{-}10^5$	$10^3\text{-}10^7$	$10^{10}\text{-}10^{12}$
Aerobic or facultative anaerobic bacteria				
Enterobacteria	$0\text{-}10^2$	$0\text{-}10^3$	$10^2\text{-}10^6$	$10_4\text{-}10^{10}$
Streptococci	$0\text{-}10^3$	$0\text{-}10^4$	$10^2\text{-}10^6$	$10^5\text{-}10^{10}$
Staphylococci	$0\text{-}10^2$	$0\text{-}10^3$	$10^2\text{-}10^5$	$10^4\text{-}10^7$
Lactobacillus	$0\text{-}10^3$	$0\text{-}10^4$	$10^2\text{-}10^5$	$10^6\text{-}10^{10}$
Fungi	$0\text{-}10^2$	$0\text{-}10^2$	$10^2\text{-}10^3$	$10^2\text{-}10^6$
Anaerobic bacteria				
Bacteroides	Rare	$0\text{-}10^2$	$10^3\text{-}10^7$	$10^{10}\text{-}10^{12}$
Bifidobacteria	Rare	$0\text{-}10^3$	$10^3\text{-}10^5$	$10^8\text{-}10^{12}$
Gram-positive cocci	Rare	$0\text{-}10^3$	$10^2\text{-}10^5$	$10^8\text{-}10^{11}$
Clostridia	Rare	Rare	$10^2\text{-}10^4$	$10^6\text{-}10^{11}$
Eubacteria	Rare	Rare	Rare	$10^9\text{-}10^{12}$

A large number of compounds ingested orally are metabolised by gut bacteria. A summary of the most important metabolic reactions carried out by intestinal bacteria is given below (Scheline, 1973).

Hydrolysis of glycosides, sulphate esters, amides, esters, sulphamates and nitrates

Reduction of C=C, azo bonds, nitro groups, aldehydes, ketones, alcohols & N oxides

Dehydroxylation (C & N dehydroxylation)

Decarboxylation

Dealkylation of O-alkyl groups and N- alkyl groups

Dehalogenation

Desamination

Heterocyclic ringfission

Acetylation

Esterification

The above metabolic actions of the microflora are influenced by numerous factors such as age, gastrointestinal disease, intake of drugs and fermentation of dietary residues (Rowland, 1988) and can lead to inactivation of drugs (Lindenbaum et al, 1981) or the enhancement of the action and side effects of the drugs (Peppercorn & Goldman, 1976).

Water absorption occurs secondary to the absorption of electrolytes and short chain fatty acids (SCFA) by solvent drag. The human colon absorbs sodium (Na^+) and chloride (Cl^-) and secretes bicarbonate (HCO_3^-) and potassium (K^+) against electrochemical gradients. Bicarbonates in the lumen neutralise the acidity caused by SCFA production. Carbohydrates that enter the colon, in any form but mostly as dietary fiber or mucopolysaccharides are fermented to SCFA mainly acetic, propionic and butyric. These SCFA are rapidly absorbed from the colon and are used by the colonic epithelial cells or are transported to the liver. The absorption of SCFA enhances the absorption of electrolytes and water. Sugars such as glucose and sucrose are poorly absorbed in the adult human colon. Lipid soluble molecules are most readily absorbed by passive diffusion. In general, organic acids, bases, and drugs are most rapidly absorbed in their lipid soluble undissociated form. The equivalent pore size of the colon was estimated as 2.3 Å when compared with jejunum (8 Å) and ileum (4 Å).

Mucins are degraded by the colonic bacteria and hence the changes in the intestinal flora may affect the mucosal environment. The mucus layer may also be affected by disease and is thinned by the action of prostaglandins. Some dietary fibers such as pectin have cation exchange properties that may bind charged molecules such as bile acids. This binding is increased at the low pH encountered in the colon and may be a factor in the immobilisation of some drugs.

5.3 DRUG ABSORPTION IN THE COLON

The colon may not be the best site for drug absorption since the colonic mucosa lacks well defined villi as found in the small intestine and this drastically reduces the absorptive surface area, despite the large diameter. Moreover, the viscosity of the colonic contents is high, especially after the hepatic plexure when chyme is processed into feces, which makes it even more difficult for a drug to diffuse from the lumen to the site of absorption. Mrsny (1992) extensively reviewed the absorption of drugs from the colon. Absorption of drugs from the colon is limited by a number of barriers. In lumen itself specific and non-specific drug binding can occur with dietary components and products released from colonic bacteria. This drug binding might facilitate longer colonic residence time and hence more enzymatic or environmental degradation. The mucus layer at the epithelial surface presents a formidable physical barrier because of specific and non-specific drug binding. For example, cephalosporin, penicillin and aminoglycoside antibiotics bind to the negatively charged mucus (Nubuchi et al, 1986). As a corollary to drug-mucus binding, drug-mucus repulsion or expulsion could also act to retard the drug from reaching the epithelial surface. Although removal of the mucus barrier using mucolytic agents might seem attractive; this may implicate in a variety of disease processes and pathological conditions due to alteration of intact mucus layer.

The space between the mucus layer and epithelial cells i.e., the unstirred water layer, presents another barrier to colonic absorption particularly for lipophilic drugs. A pH gradient may also exist across the unstirred water layer, which dramatically alters the solubility of drugs affecting the absorption of drug by the epithelial cells. The enzymatic degradation within the unstirred water layer also influences the extent of drug absorption.

Probably, the single most significant barrier to epithelial transport of drugs in colon is at the level of the epithelium (Powell, 1981). In this connection, it is to be noted that the lipid bilayer of the individual colonocytes and the occluding junctional complex between the cells provide a physical barrier to drug absorption. Drugs that intend to pass from the epical to basolateral surface of this epithelial barrier must do so by passing through either colonocytes (the transcellular route) or between adjacent colonocytes (the paracellular route). Small amphipathic drugs have a reasonable probability of transcellular transport. Transit through the cell cytoplasm may result in extensive enzymatic degradation. Therefore, successful passive transcellular transport requires a drug moiety that is stable to the multiple environments encountered on its transit through the colonic epithelial cells. Interestingly, membrane lipid fluidity of proximal colonocytes is greater than distal colonocytes, which may allow for increased passive drug absorption in the proximal colon. Carrier-mediated uptake of drugs in the colon is not extensive and usually relates to the metabolic events of the resident bacteria. Receptor-mediated endocytosis and fluid-phase endocytosis (pinocytosis) represent two active transport pathways, which could result in transcellular drug delivery. Paracellular transport may be the most promising means of general drug absorption in the colon.

For those molecules, which successfully traverse the physical and enzymatic barriers of the colonic mucosa, uptake into the blood-capillary or lymphatic sinuses can also be problematic. Local enzymatic degradation in the submucosa can also occur. Intact drug, which passes from the submucosa into venous capillaries, is transported to the liver through the hepatic portal system. A significant amount of metabolism can occur at the liver prior to the drug ever reaching the systemic circulation. Alternately, uptake into the lymphatic sinuses results in drug delivery directly into the systemic circulation which usually results in less metabolic breakdown of the absorbed drug.

The positive aspect for drug absorption is the prolonged residence time in the colon. The factors influencing the residence time are likely to affect the absorption of drugs from the colon. In spite of the unfavourable conditions for absorption, Fara (1989) concluded that a large variety of drugs is well absorbed from the colon. These include theophylline, ibuprofen, nifedipine, metoprolol, diclofenac, pseudoepinephrine, brompheniramine, isosorbide dinitrate, and oxprenolol. Colon is considered as a site for absorption of protein and peptide drugs, but the region where absorption occurs is variable depending on the number of aminoacids present in such drugs.

5.3.1 Role of absorption enhancers

The permeability of the epithelium to drugs can be modified by the use of chemical enhancers, which are compounds that promote absorption. For most potential drug molecules, particularly for protein and peptide drugs, colonic epithelial permeability is insufficient to allow for a transport rate required for therapeutic action. For this reason, a variety of methods (Fix, 1987) have been explored to enhance colonic permeability by means of absorption enhancers (Table 5.4). These enhancers increase transcellular and paracellular transport through one or other of the following mechanisms: (i) by disruption of intercellular occluding junctional complex function to open the paracellular route; (ii) by modifying epithelial permeability via denaturing membrane proteins and/ or modifying lipid-protein interactions; and (iii) by disrupting the integrity of lipid bilayer of colonic enterocytes. Mention may be made of the usefulness of the protease inhibitors such as aprotinin and bacitracin as absorption enhancers, which act by inhibiting the activity of aminopeptidases present in the colon. This action is particularly useful in the colonic absorption of protein and peptide drugs. Enhancement of colonic absorption by these agents appears to be drug-specific. For example, mixed micelles composed of either taurocholate or glycocholate with monoolein, oleic or lauric acid enhanced the absorption of 5-fluorouracil (Muranishi et al, 1979), heparin (Muranishi et al, 1980) and bleomycin (Yoshikawa et al, 1981). Since, many of these absorption enhancers are acidic in nature, local high concentrations might alter luminal pH and have significant effects on the colonic microbial flora which can result in epithelial pathologies.

These absorption enhancers also produce transport windows in colonic epithelia large enough for the passage of many bacterial toxins. Clearly, a number of concerns over the deleterious actions of absorption enhancers on the colon, must be addressed.

5.3.2 Methods for studying colonic drug absorption

Absorption of drug molecules from the colon, like other regions of the GI tract, is the result of a series of complex events. In vitro approaches, using isolated colonic epithelial cells or colonic tissue, have been used to study the role of physical and enzymatic barriers in colonic drug absorption. Relatively pure cell population, isolated from colonic crypt and surface regions, are useful in assessing the potential for metabolic modification and/or transmembrane uptake of a drug moiety (Osiecks et al, 1985). Isolated colonic epithelial cells, however, lose their epical and isolateral polarity. Incubation under certain in vitro conditions allows these cells to form monolayers and restore this polarity. Without this polarity, the sequential epical and basolateral membrane transport required for successful in vivo drug uptake can not be assessed.

Instead of using primary colonocyte isolates, most laboratories have used a *colonic carcinoma cell line* for in vitro monolayer studies with *T-84, Caco-2* and *HT-29* (Audus et al, 1990). Individually, none of these

Table 5.4 : Absorption enhancers used in colonic drug delivery

---

Nonsteroidal Anti-inflammatory Agents
    Indomethacin, Salicylates
Calcium ion chelating agents
    Ethylenediaminetetraacetic acid
Surfactants
    Polyoxyethylene lauryl ether
Saponins
Bile salts
    Taurocholate
    Glycocholate
Fatty Acids
    Sodium caprate
    Sodium caprylate
    Sodium laurate
    Sodium oleate
Mixed micelles
    Monoolein-taurocholate
    Oleic acid-taurocholate
    Oleic acid-polyoxyethylene hydrogenated castor oil
    Oleic acid-glycocholate
Other agents
    Acylcarnitine
    Phenothiazines
    Emanine
    Dicarboxylic acids

---

carcinoma cell lines model the heterogeneous nature of colonic tissue. Another in vitro method, everted sac, traces drug transport from the external mucosal surface to the internal serosal surface. This method has been used to study the physical pore size for paracellular transport of drug molecules in the colon produced by a series of permeation enhancers (Tomita et al, 1989). In situ loops of colon with a solution flushed slowly through the lumen have also been used to evaluate drug uptake by monitoring venous blood and lymph which drain the segments of the colon (Tomita et al, 1989; Riad & Sawchuk, 1991).

In vivo methods for the assessment of colonic drug absorption have been set up in a variety of animal models including the rat (Suzuka et al, 1986), the dog (Tolls, 1986) and the pig (Fujii et al, 1988). Colonoscopy is proved to be a relatively simple and well tolerated method for assessing the absorption of drugs from formulations in the man (Gleiter et al, 1985). A potentially powerful model, a xenograft of human foetal bowel, grafted and matured in nude mice was described (Winter et al, 1991). Using this model, both in vitro and in vivo colonic drug uptake could be assessed. Pharmacokinetic data can be used to indirectly evaluate the absorption (Lee et al, 1991) while the direct methods include colonoscopy and intubation (Gleiter et al, 1985) and the use of high frequency capsule (McLeod & Tozer, 1992). Gamma scintigraphy is nowadays the preferred method to study GI transit behaviour.

5.4 DRUG CANDIDATES FOR COLONIC DRUG DELIVERY

Drug delivery selectively to the colon through oral route is becoming increasingly popular for the treatment of large bowel diseases and for systemic absorption of peptide and protein drugs. Inflammatory bowel diseases

(IBD) such as ulcerative colitis and Crohn's disease require selective local delivery of drugs to the colon. Conventional rectal delivery dosage forms (suppositories and enemas) as alternatives are not always effective since a high variability in the distribution of these forms is observed (Wood et al, 1985). Suppositories are only effective in the rectum because of the confined spread (Jay et al, 1985) and enema solutions can only offer effective topical local action to the sigmoid and descending colon (Hardy, 1989). Sulfasalazine is the most commonly prescribed medication for such diseases. It is a conjugate of 5-aminosalicylic acid (5-ASA) and sulphapyridine, the active moiety being 5-ASA. When administered orally, about 20 % of the dose is absorbed in the upper part of the GI tract and remainder of the dose passes into colon, wherein the colonic azoreductases cleave the azo bond thereby liberating 5-ASA and sulphapyridine (SP). The SP gets absorbed from the colon and produces a number of side effects. Selective delivery of 5-ASA to the colon is required for therapeutic efficacy with less or no side effects.

The other drugs used in IBD are steroids such as dexamethasone, prednisolone and hydrocortisone. When these steroids are specifically delivered to the colon, they produce fewer and less intense side effects than when administered orally or intravenously. Nicotine is currently under investigation for its therapeutic role in the treatment of ulcerative colitis and hence is a promising drug candidate for colonic drug delivery (Rhodes & Thomas, 1995). Irritable bowel syndrome is another disorder of the colon. Pinaverium bromide is a drug for the local treatment of irritable bowel syndrome (Passreti et al, 1989). Advanced ulcerative colitis, if not treated, may lead to colon cancer. In such cases, anticancer drugs like 5-fluorouracil, doxorubicin and nimustine are to be delivered specifically to the colon for an effective and safe therapy. The site-specific delivery of drugs for the treatment of infectious diseases such as amoebiasis (e.g. metronidazole) would be very much useful in reducing the relapse of these diseases and for minimising the side effects associated with the systemic absorption of these drugs.

With the explosion of new peptide and protein drugs through biotechnology, there has been an increasing interest in utilising the colon as a site for systemic absorption of these drugs in view of the less hostile environment prevailing in the colon. However, there is significant protease and peptidase enzyme activity within the colon, arising from the microflora. Consequently, the stability of peptide and protein drugs within the colon is likely to be poor and the opportunities for absorption are still relatively limited.

A variety of protein and peptide drugs like calcitonin, interferon, interleukins, erythropoietin, growth hormone and even insulin are being investigated for their systemic absorption using colon-specific delivery (Mackay & Tomlinson, 1993). Most of the reports on the colonic absorption of protein and peptide drugs are in animal models (Moore et al, 1986; Kraeling & Ritschel, 1992; Rao & Ritschel, 1992; Hastewell et al, 1992; Langguth et al, 1994; Fisher et al, 1996). A few reports exist in the literature on the colonic absorption of therapeutic macromolecules in man.

Besides peptide and protein drugs, the colon is also a good site for the absorption of drugs that are not stable in the acidic environment of the stomach, cause gastric irritation (e.g. aspirin, iron supplements) or those degraded by small intestinal enzymes. Nowadays, a number of drugs are available as sustained release or delayed release or timed release tablets or capsules for oral administration. The different categories of drugs that are available in this form are anti-inflammatory drugs, anti-asthamatic drugs, anti-hypertensive drugs, etc. Unless these drugs have good absorption characteristics in the colon, their intended use in the management of respective disorders through sustained release or timed release formulations will be in question. This is due to the fact that most of these formulations are supposed to release their drug load slowly over a period of 12 hours, sometimes even 24 hours. The total residence time of these formulations in the stomach and small intestine will be not more than 5-6 hours. If the drug is not having inherent absorption properties in the colon, it will be eliminated in the faeces as it is. The drugs that are having good absorption properties from the colon include theophylline, glibenclamide (Brockmeier et al, 1985), and oxprenolol (Antonin et al, 1985; Davis et al, 1988). diclofenac, ibuprofen, brompheniramine, nitrendipine, nisoldipine, isosorbide, metoprolol, nifedipine, etc. and hence can be investigated for better bioavailability through colon-specific drug delivery (Fara, 1989). However, absorption of furosemide (Bieck, 1989), piretanide (Brockmeier et al, 1986), buflomedil (Wilson et al, 1991), atenolol, cimetidine and hydrochlorthiazide (Riley et al, 1992) are found poorly absorbed from colon.

5.5 APPROACHES TO COLON-SPECIFIC DRUG DELIVERY

The targeting of orally administered drugs to the colon is accomplished (Kinget et al, 1998; Watts & Illum, 1997; Van den Mooter et al, 1995; Rama Prasad et al, 1996) by:

(i)   Coating with pH dependent polymers

(ii) Timed release dosage forms

(iii) Delivery systems based on the metabolic activity of colonic bacteria

5.5.1   Coating with pH dependent polymers

In these systems, drugs are formulated into solid dosage forms such as tablets, capsules and pellets and coated with pH sensitive polymers as in enteric coating. Widely used polymers are methacrylic resins (Eudragits) which are available in water-soluble and water-insoluble forms. Eudragit L and S are copolymers of methacrylic acid and methyl methacrylate. Eudragit L is water soluble at pH 6 or above and is used as an enteric coating polymer. Eudragit S is water soluble at pH 7 or above and is used to deliver drugs to the end of the small bowel and large intestine. At present, 5-ASA is commercially available as an oral dosage form coated with Eudragit L100 (Claversal , Mesazal® and Colitofalk®) or Eudragit S (Asacol®). Dew et al, (1982) studied the usefulness of Eudragit S as a colonic delivery carrier. Thirty capsules filled with sulphapyridine and barium sulphate were coated with Eudragit S and validated in six convalescent patients using x-ray evidence and serum levels of sulphapyridine. After 12 hours, all the 36 capsules arrived at the colon of which 23 released their content, while 9 remained intact and 4 disintegrated in the ileum.

Although the use of Eudragit S provided reliable results, the effect of partially methylating the free carboxylic acid groups of Eudragit S was investigated by Peeters & Kinget (1993). The modified product was found to dissolve at a slightly higher pH value and its effectiveness as a coating material for colon-specific drug delivery was proved in human volunteers. Other oral drug delivery systems based on methacrylic resins are described for prednisolone (Thomas et al, 1985), insulin (Touitou & Rubinstein, 1986) and quinolones (Van Saene et al, 1986).

The disadvantage of this technique is the lack of consistency in the dissolution of the polymer at the desired site. Depending on the intensity of the GI motility, the dissolution of the polymer can be in the distal portion of the colon or at the end of the ileum. Moreover, many factors such as the presence of short chain fatty acids, residues of bile acids, carbon dioxide or other fermentation products reduce the colonic pH to approximately 6 and call its pH as a trigger into question. The lack of site-specificity of pH dependent systems was demonstrated by Ashford et al, (1993). Eudragit S, a model pH dependent polymer, was used to coat rapidly disintegrating tablets. These tablets were administered to healthy volunteers and studied for their in vivo behaviour using gamma scintigraphy. Though the polymer coat protected the tablet during its passage through the stomach and upper small intestine, its site specificity was poor. The disintegration sites varied from the ileum to the splenic flexure.

5.5.2.   Timed-release dosage forms

Small intestinal transit time is relatively constant and is hardly influenced by the nature of the formulation administered. Studies have shown that, once having left the stomach, the formulation arrives at the ileocaecal junction about 3 to 4 hours after dosing. An extension of the use of pH dependent polymers is the use of the Pulsincap® System (Rashid, 1990). This delivery system consists of a capsule, half of which is nondisintegrating and other half enteric coated. The enteric coat dissolves on entering the small intestine and a hydrogel plug, stoppering the nondisitegrating part, swells at a rate determined by the degree of cross-linking. After a predetermined time (e.g. 5 hours), the hydrogel plug swells so much that it becomes ejected from the nondisintegrating bottom half of the capsule thereby releasing the drug. It must be noted that the swelling of the hydrogel plug is pH independent. Other reports also appear in the literature on the use of pH dependent timed-release system for site specific drug release in the colon (Gazzaniga et al, 1994; Gazzaniga et al, 1994a; Pozzi et al, 1994). However, the site-specificity of timed-release dosage forms is considered poor because of large variations in gastric emptying times (Davis et al, 1984) and passage across the ileo-caecal junction (Marvola et al, 1987).

5.5.3 Delivery systems based on the metabolic activity of colonic bacteria

The colonic bacteria carry out a variety of metabolic reactions (Scheline, 1973) and the most important of them are reduction and hydrolysis. Different strategies were used to target drugs to the colon based on these actions. The main feature of these systems is their site-specificity. An excellent review was published by Rubinstein (1990) on the concepts of microbially controlled drug delivery to colon. These strategies are described below.

5.5.3.1 Coating with biodegradable azo polymers

The intestinal microflora have a large metabolic capacity and it appears that reduction of azo bonds is a general reaction of colonic bacteria. Van den Mooter et al, (1993) investigated the degradation of different types of azo polymers by colonic bacteria. The influence of the type of azo aromatic group built in the azo polymers and the degree of hydrophilicity of the azo polymer on the degradation by intestinal microflora were studied. The azopolymers having a high degree of hydrophilicity were degraded by colonic bacteria. It was also found that the chain length of the azo aromatic group in the azo polymers had no much influence on the rate of degradation. Saffran et al, (1991; 1988) developed copolymers of styrene and 2-hydroxyethyl methacrylate which were cross-linked with divinyl azobenzene and N,N^1 bis(β-styrene sulphonyl)-4,4^1-diaminoazo-benzene to coat oral dosage forms of insulin and vasopressin. On entering the colon, the coating was degraded by bacterial azoreductases thereby releasing the drug.

Colonic drug delivery systems based on the biodegradable poly(ether-ester) azopolymers were developed by Kalala et al, (1996). Since the azoploymers had poor film forming properties, a pH independent Eudragit polymer was mixed with azopolymer to coat ibuprofen capsules. Drug release studies carried out in rat caecal content medium showed that capsules coated with three layers of polymer coat containing 15% polyethylene glycol were useful for colonic drug delivery. The relationship between the swelling properties and the enzymatic degradation of azopolymers, designed for colon-specific drug delivery, was also studied (Van den Mooter et al, 1994).

An *in vivo* evaluation of theophylline capsules coated with azopolymers based upon 2-hydroxyethyl methacrylate, methyl methacrylate and methacrylic acid was carried out by Van den Mooter et al, (1995). The studies were carried out in the proximal part of the small intestine and the caecum of male rats. The plasma concentration of the drug was found higher when the capsules were ingested in the caecum as compared to the small intestine. The drug release was found to be by both diffusion of the drug and degradation of the coatings by bacterial azoreductases. However, it was felt that the reported colonic drug delivery systems were insufficient for the delivery of drugs with narrow therapeutic index for systemic action, but might be useful for drugs meant for local action in the colon.

The advantages of these pH-independent biodegradable polymers are site-specificity and scope for administering large doses of drugs. These expensive polymers have poor film forming properties, and their safety is yet to be established.

5.5.3.2 Prodrugs

A well known colon-specific prodrug, sulfasalazine, is used in the treatment of ulcerative colitis and Crohn's disease. Chemically, sulfasalazine is 5-aminosalicylic acid (5-ASA) coupled with sulphapyridine by azo bonding. On reaching the colon, the azo bond is reduced by colonic azoreductases to 5-ASA and sulphapyridine. The active moiety is 5-ASA and sulphapyridine simply acts as a carrier to deliver 5-ASA intact to the colon. Majority of side effects associated with the use of sulfasalazine are due to systemic absorption of sulphapyridine from colon. Olsalazine, consisting of two 5-ASA molecules linked by an azo bond, was developed for the purpose of delivering 5-ASA to the colon without the use of sulphapyridine.

The polymeric prodrugs of 5-ASA were also developed by coupling 5-amino group to a spacer group by means of an azo bond (Schacht et al, 1991). The spacer-5-ASA conjugate is then covalently linked to poly(methyl vinyl ether/ co-maleic anhydride) and also to chloroformate-activated derivatives of dextran and poly[(2-hydroxyethyl) aspartamine]. A very recent novel approach is the use of a water-soluble copolymer, N-(2-hydroxypropyl) methacrylamide together with a bioadhesive sugar moiety complimentary to mucus lectins of the GI tract (Kopeckova et al, 1994). In this approach, 5-ASA was linked through an azo bond to the polymeric carrier and fucosylamine (sugar moiety) serves as bioadhesive material

Glycosidases are a prominent group of enzymes produced by the intestinal microflora. The major glycosidases found in human faeces are β-D-galactosidase, α-L-arabinofuranosidase, β-D-xylo-pyranosidase and β-D-glucosidase (Friend, 1992). Prodrugs of prednisolone, dexamethasone, hydrocortisone and fludrocortisone with β-D-galactosides and β-D-glucosides were prepared, which are larger and hydrophilic and thus are not absorbed from small intestine (Friend & Chang, 1985). Other glucoside prodrugs were also prepared and studied for their efficacy in different animal models (Friend et al, 1991; Friend & Tozer, 1992). On reaching the colon, these prodrugs are split by colonic glycosidases delivering the corticosteroids at the site of action. The glucuronide prodrug of dexamethasone was prepared by Haeberlin et al (1993) and was subjected to stability studies in the homogenates of the different segments of the rat GI tract with an objective of achieving colon-specific drug delivery.

A class of macromolecules such as dextran ester prodrugs have been the focus of increasing interest in colon-specific drug delivery. These prodrugs, on reaching the colon, are acted upon by colonic dextranases resulting in the release of active moiety. Dextran ester prodrugs of naproxen were synthesized and tested for their drug release in homogenates of various segments of the pig GI tract (Larsen et al, 1989). Drug release was found to proceed 15-17 times faster in caecum and colon homogenates than in homogenates of the small intestine. The drug release was attributed to the initial depolymerisation of dextran chains by dextranases of the pig colonic bacteria and the resultant fragments served as substrates for esterases and other hydrolases. The bioavailability of naproxen after oral administration of aqueous solutions of various dextran-naproxen ester prodrugs in pigs was found to be close to 100 %. Though the study demonstrated the potential of dextran prodrugs for colon-specific delivery, it requires the presence of a carboxyl functional group in the drug.

Anti-inflammatory glucocorticoids do not possess carboxylic acid groups and must be chemically transformed in order to react with dextran. Dexamethasone and methyl prednesolone were attached to dextran using succinic acid as a spacer (McLeod et al, 1993; 1994) and the resultant prodrugs were incubated with rat GIT contents and dextranases. The study showed that dextran conjugates underwent hydrolysis in upper GIT contents, but were rapidly degraded in caecal and colonic contents. This illustrates the usefulness of the conjugates for selective delivery of glucocorticoids to the large intestine.

Prodrugs of steroids having a hydroxy group at C_{21} position were prepared using poly-L-aspartic acid as carrier (Leopold & Friend, 1995). The ester prodrug of dexamethasone with poly-L-aspartic acid when subjected to in vitro drug release studies in GIT homogenates of rats released dexamethasone because of the cleavage of the ester bond by bacterial enzymes. The in vivo performance of this prodrug was also demonstrated in rats

(Leopold & Friend, 1995a).

The prodrugs have some limitations. They need a functional group in the drugs such as carboxyl group for dextrans and hydroxy group at 21 position for poly-L-aspartic acid for the synthesis. Further, most of the prodrugs can accommodate the drugs to the extent of only 20% of their weight and hence may not be suitable for high dose drugs. The prodrugs are considered expensive.

5.5.3.3 Hydrogels

The synthesis and characterisation of hydrogels for site-specific delivery of peptide and protein drugs to the colon was described by Brondsted & Kopecek (1991). The hydrogels contain acidic comonomers and enzymatically degradable azoaromatic cross-links. In the acidic pH of the stomach, the gels have a low degree of swelling, which protect the drug against degradation by digestive enzymes. As the gels pass down the GI tract, the degree of swelling increases. On entering the colon, the gels reach a degree of swelling which makes the cross-links accessible to enzymes (azoreductases) or mediators (electron carriers). The cross-links are then degraded and the drug is released from the disintegrated gels. The performance of the hydrogels for colon-specific drug delivery was evaluated by conducting in vitro degradation studies in rat caecal content medium and in vivo degradation studies by implanting (in a nylon bag) in the stomach and caecum of male rats (Brondsted & Kopecek 1992).

5.5.3.4 Polysaccharides as carriers

Natural polysaccharides such as pectin and xylan are not digested in the human stomach or small intestine, but are degraded in the colon by resident bacteria (Salyers et al, 1977). Bacterial enzymes are capable of degrading a wide variety of polysaccharides present in the diet. The bacteria ferment polysaccharides to gases such as methane, CO_2 hydrogen and to short chain fatty acids thus accounting for the drop in the pH of the colon (Englyst et al, 1987). These dietary polysaccharides thus have the potential as non-toxic carriers for colon-specific drug delivery. A number of polysaccharides that are under investigation for colon-specific drug delivery are detailed below.

Pectin, an anionic polysaccharide extracted from plant primary cell wall was used by Ashford et al, (1993a) for developing a colonic drug delivery system. The in vitro studies demonstrated that high methoxy pectin, when applied as a compression coat, protected the core tablet from disintegration and dissolution in the upper part of the GI tract. The coat was susceptible to enzymatic attack in the colon thereby releasing the drug. In vivo gamma scintigraphic studies confirmed the in vitro findings. The same research group carried out further studies on matrix formulations with different types of pectin (high and low methoxy pectin) using different concentrations of pectinase enzyme and calcium salts (Ashford et al, 1994). It was concluded that an ideal pectin for colonic drug delivery should consist of either high methoxy pectin or low methoxy pectin with controlled calcium levels. Another promising matrix system was developed by Rubinstein et al, (1993) with calcium pectinate which was evaluated for colonic drug delivery using indomethacin as a model drug.

Pectin in the form of compression coat was evaluated for drug targeting to colon by Wakerly et al, (1996). An in vitro system for the evaluation of these formulations was developed and used to carry out the drug release studies with isolated enzymes and cultures of Bacteroides ovatus. The study showed that hydration is an important consideration with polysaccharide-based dosage forms since they must absorb water to swell before they are open to be attacked by bacterial enzymes. A biodegradable coating containing pectin and ethyl cellulose was evaluated by Wakerly et al, (1996a) for colon-specific drug delivery.

The suitability of hydrogel beads based on **amidated pectin** for potential use as colon-specific drug delivery matrices was investigated using indomethacin and sulfamethoxazole as model insoluble and relatively soluble drugs respectively by Munjeri et al, (1997). Drug release from the beads was found to be a function of media pH and drug loading. In simulated gastric and small intestinal conditions, drug release was greater with the more soluble sulfamethoxazole, but release of both drugs could be reduced to satisfactory levels by the formation of a chitosan polyelectrolyte complex around the beads. All the preparations released the drug in simulated colonic conditions within 135 minutes. Wakerly et al, (1997) also studied the potential of amidated petctins for colonic drug delivery and suggested that these materials might be of value in the form of a coating.

Chondroitin sulfate is a soluble mucopolysaccharide utilised as a substrate by the bacteroides inhabitating the large intestine, mainly by *Bacteroides thetaiotaomicron* and *Bacteroides ovatus* (Salyers, 1979). It consists of D-glucuronic acid linked to N-acetyl-D-galactosamide. Sloughed epithelial cells and dietary meat are considered as the natural sources of chondroitin sulfate in human colon. Colon-specific drug delivery systems based on chondroitin sulfate and cross-linked chondroitin sulfate were reported by Rubinstein et al, (1992; 1992a).

Inulin is a naturally occurring carbohydrate found in many plants such as onion, garlic, artichoke and chicory. It consists of a mixture of oligomers and polymers containing 2 to 60 or more D-fructose molecules which are linked by β (2-1) bonds. It is generally accepted that inulin can resist hydrolysis and digestion in upper GI tract. In the colon, it is fermented by the colonic microflora, more specifically by Bifidobacteria and Bacteroides (Roberfroid, 1993; Wang & Gibson, 1993). InulinHP (high degree of polymerisation) incorporated in Eudragit RS film was evaluated as a possible biodegradable coating for colonic drug delivery (Vervoort & Kinget, 1996). A preliminary study on the synthesis and characterisation of inulin hydrogels as carriers for colonic drug delivery was carried out by Vervoort et al, (1997).

A delivery system based on glassy amylose for colon-specific drug delivery was also reported (Milojevic et al, 1995). Chitosan is a high molecular weight cationic polysaccharide derived from naturally occurring chitin in crab and shrimp shells by deacetylation. It has been previously used as a pharmaceutical excipient in oral drug formulations to improve the dissolution of poorly soluble drugs or for the sustained release of drugs. Tozaki et al, (1997) have used chitosan in the form of a small capsule (length 3.5 mm) to deliver insulin to the colon for systemic absorption in rats. They also studied the effect of protease inhibitors and absorption enhancers on the bioavailability of insulin. The findings of the study suggested that chitosan capsules might be useful carriers for the colon-specific delivery of peptides including insulin.

A suspension of natural **polygalactomannans** in polymethacrylate solutions to form degradable coatings around the drug core was prepared by Lehmann & Dreher (1991). The polygalactomannans form a swellable layer around the drug core, thus delaying the release of the drug in the small bowel. They are destroyed enzymatically in the colon with consequent drug release. Polymethacrylate copolymers were used to improve the film forming properties of polygalactomannans. Block polymers of polyurethanes with ethylated or acetylated galactomannan segments were synthesised to form water-insoluble films (Sarlikiotis & Bauer, 1992). A significant change in the mechanical properties of these films was observed when incubated in a suspension of human faeces and pig caecal content in phosphate buffer indicating their potential use in colon-specific drug delivery. In view of these reports, Krishnaiah et al (1998a; 1998b) carried out investigations on the usefulness of guar gum, which also contains galactomannan, as a carrier for colon-specific drug delivery.

Guar gum is a natural polysaccharide derived from the seeds of **Cyamopsis tetragonolobus**, family Leguminosae. A novel tablet formulation for oral administration using guar gum as the carrier and indomethacin as a model drug has been investigated for colon-specific drug delivery using in vitro methods (Rama Prasad et al, 1998). Drug release studies under conditions mimicking mouth to colon transit have shown that guar gum protects the drug from being released completely in the physiological environment of stomach and small intestine. Studies in pH 6.8 phosphate buffered saline (PBS) containing rat caecal contents have demonstrated the susceptibility of guar gum to the colonic bacterial enzyme action with consequent drug release. The pre-treatment of rats orally with 1 ml of 2%w/v aqueous dispersion of guar gum for 3 days induced enzymes specifically acting on guar gum thereby increasing drug release. A further increase in drug release was observed with rat caecal contents obtained after 7 days of pre-treatment. The presence of 4%w/v of caecal contents obtained after 3 days and 7 days of enzyme induction showed biphasic drug release curves. The results illustrate the usefulness of guar gum as a potential carrier for colon-specific drug delivery. The study also reveals that the use of 4%w/v of rat caecal contents in PBS, obtained after 7 days of enzyme induction provide the best conditions for in vitro evaluation of guar gum.

In vivo gamma scintigraphic studies were carried out on the guar gum matrix tablets, using technetium-99m-DTPA (^{99m}Tc-DTPA) as a tracer, in healthy subjects to evaluate their in vivo performance (Krishnaiah et al, 1998a). Scintigraphs taken at regular intervals have shown that some amount of tracer present on the surface of the tablets was released in stomach and small intestine. However, the bulk of the tracer present in the tablet mass was delivered to the colon. The colonic arrival time of the tablets was found to vary from 2 to 4 hours. On entering the colon, the tablets degraded in five out of six volunteers thereby releasing more amount of the tracer. The study clearly demonstrated that guar gum, in the form of directly compressed matrix tablets, was a potential carrier for colon-specific drug delivery.

In vitro and *in vivo* studies on guar gum matrix tablets clearly demonstrated that guar gum is a potential carrier for colonic drug delivery. However, matrix tablets, released about 21% of drug or tracer present on their surface in the in vitro and in vivo studies. Such a phenomenon is undesirable for delivering certain categories of drugs such as anticancer drugs for local action in the colon and drugs meant for systemic absorption such as peptide and protein drugs. In order to prevent or minimise drug release in the upper part of the GI tract, guar gum was applied as a compression coat over the core tablets and subjected to in vitro drug release studies and in vivo gamma scintigraphic studies (Krishnaiah et al, 1998b). In vitro drug release studies have shown that guar gum in the form of a compression coat applied over indomethacin core tablets protects the drug from being released under conditions mimicking mouth to colon transit. Studies in pH 6.8 phosphate buffered saline (PBS) containing 4%w/v rat caecal contents have demonstrated the susceptibility of guar gum to the colonic bacterial enzyme action with consequent drug release. Gamma scintigraphic studies in human volunteers with technetium-99m-DTPA as a tracer in sodium chloride core tablets compression coated with guar gum have shown that gum coat protects the drug from being released in the stomach and small intestine. On entering the ascending colon, the tablets commenced to release the tracer indicating the breakdown of the gum coat by the enzymatic action of colonic bacteria. The tablets disintegrated in the ascending colon of all the volunteers, except one, resulting in the distribution of released tracer across the entire colon. The study clearly established that guar gum, in the form of compression coat, is a potential carrier for drug targeting to colon. Adkin et al, (1997) compared the carrier combination of calcium pectinate/ pectin with calcium pectinate/ guar gum for colonic drug delivery using gamma scintigraphy in healthy volunteers. The study revealed that the time and location of complete tablet disintegration was more reproducible with calcium pectinate/ pectin than with calcium pectinate/ guar gum.

In the light of the successful establishment of guar gum as a carrier for colonic drug delivery, drug delivery systems for 5-aminosalicylic acid (5-ASA) were developed by Krishnaiah et al, (1999). Core tablets containing 5-ASA were prepared by wet granulation with starch paste and were compression coated with coat formulations containing different quantities of guar gum (300, 200, 150 and 125 mg). In vitro drug release studies were carried out in simulated gastric and intestinal fluids and in pH 6.8 buffer containing rat caecal contents. The application of 175 mg of coat formulation containing 150 mg of guar gum over 5-ASA core tablets resulted in the release of less than 2% drug in simulated gastric and intestinal fluids and about 93% of 5-ASA in pH 6.8 buffer containing rat caecal contents. Differential Scanning Calorimetric studies showed the absence of any interaction between 5-ASA and the excipients on storage at 45°C for 12 weeks. The study confirmed that selective delivery of 5-ASA to the colon could be achieved using guar gum as a carrier in the form of a compression coat over the drug core.

5.6. EVALUATION OF COLON-SPECIFIC DRUG DELIVERY SYSTEMS

A successful colon-specific drug delivery system is one that remains intact in the physiological environment of stomach and small intestine, but releases the drug in the colon. Different in vitro and in vivo methods are used to evaluate the colonic drug delivery systems.

5.6.1 *In vitro* methods

The ability of the coats/ carriers to remain intact in the physiological environment of the stomach and small intestine is generally assessed by conducting drug release studies in 0.1N HCl for 2 hours (mean gastric emptying time) and in pH 7.4 Sorensen's phosphate buffer for 3 hours (mean small intestinal transit time) using USP dissolution rate test apparatus or flow through dissolution apparatus. Tablets covered with compression coats of pectin were evaluated by this method and it was found that drug was not released during the period of testing (Ashford et al, 1993). The ability of the delivery system to release the drug in the colon is tested in vitro by incubating it in a buffer medium in the presence of either enzymes (e.g. pectinase [Ashford et al, 1993], dextranase (McLeod et al, 1994) or rat (Rubinstein et al, 1992)/ guinea pig (Larsen et al, 1989)/ rabbit (Kopeckova et al, 1994) caecal contents. The amount of drug released at different time intervals during the incubation is estimated to find out the degradation of the carrier under study. Rama Prasad et al, (1998) while reporting the usefulness of guar gum as a carrier for colon-specific delivery established that a buffer medium with rat caecal contents (4%w/v) obtained after 7 days of enzyme induction provides the best conditions for in vitro evaluation. Another in vitro method involves incubation of the drug delivery system in a fermentor with commonly found human colonic bacteria like Streptococcus faecium (Kopecek, 1990) or Bacteroide ovatus (Rubinstein et al, 1993) in a suitable medium under anaerobic conditions and the amount of drug released at different time intervals is found out. This method is considered more specific since it involves the use of commonly found human colonic bacteria.

5.6.2 *In vivo* methods

5.6.2.1 Animal models

Different animal models are used for evaluating in vivo performance of colon-specific drug delivery systems. Guinea pigs were used to evaluate colon-specific drug delivery from a glucoside prodrug of dexamethasone (Friend et al, 1991). Other animal models used for the in vivo evaluation of colon-specific drug delivery systems include the rat (Van den Mooter et al, 1995; Leopold & Friend, 1995) and the pig (Harboe et al, 1989).

Techniques for monitoring the in vivo behaviour of colon-specific delivery systems in humans: A variety of techniques like (i) string technique (ii) endoscopy (iii) radiotelemetry (iv) roentgenography and (v) gamma scintigraphy were used for monitoring the in vivo behaviour of the oral dosage forms (Fell & Digenis, 1984).

5.6.2.1.1 String technique

This technique was first applied by Gruber et al, (1958) and Steinberg et al, (1965). In these studies, a tablet was attached to a piece of string and the subject swallowed the tablet, leaving the free end of the string hanging from his mouth. At various time points, the tablet was withdrawn from the stomach by pulling out the string and physically examining the tablet for the signs of disintegration. In some studies, the tablets were recovered by inducing a vomiting reflex. The presence of a foreign object, such as the string in the GI tract may alter its motility and the physicochemical environment. The psychological stress and anxiety associated with this method also affect the motility of the GI tract.

5.6.2.1.2 Endoscope technique

This technique has been employed by Hey et al, (1979). It is an optical technique in which a fibre scope (gastroscope) is used to directly monitor the behaviour of the dosage form after ingestion. This method requires administration of a mild sedative to facilitate the swallowing of the endoscopic tube. The sedative itself may alter gastric emptying and GI motility. The psychological factors also contribute to the change in the motility of the GI tract.

5.6.2.2.3 Radiotelemetry

This technique involves the administration of a capsule that consists of a small pH probe interfaced with a miniature radio transmitter which is capable of sending a signal indicating the pH of the environment to an external antenna attached to the body of the subject. So, it is necessary to physically attach the dosage form to the capsule which in turn may affect the behaviour of the dosage form being studied. Furthermore, the dosage form must contain significant amounts of buffer salts, the release of which produces a change in the gastrointestinal pH that is detected by the pH capsule indicating the change in the dosage form. This prevents the evaluation of commercially available products which do not contain buffer salts.

5.6.2.1.4 Roentgenography

The inclusion of a radio-opaque material into a solid dosage form enables it to be visualised by the use of X-rays. By incorporating barium sulphate into a pharmaceutical dosage form, it is possible to follow the movement, location and the integrity of the dosage form after oral administration by placing the subject under a fluoroscope and taking a series of X-rays at various time points. This method was first used by Losinsky & Diver (1933) and has been used by many subsequent workers (Steinberg et al, 1965; Evans & Roberts, 1981). This technique was used by Dew et al, (1982) to evaluate a capsule dosage form coated with Eudragit S® to deliver orally ingested drugs to the colon using barium sulphate as a radio-opaque material The use of X-rays involves exposing the subjects to a fairly high radiation dose as several photographs must be taken. Information can not be obtained on a continuous basis. The radio-opaque material, such as barium sulphate, has high density and may not be a good model for most pharmaceuticals.

5.6.2.1.5 Gamma scintigraphy

The most useful technique, to date, to evaluate the in vivo behaviour of dosage forms in animals and humans is external scintigraphy or gamma scintigraphy. Work in this area began in the 1970s through the modification of standard nuclear medicine methods, to monitor the in vivo behaviour of dosage forms (Casey et al, 1976). Gamma scintigraphy requires the presence of a γ-emitting radioactive isotope in the dosage form that can be detected in vivo by an external gamma camera. The dosage form can be radiolabelled using conventional labelling or neutron activation methods.

Of all these methods available, **gamma scintigraphy** is the most widely used non-invasive technique for studying the in vivo behaviour of oral dosage forms under normal physiological conditions (Wilding, 1995; Wilding et al, 1991; Davis et al, 1992; Krishnaiah et al, 1998). The advantages of gamma scintigraphy over the earlier methods are as follows: (a) gives very little radiation exposure to the participating subjects compared to roentgenography (X-rays), (b) gives both qualitative and quantitative results, which is not possible with other techniques, (c) totally non-invasive, and (d) allows for the in vivo evaluation of dosage forms under normal physiological conditions. A brief account of the gamma scintigraphy including the methodology and applications is given below.

Gamma Scintigraphy

Methodology The factors to be considered for studying the in vivo behaviour of solid dosage forms using gamma scintigraphy include (a) selection of radioisotope, (b) radiolabeling of the dosage form, and (c) choice of imaging device.

(a) Selection of radioisotopes for gamma scintigraphy The most commonly used radionuclides to correlate gastrointestinal behaviour of the dosage forms with pharmacokinetic parameters i.e., correlation of the location of the dosage form in a certain region of the GI tract to maximum plasma concentration, are technetium-99m (Tc-99m) and indium-111 (In-111). Using these two isotopes and the conventional labelling process, simple dosage forms such as direct compression tablets and capsules can be easily monitored for their in vivo behaviour. More sophisticated dosage forms (sustained release or timed release tablets and capsules) can be radiolabelled with barium-139, erbium-171 and samarium-153 employing neutron activation radiolabeling method

(Parr & Jay, 1987). The four commonly used **positron emitting isotopes** are **Oxygen-15**, **Nitrogen-13**, **Carbon-11** and **Fluorine-18**. They emit very high energy photons of 511 KeV. These cyclotron produced positron emitting radionuclides are more difficult to work with, because of their short half-lives and requirement of costly equipment like Positron Emission Tomography (PET) scanners to detect them. They are, however, useful in determining the in vivo distribution of drugs and their site of action.

(b) Radiolabeling The radiolabeling can be achieved either by (i) direct incorporation of a radioactive tracer into the preparation (conventional method), or (ii) neutron activation of a dosage form that contains a non-radioactive tracer. The quantity of tracer to be incorporated into a formulation to render it suitable for gamma scintigraphic study is very small and does not compromise the performance of the delivery system.

In **conventional method**, gamma-emitting isotope is incorporated into the dosage form of interest prior to its manufacture. The nuclide (Tc-99m or In-111) is added, in a liquid form, to an aliquot of one of the excipients present in the formulation. The resulting mixture is dried and incorporated into the formulation. This radiolabeled dosage form is administered via its appropriate route and followed externally with a gamma camera. This method is non-specific and does not involve the direct radiolabeling of the drug molecule. This method can be used to radiolabel tablets, capsules, suppositories, aerosols, liquids and enemas. However, its application is limited to simple dosage forms made in small-scale batches.

The conventional method is not suitable for more complex dosage forms such as sustained release or delayed release formulations which require long manufacturing times or unique manufacturing equipment. Production-scale batches can not be radiolabeled by conventional method because of large amount of radioactive isotopes needed and the radiation exposure to the manufacturing personnel. Hence, neutron activation method was developed by Parr et al, (1985) to radiolabel intact dosage forms. The study was carried out with barium (Ba-138), erbium (Er-170) and samarium (Sa-152) as isotopes (Digenis et al, 1991).

In **neutron activation method**, small amount (μg to mg) of an appropriate stable isotope (Ba-138, Sa-152 or Er-170) is incorporated into the formulation similar to that of any other excipient prior to the manufacture of the dosage form. Once manufactured, the dosage form is exposed to a neutron source (Nuclear Reactor) and the stable isotope is converted to a radioactive γ–emitting isotope (Ba-139, Sa-153 or Er-171) that can be easily followed by a gamma camera. This also is a non-specific method of radiolabeling. Studies by Parr et al, (1987) have shown that this procedure does not affect the physical parameters of the dosage forms such as hardness, dissolution and disintegration. This labeling procedure was found not to affect the chemical stability of erythromycin and ibuprofen (Parr et al, 1990; 1987a).

(c) Choice of imaging devices for gamma scintigraphy: Nuclear imaging is mostly conducted with Planar or SPECT cameras and by using radionuclides that emit g-radiation with energies between 100 and 250 KeV. The single photon emitting radioisotopes such as Tc-99m and In-111 are widely used with these instruments. Gamma camera is composed of an array of photomultiplier tubes coupled to a sodium iodide crystal The interaction of a gamma photon from the source with the crystal leads to the production of a flash and it is detected by photomultiplier tubes. This can be displayed on a cathode ray oscilloscope and is digitised so that it can be stored on a magnetic disc and subsequent quantitative image processing can be performed. To ensure that radiation from the source is detected in straight line, a lead collimator is placed between the subject and the crystal

The camera provides two-dimensional or planar images of the distribution of radioactivity in the subject. These planar images have the disadvantage of averaging the activity throughout the target. For example, a posterior image of the kidney includes a radiotracer in the blood and soft tissues behind the organ, particularly the intestines, which prevents actual quantification of the radioactivity in the kidney. The planar images, however, provide a good depiction of the position of the radiotracer. For this reason, radiolabelled drug delivery systems are best studied with planar camera.

Modern-day scintillation cameras employ larger detectors and are capable of generating three-dimensional images through the use of computer enhanced reconstruction algorithms. This method is called **Single Photon Emission Computed Tomography** or SPECT, because it detects and analyses radionuclides which emit a single photon per decay. In this camera, the detector moves at a controlled rate around the subject in up to a 360° arc, detecting gamma radiation emanating from the organ of interest. The information is stored in a computer which is capable of constructing 6 mm slice images through the organ in transverse (top-to-bottom), sagittal (side-to-side) and coronal (front-to-back) planes. The SPECT method is particularly useful when overlying structures are obscuring the imaging of the interested organ. The time of image acquisition is also fast because of the presence of more number of sodium iodide crystals. However, the resolution of the SPECT images is not as good as the planar camera.

Another modern imaging device is **Positron Emission Tomography (PET)**. The **PET** camera displays three-dimensional images similar to SPECT. The subject is injected with a positron-emitting radionuclide capable of producing two 511 KeV gamma photons simultaneously at 180° angle from each other. The subject is moved at a controlled rate through a circular gantry containing an array of sodium iodide detectors. The PET camera does not require a collimator and therefore is more sensitive (collimators prevent a large percentage of gamma rays from reaching the sodium iodide crystal of a gamma camera). Positron emitting radionuclides (O-15, C-11, F-18) are very expensive to purchase and operate. Further, the PET scanners cost two to three times that of most SPECT cameras. However, the information obtained with PET cameras is more quantitative than those obtained with SPECT cameras and it is also possible to label the drug of interest via isotopic substitution using positron emitting radionuclides such as Carbon-11 and Fluorine-18.

Pharmaceutical applications of gamma scintigraphy: Since its introduction, the gamma scintigraphy has been employed in the in vivo evaluation of tablets, capsules, pellets, suppositories, enemas, aerosols and parenteral preparations such as intravenous emulsions and liposomes. The in vivo information that can be obtained from gamma scintigraphic studies on solid oral dosage forms include (a) transit time through various regions of the GI tract, (b) in vivo disintegration of dosage form, (c) the ability of a dosage form to target drug delivery to specific regions of GI tract, and (d) correlation of pharmacokinetic results (Pharmaco-scintigraphy).

(a) Determination of GI transit times Gamma scintigraphic technique has been widely used to determine the GI transit times of different dosage forms. Khosla & Davis (1989) have studied the gastric emptying and small and large bowel transit of non-disintegrating tablets in healthy male volunteers under fasting conditions. Non-disintegrating tablets of ethyl cellulose containing a small quantity of cationic resin IR120 were prepared. The resin was radiolabelled with Indium-111. The tablets were administered orally with water radiolabelled with ^{99m}Tc-DTPA to get the outline of the GI tract. The tablets were monitored using a gamma camera. The tablets emptied from the stomach and traversed the small intestine as a bolus. The time of colonic transit showed a large inter-subject variation.

The GI transit of single unit dosage forms of different sizes (3 mm, 6 mm, 9 mm and 12 mm) was investigated by Adkin et al, (1993) in healthy male subjects using dual-isotope gamma scintigraphic technique. The control tablets (6 mm) were labeled with indium-111 and the other tablets with technetium-99m. Gastric emptying times, small intestinal transit times, colon arrival times and total transit times were calculated. The transit through ileocaecal junction was found to be unaffected by tablet size. The small tablets (3 mm & 6 mm) retained in the ascending colon for the longest period of time.

Hardy et al, (1988) studied the GI transit of small tablets (4 mm diameter) in patients with ulcerative colitis by carrying out gamma scintigraphic studies. Non-disintegrating ethyl cellulose tablets were prepared containing cation exchange resin, radiolabeled with indium-111 and coated with cellulose acetate. The tablets were administered with radiolabeled (^{99m}Tc-DTPA) water and were monitored using a gamma camera. The mean gastric emptying time was found to be 1.6 hours and small intestinal transit time 3-4 hours, which were almost the same as those found in healthy subjects. The tablets were found retained for 6 hours in the proximal colon.

The findings of this study indicated that small tablets could be used as controlled release drug delivery system in ulcerative colitis.

The gamma scintigraphy was also used to study the progression of a radiolabelled marker from caecal instillation to defecation in healthy male volunteers (Krevsky et al, 1986). An 8 ml solution containing ^{111}In-DTPA was instilled into the caecum via a 2 mm diameter tube, which passed orally and serial scintigraphs were obtained over 48 hours. The movement of the marker across various regions of the colon viz. caecum and ascending colon, hepatic flexure, transverse colon, splenic flexure, descending colon, sigmoid colon and rectum and finally its excretion in faecal matter was monitored. The gastric emptying and caecum arrival times of multiple theophylline pellets in fasting and fed state were investigated in human volunteers by Podczeck et al, (1995) using gamma scintigraphy.

(b) In vivo disintegration and site-specific drug delivery The GI transit and disintegration of an enteric coated modified-release oral tablet containing beclomethasone dipropionate was studied in healthy male subjects using gamma scintigraphy (Steed et al, 1994). After administration in fasted subjects, tablet integrity was maintained in the stomach and disintegration began in the small intestine. The disintegration was complete in the small intestine in 3 subjects and in proximal colon in 5 subjects. Ashford et al, (1993) evaluated the site-specificity of pH-dependent polymers meant for colon-specific drug delivery by gamma scintigraphy using ^{99m}Tc-DTPA as a tracer. The study was carried out in healthy human volunteers using Eudragit S® as pH-dependent polymer. The study demonstrated that the polymer was capable of protecting a core tablet through the stomach and upper small intestine. But, the disintegration times varied from 5 to 15 hours and the disintegration sites varied from ileum to splenic flexure showing the lack of site-specificity. Thus, the study demonstrated that pH-dependent polymers were not suitable for colon-specific drug delivery.

In vivo gamma scintigraphic studies were carried out to evaluate pectin, a polysaccharide, as a colon-specific drug delivery carrier (Ashford et al, 1993a). Compression coated tablets of pectin containing ^{99m}Tc-DTPA as radionuclide were administered to healthy human subjects and were monitored for their transit in the GI tract using a gamma camera. The study showed that pectin coat protected the activity from being released in the stomach and small intestine, but on reaching the colon, the coat disintegrated thereby releasing the activity. The study, thus, indicated that pectin was a potential carrier for colon-specific drug delivery. Hardy et al, (1985) have used gamma scintigraphy to study the transit times and disintegration sites of dosage forms meant for drug targeting to the proximal colon using indium-111 and ^{99m}Tc-DTPA as tracers (Hardy et al, 1985).

Krishnaiah et al (1998a; 1998b) used gamma scintigraphy for evaluating guar gum as a carrier for colon-specific drug delivery in the form of a matrix tablet and as a compression coat. Oral pellets of model drugs coated with amylose and ethyl cellulose were studied for their in vivo performance in healthy male subjects using gamma scintigraphy (Milojevic et al, 1995). The mean arrival time of the pellets in the caecum was found to be 3.5 hours. It was concluded from the study that the amylose-ethyl cellulose coating allowed the controlled delivery of drug pellets to the colon.

(c) In vivo performance of sustained action dosage forms In order to assess the in vivo performance of controlled release dosage forms, the pharmaceutical industry had turned to nuclear medicine methodologies. Gamma scintigraphy was used to determine the location and integrity of sustained release tablets, GI transit times of tablets and the time and site of tablet disintegration. By using multiple labeling procedures with samarium and erbium, a sustained release dosage form with a complex structure was evaluated (Heald et al, 1993). Digenis et al, (1991) evaluated a bi-layer tablet using dual-isotope studies. They labeled the dosage form with two different isotopes, one layer with Sa-153 and other layer with Er-171. Both the isotopes were monitored by the gamma camera simultaneously, thereby evaluating the behaviour of both layers of the tablet at the same time.

(d) Correlation of pharmacokinetic parameters In the scintigraphic evaluation of pharmaceutical preparations, it is now a normal practice to include the required drug within the labeled dosage form and to measure drug absorption by established analytical procedures. It is thereby possible to relate the pharmacokinetics of the drug with the derived scintigraphic information. This combined technique has been termed **Pharmacoscintigraphy** (Wilding, 1994) and has become an important means of providing information about the transit and release behaviour of oral dosage forms and subsequent drug absorption.

Wilding (1994; 1994a) has described the pharmacoscintigraphic studies carried out on enteric coated naproxen tablets, pulsed release captopril formulation, controlled release osmotic pump system, tabletted 5-aminosalicylic acid pellet preparation and diltiazem geomatrix formulation. Parr et al, (1987a) used external scintigraphy to correlate the GI transit of an ibuprofen tablet with its pharmacokinetic parameters. The study showed a strong correlation between total area under the curve and total GI transit time. It also indicated that the largest percentage of ibuprofen absorption occurred in the colon. The researchers also used the data to predict and explain unusual pharmacokinetic parameters such as poor bioavailability (rapid GI transit time) and double peaks observed in the plasma profile (the second peak was associated with the complete disintegration of the dosage form and the release of drug).

In pharmaceutical industry, both beta and gamma emitting isotopes are being used to evaluate the metabolic fate of drugs i.e. absorption, distribution, metabolism and elimination, DNA sequencing and receptor localisation and binding. In addition, pharmaceutical scientists used radiopharmaceuticals to evaluate the effect of drugs on various physiological factors such as cardiac output. Gamma scintigraphy also finds application in other areas such as in vivo melting and rate of dissolution of drug from a suppository (Jay et al, 1983), in vivo migration of enemas (Hay et al, 1979) and transcervical migration of polylactic acid microspheres after intravaginal administration (Digenis et al, 1984). This technique was used to assess the performance of commercial aerosol inhalation devices by Gaddipati et al (1996). The study in two groups of 9 male healthy volunteers by gamma scintigraphy demonstrated the superior performance of the cylindrical prototype aerosol inhalation device over compact prototype device. The application of gamma scintigraphy in clinical studies for monitoring the drug distribution from dosage forms administered by the non-enteral routes such as parenteral, rectal, buccal, nasal, pulmonary and ophthalmic was reviewed by Meseguer et al (1994).

The limitations of gamma scintigraphy include (a) inability to accurately quantify the activity in the small bowel because of its coiled nature, (b) it is not possible to label all the compounds/ drugs of interest, (c) the gamma scintigraphic assembly is expensive, and (d) requires qualified personnel for operation.

The radiation safety involved in gamma scintigraphy needs a mention. Human beings have been continuously exposed to natural sources of radiation namely cosmic rays and naturally occurring radionuclides. The average radiation dose due to this background radiation is estimated to be about 0.1 rem/year, although there are places where the background dose may be 10-30 times higher than this value. The International Commission on Radiological Protection (ICRP) recommended an average permissible whole body radiation dose of 0.1 rem/ week and 5 rem/ year (Radiation protection procedures, International Atomic Energy Agency, Safety Series, No. 38, pp 40-45, 1978). These limits still hold valid and are considered to be safe from the health point of view of the individuals. The level of radioactivity used in gamma scintigraphy is very low and it gives a radiation dose to participating subjects which is well below the maximum permissible dose. Hence, it can be considered that the radionuclides used in gamma scintigraphy are harmless at the level they are used.

5.7. CONCLUSION

A considerable amount of research work has been carried out on the development of colon-specific drug delivery systems for the last two decades. The large inter- and intra-subject variation in GI pH makes the approach of delivery systems based upon pH dependent polymers less suitable. The preferred colon-specific delivery systems are those which rely on conditions which are only encountered in the colon, since such systems will give true site-specificity. In this respect, systems, which can be degraded by colonic bacteria, are very attractive and promising. Of the colon-specific carriers so far tested, the natural polymers such as dextran, pectin, guar gum, etc. are more favourable with respect to safety. However, the disadvantage of the most naturally occurring polymers is the inherent water solubility, which has to be decreased by chemical derivatisation, but which can lead to decreased biodegradability.

It is now appreciated that colon can be another important site for the absorption and delivery of drugs. In the case of sustained release dosage forms, they spend a large proportion of their time in the GI tract within the colon, and therefore an understanding of colonic drug absorption is important. Although the surface area in the colon is low compared to the small intestine, suggesting relatively poor drug absorption, this is compensated for by the markedly slower rate of transit. However, colon is a selective site for the absorption of hydrophobic drugs, which are absorbed by transcellular transport. It has often been claimed that colon targeting is one of the best alternatives for the oral administration of peptides and proteins. Many more studies need to be conducted to confirm such a fantastic possibility of oral delivery of biopharmaceuticals.

5.8 SUGGESTIONS FOR FURHTER STUDY

The colon appears to be a promising site for absorption of peptides and proteins. However, overcoming degradation by bacterial protease and peptidase enzymes and low permeability of the colonic epithelium remain major challenges. By the use of absorption enhancing agents which increase the permeability of the colonic epithelium, therapeutically effective amount of low molecular weight peptides can be absorbed, although the overall bioavailability is still relatively low. A lot of research remains to be conducted to find out to what extent these molecules can be absorbed after oral administration. It is probable that such formulations will reach the market in the coming years.

Local therapy of pathologies of the large intestine and reduced drug availability due to degradation by digestive or mucosal enzymes can benefit from colon delivery. Still, a substantial amount of research remains to be conducted in order to find out to what extent drugs, and more specifically peptides and proteins, could be absorbed, since it has often been claimed that colon targeting is one of the best alternatives for the oral administration of peptides and proteins. A major problem in comparing different delivery systems is the fact that degradation studies are performed under different conditions. In this respect, the use of simulated human intestinal microbial system, developed by Molly et al (1993), might offer the possibility to standardize drug release studies and will permit to correlate the results with in vivo situations.

An area, which needs more investigation, is the performance of the colonic delivery system in patients with colonic diseases, especially those diseases that may have an impact on their dissolution and disintegration characteristics via changes in colonic pH or transit. In addition, it needs special emphasis on the performance of bacterially triggered colon-specific drug delivery systems in patients receiving antibiotics and antibacterial drugs concomitantly.

5.9 ACKNOWLEDGEMENT

The authors greatly acknowledge the receipt of research grant from University Grants Commission, Government of India, New Delhi for developing colon-specific drug delivery systems. The research funding from All India Council of Technical Education under TAPTEC and MODROBS schemes is highly acknowledged. The authors also thank Council of Scientific and Industrial Research (CSIR) for sanction of a senior research fellowship to work on colon-specific drug delivery systems.

REFERENCES

Adkin, D.A.; Kenyon, C.J.; Lerner, E.I.; Landau, I. Wilding, and I.R. et al (1997) "Use of scintigraphy to provide proof of concept for novel polysaccharide preparations designed for colonic drug delivery." Pharm Res., 14: 103-107.

Adkin, D.A.; Davis, S.S.; Sparrow, R.A.; and Wilding, I.R. (1993) "Colonic transit of different sized tablets in healthy subjects." J. Control. Rel., 26: 147-156.

Antonin, K.H.; Bieck, P.; Scheurlen, M.; Jedrychowski, M. and Malchow, H. (1985) "Oxprenolol absorption in man after single bolus dosing into two segments of the colon compared with that after oral dosing." Br. J. Clin. Pharmacol, 19: 137S-142S.

Ashford, M.; Fell, J.T.; Attwood, D.; Sharma, H. and Woodhead, P.J. (1993) "An in vivo investigation into the suitability of pH dependent polymers for colonic targeting." Int. J. Pharm., 95: 193-199.

Ashford, M.; Fell, J.; Attwood, D.; Sharma, H.; Woodhead, P. (1993a) "An evaluation of pectin as a carrier for drug targeting to the colon." J. Control. Rel., 26: 213-220.

Ashford, M.; Fell, J.; Attwood, D.; Sharma, H.; Woodhead, P. (1994) "Studies on pectin formulations for colonic drug delivery." J. Control. Rel., 30: 225-232.

Audus, K.L.; Bartel, R.L.; Hidalgo, I.J. and Borchardt, R.T. (1990) "The use of cultured epithelial and endothelial cells for drug transport and metabolism studies." Pharm. Res., 7: 435-451.

Bararow, L.; Spiller, R.C.; Wilson, C.G. (1991) "Pathological influences on colinic motility: implications for drug delivery." Adv. Drug Del. Rev., 7: 201-220.

Bieck, P.R. (1989) "Drug absorption from the human colon, Chapter 12 In: Drug Delivery to the gastroinetstinal tract." (Hardy, J.G., Davis, S.S. and Wilson, C.G. eds.), Ellis Horwood, Chichester.

Binder, H.J.; Foster E.S.; Budinger, M.E. and Hayslett, J.P. (1987) "Mechanism of electroneural sodium chloride absorption in distal colon of the rat." Gastroenterology, 93: 449-455.

Brockmeirer, H.G.; Grigoleit, H.G.; Leonhardt, H. (1985) "Absorption of glibenclamide from different sites of the gastrointestinal tract." Eur. J. Clin. Pharmac., 29: 193-197.

Brockmeirer, H.G.; Grigoleit, H.G.; Leonhardt, H. (1986) "The absorption of piretanide from the gastrointestinal tract is site-dependent." Eur. J. Clin. Pharmacol., 30: 79-82.

Brown, R.L.; Gibson, J.A.; Sladen, G.E.; Hicks, B. and Dawson, A.M. (1974) "Effects of lactulose and other laxatives on ileal and colonic pH as measured by a radiotelemetry device." Gut, 15: 999-1004.

Brondsted, H. and Kopecek, J. (1991) "Hydrogels for site-specific oral drug delivery: Synthesis and characterisation. Biomaterials." 12: 584-592.

Brondsted, H.; Kopecek, J. (1992) "Hydrogels for site-specific drug delivery to the colon: In vitro and in vivo degradation." Pharm. Res., 9: 1540-1545.

Cann, P.A.; Read, N.W.; Brown, C.; Hobson, N. and Holdsworth, C.D. (1983) "Irritable bowel syndrome: Relationship of disorders in the transit of a single solid meal to symptom patterns." Gut, 24: 405-411.

Casey, O.L.; Beihn, R.M.; Digenis, G.A. and Shambu, M.B. (1976) "Methods for monitoring hard gelatine capsule disintegration times in humans using external scintigraphy." J. Pharm. Sci., 65: 1412-1413.

Davis, S.S.; Hardy, J.G.; Taylor, M.J.; Stockwell, A.; Whatley, D.R. and Wilson, C.G. (1984) "The in vivo evaluation of an osmotic device (Osmet) using gamma scintigraphy." J. Pharm. Pharmacol., 36: 740-742.

Davis, S.S.; Hardy, J.G. and Fara, J.W. (1986) "Transit of Pharmaceutical dosage forms through the small intestine." Gut, 27: 886-892.

Davis.S.S.; Washington, N.; Parr, G.D.; Short, A.H.; John, V.A.; Lloyd, P. and Walker, S.M. (1988) "Relationship between the appearance of oxprenolol in the systemic circulation and the location of an oxprenolol 16/260 drug delivery system within the gastrointestinal tract as determined by scintigraphy." Br. J. Clin. Pharmacol., 26: 435-443.

Davis, S.S.; Hardy, J.G.; Newman, S.P. and Wilding, I.R. (1992) "Gamma scintigraphy in the evaluation of pharmaceutical dosage forms." Eur. J. Nucl. Med., 19: 971-986.

Dew, M.J.; Hughes, P.J.; Lee, M.G.; Evans, B.K. and Rhodes, J. (1982) "An oral preparation to release drugs in the human colon." Br. J. Clin. Pharamacol., 14: 405-408.

Digenis, G.A.; Jay, M. Beihn, R.M. et al, (1984) "External scintigraphy in the study of long acting contraceptive delivery systems." In: Long acting contraceptive delivery systems, Hayerstown, Harper and Row, pp.173-177.

Digenis, G.A. and Sandefer, E. (1991) "Gamma Scintigraphy and neutron activation techniques in the in vivo assessment of orally administered dosage forms." Crit. Rev. Ther. Drug Carrier Syst., 7: 309-345.

Digenis, G.A.; Sandefer, E., Beihn, R.M. and Parr, A.F. (1991) "Dual-isotope imaging of neutron activated erbium-171 and samarium-153 and in vivo evaluation of a dual-labeled bilayer tablet by gamma scintigraphy." Pharm. Res., 8: 1335-1340.

Drasar, B.S. and Hill, M.J. (1974) "Human intestinal flora." Academic Press, London, pp. 9-50.

Englyst, H.N.; Hay, S. and Macfarlane, G.T. (1987) "Polysaccharide breakdown by mixed populations of human faecal bacteria." FEMS Microbiol. Ecol., 95: 163-171.

Evans, K..T.; Roberts, G.M. (1981) "The ability of patients to swallow capsules." J. Clin. Hosp. Pharm., 6, 207-208.

Evans, D.F.; Pye, G.; Bramely, R.; Clark, A.G. and Dyson, T.S. (1988) "Measurement of gastro-intestinal pH profiles in normal ambulant human subjects." Gut, 29: 1035-1041.

Fara, J.W. (1989) "Colonic drug absorption and metabolism." In: Novel Drug Delivery and its Therapeutic Application, Prescott L.F.; Nimmo W.S. (Eds.), , Wiley, Chichester, 103-122.

Fell, J.T. and Digenis, G.A. (1984) "Imaging and behaviour of solid oral dosage forms in vivo." Int. J. Pharm., 22: 1-15.

Fisher, A.N.; Illum, L.; Davis, S.S.; Haresign, W.; Jabbal-Gill, J. and Hinchcliffe, M. (1996) "Use of a pig model for colon-specific delivery of peptides, proteins and other drugs." In: Minutes from European Symposium on Formulation of poorly-available drug for oral administration. Editons de Sante, Paris, pp 183-186.

Fix, J.A. (1987) "Absorption enhancing agents for the GI system." J. Control. Rel., 6: 151-156.

Friend, D.R. and Chang, G.W. (1985) "Drug glycosides: Potential prodrugs for colon-specific drug delivery." J. Med. Chem., 28: 51-57.

Friend, D.R. (1991) "Colon-specific drug delivery." Adv. Drug Del. Rev., 7: 149-199.

Friend, D.R.; Philips, S. and Tozer, T.N. (1991) "Colon-specific drug delivery from a glucoside prodrug in the guinea pig. Efficacy study." J. Control. Rel., 15: 47-54.

Friend, D.R. and Tozer, T.N. (1992) "Drug glycosides in oral colon-specific drug delivery." J. Control. Rel., 19:109-120.

Friend, D.R. (1992) "Glycosides in colonic drug delivery." In: Oral colon-specific drug delivery, Friend, D.R. (Ed.),. CRC Press, London, pp. 153-187.

Fujii, T.; Yanagisawa, J. and Nakayama, F. (1988) "Absorption of bile acids in dogs as determined by portal sampling: Evidence for colonic absorption of bile acid conjugates." Digestion, 41: 207-214.

Gaddipati, N. Graziosi, M.; Ellway, K.; Ganesan, M. and Schreier, H. (1996) "Novel aerosol inhalation device for pressurised metered dose inhalation aerosols: Gamma scintigraphic evaluation of pulmonary deposition profiles and comparison with commercial inhalation devices." Int. J. Pharm., 128: 55-63.

Gazzaniga, A.; Giordana, F.; Sangalli, M.E. and Zema, L. (1994) "Oral colon-specific drug delivery: design strategies." STP Pharma Sci., 4: 336-343.

Gazzaniga, A.; Sangali, M.E. and Giordano, M. (1994a) "Oral Chronotopicâ drug delivery systems: achievement of time and/or site specificity." Eur. J. Pharm. Biopharm., 40: 246-250.

Gingell, C.H.; Davis, M.W. and Shields, R. (1968) "Effect of synthetic gastrin-like pentapeptide upon the intestinal transport of sodium, potassium and water." Gut, 9: 111-115.

Gleiter, C.H.; Antonin, K.H.; Bieck, P.; Godbillan, J.; Schonleber, W. and Malchow, H. (1985) "Colonoscopy in the investigation of drug absorption in healthy volunteers." Gastrointest. Endosc., 31: 71-73.

Gruber, C.M.; Ridolfo, A.S. and Rosick, W.A. (1958) "An enteric compression coating II." J. Am. Pharm. Assoc. Sci. Ed., 47: 862-866.

Gustafsson, B.E. (1982) "The physiological importance of the colonic microflora." Scand. J. Gastroenterol., Suppl., 77: 117-131.

Haeberlin, B.; Rubas, W.; Nolen, H.W. and Friend DR. (1993) "In vitro evaluation of dexamethasone-b-D-glucoside for colon-specific drug delivery." Pharm. Res., 10: 1553-1562.

Harboe, E.; Larsen, C.; Johansen, M. and Olesen, H.P. (1989) "Macromolecular prodrugs. XV. Colon-targeted delivery-Bioavailability of naproxen from orally administered dextran-naproxen ester prodrugs varying in molecular size in the pig." Pharm. Res., 6: 919-923.

Hardy, J.G.; Wilson, C.G. and Wood, E. (1985) "Drug delivery to the proximal colon." J. Pharm. Pharmacol., 37: 874-877.

Hardy, J.G.; Davis, S.S.; Khosla, R. and Robertson, C.S. (1988) "Gastrointestinal transit of small tablets in patients with ulcerative colitis." Int. J. Pharm., 48: 78-82.

Hardy, J.G. (1989) "Colonic transit and drug delivery." In: Drug Delivery to the Gastrointestinal Tract, Hardy, J.G.; Davis, S.S.; Wilson, C.G. (Eds.), Ellis Horwood, Chichestea, pp. 75-81.

Hastewell, J.; Lynch, S.; Williamson, I.; Fox, R. and Mackay, M. (1992) "Absorption of human calcitonin across the rat colon in vivo." Clin. Sci., 82: 589-594.

Hawker, P.C.; Mashier, K.E. and Turnberg, L.A. (1978) "Mechanism of transport of sodium chloride and potassium in human colon." Gastroenterology, 74: 1241-1247.

Hay, D.J.; Sharma, H. and Irving, M.H. (1979) "Spread of steroid containing foam after intrarectal administration." Br. Med. J., 1: 1751-1753.

Heald, D.L.; Ziemiak, J.A. and Wilding, I.R. (1993) "The gastrointestinal transit and systemic absorption of diltiazem HCl from a modified-release dosage form". In: Nuclear imaging in drug discovery, development and approval Birkhauser, M. (Ed.), Boston-New York, 301-320.

Hey, H.; Matzen, P. and Thorup, A.J. (1979) "A gastroscopic and pharmacological study of the disintegration time and absorption of pivampicillin capsules and tablets". Br. J. Clin. Pharmacol., 8: 237-242.

Hill, M.J. (1981) "Diet and the human intestinal bacterial flora". Cancer Res., 41: 3778-3780.

Ikesue, K.; Kopeckova, P. and Kopecek, J. (1991) "Degradation of proteins by enzymes of the gastrointestinal tract". Proc. Int. Symp. Control. Rel. Bioact. Mater., 18: 580-581.

Jay, M.; Beihn, R.M.; Snyder, G.A.; et al (1983) "In vitro and in vivo suppository studies with perturbed angular correlation and external scintigraphy". Int. J. Pharm., 14: 343-347.

Jay, M.; Beihn, R.M.; Digenis, G.A.; Deland, F.H.; Caldwell, L.; Mlodozeniec, A.R. (1985) "Disposition of radiolabelled suppositories in humans". J. Pharm. Pharmacol., 37: 266-268.

Kalala, W.; Kinget, R.; Van den Mooter, G. and Samyn, C. (1996) "Colonic drug targeting: in vitro release of ibuprofen from capsules coated with poly(ether-ester) azopolymers". Int. J. Pharm., 139: 187-195.

Khosla, R. and Davis. S.S. (1989) "Gastric emptying and small and large bowel transit of non-disintegrating tablets in fasted subjects". Int. J. Pharm., 52: 1-10.

Kinget, R.; Kalala, W.; Vervoort, L. and Van den Mooter, G. (1998) "Colonic drug targeting". J. Drug Target., 6: 129-149.

Kopecek, J. (1990) "The potential of water-soluble polymeric carriers in targeted and site-specific drug delivery". J. Control. Rel., 11: 279-290.

Kopeckova, P.; Rathi, R.; Takada, S.; Rihova, B.; Berenson, M.M. and Kopecek, J. (1994) "Bioadhesive N-(2-hydroxypropyl) methacrylamide copolymers for colon-specific drug delivery". J. Control. Rel., 28: 211-222.

Kraeling, M.E.K. and Ritschel, W.A. (1992) "Development of colonic release capsule dosage form and the absorption of insulin". Meth. Find. Exp. Clin. Pharmacol., 14: 199-209.

Krevsky, B.; Malmud, LS.; D'Ercole, F.; Maurer. A.H. and Fisher, R.S. (1986) "Colonic transit scintigraphy: a physiologic approach to the quantitative measurement of colonic transit in humans". Gastroenterology, 91:1102-1112.

Krishnaiah, Y.S.R.; Satyanarayana, S. and Rama Prasad, Y.V. (1998) "Gamma scintigraphy: an imaging technique for non-invasive in vivo evaluation of oral dosage forms". Indian Drugs, 35: 387-399.

Krishnaiah, Y.S.R.; Satyanarayana, S.; Rama Prasad, Y.V. and Narasimha Rao, S. (1998a) "Gamma scintigraphic studies on guar gum matrix tablets for colonic drug delivery in healthy human volunteers". J. Control. Rel., 55: 245-252.

Krishnaiah, Y.S.R.; Satyanarayana, S.; Rama Prasad, Y.V. and Narasimha Rao, S. (1998b) "Evaluation of guar gum as a compression coat for drug targeting to colon". Int. J. Pharm., 171: 137-146.

Krishnaiah, Y.S.R.; Satyanarayana, S. and Rama Prasad, Y.V. (1999) "Studies of guar gum compression-coated 5-aminosalicylic acid tablets for colon-specific drug delivery". Drug Dev. Ind. Pharm., 25: 651-657.

Langguth, P.; Breves, G.; Stockli, A.; Merckle, H.P. and Wolffram, S. (1994) "Colonic absorption and bioavailability of the pentapeptide metkephamid in the rat". Pharm. Res., 11: 1640-1645.

Larsen, C.; Harboe, E.; Johansen, M. and Olesen, H.P. (1989) "Macromolecular prodrugs. XVI. Colon-targeted delivery-Comparison of rate of release of naproxen from dextran ester prodrugs in homogenates of various segments of the pig gastrointestinal (GI) tract". Pharm. Res., 6: 995-999.

Lee, V.H.L. (1991) "Changing needs in drug delivery". In: Peptide and protein drug delivery, Lee, V.H.L. (Ed.), Marcel Dekker, New York, pp. 1-56.

Lehmann, K.O.R. and Dreher, K.D. (1991) "Methacrylate-galactomannan coating for colon-specific drug delivery". Proc. Int. Symp. Control. Rel. Bioact. Mater., 18: 331-332.

Leopold, C.S. and Friend, D.R. (1995) "In vitro study for the assessment of poly(L-aspartic acid) as a drug carrier for colon-specific drug delivery". Int. J. Pharm., 126: 139-145.

Leopold, C.S. and Friend, D.R. (1995a) "In vivo pharmacokinetic study for the assessment of poly-L-aspartic acid as a drug carrier for colon-specific drug delivery". J. Pharmacokinet. Biopharm., 23: 397-406.

Lindenbaum, J.; Rund, D.G.; Butler, V.P. Jr.; Tse-Eng, D. and Shah, J.R. (1981) "Inactivation of digoxin by the gut flora: Reversal by antibiotic therapy". N. Engl. J. Med., 305: 789-794.

Losinsky, E. and Diver, G.R. (1933) "A direct method for studying efficiency of enteric coated tablets". J. Am. Pharm. Assoc. Sci. Ed., 22: 143-145.

Mackay, M. and Tomlinson, E. (1993) "Colonic delivery of therapeutic peptides and proteins". In: Colonic drug absorption and metabolism, Bieck, P. (Ed.), Marcel Dekker, New York, pp. 159-176.

Marvola, M.; Aito, H.; Ponto, P.; Kanniksoki, A.; Nykanen, S. and Kokkonen, P. (1987) "Gastrointestinal transit and concomitant absorption of verapamil from a single unit sustained release tablet". Drug Dev. Ind. Pharm., 13: 1593-1609.

McLeod, A.D. and Tozer, T.N. (1992) "Kinetic perspectives in colonic drug delivery". In: Friend, D.R. (ed.) Oral Colon-Specific Drug Delivery (Boca Ration: CRS Press), pp 85-114.

McLeod, A.D.; Friend, D.R. and Tozer, T.N. (1993) "Synthesis and chemical stability of glucocorticoid-dextran esters: Potential prodrugs for colon-specific delivery". Int. J. Pharm., 92: 105-114.

McLeod, A.D.; Friend, D.R.; Tozer, T.N. (1994) "Glucocorticoid-dextran conjugates as potential prodrugs for colon-specific delivery: Hydrolysis in rat gastrointestinal tract contents". J. Pharm. Sci., 83: 1284-1288.

Meldrum, S.J.; Watson, B.W.; Riddle, H.C.; Bown, R.L.; Sladen, G.E. (1972) "pH profile of gut as measured by radiotelemetry capsule". Br. Med. J., 2: 104-106.

Meschan, I. (1975) "Small intestine, colon and biliary tract". In: An atlas of basic anotomy to radiology, Meschan, I. (Ed.), Philadelphia: W.B. Saunders Co., pp. 843-925.

Meseguer, G.; Gurny, R. and Buri, P. (1994) "In vivo evaluation of dosage forms: Application of gamma scintigraphy to non-enteral routes of administration". J. Drug Target., 2: 269-288.

Milojevic, S.; Newton, J.M.; Cummings, J.H.; et al (1995) "Amylose, the new perspective in oral drug delivery to the human large intestine". S.T.P. Pharma Sci., 5: 47-53.

Molly, K.; Vande Woestyne, M. an]\=74 Verstracte, W. (1993) "Development of a 5-step multi chamber reactor as a simulation of the human instestinal microbial ecosystem". Appl. Microbiol. Biotechnol., 39: 254-258.

Moore, J.A.; Pletecher, S.A.; Ross, M.J. (1986) "Absorption enhancement of growth hormone from the gastrointestinal tract of rats". Int. J. Pharm., 34: 35-43.

Mrsny, R.J. (1992) "The colon as a site for drug delivery". J. Control. Rel., 22: 15-34.

Munjeri, O.; Collett, J.H.; Fell, J.T. (1997) "Hydrogel beads based on amidated pectins for colon-specific drug delivery: Role of chitosan in·modifyıng drug release". J. Control. Rel., 46: 272-278.

Muranishi, S.; Yoshikawa, H.; Sezaki, H. (1979) "Absorption of 5-fluorouracil from various regions of the gastrointestinal tract in rat: Effect of mixed micelles". J. Pharmacobio-Dyn., 2: 286-294.

Muranishi, S.; Yoshikawa, H.; Sezaki, H. (1980) "Enhanced intestinal permeability to macromolecules II. Improvement of the large intestinal absorption of heparin by lipid-surfactant mixed micelles in rat". Int. J. Pharm., 4: 219.

Nord, C.E.; Heimdahl, A. (1986) "Impact of orally administered antimicrobial agents on human oropharyngeal and colonic microflora". J. Antimicrob. Chemother., 18: 159-169.

Nubuchi, J.J.; Aramaki, Y.; Tsuchiya, S. (1986) "Binding of antibiotics to rat intestinal mucin". Int. J. Pharm., 30: 181-188.

Osiecka, I.; Porter, P.A.; Borchardt, R.T.; Fix, J.A.; Gardner, C.R. (1985) "In vitro drug absorption models I. Brush border membrane vesicles, isolated mucosal cells and everted intestinal rings: characterisation and salicylate accumulation". Pharm. Res., 2: 284-293.

Ovesen, L.; Bendsten, F.; Tage-Jensen, U.; Pedersen, N.T.; Gram, B.R.; Rune, S.J. (1986) "Intraluminal pH in the stomach, duodenum and proximal jejunum in normal subjects and patients with exocrine pancreatic insufficiency". Gastroenterology, 90: 958-962.

Parr, A.; Jay, M.; Digenis, G.A.; Beihn, R.M. (1985) "Radiolabeling of intact tablets by neutron activation for in vivo scintigraphic studies". J. Pharm. Sci., 74: 590-591.

Parr, A.; Jay, M. (1987) "Radiolabeling of intact dosage forms by neutron activation: Effects on in vitro performance". Pharm. Res., 4: 524-526.

Parr, A.; Beihn, R.M.; Franz, R.M.; Szupunar, G.J.; Jay, M. (1987a) "Correlation of ibuprofen bioavailability with gastrointestinal transit by scintigraphic monitoring of 171Er-labeled sustained release tablets". Pharm. Res., 4: 486-489.

Parr, A.; Digenis, G.A.; Sandefer, E.P.; et al (1990) "Manufacture and properties of erythromycin beads containing neutron activated erbium-171". Pharm. Res., 7: 264-269.

Passaretti, S.; Sirghi, M.; Colombo, E.; Mazzotti, G.; Tittobello, A.; Guslandi, M. (1989) "Motor effects of locally administered pinaverium bromide in the sigmoid tract of the patients with irritable bowel syndrome". Int. J. Clin. Pharmacol. Ther. Tax., 27: 47-50.

Peeters, R.; Kinget, R. (1993) "Film-forming polymers for colonic drug delivery. I. Synthesis and physical and chemical properties of methyl derivatives of Eudragit S". Int. J. Pharm., 94: 125-134.

Peppercorn, M,A.; Goldman, P. (1976) "Drug bacteria interactions". Rev. Drug Metab. Drug Interactions, 2: 75-88.

Podczeck, F.; Newton, J.M.; Yuen, K.H. (1995) "Description of the gastrointestinal transit of pellets assessed by gamma scintigraphy using statistical moments". Pharm. Res., 12: 376-379.

Powell, D.W. (1981) "Barrier function of epithelia". Am. J. Physiol., 241: G275-G288.

Pozzi, F.; Furlani, P.; Gazzaniga, A.; Davis, S.S.; Wilding, I.R. (1994) "The time clock system: a new oral dosage form for fast and complete release of drug after a predetermined lag time". J. Control. Rel., 31: 99-108.

Quadros, E.; Cassidy, J.; Hirschberg, Y.; et al(1995) "Evaluation of a novel colonic delivery device in vivo". STP Pharma Sci., 5: 77-82.

Raimundo, A.H.; Evans, D.F.; Rrogers, J.; Silk, D.B.A. (1992) "Gastrointestinal pH profiles in ulcerative colitis". Gastroenterology, 104: A681

Rama Prasad, Y.V.; Krishnaiah, Y.S.R.; Satyanarayana, S. (1996) "Trends in colonic drug delivery: A review". Indian Drugs, 33: 1-10.

Rama Prasad, Y.V.; Krishnaiah, Y.S.R.; Satyanarayana, S. (1998) "In vitro evaluation of guar gum as a carrier for colon-specific drug delivery". J. Control. Rel., 51: 281-287.

Rao, S.S. and Ritschel, W.A. (1992) "Development and in vitro/ in vivo evaluation of a colonic release capsule of vasopressin". Int. J. Pharm., 59: 35-41.

Rashid, A. (1990) "Dispensing Device". Br. Patent Application 223030441A.

Rhodes, J. and Thomas, G. (1995) "Nicotine treatment in ulcerative colitis, current status". Drugs, 49: 157-160.

Riad, L.E. and Sawchuk, R.J. (1991) "Effect of polyethyleneglycol 400 on the instestinal permeability of carbamazepine in the rabbit". Pharm. Res., 8: 491-497.

Riley, S.A.; Kim, M.; Sutcliffer, F.; Rowland, M. and Turnberg, L.A. (1992) "Absorption of polar drugs following caecal instillation in healthy volunteers. Aliment". Pharmacol. Ther., 6: 701-706.

Roberfroid, M. (1993) "Dietary fibre, inulin and oligofructose: a review comparing their physiological effects". Crit. Rev. Food Sci. Nutr., 33: 103-148.

Rowland, I.R. (1988) "Factors affecting metabolic activity of the intestinal microflora". Drug Metabol. Rev., 19: 243-261.

Rubinstein, A. (1990) 'Microbially controlled drug delivery to the colon". Biopharm. Drug. Dispos., 11: 465-475.

Rubinstein, A.; Nakar, D. and Sintov, A. (1992) "Chondroitin sulfate: A potential biodegradable carrier for colon-specific drug delivery". Int. J. Pharm., 84: 141-150.

Rubinstein, A.; Nakar, D. and Sintov, A. (1992a) "Colonic drug delivery: Enhanced release of indomethacin from cross-linked chondroitin matrix in rat caecal content". Pharm. Res., 9: 276-278.

Rubinstein, A.; Radai, R.; Ezra, M.; Pathak, S. and Rokea, J.S. (1993) "In vitro evaluation of calcium pectinate: A potential colon-specific drug delivery carrier". Pharm. Res., 10: 258-263.

Saffran, M.; Kumar, G.S.; Neckers, D.C.; et al(1988) "New approaches to the oral administration of peptide drugs". Pharm. Weekbl. Sci. Ed., 10: 159-176.

Saffran, M.; Bedra, C.; Kumar, G.S. and Neckers, D.C. (1988a) "Vasopressin: A model for the study of the effects of additives on the oral and rectal administration of peptide drugs". J. Pharm. Sci., 77: 33-38.

Saffran, M.; Field, J.B.; Pana, J.; Jones, R.H.; Okuda, Y. (1991) "Oral insulin in diabetic dogs". J. Endocrinol., 131: 267-278.

Salyers, A.A.; Vercellotti, J.R.; West, S.H.E.; Wilkins, T.D. (1977) "Fermentation of mucin and plant polysaccharides by strains of bacteroides from the human colon". Appl. Environ. Microbiol., 33: 319-322.

Salyers, A.A. (1979) "Energy sources of major intestinal anaerobes". Am. J. Clin. Nutr., 32: 158-163.

Sarlikiotis, A.W. and Bauer, K.H. (1992) "Synthese und untersuchung von polyurethanen mit galactomannan-segmenten als hilfsstoffe zur freizetzung von peptid-arzneistoffen im dickdarm". Pharm. Ind., 54: 873-880.

Schacht, E.; Callant, D. and Verstrasct, W. (1991) "Synthesis and evaluation of polymeric prodrugs of 5-aminosalicylic acid". Proc. Int. Symp. Control. Rel. Bioact. Mater., 18: 686-687.

Scheline, R.R. (1973) 'Metabolism of foreign compounds by gastrointestinal microorganisms'. Pharmacol. Rev., 25: 451-523.

Simon, G.L. and Gorbach, S.L. (1983) 'Bacteriology of the colon". In: Colon, structure and function, Bustos-Fernandez, L. (Ed.), Plenum Press, New York, 103-114.

Simon, G.L. and Gorbach, S.L. (1984) "Intestinal flora in health and disease". Gastroenterology, 86: 174-193.

Smith, M.B.; Goradia, V.K.; Holmes, J.W.; McCluggage, S.G.; Smith, J.W. and Nicholas, R.L. (1990) "Suppression of the human mucosal related colonic microflora with prophylactic parenteral and/or oral antibiotics". World J. Surg., 14: 636-641.

Steed, K.P.; Hooper, G.; Ventura, P.; Musa. R. and Wilding, I.R. (1994) "In vivo behaviour of a colonic delivery system: A pilot study in man". Int. J. Pharm., 112: 199-206.

Steinberg, W.H.; Frey, C.H.; Masci, J.N. and Hutchins, H.H. (1965) "Methods for determining in vivo tablet disintegration". J. Pharm. Sci., 54: 747-752.

Suzuka, T.; Furuya, A.; Kamada, A. and Nishihata, T. (1986) "Effects of phenothiazines and N-(6-aminohexyl)-5 chloro-1-napthalene sulphonomide on rat colonic absorption of cefmetazole". J. Pharmacobiodyn., 9: 460-465.

Taniguchi, K.; Muranishi, S. and Sezaki, H. (1980) "Enhanced intestinal permeability through macromolecules. II. Improvement of the large intestinal absorption of heparin by lipid-surfactant mixed micelles in rat". Int. J. Pharm., 4: 219-228.

Thomas, P.; Richards, D.; Richards, A.; Rogers, L.; Evans, B.K.; Dew, M.J. and Rhodes, J. (1985) "Absorption of delayed release prednisolone in ulcerative colitis and Crohn's disease". J. Pharm. Pharmacol., 37: 757-758.

Tolls, R.M.; Imamovic, M.A. and McGarry, M.P. (1986) "Enteral perfusion in the pig". Lab. Anim. Sci., 36: 400-401.

Tomita, T.; Hayashi, M.; Toshihane, H.; Ishizawa, T. and Awazu, S. (1989) "Enhancement of colonic drug absorption by the transcellular permeation route". Pharm. Res., 5: 786-789.

Tomlin, J. and Read, N.W. (1988) "The relation between bacterial degradation of viscous polysaccharides and stool output in human beings". Br. J. Nutr., 60: 467-475.

Touitou, E. and Rubinstein, A. (1986) "Targeted enteral delivery of insulin to rats". Int. J. Pharm., 30: 95-99.

Tozaki, H.; Komoike, J.; Tada, C.; Maruyama, T.; Terabe, A.; Suzuki, T.; Yamamoto, A. and Muranishi, S. (1997) "Chitosan capsules for colon-specific drug delivery: Improvement of insulin absorption from the rat colon". J. Pharm. Sci., 86: 1016-1021.

Van den Mooter, G.; Samyn, C. and Kinget, R. (1993) "Azo polymers for colon-specific drug delivery. II: Influence of the type of azo polymer on the degradation by intestinal microflora". Int. J. Pharm., 97: 133-139.

Van den Mooter, G.; Samyn, C. and Kinget, R. (1994) "The relation between swelling properties and enzymatic degradation of azo polymers designed for colon-specific drug delivery". Pharm. Res., 11: 1737-1741.

Van den Mooter, G.; Samyn, C. and Kinget, R. (1995) "In vivo evaluation of a colon-specific drug delivery system: An absorption study of theophylline from capsules coated with azo polymers in rats". Pharm. Res., 12: 244-247.

Van den Mooter, G. and Kinget, R. (1995) "Oral colon-specific drug delivery: A review". Drug Delivery, 2: 81-93.

Van Saene, J.J.M.; Van Saene, H.F.K.; Geitz, J.N.; Tarko-Smith, N.J.P. and Lerk, C.F. (1986) "Quinolones and colonisation resistance in human volunteers". Pharm. Weekbl. Sci. Ed., 8: 67-71.

Vervoort, L. and Kinget, R. (1996) "In vitro degradation by colonic bacteria of inulinHP incorporated in Eudragit RS films". Int. J. Pharm., 129: 185-190.

Vervoort, L.; Van den Mooter, G.; Augustijns, P.; Busson, R.; Kinget, R.; et al (1997) "Inulin hydrogels as carriers for colonic drug targeting. Part 1. Synthesis and characterization of methacrylated inulin and hydrogel formation". Pharm. Res., 14: 1750-1737.

Wakerly, Z.; Fell, J.T.; Attwood, D. and Parkins, D.A. (1996) "In vitro evaluation of pectin-based colonic drug delivery systems". Int. J. Pharm., 129: 73-77.

Wakerly, Z.; Fell, J.T.; Attwood, D. and Parkins, D.A. (1996a) "Pectin/ethyl cellulose film coating formulations for colonic drug delivery". Pharm. Res., 13: 1210-1212.

Wakerly, Z.; Fell, J.T.; Attwood, D. and Parkins, D.A. (1997) 'Studies on amidated pectins as potential carriers in colonic drug deivery". J. Pharm. Pharmacol., 49: 622-625.

Wang, X. and Gibson, G.R. (1993) "Effects of the in vitro fermentation of oligofructose and inulin by bacteria grouping in the human large intestine". J. Appl. Bacteriol., 75: 373-380.

Watts, P.J. and Illum, L. (1997) "Colonic drug delivery". Drug Dev. Ind. Pharm., 23: 893-913.

Wilding, I.R.; Coupe, A.J. and Davis, S.S. (1991) "The role of gamma scintigraphy in oral drug delivery". Adv. Drug Del. Rev., 7: 87-117.

Wilding, I.R. (1994) "Pharmacoscintigraphic evaluation of oral delivery systems: Part I". Pharm. Tech. Eur., March,: 19-26.

Wilding, I.R. (1994a) "Pharmacoscintigraphic evaluation of oral delivery systems: Part II". Pharm. Tech. Eur., April: 32.

Wilding, I.R. (1995) "Scintigraphic evaluation of colonic drug delivery systems". STP Pharma Sciences., 5: 13-18.

Wilson, C.G. and Washington, N. (1989) "Physiological Pharmaceutics, Biological Barriers to Drug Absorption". Ellis Horwood Ltd., Chichester, UK.

Wilson, C.G.; Washington, N.; Greaves, J.L.; Wasshington, C.; Hoadley, T. and Sims, E.E. (1991) "Predictive modelling of the behaviour of a controlled release buflomedil HCl formulation using scintigraphic and pharmacokinetic data". Int. J. Pharm., 72: 79-86.

Winter, H.S.; Hendren, R.B.; Fox, C.H.; Russel, G.J.; Perez-Atayde, A.; Bhan, A.K. and Folkman, J. (1991) "Human intestine matures as nude mice xenograft". Gastroenterology, 100: 89-98.

Wood, E.; Wilson, C.G. and Hardy, J.G. (1985) "The spreading of foam and solution enemas". Int. J. Pharm., 25:191-197.

Yoshikawa, H.; Muranishi, S.; Kato, C. and Sezaki, H. (1981) "Bifunctional delivery system for selective transfer of bleomycin into lymphatics via enteral route". Int. J. Pharm., 8: 291-302.

Chapter 6

Advances in Pulmonary Drug Delivery

A. N. Misra

6.1 INTRODUCTION

The airways represent a unique organ system in the body, their structure allowing air to come into close contact with blood, is one of the principal adaptations permitting the existence of terrestrial life. This adaptation also makes the airways a useful route of administration of drugs in the inhaled or aerosol form. Numerous techniques have been developed to aerosolize liquids, resuspend particles, or generate aerosol particles. Physicochemical properties, such as size, shape, and structure, of the aerosol particle and the number or mass concentration is prerequisite for the accurate determination of the effective dose and targetting drug at specific site in a lung in the aerosol therapy. Inhalation therapies have until now primarily provided fast acting treatment for respiratory illnesses such as asthma and chronic obstructive pulmonary disease (COPD). Relative to oral delivery, inhalation of bronchodilators, corticosteroids, and other anti-inflammatory agents to the airways often produce therapeutic levels in the respiratory tract while maintaining low systemic concentrations and thereby minimizing side effects (Taylor, 1987). More recently, inhalation therapies for the systemic delivery of proteins and peptides to the body have made important advances in human clinical trials, notably owing to the success with which many macromolecules permeate the alveolar/blood barrier once inhaled (Service, 1998). For these inhalation therapies, inhalation systems are often required that achieve high reproducibility and efficiency, this need has propelled active research and development in the inhalation drug delivery field.

The heightened scientific and industrial attention paid to inhaled drug delivery has exposed an unmet need for the controlled release of inhaled drug (Zeng et al,1995). A logical strategy to achieve sustained release of these drugs in the respiratory tract involves encapsulating drugs in slowly degrading/releasing particles that can be inhaled. Efforts are therefore underway to create sustained release particles that safely avoid respiratory clearance mechanisms, thereby permitting the development of practically useful controlled drug release in the lungs (Ben-Jebria et al, 1999).

The chapter elaborates on the advances in design considerations, therapeutic applications and delivery systems of inhalation aerosols. To understand how aerosolized drugs can be targeted to relatively well defined regions within the human respiratory tract, it is necessary to appreciate the relative roles of various factors affecting the air borne motions (aerodynamics) and action of inhaled drugs (biological considerations).

6.2 DESIGN CONSIDERATIONS

6.2.1   Aerodynamic behaviour

Aerodynamics behavior of drug particles is discussed to understand the deposition mechanics, thermodynamics of inhaled hydrophilic drugs, and mathematical models used in predicting drug distribution.

6.2.1.1 Deposition mechanics of pharmaceutical particles in human airways

The deposition of inhaled aerosolized particles to the targeted regions within the human respiratory tract depends on the relative roles of various factors affecting the airborne motion. Undoubtedly, deposition of inhaled particles is affected by three factors: aerosol characteristics, ventilatory parameters, and respiratory tract morphologies. Clinical personnel can effectively regulate particle deposition pattern within the lung by manipulating these factors governing the efficiencies of the different deposition mechanisms of inertial impaction, sedimentation and diffusion.

Massive doses of the drugs are required to the whole lung in order to achieve a required quantity of the prescribed drug to airway cells at desired sites and thereby elicit a therapeutic response. The benefits of selectively deposited inhaled drug are elimination of proportionate adverse/side effects often experienced by patient following such high doses and reduction in the waste (i.e. lung over doses) to requisite amount to a desired location rendering more cost effective therapy. Thus, the aerosol therapy delivering predetermined quantities of drugs to desired sites (e.g., to receptors in the treatment of asthma and malignant tumors) is now being demanded by the physicians to offer patients, a well defined therapy.

6.2.1.2 Deposition model for aerosolized drugs

6.2.1.2.1 Elements of biology and physiology

Head and throat airways: The filtering efficiency of the upper respiratory tract is important while delivering the drugs to the lung. If the inhaled aerosol mass is Mi , the quantity that penetrates to the trachea, M, may be written as :

$$M = M_i \, [1\text{-}p(m)] \, [1\text{-}p(\ell)] \tag{1}$$

where, p(m) and p(l) are the particle deposition efficiencies within the oropharyngeal region and larynx respectively. Many formulae for such losses under passive breathing conditions have been presented by Martonen (1983a) by various experiments. The formulae are true for drugs delivered by metered dose inhalers (MDIs) when used with spacers, dry powder inhalers (DPIs), and nebulizers.

The deposition of inhaled particles in the airways of human head and throat can be considerable even during breathing under normal, ambient conditions (Stahlhofem et al,1989). There is great loss of drug, if administered by pressurized devices, may be >70% and can exceed 90%. The situation is somewhat better (i.e., particles losses are not as great) when using DPIs that are activated by patients inhalation and nebulizers.

Many developments have been continued to evolve in both design of hardware and techniques of delivery in reducing the particle deposition during inhalation. For example, spacer devices with MDIs (Rodrigo and Rodrigo,1993) and new kinds of mechanical instruments have been designed (Hanania et al, 1994).

Lung morphology : McBride (1992) has presented a review of various syμmetric and asyμmetric morphologies for human lungs. It is noted that human lungs do not exhibit the marked degree of asyμmetry documented in the lungs of experimental animals (Martonen and Yang, 1994a). Laboratory surrogates such as dogs, rats, and guinea pig possess very monopodial structures.

A syμmetric, dichotomously branching model is used for this work. The TB airways are numbered in sequential order from the trachea (generation I = 0) to the terminal bronchioles (I = 16). Generations I = 1, 2, 3, and 4 correspond to the main, lobar, segmental, and first subsegmental bronchi respectively. The pulmonary

(P) region, consisting of generation I = 17-23, out of which three generations are of partially alveolated respiratory bronchioles, three generations of alveolar ducts, and final alveolar sacs. The bifurcation and gravity angles among the airway network will be assumed to be 70° (Horsfield and Cumming, 1967) and 45° (Heyder, 1977a) respectively. There are 2^I identical airways in each generation. The dimensions of each generation of the lung are presented in Fig 6.1.

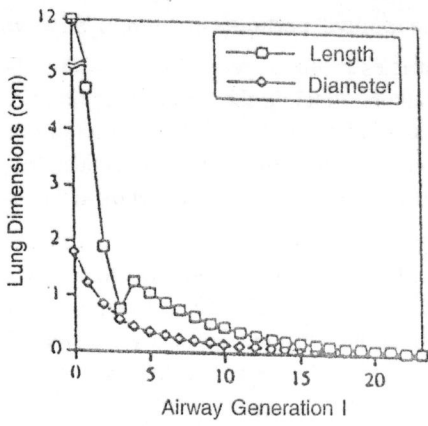

Fig 6.1: Dimensions of airways within the adult human lung.

Respiratory parameters :An appropriate range of ventilatory conditions must be addressed to evaluate effects of inter-subject variability in aerosol therapy regimens. The parameters associated with prescribed respiratory intensities, as recommended by Hofmann et al (1989), are given in Table 6.1 :

Table 6.1 : Breathing patterns for human subjects at prescribed levels of activity.

Ventilatory parameters	Physical state				
	Sedentary	Low	Light	Heavy	Maximal
Tidal volume (ml)	500	793	1291	2449	3050
Breathing frequency (min^{-1})	14.0	12.6	15.5	24.5	40.0
Minute volume (ml)	7000	9992	20011	60001	122000
Flow rate(ml sec^{-1})	233.3	333.1	667.0	2000.0	4066.7

The corresponding average velocities in each airway are described in Fig 6.2.

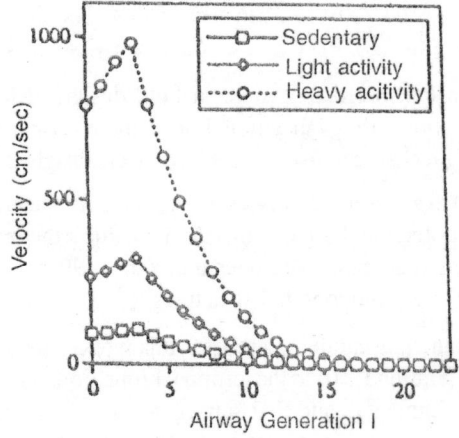

Fig 6.2 : Air velocity profile within the lung as a function of subject activity levels.

6.2.1.2.2 Elements of physics and mathematics

Nomenclature

D_g	=	Particle geometric diameter, cm
ρ	=	Particle density, gm/cm^3
λ	=	Mean free path of air = 7.0 ´ 10-6, cm.
G	=	Gravitational constant = 980 cm/sec^2
T	=	Absolute temperature = 293° K
K	=	Boltzmann constant = 1.38 ´ 10-16 g cm^2 /sec^{-2} molecule °K
L(I)	=	Length of generation I airway, cm
D(I)	=	Diameter of generation I airway, cm
η	=	Air kinematic viscosity = 1.5 ´ 10^{-1} cm^2/sec
μ	=	Air absolute viscosity = 1.84 ´ 10^{-4} gm/cm sec
U(I)	=	Mean air velocity in generation I airway, cm/sec
ϕ(I)	=	Inclination of generation I airway with respect to horizontal, degrees
θ(I)	=	Angle of bend of generation I, degrees
Re(I)	=	Airflow Reynolds number in generation I airway = D(I)U(I)/h, dimensionless.
m	=	Particle mass, g
$C(D_g)$	=	Particle slip correction factor=1+A(2l/Dg),dimensionless
		where A 1.257+0.4 exp {-1.1Dg/(2l)}
τ	=	Particle relaxation time = mC (Dg)/(3pmDg), sec
V	=	Particle stokes terminal settling speed = Gt, cm/sec
d	=	Particle diffusion coefficient = k Tt/m,cm^2/sec
t(I)	=	L(I) / U(I) ± V sinf (I),residence time of particles in generation I airways, sec.

[Note : – or +, denotes downhill, or uphill, flow in an airway when V has a component with, or against, fluid motion (Martonen et al,1982a)].

Primary deposition mechanisms : The major deposition processes are shown in Fig 6.3. There are three mechanisms governing particle behavior at the bronchial branching. They are inertial impaction, Sedimentation, and Diffusion.

Inertial impaction : Particles of sufficient momentum (product of mass and velocity) will be affected by the considerable centrifugal forces generated where the airway network, and thus convective fluid motion, changes direction abruptly.

Sedimentation : Particles of sufficient mass may be deposited by the action of gravity when residence times within airways are large.

Diffusion : Particle deposition can be a consequence of random Brownian motion. The efficiencies of these mechanisms will obviously depend on local respiratory tract geometries, particle parameters, and air stream characteristics. For this reason inhalation therapy is restricted to given patient (i.e., fixed morphology) and drug (i.e., prescribed aerosol), breathing is the only parameter that can be regulated. The velocity distribution of air within the lung is determined by the tidal volume and breathing frequency parameters. Hence deposition probability formulae must be indicative of the character of convective air movement. Diffusion is most effective for submicrometer-size particles. For larger particles, the inertial impaction deposition mechanism is dominant in upper TB airways where velocities are maximum, and the effect of gravitational settling is most pronounced in distal airways where velocities are minimum. The fluid dynamics environment of upper TB tree is characterized by flow instabilities initiated at the vibrating glottic aperture of the larynx. An air stream will enter the trachea as a laryngeal jet (Martonen et al,1983b). Additional air stream instabilities may be attributed to the branching nature of the lung and neighborhood airway surface irregularities (Pedley et al,1979). The unstable motion will be dampened with progression to distal airways. Within such bifurcation localized airflow patterns have been studied (Chang and Masry, 1982). Laminar but asyµmetric primary flow patterns were observed. In other experimental studies (Isabey and Chang, 1982), secondary (double-vortex) currents have been observed.

Many formulae have been used (Martonen,1982b) to derive particle deposition in human airway (Table 6.2)

Table 6.2 : Particle deposition formulae for human airway

Flow	Deposition mechanisms		
Condition	Inertial impaction P(I)	Sedimentation P(S)	Diffusion P(D)
Laminar	$2/\pi\ [e(1-e^2)^{1/2} + \arcsin(e)]^a$	$2/\pi\ [f(1-f^2)^{1/2} + \arcsin(f)]^b$	$4(K/p)^{1/2} - K^c$
		$1 - \exp\left[\dfrac{(-8rGt(I)\cos(\phi(I)))}{\pi\ D(I)}\right]$	$1 - \exp\left[\dfrac{-0.088d^{3/4}\ Re(I)^{7/8}L(I)}{U(I)D(I)^2}\right]^{3/4}$
Turbulent	$1 - \exp(-4e/\pi)^a$		

$^a e = q\ (I)\tau U(I)/D(I)$

$^b f = t(I)V\cos(\phi(I))\ /\ D(I)$

$^c K = 4dL(I)/\ U(I)D(I)^2$

Miscellaneous deposition processes : Other forces may become significant under special circumstances. The most prominent of these that are appropriate to particles within the human respiratory tract are represented below :

Cloud motion : A theory of cloud motion was developed employing the concept of Smoluchowski (1912). Cloud motion will take place when the stokes settling velocity of an array, U_c, exceeds that of an isolated particle, U_r or $U_c > U_r$; conversely, individual particle motion occurs when $U_r > U_c$. This situation may be mathematically described as:

$$\rho_c\ \text{«}1/\text{»}6\ \rho_c\ (D_g)\ [\ D_g\ /\ D_c\ ]^2\ (6 + Re_c^{\ 2/3}) \qquad (2)$$

Where the upper inequality depicts the condition necessary for single particle settling to occur and the lower inequality signifies cloud motion. Dc and Rec denote the cloud diameter and Reynolds number within the human lung.

Interception : This is the most effective deposition mechanism for aggregates and fibres. For such shapes, deposition can occur when a particle contacts an airway wall although its center of mass remains on a fluid streamline. Particle orientation is a critical factor in describing interception (Martonen,19 92).

Electric charge effects : During the mechanical generation of aerosols electric charges may be produced on particles. Electric charge effects have been studied using surrogate airway systems and human subjects (Melandri et al,1983). The data indicate that the effect will be most pronounced for sub-micron particles which

which possess correspondingly greater mobilities than larger (i.e., > 1μm) ones. Electric charges may be of two types, (a) image charge field, and (b) space charge forces.

Image charges field is the response between charges of opposite sign on an airway surface and a particle that create attraction and subsequent deposition. Space charge is the repulsion between like charged inhaled particles that may direct their motion toward airway walls resulting in deposition. Either effect may result in deposition being enhanced relative to an uncharged particle. It has been suggested (Chen, 1978) that space charge forces are of less significance than image forces.

To reduce effects on deposition during controlled human subjects exposures, it is standard operating procedure for aerosols to pass through an electric charge deionizer and thereby attain a Boltzmann equilibrium (i.e., no net electric charge) prior to inhalation.

6.2.1.2.3 Simulation of inhaled aerosols

To describe particle deposition in the lung we shall follow an inhaled bolus of aerosol throughout the TB and P airways. The method is depicted in Fig 6.3.

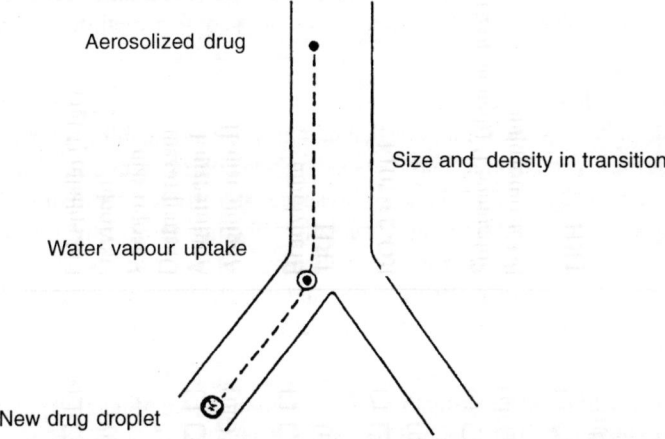

Fig 6.3 : Simulation of hygroscopic growth in the lung.

The bolus designates an incremental volume of inhaled aerosol. Particles are continuously removed from the bolus (i.e., deposited on airway surfaces) as it travels throughout the lung during a cycle of breathing. This simulates popular experimental protocols for human exposures (Scheuch et al, 1988). The superposition principle advocated by Landahl (1950a) may be used to determine cumulative deposition:

$$P(C) = P(I) + P(S) + P(D) + P(I)P(S)P(D) - P(I)P(S) - P(I)P(D) - P(S)P(D) \qquad (3)$$

P(C) considers interactive effects between deposition processes that have been simulated as being independent in the derivations of the equations in Table 6.2.

Alternative way to account for interactive effects between deposition process have been presented as various investigators have attempted to isolate conditions where only selected mechanisms need be addressed. For instance, let us consider two mechanisms, sedimentation and diffusion, which have received considerable attention in the literature. Simple superposition would indicate that:

$$P(C) = P(D) + P(S) - P(D)P(S) \qquad (4)$$

For long straight, smooth-walled tubes of circular cross section Heyder et al (1985) have presented an empirical equation:

$$P(C) = P(D) + P(S) - P(D)P(S) / [P(D) + P(S)] \qquad (5)$$

For idealized tubes, Chen and Yu (1993) have predicted that:

$$P(C) = \{P(S)2 + P(D)2 - [P(S)\,P(D)2]^{1/2} \qquad (6)$$

The latter formulae were proposed for the peripheral regions of the lung where diffusion and sedimentation are relatively effective. It must be emphasized, however, that those mechanisms are most relevant to particles of vastly different sizes.

6.2.2 Thermodynamics of inhaled hydgroscopic drugs

The implications of hygroscopicity to drug delivery are elementary in concept and straightforward in practice. The role of hygroscopicity is so fundamental to the administration of inhaled pharmaceuticals, especially for the success of targeted drug delivery; that it is difficult to comprehend the extent to which it has been neglected in the literature. It is fact that the deposition pattern of inhaled hygroscopic drugs may not be related to particle sizes and densities as measured at the sites of aerosol generation. Specifically, the aerosol characteristics of mass median aerodynamic diameter (μMAD) and geometric standard deviation (GSD) determined at a nebulizer, metered dose inhaled (MDI), or dry powder inhaler (DPI) are not relevant parameters in estimating the dose delivered to the lung unless hygroscopic growth following inhalation is considered.

Ferron and colleagues (1993) have developed mathematical models describing processes of hygroscopic growth. The models have two rather severe limitations that compromise applicability to human airways. First of all, they ignored coupling effects (i.e., interactions) between inhaled particles and surrounding air. Eisner et al (1990), however, clearly demonstrated that the very presence of particles can indeed have a profound influence on thermodynamic conditions in the lung, especially affecting aerosol hygroscopicity. Secondly, they assumed that heat and mass transfer processes are controlled by molecular diffusion. It has been explained that convection is likely the salient mechanism affecting heat and mass transfer processes in airways, and may therefore be the more important factor (i.e. rather than molecular diffusion) regulating the behavior of inhaled hygroscopic pharmacologic drugs.

A mathematical model describing factors affecting the behavior and fate of inhaled pharmacologic drugs has been defined (Martonen,1993a). Particle deposition patterns have been examined as functions of : (a) patient's ventilatory parameters (Martonen et al,1993b); (b) aerosol polydispersity (Martonen et al,1993d); and (c) airway morphologies (Martonen et al,1994b). The model has been validated by comparisons of predicted deposition pattern with data from inhalation exposures with healthy volunteer human subjects (Martonen,1993a) and clinical data from patients with respiratory tract diseases (Martonen et al, 1993c & Martonen et al,1994b).

Most recently, the model has been employed in an investigation of the effects of disease induced changes in airway morphologies upon the targeted delivery of inhaled drugs used in their treatment (Martonen et al,1995). It should be recognized that the atmospheres within the passages of the head, throat, and lung can exert a great influence upon the deposition of pharmacologic drugs. The effect of hygroscopicity and drug delivery has established that the effect of hygroscopicity is quite complex. For instance, in the medical coμmunity, it is widely assumed that the effects of water vapor uptake are to increase the aerodynamic diameters of inhaled particles. However, for bronchodialator, it has been clearly shown (Martonen et al,1983c) that, they may not be the case. To be specific, aerodynamic sizes of inhaled drugs may actually decrease upon the absorption of water vapor, depending on the chemical formulation of the drug and the initial sizes of inhaled particles.

Moreover, the extent to which hygroscopic growth can occur within an airway depends on its residence time therein. Therefore, drug hygroscopicity is a direct function of localized fluid dynamics profiles. In a recent sequence of simulations using the Cray Y-MP supercomputer, the kinetics of air within the human lung has been systematically investigated. The effects of naturally occurring anatomical features, ignored in other drug deposition models in the current literature, have been quantitated. In the order that they are experienced by an inhaled bolus of drug, the effects of the laryngeal jet (Martonen et al, 1993c), cartilaginous rings (Martonen et al, 1994a), and carnial ridge shapes (Martonen et al, 1994c) have been formulated. The subject of air motion has been recently reviewed by Martonen et al (1994d)

Therefore, it is necessary to identify the factors affecting hygroscopicity within the human lung. It is assumed that particle growth can be controlled to target delivery of inhaled pharmacologic drugs. Thus, efficiencies of the drug would be enhanced.

6.2.3 Mathamatical model predicting distribution of inhaled therapeutic aerosols

The purpose of mathematical models is to predict the deposition of inhaled aerosol particles in the human respiratory tract. The early deposition models assumed relatively simple lung morphologies, a small number of breathing conditions and a limited range of particle sizes. Models for specific respiratory zone, such as the nasal-pharyngeal-laryngeal-tracheal zone or the tracheo-bronchial zone, were often presented rather than models for the entire respiratory tract. With improvement of techniques for determining the morphology of the lung, measuring breathing conditions, and calculating deposition based on fluid flow in the airways, the models have become more sophisticated. Simultaneously, techniques for measuring both overall and regional deposition of aerosols have improved, so that experimental verification of models is more readily accomplished.

6.2.3.1 Early models (1935-1966)

Although experimental measurement of respiratory deposition of aerosols were reported by Drinker et al (1928) and Brown (1931), the first mathematical model was presented by Findeisen (1935). He divided the respiratory tract into nine generations, beginning with the trachea, progressing through three orders of bronchi and two orders of bronchioles, and terminating with alveolar ducts and sacs. Findeisen (Table 6.3), assumed branching factors, dimensions, flow speeds, and transit times for each generation. The latter values were based on his assumed breathing pattern of 2 sec inspiration and 2 sec expiration with a tidal volume of 400 cm^3, resulting in a constant flow rate of 200 cm^{3}sec^{-1}.

Table 6.3 : Schematic representation of the respiratory tract

Generation	Branching	Number Factor	Diameter (cm)	Length (cm)	Cross-sec. area (cm^2)	Velocity (cm sec^{-1})[a]	Residence time (sec)[a]
Trachea	1	1	1.3	11.0	1.3	150	0.07
Main bronchi	2	2	0.75	6.5	1.1	180	0.04
1st bronchi	6	12	0.4	3.0	1.5	130	0.02
2nd bronchi	8	100	0.2	1.5	3.1	65	0.02
3rd bronchi	8	770	0.15	0.5	14.0	14	0.04
Term. bron.	70	54000	0.06	0.3	150.0	1.3	0.22
Resp. bron.	2	1.1x10^5	0.05	0.15	220.0	0.9	0.17
Alv. Ducts	240	2.6x10^7	0.02	0.02	8200.0	0.025	0.82
Alv. Sacs	2	5.2x10^7	0.03	0.03	1.47x10^5	0	1.2

[a]For ventilatory flow rate of 200 cm^{3}sec^{-1}.

Findeisen assumed simple expression for the deposition of particles in each generation resulting from three mechanisms: Brownian motion, sedimentation, and impaction. He also assumed that the particles were spherical shaped and there density was 1 gm cm^{-3}. He calculated deposition in each generation for seven particle diameters, 0.03, 0.1, 0.3, 1.0, 3.0, 10 and 30 μm. For the three smallest sizes the total deposition fraction in the respiratory tract (% of inhaled aerosol mass) was, respectively, 68%, 35%, and 34%, the deposition being essentially confined to the last two generations. For 1.0 μm diameter particles, he calculated 97.4% total deposition, while for two largest diameters, the deposition was 100%. For 1μm diameter, deposition was still primarily in the last two generation, but as particle diameter increased, the site of deposition moved proximal, the 30 μm diameter particles all being deposited in the trachea and first bifurcation (carina). Shortcoming of Findeisen model is that, it neglected the airways above the trachea and in the nasal and oral passages. He assumed a very simple anatomical generation scheme, the calculation was limited to a single breathing pattern that was not physiologically reasonable.

The next model was assumed by Landahl (1950a). This model was modified by Findeisen(1964) in several important respects. He added two upper airway compartments, the mouth and pharynx, and additional alveolar duct generation. Quantitatively results of Landahl's calculations were not greatly different from those of Findeisen, with some exceptions. For largest particles, deposition is still predominantly in the upper airways but because the mouth and pharynx are included, a significant fraction of these particles is deposited in these airways as well as in the first few broncheal generations. As with Findeisen's model, deposition shifted more distally as the particle diameter decrease from 20 μm to 0.2 μm for all breathing conditions. For the largest diameter, 20 μm, no particles penetrated beyond the eight generations, the terminal bronchioles. Twelve generations at sites are considered:

Generation	Site
First	Mouth
Second	Pharynx
Third	Trachea
Fourth	1st Bronchi
Fifth	2nd Bronchi
Sixth	3rd Bronchi
Seventh	4th Bronchi
Eighth	Terminal bronchiole
Ninth	Respiratory bronchiole
Tenth	Alveolar ducts
Eleventh	Alveolar sacs
Twelveth	Total deposition (%)

Landahl's model (1950b) was further modified by the addition of the nasal passage as an alternative upper airway path. Nasal passage was assumed to be more efficient than the oral passage as a particle filter, aerosols that passed through the nasal passage had less penetration than those that passed through the oral passage for similar conditions.

Becknams (1965) presented a deposition model that assumed three mechanisms of particle deposition: Brownian diffusion, sedimentation, and impaction.

A scheme of the human respiratory tract was presented by Davies (1961), containing 15 generations, beginning with the mouth and ending at the alveolar sacs. However, there were no depositional models published employing this anatomical arrangements. The lung anatomical schemes published by Weibel (1963) were used in many subsequent lung deposition models, especially the syµmetric model A shown in Table (6. 4). It and the nonsyµmetrical model (more difficult to use in deposition models) were based on very detailed anatomical examination of several excised normal adult human lungs inflated to approximately 75% of their vital capacity (Vc).

Table 6.4 : Dimensions of dichotomous human airway model A by Weibel

Name of airway	Generation	Number per generation	Diameter (cm)	Length (cm)	Total cross Section (cm^2)	Total vol. (cm^3)	Accum. Vol (cm^3)
Trachea	0	1	1.8	12.0	2.54	30.5	30.5
Main bronchus	1	2	1.22	4.76	2.33	11.25	41.8
Lobar bronchus	2	4	0.83	1.90	2.13	3.97	45.8
Lobar bronchus	3	8	0.56	0.76	2.00	1.52	47.2
Seg. Bronchus	4	16	0.45	1.27	2.48	3.46	50.7
Seg. Bronchus	5	32	0.35	1.07	3.11	3.30	54.0
Bronchus	6	64	0.28	0.90	3.96	3.53	57.5
Bronchus	7	128	0.23	0.76	5.10	3.85	61.4
Bronchus	8	256	0.186	0.64	6.95	4.45	65.8
Bronchus	9	512	0.154	0.54	9.65	5.17	71.0
Bronchus	10	1024	0.130	0.46	13.4	6.31	77.2
Term. Bronchus	11	2048	0.109	0.39	19.6	7.56	84.8
Term. bronchus	12	4096	0.095	0.33	28.8	9.82	94.6
Bronchiole	13	8192	0.082	0.27	44.5	12.45	106.0
Bronchiole	14	16384	0.074	0.23	69.4	16.40	123.4
Bronchiole	15	32768	0.066	0.20	113.0	21.70	145.1
Ter. Bronchiole	16	65536	0.060	0.165	180.0	29.70	174.8
Res. Bronchiole	17	1.31×10^5	0.054	0.141	300.0	41.80	216.6
Res. Bronchiole	18	2.62×10^5	0.050	0.117	534.0	61.10	277.7
Res. Bronchiole	19	5.24×10^5	0.047	0.099	944.0	93.20	370.9
Alv. duct	20	1.49×10^6	0.045	0.083	1600	139.50	510.4
Alv. duct	21	2.10×10^6	0.043	0.070	3220	224.20	734.7
Alv. duct	22	4.19×10^6	0.041	0.059	5880	350.00	1084.7
Alv. sac	23	8.39×10^6	0.041	0.050	11800	591.00	1675.0

A model of lung deposition that has been used is contained in the report of Task Group of Lung Dynamics (TGLD) to the International Commission on Radiation Protection (ICRP), and later published (1966). This model was a modification of the Findeisen anatomical scheme containing an additional compartment, the nasopharyngeal (N-P) airway. For the purpose of calculating the deposition of aerosol in this airway, the empirical equation of Pattle (1961) for the inspiratory nasal deposition fraction, hNl, was employed:

$$\eta_{NI} = -1.200 + 0.475 \ \log \ (\rho d_p^2 Q) \qquad \qquad (7)$$

Where r = particle density, gm cm^{-3} , dp = particle diameter, μm , and Q = flow rate, cm^{3}sec^{-1}

Equation (7) represents nasal deposition by impaction and is important for particle diameter > 1 μm. The quantity $(\rho d_p^2 Q)$ is an impactive parameter that appears in deposition efficiency equation for the nasal passage, the oral passage, and the bronchial airways, where velocities are relatively large.

Calculations were performed for particle diameters ranging from 0.01 to 100 μm for three tidal volumes (750,1450,and 2150 cm^3) and a breathing rate of 15 bpm. It was assumed that the aerosols were breathed through the nasal airways. The deposition fractions were grouped into three zones - the N-P (nasopharyngeal), T-B (tracheobronchial), and P (pulmonary). The results of the calculations are shown in Fig 6. 4 .

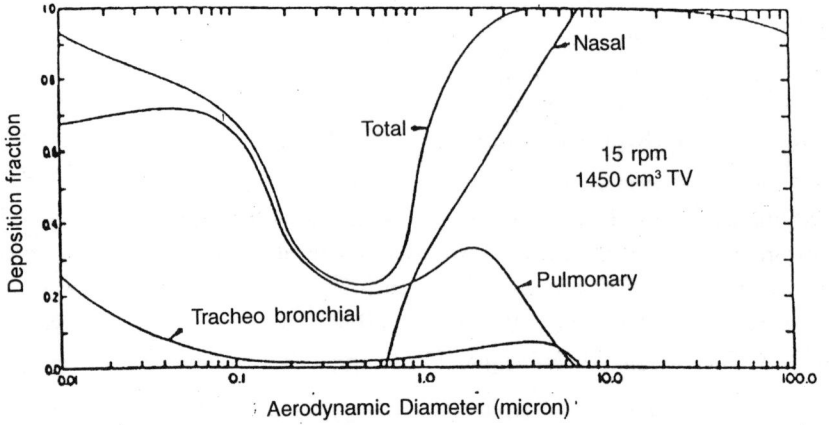

Fig 6.4 :   Regional deposition fraction curves of the task group on lung dynamics (1966) as a function of particle diameter.

As with previous deposition models, the total deposition fraction demonstrated minimum at a particle diameter of approximately 0.3 μm, and increased monotonically as particle diameter increased or decreased from this minimum.

In this deposition model, it was also assumed that the particle were spherical, non-hygroscopic, non-evaporating, and non-reactive, and that behaved inertially as isolated particles (no "cloud effect").

6.2.3.2 More recent deposition models (1964 - 1991)

Following the Task Group model and prior to the most recent NCRP* and ICRP* models, almost all the mathematical models that covered the entire respiratory tract have employed the Weibel symmetrical model A. It was described as having 23 generations: generation zero denoted for trachea, generation 1 to 16 for the bronchial airways (large bronchi, small bronchi, and bronchioles), and generation 17 to 23 for the gas exchange region (respiratory bronchioles, alveolar ducts, and alveolar sacs). The dimensions of each airway generation were given, allowing for calculation of deposition for each generation for the major mechanisms.

An alternative approach was presented by Taulbee and Yu (1975) and later by Egan and Nixon (1988), in which the human respiratory tract is treated as a continuously expanding duct ("trumpet model") as one moves more distally into the lungs. This approach shows the phenomena of mixing between the tidal and residual air in the lung and as a result aerosol deposition is a non steady process at the onset of aerosol exposure.

6.2.3.3 Regional or local deposition models

This model is to focus on a particular region or subregion of respiratory tract such as the nasal passage, the large bronchi or the alveolar spaces. The long-term objectives of these modeling efforts is to piece the region together to achieve an overall model of aerosol deposition. This attempt has been done to model a particular respiratory region over a range of particle diameters and breathing conditions, seeking to obtain a deposition efficiency expression that can be used in a larger model.

As an example, we consider the deposition models for the nasal passage, beginning with the work of Landahl & Black (1947), where experiments consisted of drawing aerosol of several materials into the nasal passages and out the mouth at four constant flow rates. The inlet and outlet size distribution were measured, from which deposition efficiency as a function of particle diameter was calculated. As a follow-up to this study, Landahl (1950a) developed a theoretical expression for particles in the diameter range 1-40 μm, where the mechanisms of deposition for particles were assumed to be impaction and sedimentation. The nasal passage was assumed to consist of four zones, which were modeled as simple geometric shapes. These zones were combined to give a total nasal removal efficiency curve.

Equation (7) presented by Pattle (1961) and used by the Task Group, have been extended to include wider particle diameter range and flow rates, and improved based on more subjects studied. Experimental data from five studies were summarized by Heyder & Rudolf (1977b), who presented separate empirical equations for inspiration and expiration. Using more recent data from nasal replicate models, Cheng et al. (1991) extended the diameter range through the ultrafine particle range to 1 nm diameter, so that an empirical equation covering 5 orders of magnitude of particle diameter can be employed for predicting nasal inspiratory and expiratory deposition efficiency. Tl.eir expression for nasal inspiratory deposition efficiency hNI , was :

$$\eta_{NI} = 1 - \exp(-0.00168\, d_{ar}^2\, Q - 12.8\, D^{0.5}\, Q^{-0.125}) \qquad (8)$$

Where d_{ar} = aerodynamic particle diameter, μm; Q = flow rate, Lmin-1; and D = particle diffusivity, $cm^2 sec^{-1}$. A similar expression was used to describe expiratory deposition efficiency with different constants. The exponential term containing $d_{ar}^2\, Q$ represents the impactive mechanism. The terms are multiplicative, but each term is of negligible effect where the other term is significant.

NCRP (National council on Radiation Protection and Measurement) Lung Deposition Model : U.S. NCRP appointed a task group (TG2) to prepare a new lung deposition and clearance model for radiation protection purposes. Although the model has not been formally adopted by NCRP and published, the features of the proposed model have been presented by Phelan et al.(1991). The model consists of a description of the respiratory tract region (Fig 6.5) which contains the clearance pathways, a morphometric model of the adult human nasal and oral airways, a morphometric model of the tracheobronchial and pulmonary regions (Yeh & Schum, 1980) , and a regional deposition curve (Fig 6. 6) based on equation for sedimentation, impaction and diffusion of particles onto airway surfaces.

ICRP (International Coumission on Radiation Protection) Lung Deposition Model: This model was presented by Bair (1991). He considered the dose calculation to the nasal and oral passage radioactive gases, ultrafine particles (dp < 0.01 μm) and clearance of particles which were omitted by Task Group model. ICRP model took advantage of new developments in lung macro- and micromorphology, new information in respiratory physiology, and progress in computer technology, making complex computation possible on PCs.

All existing models rest on a set of assumptions that must be made to arrive at simple predictive equations, but these assumptions are not met for many therapeutic aerosols. It can therefore be concluded that efforts to

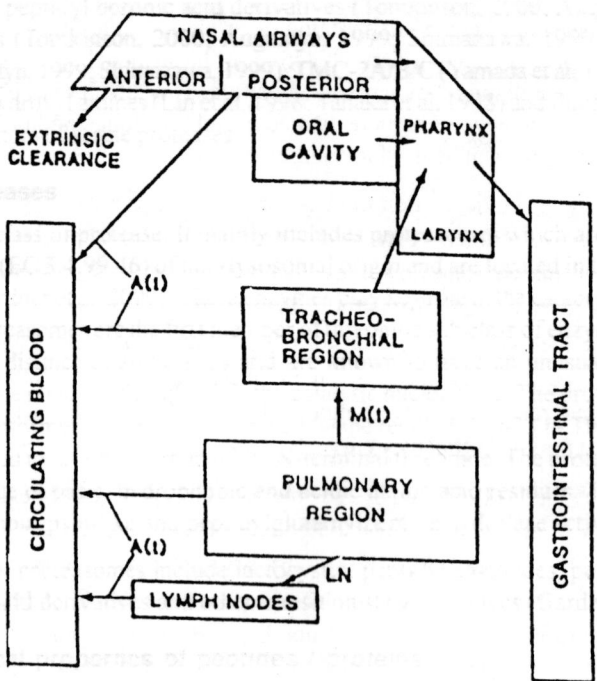

Fig 6.5 : Functional diagram of deposition region and clearance pathway definitions for the NCRP respiratory tract model (Phelan et al,1991).

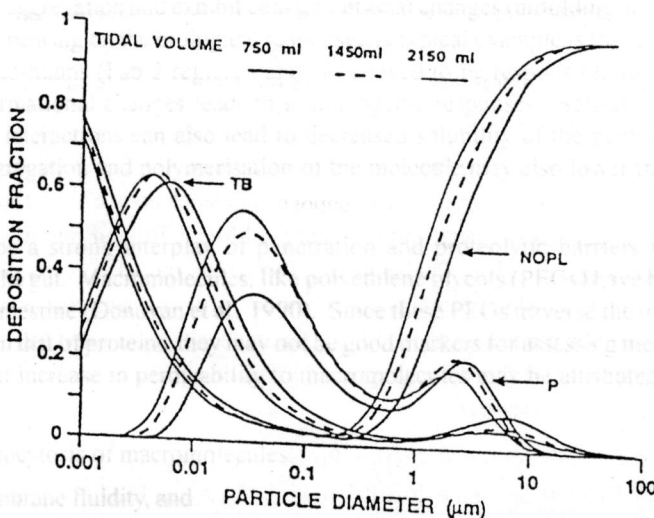

Fig 6.6 : Regional deposition fraction curves of the NCRP model (Phelan wt al,1991) as a function of particle diameter.

improve the predictive models for environmental aerosols should be matched by similar efforts for therapeutic substances in aerosol form.

Thus, a challenge is ahead for deposition modelers and pharmaceutical scientists to collaborate in the development of models that will both predict behavior of existing aerosol systems and lead to improved design of new systems that can better target specific drugs in known quantity to desired sites in the respiratory tract.

6.3   BIOLOGICAL CONSIDERATIONS

6.3.1 Physiology and pharmacology of the airways

Knowledge of lung function, particularly as it relates to mechanical properties of the lungs during the process of ventilation, is essential to understand inhalation aerosol therapy. The discussion has been classified into two major sections. In the first section, emphasis is placed on physiological aspects of lung function, including lung structure and function, pulmonary ventilation, mechanical properties of the lungs, pulmonary function tests and altered lung function in several prominent pulmonary diseased conditions. The second section of pulmonary pharmacology considers basic pharmacodynamics and explores briefly the pharmacology of agents affecting airway smooth muscle and mucus secretion.

6.3.1.1 Phisiology of lung

Structure and function of the lung : Lung function is intimately linked with the structural features of the airways and lung parenchyma. The airways of the lungs provide a pathway of normally low resistance to the bulk flow of air into and out of the lung periphery where alveoli perform the essential function of gas exchange. Based on this concept, the lungs have been divided into two general compartments or zones - the conduction zone and the respiratory zone (Fig 6.7) (Weibel,1989).

The conducting zone consists of first 16 generations of airway comprised of the trachea (generation 0), which bifurcates into the two mainstem bronchi, which further subdivides into bronchi that enter two left and three right lung lobes. The intrapulmonary bronchi continue to subdivide into progressively smaller-diameter bronchi and bronchioles. The conducting zone ends with terminal bronchioles, which are devoid of alveoli. Accordingly, the function of the conducting zone is to move air by bulk flow into and out of the lungs during each breath. The respiratory zone consists of all structures that participate in gas exchange and begins with respiratory bronchioles containing alveoli. These bronchioles subdivide into additional respiratory bronchioles, eventually giving rise to alveolar ducts and finally to alveolar sacs. The acinus is defined as the unit comprised of a primary respiratory bronchiole, alveolar ducts, and alveolar sacs.

Several models of airway branching have been developed (Weibel, 1989). As the airways branch, they become smaller in diameter and length but greater in number and cross sectional area. The total alveolar surface area approaches 140-160 m^2 in the adult human (Gehr et al,1978). As a result of the enormous increase in surface area, bulk flow of air decreases rapidly with movement of air within alveoli occurs entirely by diffusion (Figure 6.8) (Paiva, 1985).

The presence or absence of cartilage is another structural feature if the airways that undergo significant change along the tracheobronchial tree and influences airway function . The presence of channels for collateral flow between acini and between alveoli (Menkes and Macklem, 1986) is another structural feature of the distal airway within the respiratory zone .

Other morphological and histological features of the airways change along the tracheobronchial tree and can have important influences on lung function under normal and pathophysiological conditions. Numerous cell types contribute to the characteristic features of different regions of the airways, glands that surrounds airways, nerves, blood vessels; and resident cells within the airways.

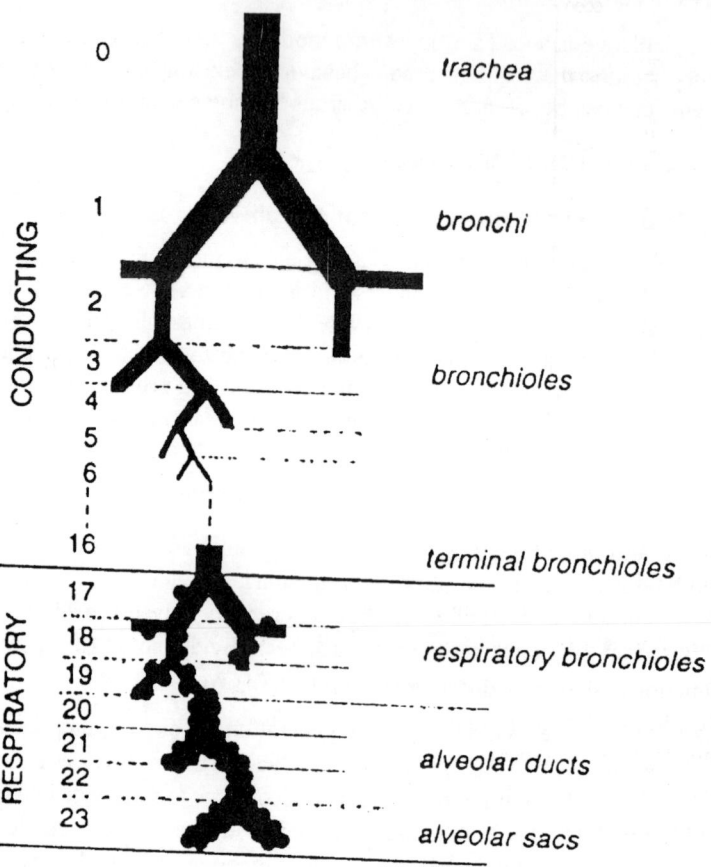

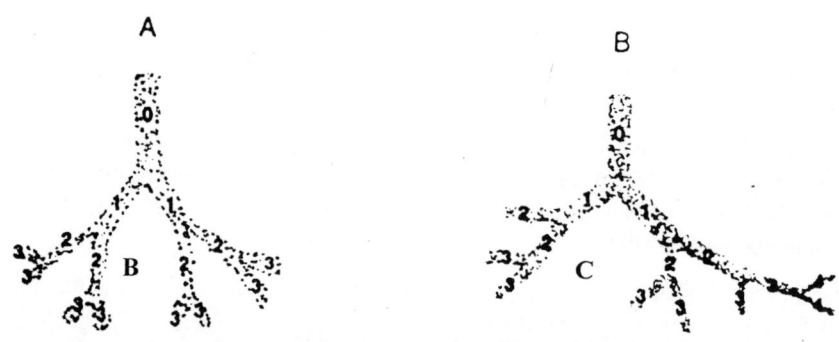

Fig 6.7 : Model of airway morphology.

Upper figure: Conducting (treachea-terminal bronchioles) and (respiratory bronchioles-alveolar sacs) zones of the airways.

Lower figure: Regular dichotomy (B) and irregular dichotomy (C) of airway branching.

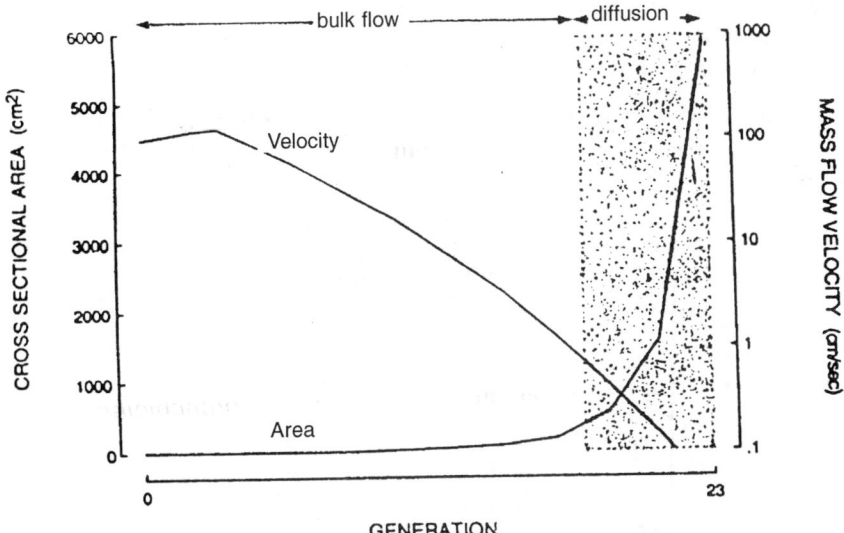

Fig 6.8 :   Generation dependent changes in airway cross-sectional area and flow of air. As the generation of airway increases (i.e., diameter decreases but number of airway increases), the velocity of air flow (as measured by mass flow velocity) decreases and airway cross-sectional area increases. The respiratory zone is identified by the shaded area .

Lung functions can be broadly subdivided into two principle categories- respiratory and non respiratory functions. Respiratory functions include the two principal respiratory activities of gas exchange and acid-base balance (Staub, 1991). Non respiratory functions include all other aspects of lung function, such as endocrine and metabolic activities.

Evaluation of pulmonary function Tests of pulmonary functions provide objective, quantifiable measurements of lung function and are utilized for various purposes (Nunn, 1993). They are used diagnostically to evaluate diseases that affect heart and lung function, to screen persons at risk for pulmonary disease, to assess prognosis, and to assess preoperative risks. Pulmonary tests are also used to monitor the effectiveness of drug with known pulmonary toxicity.

Measurements of various pulmonary functions include peak flow measurements, expiratory flow measurements, forced expiratory flow rate, flow - volume curve, lung volumes, ventilation - perfusion ratios and airway resistance and compliance.

(i) Peak Flow Measurements: These are the simplest tests of expiratory airflow to determine airway func tion. Subjects inhale completely (to TLC i.e., total lung capacity), then expire forcefully (both rapidly and completely) into a peak flowmeter which records the maximal flow rate of expiration.

(ii) Forced Expiratory Flow Measurements : A useful and simple test of pulmonary function is the measurement of a single forced expiratory maneuver, spirometeric methods are used to measure the time course of the forced expiratory volumes. The subject starts of TLC and exhales as rapidly and as compeltely as possible into the mouthpiece of a spirometer, which records the volume of air expired over time. The volume of air exhaled in the first second is termed the force expiratory volume ($FEV_{1.0}$), and the total volume exhaled is the forced vital capacity (FVC). The $FEV_{1.0}$ is normalised to body size, age and sex for comparison with standardized values. Additionally the $FEV_{1.0}$ / FVC ratio is useful in interpreting these pulmonary function tests.

(iii) Forced Expiratory Flow Rate: A related measurements is the force expiratory flow rate (FEF 25-75%) which represents the average flow rate determined over the midportion of the expiration. Generally, FEF25-75% is closely related to $FEV_{1.0}$.

(iv) Flow Volume Curve: Another useful measure of pulmonary function is the Flow-volume curve (Fig 6.9) (West, 1990), for normal lung functions and for obstructive and restrictive lung diseases.

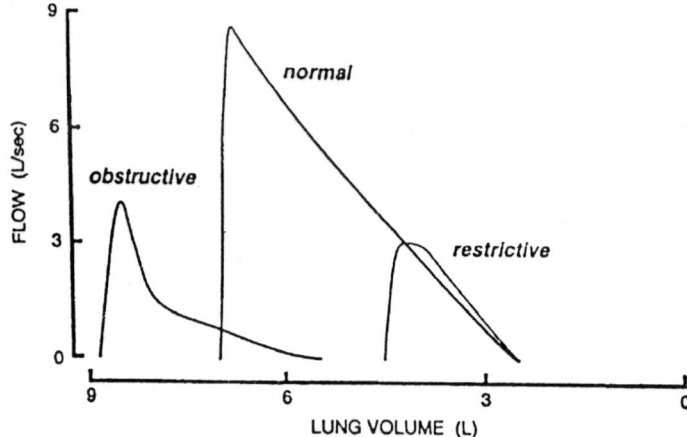

Fig 6.9 : Flow-volume measurements under normal, obstructive, and restrictive airway conditions.

In normal function, flow rate upon forced expiration rapidly reaches a peal at which point airway compression occurs. From this point onward, expiration is effort independent because greater effort simply compresses more airways and does not expel air at a greater rate. Thus, expiration depends on lung elastic recoil and resistance of airway upstream from the collapsed points in the airway.

Obstructive lung disease causes the curve after the maximal flow rate to assume a concave appearance or a reduced maximal flow and a curve shifted to higher lung volumes. These changes occur because of early airway closure, which may result from enhanced airway constriction caused by smooth muscle spasm in asthma, excessive mucus narrowing the airway lumen, or reduced radial fraction caused by loss of parenchyma in emphysema. Conversely, restrictive lung disease could result in more rapid exhalation due to increased lung elastic recoil without obstructed airways.

Maximal flow rate is also reduced in restrictive disease, and expiration occurs at lower lung volumes caused by decreased compliance and the inability to inflate the lungs normally.

(v) Lung volumes :Measurements of lung volumes by spirometry, gas dilution, and plethymography can also yield valuable information about lung function.

(vi) Ventilation-Perfusion Ratios: More sophisticated tests can determine matching of ventilation-perfusion ratios and estimate physiologic dead space.

(vii) Airway resistance and compliance :These tests are more complex then simple expiratory flow measurements and could require invasive methods, such as placement of an intraesophageal balloon. Nevertheless, they offer a more reliable measure of airway caliber and peripheral lung function.

6.3.1.2 Pharmacology of airways

Many agents influence airway caliber by regulating smooth muscle tone and mucus secretion. Receptors are protein based, a macromolecular complex existing within cell membranes, which, upon interaction with specific agents, change conformation and lead to the triggering of the cellular response, such as smooth muscle cell contraction or relaxation. A receptor shows considerable selectivity in the nature of the agent that interacts with it. As evidence of this, the nomenclature of receptors generally reflects the name of the agents that activates it. For example, cholinergic receptors are stimulated by acetylcholine. Muscarine activates muscarinic receptors, and nicotine stimulates nicotinic receptors. Acetylecholine acts on both the latter receptor types, leading to the definition that these are subtypes of cholinergic receptors. Agonist interacts with the receptors to produce a cellular response, the magnitude of which will be determined by the number of receptors occupied by the agonist and the intrinsic efficacy of the agonist (or the ability of the agonist to "activate" the receptor during occupation). Full agonists are the agents that can produce a maximal receptors-mediated tissue response. Agents with zero intrinsic efficacy bind to the receptors but do not produce a response. These agents, by definition, are receptor antagonists. The fraction of total receptors (of a specific receptor type) required to be activated to produce a maximal tissue response, varies from agonist to agonist. For example, full agonists may need occupy all or only a small fraction of the total receptor population to produce a maximal tissue response. Partial agonists, on the other hand, have a lower intrinsic efficacy and require occupation to produce a maximum effect, the magnitude of which is less than that induced by full agonist (Fig 6.10).

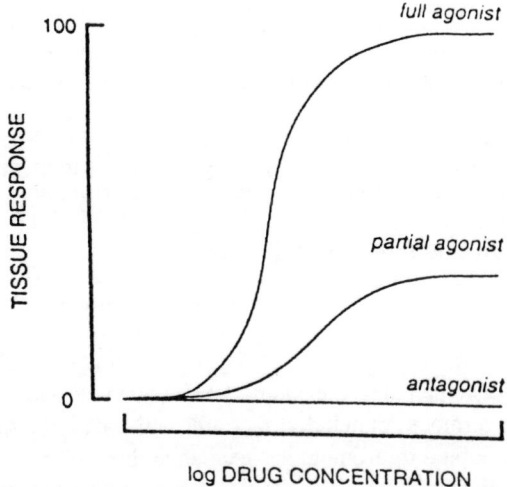

Fig 6.10 : Theoretical concentration-response curve for drugs with different intrinsic efficacies.

Bronchoactive agents may be classified mainly into three classes:

Neurotransmitters

i. Cholinergic innervations

ii. Nonadrenergic noncholinergic inhibitory (NANCI) nerves (Doidge and satchell, 1980)

iii. Adrenergic innervations (Wanger, 1992)

iv. Sensory neuropeptides (Molinard et al,1994)

Inflammatory mediators

i. Release of histamine from mast cells (White et al,1987)

ii. Release of chymase from mast cells (Sommerhoff et al,1989)

iii. Kininogenase like activity may be released form mast cells (Proud et al,1985)

iv. Effects of adenosine (Crimini, 1992), cyclo-oxygenase metabolites (Gardiner and Callier, 1980), platelet acitivating factor (PAF) (Snyder, 1990)

Others I) Xanthines like theophylline and enpropylline (Persson, 1985)

6.3.2 Solute transport following aerosol deposition in lungs

The movement of solutes between compartments in the lungs has been derived from the clearance of radioaerosols (Hayes et al, 1979). This observation can be utilized in detecting abnormalities in the permeability of the pulmonary epithelial barrier (Rinderknecht et al,1980). Indicators such as $99m_{Tc}$-DTPA and $99_{mTc}O4-$ are lost quite rapidly from the lungs of many patients, suggesting that they had diffused across the pulmonary epithelial surfaces of the lungs and been carried away in the blood. Most studies of the pulmonary epithelium have been conducted with a single indicator, 99mTc-DTPA. However there are many other indicators that could be used to define a variety of epithelial properties. Such studies are diagnostically useful for studying alteration in the pulmonary epithelium. Active transport of $Na+$, glucose, and amino acids have been studied using this technique (Effros and Chang, 1994a).

Various factors affect solute transport after aerosol deposition in the gas-exchange area of the lungs such as : surface area and droplet size (Weibel,1986), lipid solubility of solutes (Chinard et al,1962), pH of epithelial fluid (Nielson et al,1981), osmotic drug between the air spaces to the pulmonary vasculature , redox indicators in the air spaces (Effros et al, 1994b), and molecular size of solute (Effros et al, 1994b).

It is expected that the new indicators will be developed, which will permit measurements of additional properties of epithelial lining fluid and the epithelium itself along with measurements of the distribution of ventilation within the lungs and the permeability of the epithelium to relatively inert solutes.

6.3.3 Drug metabolism and enzyme kinetics in the lung

Inhalation as an alternate to oral drug administration offers several advantages in drug absorption. The lung is the only organ through which the entire cardiac output passes. Drug absorption is regulated by a thin alveolar-vascular permeability barrier, which, in parts of alveolar region, shows an air-blood pathway of less than 0.5 µm (Weibel, 1973). In the adult human lung, the number of alveoli in the deep airway ranges from 200 million to 600 million, resulting in an enormous epithelial surface area which has an estimated value of 140 m^2. While these properties are uniquely adopted to promote gas exchange through passive diffusion, they also provide a mechanism for efficient transport of drugs from the circulation to lung tissues and from lung tissues to the blood stream. Drugs that are administered intravenously may accumulate in high concentration in the lung following the first passage. On the other hand, the pulmonary epithelium may allow systemic absorption of aerosolized drugs manifolds faster than the GI tract (Enna and Schanker, 1972).

Thus, there is a great potential that many drug therapies may be improved via inhalation drug delivery, but requires further advances in aerosol technology.

The knowledge of drug metabolism is important criteria to be evaluated in order to fully appreciate the lung as an alternative route for drug delivery, which leads to dosage-related problems, associated with inhalation aerosols. The lung plays a very important role beyond the exchange of gases. Its metabolic function can result in the conversion of compounds to reactive products or inactivation of bioactive agents. The lung is a complex organ comprised of over 40 different cell types. There is a scanty knowledge available about the drug-metabolizing activities of the lung. Most of these studies are focussed on the role of pulmonary cytochrome P_{-450} (CYP_{-450}) isozyme, a group of enzymes known to convert lipophilic agent into more polar, water-soluble metabolites. This knowledge is mostly applicable to the metabolic fate of lipophilic drugs.

There is an increase in the development of protein and peptide drugs. The use of these agents may replace current low-molecular-weight drug therapy and/or introduce innovative form of treatment by countering a disease at the molecular level. Protein and peptides, which are susceptible to a variety of enzymatic degradation, are good candidates for the development of aerosol delivery systems. In addition to the monolayer nature of the alveolar epithelium and its large surface area, which are more conducive for peptide absorption. The lung may also have a relatively more manageable enzymatic effect toward protein and peptide drugs. Studies by Wang et al (1993) showed that the degradation of enkephalins by peptidases in the alveolar epithelium was significantly less than observed in other tissues.

Metabolizing enzymes found in the liver include phase-I reactive CYP_{-450s}, flavin-containing mono-oxygenases (FMO), monoamine oxidase (MAO), aldehyde dehydrogenase, NADPH-cytochrome P_{-450} reductase, esterases, and epoxide hydrolase; and phase-II conjugating enzymes glutathiones-transferase (GST), UDP-glucuronyl transferase (UDP-GT), sulfotransferase, N-acetyl transferase, and methyl transferase.

The phase-I reactions involve substrate modification by attachment or alteration of reactive functional groups such as -OH, -NH2, or -COOH, through oxidation, reduction, and hydrolysis. The phase-II pathways involve reaction of phase-I metabolites with endogenous molecules such as glucuronic acid, to yield highly polar, readily excretable conjugates. These enzyme systems are located at various subcellular sites e.g. the cytosol, mitochondria, and smooth endoplasmic reticulum. Table 6. 5 depicts various enzyme systems in the lungs

Table 6.5 : Enzyme system in lungs

Enzyme System	Involved in the metabolism of
1) Pulmonary CYP_{-450} mono-oxygenase system	Fatty acids, steroids, and lipid soluble xenobiotics.
2) Pulmonary NADPH cytocrome P_{-450} reductase	Drugs containing nitro groups, yielding a free radical which reacts with molecular oxygen to regenerate the parent drug and superoxide anion e.g. nitrofurantoin (Holtzman et al,1981).
3) Flavin-containing Mono-oxygenase (FMO)	Secondary and tertiary amines and sulphur-containing compounds e.g.; cocaine (Kloss et al,1982), phenothiazines (Williams et al,1985).
4) Esterase	Esters, amides, and thioesters, e.g.hydrolysis of beclomethasone dipropionate to its monopropionate and beclomethasone (Andersson et al,1984).
5) UDP-GT and sulfotransferase	Phenols, thiols and amines e.g.; 1-napthol (Gibby and cohen,1984).

Since the entire cardiac output perfuses through the lung the pulmonary vascular bed can be regarded as a gate for controlling the levels of bioactive agents allowed to enter the blood circulation. Studies have shown that the lung selectively removes endogenous norepinephrine (NE) and 5-hydroxytryptamine (5-HT), and b-phenyl ethylamine (PEA) from the blood and converts angiotensin-I to angiotensin-II .This implies that drugs with properties similar with the endogenous compounds may also be candidates for sequestration and metabolism by the lung. Knowledge of the combined effects of uptake and metabolism may prove useful in the elucidation of the therapeutic/toxic outcome of bioactive agents and in the design of drugs to be targeted to the lung.

Aerosol drug delivery has also been affected by the gross anatomical structure of the lung. The tracheobronchial airways are protected by a mucocilliary apparatus which serves to entrap and eliminate particles from the lung via a combined activity of mucous secretion from the submucosal glands and goblet cells, and the beating of cilia protruding from the luminal surface of the columnar epithelial cells (Sleigh et al,

1988). Mucin is stored in a dehydrated state but is spontaneously hydrated upon secretion to produce a gel, which floats atop a layer of periciliary fluid. The complex by coordinated beating pattern of the cilia moves this mucous layer toward the pharynx, thereby providing a clearance mechanism for the lung.

The alveolar wall consists of a specialized epithelium and closely apposed network of capillaries supported by a delicate interstitial matrix. Nearly, a single layer of epithelial type I pneumocytes joined by tight junctions covers 95% of the alveolar surface area. These terminally differentiated cells are vulnerable to a variety of injuries, and have little, if any, regenerative or replicative potential. In contrast, type II cells are more resistant to oxidative injury (Freeman et al,1986) and are capable of proliferating and repairing the epithelial lesion (Bowden,1981). Alveolar macrophages are residents of the alveolar spaces and are primarily responsible for the host defense mechanism in the deep lung.

The pulmonary endothelium is composed of metabolically active, functionally responsive cells that serve to monitor the circulating bioactive agents (Ryan, 1986). In addition, the permeability of the endothelium for hydrophilic compounds is at least 10 times greater than that of the alveolar epithelium (Staub,1974). Aerosolized drugs, especially those meant for systemic delivery, will come into contact with the endothelium. A number of drugs such as bleomycin and monocrotaline have been shown to damage the pulmonary vasculature either through their oxidative properties or the generation of toxic metabolites (Lafranconi and Huxtable, 1984). Other drugs known to cause interference in the localized metabolic activity include desmethylimipramine (DMI), a tricyclic antidepressant drug that has been shown to decrease pulmonary clearance of 5-HT and PEA in a dose-dependent manner (Minchin et.al, 1982). The PEA metabolism was diminished entirely owing to inhibition of pulmonary MAO by DMI, while the clearance in both drug uptake and MAO activity (Minchin et al,1982). Hence, the possibility of drug interactions with the endothelial components can not be overlooked. Various experimental in vivo and in vitro models in lung metabolism studies have been worked out. A researcher must go through the literature to understand the utility of these models.

Thus, in a nutshell, we can conclude that various protease inhibitors and absorption enhancers can be used to promote pulmonary absorption of peptides for systemic drug effect. Aerosolized insulin and other drugs have already been studied in human (Laube et al,1993). Although aerosol delivery is associated with variability in the fraction of the administered dose deposited, this may not be an obstacle in the future, pending further improvement in inhaler devices and aerosol formulation. The capacity of the lung to metabolize drugs is not as high as that of the liver. This, in conjunction with vast surface area and thin nature of the alveolar epithelial barrier, makes the lung a highly feasible route for the delivery of aerosolized drugs.

6.4 MEDICAL DEVICES FOR THE DELIVERY OF THERAPEUTIC AEROSOLS TO THE LUNGS

Despite the numerous methods that can be employed to generate aerosols in therapeutically useful size ranges and concentrations, only three basic aerosol delivery systems have found their way into coμmercially marketed drug products. Specifically, these are metered-dose inhalers (MDIs), dry powder inhalers (DPIs), and nebulizers. These three classes of devices do not represent optimal delivery systems in terms of their ability to produce monodisperse aerosols that can be precisely dosed in a single breath, but rather are examples of delivery systems that achieve minimally acceptable characteristics in a simple, convenient, inexpensive, and portable format. To be acceptable for clinical use, an inhalation delivery system must meet certain criteria:

1. It must generate an aerosol with most of the drug carrying particles less than $10\mu m$ in size, and ideally in the range 0.5 to $5\mu m$, the exact size depending on the intended application.

2. It must produce reproducible drug dosing.

3. It must protect the physical and chemical stability of the drug.

4. It must be relatively portable and inconspicuous during use.

5. It must be readily used by a patient with minimal training.

These minimal requirements alone do not guarantee coµmercial success. Most coµmercial products currently under development aimed to provide multiple dosing (typically 200 doses) with minimal excipients inhalation (which can lead to poor organoleptic properties in the mouth, and oropharyngeal irritation). Patient convenience, competitive manufacturing cost and added value features such as dose counters or an indication of appropriate inhalation flow rates, are also considered desirable.

6.4.1 Metered Dose Inhalers

Since the 1950s, MDIs have been the mainstay of inhalation therapy, ostensibly because they were perceived to meet most of the criteria outlined above. However, over the years a number of deficiencies have been identified. Only a small fraction of the drug escaping the inhaler penetrates the patients lung (Newman et al, 1981) due to a combination of high particle exit velocity and poor co-ordination between actuation and inhalation. The unstable physical nature of the suspended drug particles in propellants, combined with suboptimal valve designs, has lead to reports of irreproducible dose metering following a period of rest (Cyr et al,1991). Low concentrations of potentially carcinogenic compounds were found to be extracted from valve components by the propellant system (Sethi et al,1992) and inhaled by the patient. However, the largest threat to the continued availability of pressurised MDIs is their dependence on Chloro-fluoro carbon (CFC) propellents, which have been linked to the depletion of stratospheric ozone and are now scheduled to be phased out under the terms of the " Montreal Protocol On Substances that Depletes the Ozone Layer" (Dalby et al,1990). Despite these concerns new device designs, improved formulations and valves, and a switch to "environmentally friendly" propellants are likely to keep MDIs in coµmon use.

The modern MDI shown in (Fig 6.11) is little different from its predecessors, and contains the same three basic ingredients: drug, one or more propellants, and in most cases, a surfactant. A liquefied propellant serves both as an energy source to expel the formulation from the valve in the form of rapidly evaporating droplets and as a dispersion medium for the drug and other excipients. A surfactant is typically present to aid with the dispersion of suspended drug particles or dissolution of a partially soluble drug, and to lubricate the metering value mechanism.

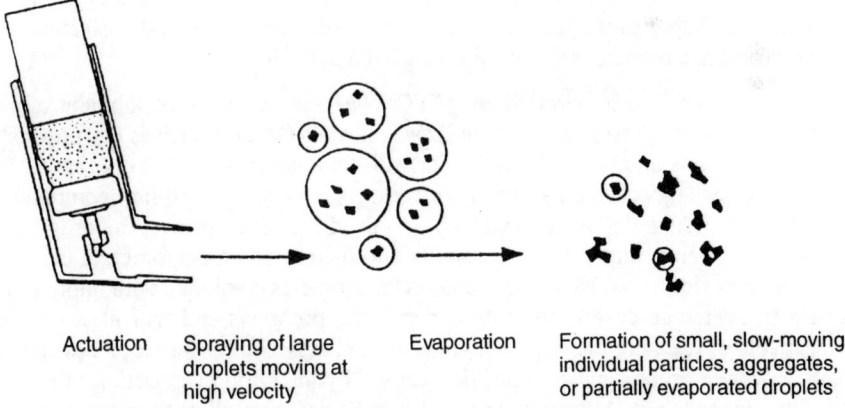

| Actuation | Spraying of large droplets moving at high velocity | Evaporation | Formation of small, slow-moving, individual particles, aggregates, or partially evaporated droplets |

Fig 6.11: Diagram of a typical pressurized-metered dose inhaler showing mechanism of particle formation.

In some formulations a surfactant is reported to be unnecessary (Atkins, 1990). Drug can be dissolved in the liquefied propellant/surfactant combination, with or without the aid of a less volatile cosolvent (Dalby et al, 1988), or suspended in the form of micronized particles (Dalby, 1992). In all currently marketed formulations, drug dissolution necessitates the use of an ethanolic cosolvent. Flavors (such as dissolved mint extracts) and suspended sweeteners (for example, micronized saccharine) may be present to combat the unpleasant taste associated with significant orophayngeal deposition following inhalation. To enhance chemical stability, antioxidants (ascorbic acid) or chelating agents (EDTA) may be present in formulations in which the drug is dissolved.

Propellants : The popularity of traditional CFC propellants has steµmed from their low pulmonary toxicity, high chemical stability and purity, and compatibility with coµmonly used packaging materials. In addition, they are nonflaµmable. Combinations of the three most widely used CFCs, trichlorofluoromethane (CFC-11), dichlorodifluoromethane (CFC-12), and 1,2-dichlorotetrafluoromethane (CFC-114), are typically combined in varying ratios to achieve a desirable combination of vapor pressure, liquid density, and solvency (Byron, 1990). Following a long search for alternative propellants with similar characteristics to CFCs, 1,1,1,2-tetrafluoroethane (HFC-134a) has emerged as the primary replacement, and coµmercial formulations containing this propellant have recently gained or are awaiting marketing approval in several countries (SanGiovanni, 1993). In addition, 1,1,1,2,3,3,3-heptafluoropropane (HFC-227) is being actively investigated. In the recent past, numerous other propellants have been investigated (Dalby,1993), and formulations containing them have been described in the patent literature (Whithman and Eagle, 1994). However, the expense of coµmercial development, primarily due to chronic toxicity testing, appears to have reduced the interest of many companies in these propellants.

Formulation : The propellant blend also dictates the product density since the other excipients are present at low concentrations. Large density differences between propellant blend and the true density of suspended drug particles are known to cause erratic dosing if there is a delay between shaking and actuation of the MDI (Dalby, 1992), owing to the nonhomogeneous drug distribution within the canister due to drug sinking or floating in the propellant. This can be minimized by matching the drug and propellant density, or by facilitating deflocculation of the bulk suspension with an appropriate surfactant. Propellant blending also allows the solubility of a drug or surfactant in the propellant system to be manipulated since some propellants (such as CFC-11) are often better solvents than others (CFC-12). However, it is important to remember that density and solvency cannot be manipulated independently of vapor pressure, so in practice the changes that can be made are limited. One problem with the availability of only one alternative propellant (HFC-134a) is the loss of flexibility associated with the use of blends. Several papers and patents address this issue with the inclusion of ethanol as a cosolvent (Whitham and Eagle,1994). While this facilitates slurry production during manufacturing, reduces the vapor pressure, and enhances the solubility of several surfactants in HFC-134a, it may result in a reduced fine particle fraction following MDI actuation.

The phase-out of chlorofluorocarbons (CFCs) has spurred the development of alternative pulmonary drug delivery systems to pressurized metered dose inhalers (MDIs), such as dry powder inhalers and pocket size nebulizers. Reformulation of CFC-MDIs with hydrofluoroalkanes (HFAs) 134a and 227 is also an opportunity to improve these widely accepted systems with respect to ease of handling, compliance, dosing, and more reliable and efficient lung deposition. MDIs have the advantage to protect the drug substance from external parameters such as temperature and humidity and to meter and de-agglomerate the drug independent from patients inspiratory flow rates. Novel formulation technologies combined with improved valves and actuators should help to overcome dose uniformity and priming problems and will increase the percentage of fine particles capable of reaching the deeper regions of the lungs. Spacer mouthpieces can reduce the cold freon effect and undesired orophayngeal deposition caused by the rapid evaporation of the propellant and plume velocity of the aerosol cloud. More advanced delivery devices may allow the patient to inhale at predetermined flow rates (fast/slow) to target the deposition of fine drug particles (1-6 micron) to specific sites into the lungs. Breath-actuated devices make these systems more effective and patient friendly. The above features in combination with numerical counters showing the remaining number of shots, and built-in blocking mechanisms to avoid tail-off dependent dose uniformity problems of the last labeled shots, should help to improve both acceptance and compliance of pMDIs compared to other inhalation devices. However, only those inhalation systems, which are accepted and appreciated by patients and offering an ambulatory treatment at reasonable cost, will be successful in a more and more competitive market. These issues must be considered in the development of future devices and formulations (Keller, M; 1999).

Oleic acid, soya-derived lecithin, and sorbitan trioleate have been widely used as surfactants in CFC-based formulations. The choice of concentration (up to 2%) is usually determined by experimentation in an attempt to maximize the fine particle fraction and dosing reproducibility. The patent literature contains numerous references to potentially useful surfactants for use with HFC-134a. These include polyethylene glycol, propoxylated polyethylene glycols, perfluoroalkanoic acids, and numerous others all of which exhibit enhanced solubility.

Drug is either dissolved or suspended in a MDI formulation. The equilibrium size of a sprayed droplet containing dissolved drug depends on the starting droplet size and the concentration and density of the dissolved, nonvolatile ingredients it initially contained. In such a system, it is theoretically possible to alter the drug concentration to achieve a wide range of sizes. If the droplet does not evaporate to dryness, which is likely if it contains a nonvolatile co-solvent, then the evaporation rate becomes the primary determinant of droplet size. In such formulations it is not necessary to reduce the size of the drug particles prior to incorporation into the formulation. Solution formulations are also easier to manufacture and do not exhibit the drug-sedimentation-related problems described above. Because of the intimate molecular interaction between the dissolved drug and excipients, reduced chemical stability compared to a suspension formulation has been observed. Thus, supersaturation and precipitation at low temperatures must be avoided. Partitioning of drug into valve elastomers has also been noted with a corresponding decrease in dose delivery per actuation (Atkins, 1991).

Valve and Conainer : As with other inhalation delivery systems, it is inappropriate to evaluate the formulation independently of the "packaging". The essential components are the container, metering valve, and actuator. Containers for suspensions are typically one-piece aluminum canisters, with a 20-μm external crimp (cut edge or rolled top) neck. Some products (e.g., Azmacort) utilize more attractive epoxy-coated aluminum canisters. Some suppliers recoµmend anodized aluminum canisters for solution formulations, although most of these products are packaged in plastic-coated glass bottles. While aluminum is inherently opaque, the coating on glass bottles is usually opacified when used with light- sensitive drugs such as epinephrine. The container is typically required to withstand internal pressures up to 180 psig without distortion. The formulation type, labeling, aesthetic requirements, and need for in-process fill weight monitoring usually dictate the choice of container. Plastic containers are also available, but are not utilized in any marketed inhalation products.

Metering valves (Fig 6.12) are designed to release a fixed volume of product during each actuation. Assuming that the valve fills with a homogeneous drug solution or suspension, the metered dose is the product of the valve volume and drug concentration. Usual valve volumes range from 25 to 100 ml, although larger volumes are available. Typically, valves contain a prefilled metering chamber that is isolated from the bulk reservoir as the chamber empties through the valve stem. This is initiated by pressing the stem into the body of the valve. When pressure on the stem is released, an internal spring returns the stem to its rest position, and the metering chamber refills through one or more channels from the reservoir. Such a valve is described as "holding its prime," indicating that the product that will be sprayed next is already located in the metering chamber prior to actuation, and must be retained there if the next dose is to be complete. If drug escapes from the metering chamber during a period of quiescence (perhaps due to propellant drainage or suspension instability), the following actuation will release a smaller dose. Drug escape from the metering chamber of MDIs during periods of nonuse has been associated with a low subsequent dose of albuterol. For this reason, alternative valve designs are available, though not without their own limitations (Schultz et al, 1994). While drug concentrations present in the canister are altered by temperature-dependent changes in propellant density and propellant leakage, the past history of under or over dosing by the valve should also be considered. Valve volumes are approximate due to propellant-induced swelling of the metering chamber elastomers and mechanical distortion during crimping and repeated use. It is therefore prudent to assess valve performance with specific formulations and not infer their reliability from successful use with a previous product. All metering valves on inhalation products are designed to operate in the "valve down" or "inverted" position and do not utilize a dip tube. This is because it is difficult to redisperse drug particles that sediment or float in a narrow tube. In addition, the valve must contain the pressurized product and retard the ingress of moisture or oxygen.

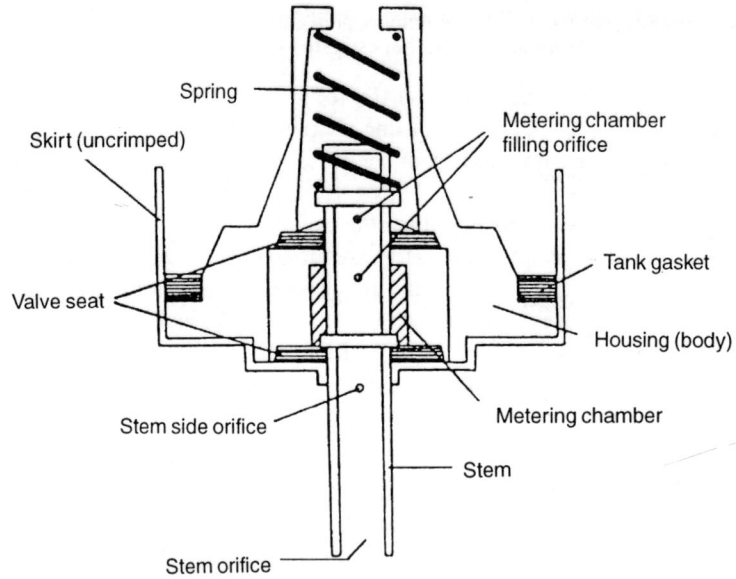

Fig 6.12 : Schematic diagram of a metering valve

Most valve bodies are constructed from plastics and resins, although metal body valves do exist. An aluminum ferule allows the valve skirt to be crimped on the canister. Return springs are usually stainless steel. Valves contain elastomeric seals in the metering chamber, and between the canister and the valve. Elastomer composition is frequently proprietary, and sometimes unknown to even the valve manufacturer. Low concentrations of several potentially harmful chemicals are known to be extracted from valve elastomers by propellant systems (Sethi et al, 1992). This has led to the use of elastomer extraction procedures to reduce the concentration of these materials prior to valve assembly and in the development of "cleaner" elastomers. Elastomer performance is critical to the functioning of a valve, since in combination with other factors, it determines the propellant leakage rate, metering reproducibility, and the speed and reliability of stem return following actuation. Limited elastomer swelling may be considered beneficial since it helps ensure a good seal. However, excessive swelling results in a nonfunctional valve. For this reason, the advent of new propellant systems has necessitated the development of new elastomers.

The actuator is frequently the most visible part of the MDI. Its function is to make actuation of the valve easier, direct the spray into the patient's mouth, and provide the orifice through which the metering valve discharges its spray. A well-designed actuator with a separate or integral (to prevent loss or accidental inhalation) dust cap protects the valve stem from damage and keeps it aligned with the seat. This prevents the accumulation and subsequent inhalation of dust, and provides a place for patient use information and product identity. The spray orifice and valve stem seat are arguably the most critical parts of the actuator. Larger spray orifices are often used in combination with large volume metering valves to spray concentrated suspensions with a minimized likelihood of blockage. Large orifices ensure fast emptying. When small volumes of dilute solutions and suspensions are sprayed, smaller spray orifice diameters may be preferred since they generate smaller droplets (Clark, 1994). To avoid leakage, a tight fit between valve stem and actuator seat is essential. Additionally, it is essential to minimize sharp turns and blind ends in the path the product follows from the valve stem to the spray orifice to prevent accumulation, and subsequent blockage, by nonvolatile drug and excipients.

With the exception of Rhone-Poulenc Rorer's Azmacort (Collegeville, PA), and Astra's Breathancer (Lund, Sweden), all MDIs are supplied with a molded plastic actuator, which positions the patient's lips very close to the spray orifice (if they use th closed-mouth method of inhaler use). This provides a short distance between the spray orifice and oropharynx and necessitates excellent coordination between actuation of the MDI and inhalation by the patient if almost complete oropharyngeal deposition is to be avoided. Spacer devices (Fig 6.13) were developed to increase this distance, allowing the rapidly advancing aerosol cloud to decelerate before reaching the throat (Byron, 1990). This makes perfect synchronization between actuation and inhalation slightly less important.

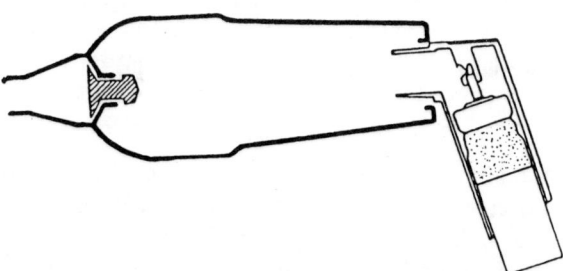

Fig 6.13: Schematic diagram of a metered dose inhaler and reservoir device (Nebuhaler).

In addition, spacers allow more time for propellant evaporation, resulting in the formation of smaller droplets or particles and less reflex coughing and exhalation due to local cooling of the throat by impacted, evaporating droplets. A large proportion of drug that would otherwise deposit in the oropharynx is retained in a spacer. This reduces systemic drug levels and minimizes local side effects. A distinction between spacers and holding chambers (also called reservoirs) is increasingly drawn. Spacers are essentially hollow tubes through which a patient should have started inhaling prior to actuating the MDI. They are designed to empty in a single inhalation. Reservoirs are typically larger in diameter, frequently conical or pear-shaped devices, and are designed to permit actuation of the MDI prior to initiating an inhalation. Their larger size is designed to reduce drug losses on the interior wall of the reservoir due to impaction and sedimentation. Reservoirs usually contain a one-way valve to prevent an inadvertent exhalation from flushing a previously aerosolized dose from the device. Delays between actuation and inhalation, making multiple actuations in the reservoir, and emptying the reservoir over several inhalations all reduce the efficiency of aerosols delivery to the lung.

Because larger spacers and reservoirs more effectively enhance lung delivery compared to smaller ones, collapsible designs are coµmon (e.g., Inspirease, Schering Corporation, Kenilworth, NJ). Other designs direct the emerging aerosol spray in the opposite direction to the inhaled airstream in an attempt to increase the flight time while minimizing device size (Opti-Haler, Healthscan Products, Cedar Grove, NJ). Spacers and reservoirs may also contain flow restrictors to control the patient's inhalation rate and have mechanisms to coordinate inhalation with MDI actuation (OptiHaler). Many audibly warn the patient when they are inhaling too fast [Aerosol Cloud Enhancer (ACE), DHD Diemolding Healthcare Division, Canastota, NY; Aerochamber, Monoghan Medical Corporation, Plattsburgh, NY; Inspirease]. Newer devices are typically transparent to encourage regular cleaning and some are designed to fit into ventilator circuits. Baffles located within several small actuators have been shown to yield many of the same advantage (Bryon et al, 1989). Because spacers and reservoirs are often designed to fit multiple MDIs (which may have significantly different compositions, valves, and actuators), their ability to equally enhance the delivery of all products has been questioned.

The Autohaler (3M Pharmaceuticals, St. Paul, MN) is a small device that uses a mechanical vane to detect when a patient's inhalation rate is appropriate for automatically firing the proprietary MDI it contains.

While achieving excellent coordination between inhalation and actuation, it does not produce the other advantages associated with a spacer or reservoir. MDIs from other manufacturers can not be used in the Autohaler. Electronic devices capable of more sophisticated flow monitoring by programming actuation at different flow rates or points in the breathing cycle, and which can record the history of patient compliance, are under development.

6.4.2 Dry powder inhalers

Dry powder inhalers offer a unique opportunity for the delivery of drugs to the lung as aerosols. These devices combine powder technology with device design in order to disperse dry particles as an aerosol in the patient's inspiratory airflow (Ganderton and Kassem,1992). Powders have been insufflated for medical purposes throughout history (Morley et al,1981). It is only recently that efforts have been made to establish the dispersion properties of particles and their impact on therapeutic effect . A great deal of progress has been made in recent years as the emphasis has changed from unit dose systems employing only the patient's breath to generate the aerosol, to multiple-dosing reservoir devices that actively impart energy to the powder bed to introduce drug particles into the inspiratory airflow.

All DPIs have four basic features: (1) a dose-metering mechanism, (2) an aerosolization mechanism, (3) a deaggregation mechanism, and (4) an adaptor to direct the aerosol into a patient's mouth. The major components of a dry powder inhaler are the drug powder, and other powdered excipients where necessary, a drug reservoir or premetered individual doses, the body of the device, and a cover to prevent ingress of dust or moisture.

To introduce drug particles into the lung, they must be < 5μm in aerodynamic diameter (Gonda, 1990). This is generally achieved by milling the powder prior to formulation. In recent years there has also been some interest in spray drying powders to achieve the same end (Pillai et al,1994). Small particles are notoriously difficult to disperse (Hickey et al,1994). The forces governing dispersion are well documented and consist mainly of electrostatic, Van der Walls, and capillary forces (Rietema, 1991). Knowing that these forces exist has not facilitated aerosol generation to any great extent. One approach that has been taken to improve the dispersion of dry powders is the inclusion of an excipient, notably lactose (Byron, 1990). The lactose particles are intended to act as carrier particles for the drug and as such are in a much larger size range, 60-80 μm (Bell et al,1971). Drug particles are theoretically stripped from the surface of the lactose particlés, to which they are loosely attached, during the generation process (Ganderton, 1992). This process is illustrated schematically in (Fig 6.14).

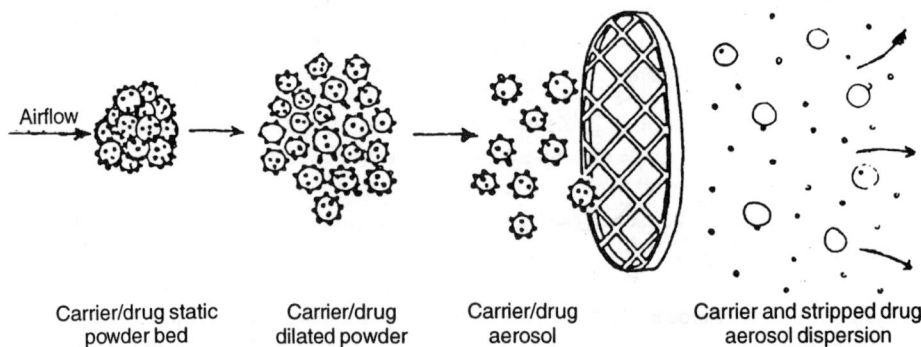

| Carrier/drug static powder bed | Carrier/drug dilated powder | Carrier/drug aerosol | Carrier and stripped drug aerosol dispersion |

Fig 6.14 : Schematic diagram of the stripping of drug particles from carrier particles on the inhaled airstream.

The DPIs currently available, the driving forces governing new designs, and the claimed advantages of DPIs in the development pipeline have been recently reviewed (Ashurst et al., 2000).

DEVICES : In the devices that have been approved for use in the United States, the Spinhaler (Fisons, Rochester, NY) and Rotahaler (Glaxo Wellcome, Inc., Research Triangle Park, NC) unit doses of Intal (disodium cromoglycate) and Ventolin (albuterol sulfate), respectively, are packaged in hard gelatin capsules. The dose of powder itself is delivered from the gelatin capsule by different mechanisms. The Spinhaler has a mechanism for piercing the capsule (Hickey, 1992). The cap of the capsule fits into an impeller, which rotates as the patient breathes through the device projecting particles into the airstream, as illustrated in (Fig 6.15).

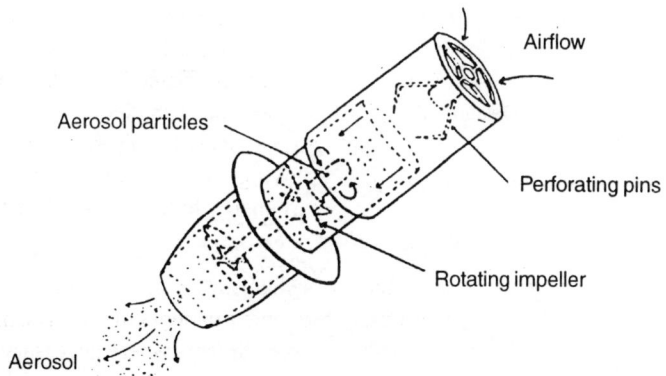

Fig 6.15: Diagram indicating the essential components of a Spinhaler.

The Rotahaler, shown in (Fig 6.16), has a mechanism for breaking the capsule in two pieces. The capsule body containing the dose falls into the device, while the cap is retained in the entry port for subsequent disposal. As the patient inhales the portion of the capsule containing the drug experiences erratic motion in the airstream, causing dislodged particles to be entrained and subsequently inhaled.

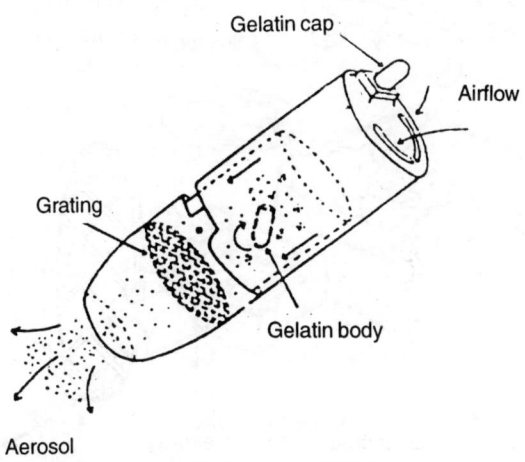

Fig 6.16 : Diagram indicating the essential components of a Rotahaler.

A number of other devices are approved for use in other countries. The Inhalator (Boehringer Ingelheim, Ridgefield, CT) has a mechanism for piercing the ends of a hard gelation capsule containing the dose of fenoterol, (Ribiero and Wiren, 1990) as shown in (Figure 6.17). The inspiratory flow then passes through the capsule. The Diskhaler (Glaxo Wellcome, Inc., Research Triangle Park, NC), shown in (Figure 6.18), employs packaging consisting of individual doses of albuterol sulfate in blister packs on a disk cassette. Following piercing, inspiratory flow through the packaging depression containing the drug induces dispersion of the powder. One of the more sophisticated systems approved for use in Europe is the Turbuhaler (Astra Pharmaceuticals, Lund, Sweden), shown in (Figure 6.19) (Wetterlin et al, 1988). This device employs a multidose reservoir of terbutaline sulfate. The dose is metered into small conical cavities by twisting a grip at the base of the device. When the patient inhales, air ducted through the cavities dislodges a dose of drug.

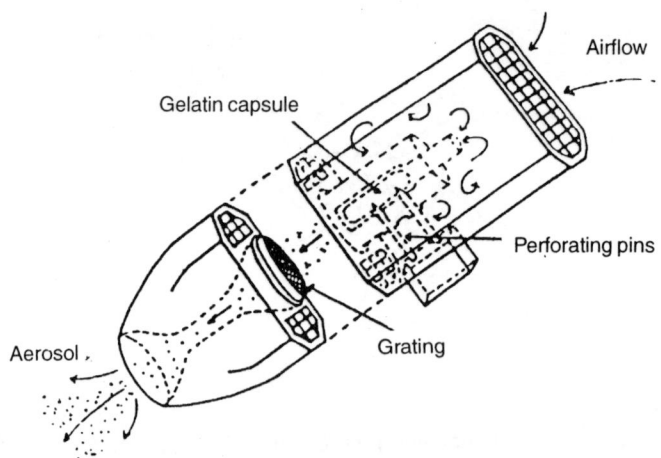

Fig 6.17 : Diagram indicating the essential components of an Inhalator.

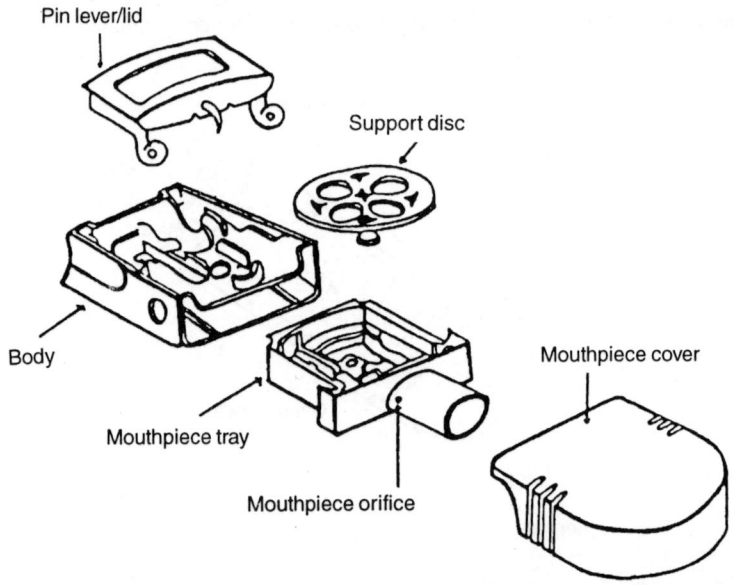

Fig 6.18: Diagram indicating the essential components of a Diskhaler

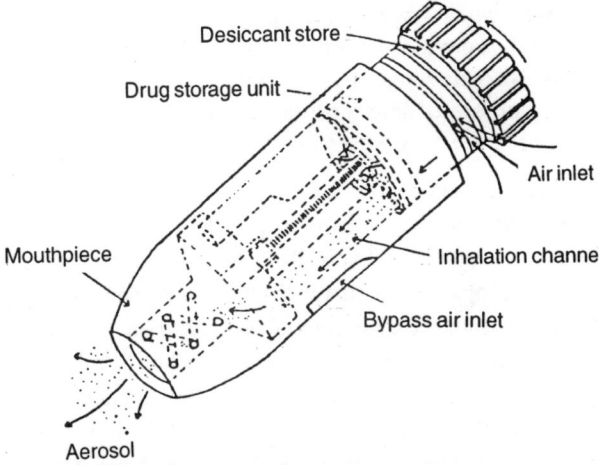

Fig 6.19: Diagram indicating the essential components of a Turbuhaler.

In addition to the devices mentioned above, many others are patented for use are described in the literature (though none have so far received regulatory approval in the United States). However, the novelty of these systems is typically associated with their mechanism for aerosolizing the powder rather than the way a unit dose is packaged or separated from a bulk reservoir. Reproducible dose metering remains the most difficult challenge in device design. For this reason, prefilled doses in gelatin capsules or multiple depression blister packages, or extraction of a specified volume of free flowing powder from a multi-dose reservoir are likely to remain common. The volumetric metering of powder poses some unique problems since powder flow and dispersion behavior is complex (Van Cleef, 1991). There are many factors related to the powder itself that influence the clinical effect of the product. Particle size is of primary importance in defining the location of lung deposition of aerosols and hence their effectiveness (Curry et al,1974). Metering and dispersion characteristics are affected not only by particle size, but also by rugosity (Whitham and Eagle, 1994), shape (Mullin et al, 1992) moisture content (Kontny et al,1994), surface chemical composition (Al-Chalabi et al,1990), and charge (Hickey, 1994). Reported exceptions to the above metering mechanisms are the Easyhaler, which has a rachet metering system to remove discrete doses from a powder bed (Vidgren et al,1991), as shown in Fig 6.20., Fig 6.21

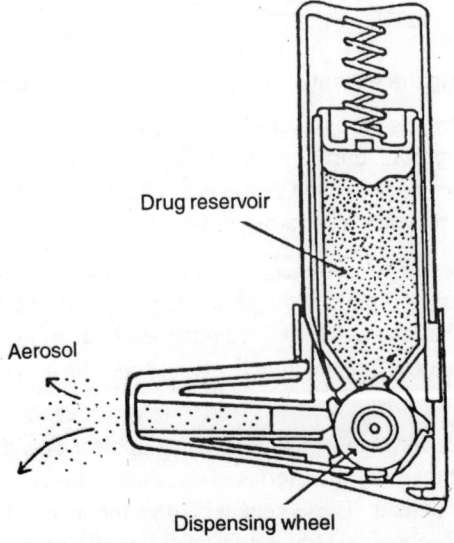

Fig 6.20: Diagram indicating the essential components of an Easyhaler.

illustrates a rotary planar device, which has a compact powder bed from which a helical blade removes a dose of drug (Wolff and Niven,1994). A device that involves dislodging powder from a specific length of dimpled tape (Anonymous, 1994) has also been suggested. To protect the drug reservoir from aggregation or chemical degradation, a desiccant is incorporated into most devices that contain bulk drug, rather than individually protected doses. Safeguards are necessary to ensure that the desiccant cannot be inhaled.

All dry powders require a mechanism to disperse the drug as an aerosol. For example, the Bernoulli, or Venturi effect has received some attention (Cheng et al,1989), as has compressed gas propulsion (Jager-Waldau et al,1994). Large, excipient particles (typically lactose), to which drug is loosely bound, are used to aid dispersion. Their improved flow properties compared to cohesive powder beds of smaller particles allow easier separation of individual particles into the airstream. Most devices have additional, mechanical methods of introducing energy into the powder bed to facilitate dispersion. The Spinhaler has an impeller that rotates to aid dispersion. Clearly, the rotation speed will vary according to patient effort (airflow rate) and through the breathing cycle (Clark and Eagan, 1994). The Rotahaler to some extent employs rotation as a means of dispersion since the capsule containing drug rotates, albeit erratically, in the device (Pederson, 1986). The Inhalator is based on the principle that a large volume of air will pass through the powder bed by inducing a large pressure

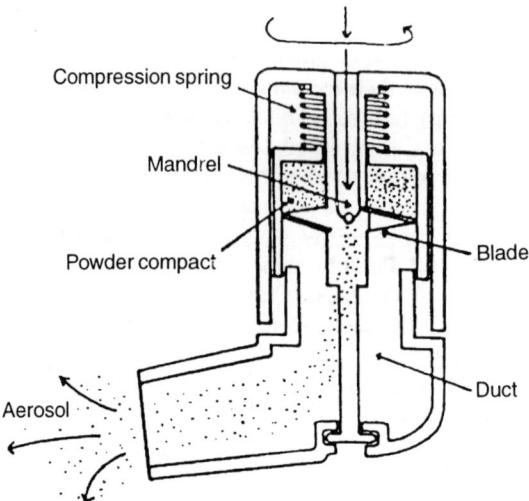

Fig 6.21: Diagram indicating the essential components of a rotary planar device

drop across the capsule. This pressure drop is brought about by the patient's inspiratory flow. Consequently, the patient's inspiratory effort and inspiratory duration may influence aerosol generation (Pederson and Steffenson, 1986). The Diskhaler (Spiro et al, 1992) and Turbuhaler (Pederson, 1994) also employ a pressure drop to introduce drug particles into the patient's inspiratory flow.

Novel approaches have been suggested to put energy into the powder bed for dispersion. Increased dose delivery has been achieved by tapping a dimple in the packaging material or by using compressed gases to assist in the generation of powder (Schultz et al,1992). Two other methods of note involve the continuous input of energy. One method employs a small motor and impeller to disperse the powder (Hill, 1994). A second method utilizes a gas-assisted approach .

The mouthpiece can simply be a tube through which the patient inhales, as is the case with the majority of dry powder inhalers. The Turbuhaler, however, has a series of tortuous channels through which the aerosol passes before entering the mouth of the patient. These channels offer the advantage that poorly dispersed particles will either impact in transit and become reentrained as smaller particles, or be permanently removed from the airstream. Provided dose uniformity is maintained, either of these options is desirable. Impaction followed by reentrainment helps ensure the correct particle size for lung deposition, while permanent impaction will remove particles destined to deposit in the mouth or throat of the patient. The induction of turbulent flow in narrow tubes is also associated with enhanced deaggregation. However, narrow tubes may produce a high resistance device through which patients may find it difficult to breath.

It has been demonstrated that, the material that the drug powders comes into contact with during processing have a significant impact on its electrostatic properties (Staniforth, 1994). Indeed, these acquired properties may influence their subsequent interaction with construction material present in the device. In extreme cases drug powders may fail to leave the device. With a growing acceptability of refillable devices, the appearance of metal devices or those composed of conductive plastics would not be surprising.

The internal geometry of the device is of great importance to the generation of the aerosol. The dimensions of the channels through which the inspired airflow passes dictate the pressure drop across the device. Accumulation of the drug particles is often associated with severe changes in the direction of the airflow. In addition device design determines whether the dose will empty as a bolus or as a continuous stream of powder over course of an entire inhalation. This has implications both for the ultimate location of drug deposition within the lung and for defining the flow rate at which the device should be tested.

6.4.3 Nebulizers

There are two coµmon types of nebulizers, air-jet and ultrasonic, with numerous coµmercially available examples of each type. The operation of an air-jet nebulizer requires an external gas supply (usually compressed air or oxygen). This gas supply is the driving force for liquid atomization. Figure 6.22 shows the typical component of the air-jet nebulizing device.

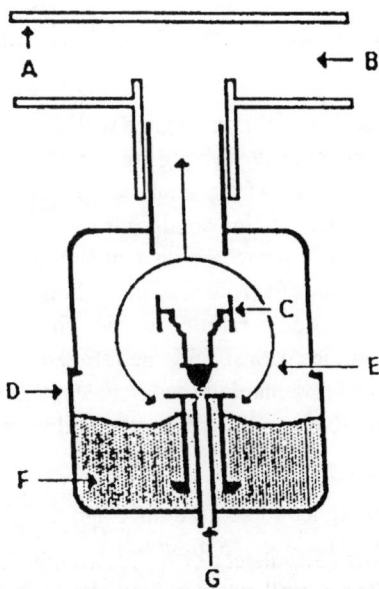

Fig 6.22 : Schematic of a typical air-jet nebulizers. (A) "t" piece; (B) dilution or makeup air (xL/min); (C) baffle; (D) reservoir; (E) recirculating droplets; (F) respiratory solution or suspension; (G) compressed gas (yL/min).

Respiratory solutions and suspensions are placed in the reservoir. Minimization of the "dead volume" (solution that will not exit the nebulizer) is of critical importance since dose volumes of 1 to 3 ml are typical, while dead volumes of 0.5 to 2 ml or more have been reported (Kendrick et al, 1995). This accounts for the conical designs of many reservoirs. Compressed gas is forced through the jet, causing a region of negative pressure to develop as the gas is expelled at high velocity through the spray orifice. This low pressure, aided by capillary action, causes the solution to travel up channels parallel to the gas supply tube where it becomes entrained in the gas stream and is sheared into a liquid film. The film is unstable and collapses under surface tension to form droplets. The larger droplets (50-500 μm in diameter) return to the reservoir to be re-circulated. This is achieved by placing a baffle or the reservoir wall in the path of the air-liquid stream to induce droplet impaction and coalescence. This accounts for the majority of the nebulized solution. It is important to minimize the internal surface area of the nebulizing chamber since a large percentage of the filled volume can adhere to the wall and be unavailable for the re-circulation. The smaller droplets (1-10 μm in diameter) that escape impaction on the baffle leave the nebulizer through a connecting "t" piece carried by the nebulizing air flow out of the nebulizer (Nerbrink et al,1994). The separation between the spray nozzle and the baffle, and the droplet exit velocity from the nozzle, are of primary importance in defining the size of droplets that escape impaction. The "t" piece allows for the introduction of dilution or 'make-up' air and provides a place to attach auxiliary tubing, facemasks, or mouth pieces, which aid in diverting the aerosol to the patient. The use of dry compressed nebulizing gases and make-up air accelerates droplet evaporation, aiding in reducing the droplet size. In some nebulizers, a large evaporation chamber further enhances the droplet drying. Evaporation also extracts heat from the recirculating droplets causing solution remaining in the reservoir to cool (a drop of approximately 5-9°C from the initial temperature). Solvent losses due to evaporation cause solution remaining in the reservoir to concentrate (Phipps and Gonda, 1990). This increase in concentration can potentially lead to drug or excipient crystallization within the reservoir, which could theoretically clog the nebulizing air jets and reduce the total aerosolized output of drug. In most situations crystallization dose not occur since reservoir fill volumes are small and rapidly exhausted, and drugs are typically hydrophilic and exhibit high solubility (Mercer et. al.,1968). However, it has been reported that increase in solution concentration may change the total output and output rate of aerosolized drug, as well as influence the equilibrium droplet size of the aerosol (Clay et al,1983).

The major controllable operating variable associated with air-jet nebulizers is the airflow rate through the nebulizers which is critically dependent on the driving pressure, except when the spray orifice acts as a critical orifice. Since most nebulizers are operated from small compressors that do not permit selection of specific driving pressures or flow rates, the nebulization conditions are usually not well defined. Additionally, many marketed compressors for domicilary use are incapable of attaining adequate pressures or flow rates to produce an aerosol from demanding air-jet nebulizers (Newman and Pallow, 1987). These problems are compounded by a lack of manufacturer-supplied specific operating condition for most nebulizers and have led to the recent trend of approving respiratory solutions with specific nebulizers/compressor combinations, as in the case of rhDNase. Other variables, such as relative humidity, ambient temperature, and inspiratory flow rate, are known to influence nebulizer performance, but are difficult to standardize under patient use conditions.

Air-jet systems are further subdivided into 'single-use' and 'multi-use' categories. Most marketed nebulizers fall into the single-use category designed to be used once and then discarded, and as such are molded from inexpensive plastics at high speed. However, to minimize costs, patients typically reuse these devices even though it is unclear to what extent a nebulizer can be considered reliable if reused (Childs and Dezateux, 1991). One study reported that patients reuse a disposable air-jet nebulizer in excess of 100 times before obtaining a new one (Allen et al,1994). Recently, nebulizer manufacturers have introduced multi-use nebulizers, which are designed for repeated use and are easy to clean and assemble reproducibly. This is significant because cleaning regimens, manufacturer specified or otherwise, and alterations in baffle or capillary feed tube position within the nebulizer have been reported to significantly alter nebulizer output characteristics (Caldwell and Milroy,1995). Other innovations include the development of dose-sparing mechanisms such as interrupters, which manually or automatically block airflow to the nebulizer, and therefore aerosol generation, during patient exhalation. This increases the total inhaled dose received by patient. Other designs divert the inspiratory airflow of the patient through the nebulizer, to enhance the volume of air available to entrain aerosolized droplets, or use valves in the mouthpiece to prevent exhaled air from passing through the nebulizer and carrying the aerosol to waste. Yet another modification collects aerosol generated during exhalation in a rubber balloon. Droplets in the balloon augment newly generated droplets during the next inhalation. While in most nebulizer systems, droplets are unlikely to evaporate to dryness prior to inhalation, systems employing dilution air and producing small droplets may have their equilibrium size limited by concentration of solutes in the initial respiratory solution, rather than the evaporation rate of the droplets. Air-jet nebulizers are known to be capable of successfully delivering respiratory suspensions (Leflein et al,1995).

Unlike the air-jet devices, an external gas supply is not required for operation of electrically or battery driven ultrasonic nebulizers. Fig 6.23 shows the typical components of an ultrasonic nebulizing device. Respiratory solution or suspension is atomized by means of a piezoelectric crystal transducer. An alternating current causes the shape of the crystal to alternately shrink and expand, causing a vibration that is amplified by a stainless steel shim. This vibration is then transferred to the solution or suspension in the nebulizer reservoirs. Two mechanisms have been proposed to explain how these oscillatory waves travelling through the bulk liquid generate an aerosol cloud. The first mechanism (Figure 6.24A) proposes that the crystal transducer, operating at a low frequency, vibrate the bulk liquid causing the formation of cavitation bubbles. As air bubbles, which have a short life span, rise toward the air-liquid interface, the internal pressure of the cavitation bubbles equilibrates with the atmosphere, causing the bubbles to implode. As the bubble bursts at the air-liquid surface, portions of the bulk liquid break free from the turbulent bulk liquid and form droplets. The second mechanism (Figure 6.24B) involves high frequency crystal vibration causing formation of capillary waves in the bulk liquid. The capillary waves constructively interfere to form peaks and a central geyser. The geyser increases in amplitude until it becomes unstable under the influence of continuing excitatory vibrations, and portions of the peak break loose from the bulk liquid and are rejected into the air as droplets (Boucher and Kreuter,1968).

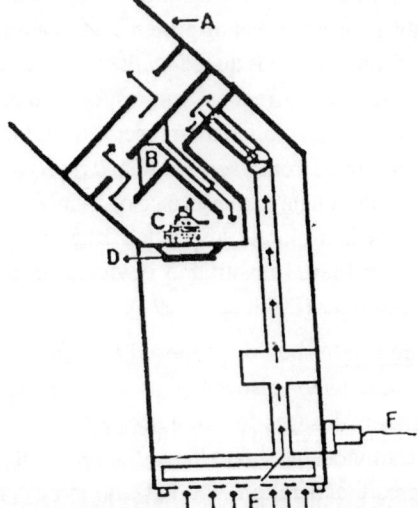

Fig 6.23 : Schematic of a typical ultrasonic nebulizer (A) Face mask or mouthpiece; (B) baffles; (C) geyser of respiratory solution or suspension; (D) piezoelectric crystal; (E) internal fan; (F) battery or electrical source.

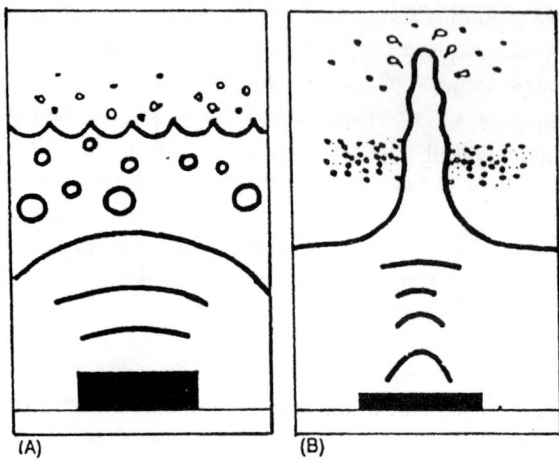

(A)   (B)

Fig 6.24 : Proposed ultrasonic nebulizer aerosolization mechanisms.
(A) Cavitation bubble formation at low frequency;
(B) Capillary wave formation at high frequency.

Regardless of the mechanism, once liquid breaks free from the bulk liquid and forms a droplet cloud, larger droplets either impact on baffles or return to the reservoir surface under the influence of gravity, to be re-circulated. Smaller droplets leave the nebulizer aided by an internal fan. Fan speed and adjustable flow restrictors can alter the air velocity over the reservoir surface, influencing both the droplet size and aerosol output rate. The reduced volume of dilution air compared to that passing through an air-jet nebulizer results in a more concentrated aerosol cloud with less evaporative capacity. What evaporative cooling does occur is more than offset by heat conducted to the reservoir from the vibratory system. This heat results from frictional forces induced by movement of the transducing crystal. The increased reservoir temperature has not been associated with altered aerosolization characteristics over short nebulization intervals (Niven et al, 1995). However, heating may be detrimental to thermolabile formulations of proteins and cause odor changes in antibiotic solutions (Dennis et al, 1992). Excessive heating can be reduced by the presence of substantive heat sinks and sensory feedback systems that reduce the oscillation frequency in response to higher temperatures. Such systems can automatically turn off nebulizers that have emptied their reservoirs. Other systems under development include multiple-dose nebulizers that are atomized from a self-contained reservoir for inhalation in a single breath. This can be achieved by dropping drug solution on to the surface of a vibrating platform or through a vibrating grid. Ultrasonic nebulizers do not reliably incorporate suspended drug particles into the aerosolized droplets they produce and may therefore be considered unsuitable devices for aerosolizing respiratory suspensions, microspheres, and other colloidal systems (Dahlback, 1994).

Unlike MDIs and DPIs, there are established or proposed USP functionality standards to characterize the nebulized output of a respiratory solution or suspension used in combination with a nebulizer. By anology to testing prescribed for other inhalation dosages forms, it seems appropriate to develop methods and agree on specifications for nebulizers. It is obviously vital to know the dead volume, quantity of aerosol emitted from the nebulizer, the duration of aerosol generation, and have an indication of the aerosol size or fine droplet fraction. Standardization of the methods necessary to perform these tests would represent substantial steps in the future utilization and development of nebulizers.

6.5 THERAPEUTIC APPLICATION OF AEROSOL

At present the main uses of aerosols designed for delivery of medications to the lungs are the iμmediate and prophylactic treatment of asthma and chronic irreversible obstructive lung diseases. In addition to these diseases the value of lung aerosol medications for cystic fibrosis and pulmonary infection has been demonstrated. Specific drugs used for pulmonary drug delivery include:

1. For asthma :

    I) β-adrenergic agents (e.g. salbutamol, terbutaline, ephedrine, albuterol etc.).

    II) Anticholinergics (e.g. ipratropium bromide).

    III) Steroids and other anti-inflammatory agents (e.g. beclomethasone, dexamethasone, budesonide, cromolyn and nedocromil sodium)

2. Pulmonary infections : (Legionnaires's disease and pulmonary aspergillosis)

    I) Antibiotics (e.g. tobramycin, amikacin sulphate, erythromicin and amphotericin B etc.)

    II) Antibacterial agents (e.g. ciprofloxacin, ofloxacin).

3. For chornic obstructive pulmonary diseases :

    I) Anticholinergic agents

    II) β_2-adrenergic agents

    III) Corticosteroids

    IV) Antiproteases (e.g. a1-antitrypsin)

    V) Mucolytics (e.g. iodine)

    VI) Cystine derivatives (e.g. acetylevestein)

4. Cardiovascular agents

    I) Antianginal agents (e.g. nitroglycerine)

    II) Antihypertensives (e.g. nifedipine)

5. Blood glucose modifiers

    I) Antidiabetics (e.g. insulin)

    II) Hyperglycemic agents (e.g. glucagoan)

6. Hormones

    I) Antidiuretic hormone (e.g. desmopressin)

    II) Gonadotropine releasing hormone

    III) Growth hormone releasing hormone

    IV) Leutinizing hormone (female contraception)

    V) Premenstrual tension formulations (e.g. progesterone, vasopressin)

    VI) Memory enhancers

7. Antidotes

8. Antivirals (e.g. rebaverin, zenamivir etc.)

9. Anti histaminics (low dose)

10. Immunizing agents (e.g. Measles vaccine)

11. Cystic fibrosis (e.g. antibiotics)

12. Gene therapy (e.g. specific vectors viz., Non-infective adenovirus)

Drugs, which are in active research for pulmonary delivery, are insulin (Inoue Yoshioka,1999) and insulin - DL lactide/glycolide co-polymer (PLGA) nanospheres to prolong hypoglycemic effect (Kawashima et al,1999), anti-cancer agents such as camptothecin, all trans retinoic acid, interleukin-II etc. (in liposomal carrier or alone)

(Koshkina et al,1999;Parthasarthy et al,1999 & Khanna et al,1997), antiviral drugs such as zenamivir etc (Cass et.al.,1999), glucocorticoids for pulmonary inflaµmations (Saari et al,1998 & Suntres and Sheck.,1998), gene delivery (Barron et al,1999), analgesics for patient controlled analgesia (Mather et al,1998 & Ward et al,1997), vaccines (LiCalsi et al, 1999) etc.

Schreier et al (1993) presented an overview of current data on pulmonary delivery of liposomes, including fate of aerosols in the respiratory tract, physico-chemical characterization of liposome aerosols, their therapeutic applications, pulmonary fate and kinetics and pulmonary safety. Pulmonary deposition and kinetics of drugs delivered via liposome aerosols and targetting strategies to deliver the drugs selectively to infected or impaired phagocytic and non-phagocytic cells in the lung were outlined.

A review (Taylor & Farr, 1993) of pulmonary delivery of liposomes including devices for liposome administration, fate of liposomes in the lungs following pulmonary administration and modification of pharmacokinetics of drugs entrapped in pulmonary deposited liposomes was presented. Schreier (1994) concluded that liposomes are a promising innocuous aerosol delivery system for drugs to achieve prolonged localized drug concentrations in the lung or intracellular drug targeting to alveolar macrophages.

6.6 FUTURE DEVELOPMENTS

Next-generation devices will probably include features that indicate how many doses remain to be inhaled or when a dose is due. They could easily measure and record the flow rate and inspired volume under which doses were inhaled, as an aid to monitoring disease progression or patient compliance. Devices that will actuate a pressurized MDI at a specific point in the breathing cycle if preset parameters are achieved already exist. Single use DPIs are under development.

Beyond these innovations, new methods of aerosol generations are likely to be developed or existing ones miniaturized to clinically useful sizes. One can easily envisage hybrids of MDIs and ultrasonic nebulizers, in which large propellant droplets are broken into more respirable sizes by impaction on a vibrating transducer or grid, rather than simply being wasted within the actuator. MDI valve stems could be trapsiently heated iµmediately before actuation to expel droplets at higher pressures and facilitate faster evaporation, without causing drug degradation. Manual pumps capable .of generating respirable sprays from aqueous solutions are closer to reality every year. Dry powders could be de-aggregated by vibrational elements, rather than relying on turbulent airstream, or generated electrostatically. Inhalers employing environmentally acceptable supercritical solvents to dissolve and atomize drugs at enormous pressures have already been described in the patent literature (Sievers et al, 1994). These opportunities, combined with the increasingly precise identification of pulmonary target regions, the prevalence of respiratory disease and a continuing need for a viable delivery system for potent biotechnologically derived drugs are likely to drive development of inhalation systems into the current century. Localized therapy in the lung will be improved by a rationale design of new drug entities or effective formulations of currently available drugs. The role of the lung as route for systemic delivery of a variety of drugs, such as, proteins and peptides has to be realized. Recently Davis (1999) reviewed the delivery of peptide and non-peptide drugs through the respiratory tract and made a comparison between nasal and pulmonary delivery. Current limitations and future directions for the development of these cell lines as models of the airway epithelium are also discussed.

REFERENCES

Al-Chalabi, S.A.M.; Jones, A.R. and Lukckham, P.F. (1990) "A simple method for improving the dispersability of micron-sized solid spheres." J Aerosol Sci. 21:821.

Allen, T.L.; Dalby, R.N. and McPherson, M.L. (1994) "Evaluation of patient nebulizer use, measurement of nebulizer flow rate and output." Poster presented at the American Pharmaceutical Association Annual Meeting, Orlando, FL.

American Thoracic Society (1987) "Standardization of spirometry 1987 update: statement of the American Thoracic Society." Am Rev Respir Dis. 136:1285

Andersson, P. and Ryrfeldt, A. (1984) "Biotransformation of the topical glucocorticoids budesonide and beclomethasone 17a,21-dipropionate in human liver and lung homogenate." J Pharm Pharmacol. 36:763.

Anonymous, (1992) "Dry powder inhalers-the shape of things to come?" Pharm J. 248:816.

Ashurst, I.; Malton, A.; Prime, D. and Sumby, B. (2000) "Latest advances in the development of dry powder inhalers, Pharm. Tech. & Sci. Today, 3(7), 246-256

Atkins, P.J. (1990) "The development of new solution metered dose inhaler delivery systems." Proceeding of the Second Annual Respiratory Drug Delivery Symposium, University of Kentucky College of Pharmacy. 416.

Atkins, P. J. (1991) "The development of new solution metered dose inhaler delivery systems." In Dalby R.N, Evans R. (eds.) Proceedings of the Second Annual Respiratory Drug Delivery Symposium. Continuing Pharmacy Education, University of Kentuky, Lexington, pp. 416.

Bair, W.J. (1991) "Overview of ICRP respiratory tract model". Rad Prot Dos. 38:147.

Barron, L.G.; Gagne, L. ; Szoka, F.C Jr. (1999) "Lipoplex-mediated gene delivery to the lung occurs whithin 60 minutes of intravenous administration." Hum. Gene Ther. 10 : 1683.

Beeknams, J.M. (1965) "The deposition of aerosols in the respiratory tract." Can J Physiol Pharmacol. 43:157.

Bell, J.H.; Hartley, P.S. and Cox, J.S.G. (1971) Dry powder aerosols. I. "A new powder inhalation device. Pharm Sci." 60:1559.

Ben- Jebria, A.; Chen, D.; Langer, R. and Edwards, D.A. (1999) "Large porous particles for sustained protection from carbochol induced bronchoconstriction in guinea pig." Pharm Res. 16:555.

Boucher, R.M.G.; Kreuter, J.; (1968) "The fundamentals of the ultrasonic atomization of medicated solutions." Ann Allergy .26:591.

Bowden, D.H. (1981) "Alveolar response to injury." Thorax . 36:801.

Brown, C.E. (1931) "Quantitative measurements of the inhalation, retention, and exhalation of dusts and fumes by man:II. Concentration below 50 mg per cubic meter." J Ind Hyg Toxicol. 13:285.

Bryon, P.R.; Dalby, R.N. and Hickey, A.J. (1989) "Optimized inhalation aerosols. I. The effects of spherical baffle size and position upon the output of several pressurized nonaqueous suspension formulation." Pharm Res .6:225.

Byron, P.R. and Jashnani, R. (1990) "Efficiency of aerosolization from dry powder blends of terbutaline sufate and lactose NF with different particle size distributions." Pharm Res . 7::881.

Byron, P.R. (1990) "Aerosol formulation, generation and delivery using metered systems." In Byron P.R. (ed.) Respiratory Drug Delivery. Boca Raton, FL:CRC Press, pp. 167.

Caldwell, N.A. and Milroy, R. (1995) "Optimizing nebulization practice within a large teaching hospital: easier said than done." Respir Med. 89:57.

Cass, L.M.; Brown, J.; Pickford, M.; Fayinka, S.; Newman, S.P.; Johansson, C.J. and Bye, A. (1999) "Pharmacoscintigraphic evaluation of lung deposition of inhaled zanamivir in healthy volunteers." Clin Pharmacokinet. 36 1:21.

Chang, H.K. and El Masry,; O.A. (1982) "A model study of flow dynamics in human central airways." Part I: Axial velocity profiles. Respir Physiol.. 49:75.

Chen, R.Y. (1978) "Deposition of charged particles in tubes." J Aerosol Sci. 9:449.

Chen, Y.K. and Yu, C.P. (1993) "Particle deposition from duct flows by combined mechanisms." Aerosol Sci Tech. 19: 389.

Cheng, Y.; Barr, E.B. and Yeh, H.C. (1989) "A Venturi disperser as a dry powder generator for inhalation studies." Inhal Toxicol .1:365.

Cheng, Y-S.; Yeh, H-C. and Swift, D.L. (1991) In: Walton WH, ed. "Aerosol deposition in human nasal airway for particles 1 nm to 20 μm: a model study." Rad Prot Dos. 38:41.

Childs, H.J. and Dezateux, C.A. (1991) A national survey of nebulizer use. Arch Dis Child. 66:1351.

Chinard, F.P.; Enns, T. and Nolan, M.F. (1962) "The permeability characteristics of the alveolar capillary barrier." Trans Assoc Am Physicians. 75:253.

Clark, A.R. (1994) "The physics of aerosol formation by MDIs-limitations of the current approach." J Biopharm Sci. 3:69.

Clay, M.; Pavia, D.; Newman S.P. and Clarke S.W. (1983) "Factors influencing the size distribution of aerosols from jet nebulizers." Thorax. 29:66.

Crimini, N.; Palermo, F.; Pliveri, R.; Polosa, R.; Settiniere, I. and Mistretta, A. (1992) "Protective effects of inhaled ipratropium bromide on bronchoconstriction induced by adenosine and methacholine in asthma." Eur Respir J. 5: 560.

Clark, A.R. and Egan, M. (1994) "Modelling the deposition of inhaled powdered drug aerosols." J Aerosol Sci. ;25:175.

Curry, A.H.; Taylor, A.J.; Evans, S.; Godfrey, S. and Zeidifard, E. (1974) "Disposition of disodium cromoglycate administered in three particle sizes." J Pharm Pharmacol. 26 : 79.

Cyr, T.D.; Graham, S.J.; Li, K.Y.R. and Lovering, E.G. (1991) "Low first spray drug content in albuterol metered dose inhalers." 8 : 658.

Dahlback, M. (1994) "Behavior of nebulizer solutions and suspensions." J Aerosol Med .7: 13.

Dalby, R.N.,and Byron, P.R. (1988). "Comparison of output particle size distributions from pressurized aerosols formulated as solutions and suspensions." 5:36.

Dalby, R.N.; Byron, P.R.; Shepard H.R. and Papadopoulos E. (1990) "CFC propellant substitution : P-134a as a potential replacement for P-12 in MDIs." Pharm Technol. 14 : 26.

Dalby, R.N. (1992) "Special considerations in the formulation of suspension type metered dose inhalers."Aerosol Age. 1992 :22.

Dalby, R.N. (1993) "Halohydrocarbons: pharmaceutical uses." In Swarbrick J, Boylan JC, eds. Encyclopedia of Pharmaceutical Technology, Vol 7. New York:Marcel Dekker.

Davies, C.N. (1961) "A formalized anatomy of the human respiratory tract.". In: Davies, C.N., ed. Inhaled particles and vapours. Oxford: Pergamon Press. 82.

Davis, S.S. (1999) "Delivery of peptide and non-peptide drugs through the respiratory tract." Pharma. Technol. Sci. Today, 2(11): 450-456

Dennis, J.H. and Hendrick, D.J. (1992) "Design characteristics for drug nebulizers." J Med Eng Technol . 16:63.

Doidge, J.M. and Satchell, D.G. (1980) "Adrenergic and non-adrenergic inhibitory nerves in maμmalian airways." J Autonom Nerv syst. 5:83-99.

Drinker, P.; Thompson, R.M.; Finn, J.L. (1928) "Quantitative measurements of the inhalation, retention and exhalation of dust and fumes by man." I. Concentration of 50 to 450 mg per cubic meter. J Ind Hyg Toxicol .10:13.

Effros, R.M. and Chang, H.K., (1994a) "Fluid and solute transport in the airspaces of the lungs." Vol.70 of Lung Biology in Health and Disease (Claude Lenfant, ed), New York: Marcel Dekker.

Effros, R.M.; Murphy, C.; Hacker, A.; Schapira, R.M. and Bongard, R. (1994b) "Reduction and uptake of methylene blue for rat airspaces." J Appl Physiol. 77:1460.

Egan, M.J. and Nixon, W. (1988) "A modeling study of regional deposition of inspired aerosols with reference to dosimetric assessments." In: Dodgson, J., McCallum, R.I., Bailey, M.R., Fisher, D.R. (eds.) Inhaled Particles VI. Oxford: Pergamon Press, pp. 909.

Eisner, A.D.; Graham, R. and Martonen, T.B., (1990) "Coupled mass and energy transport phenomena in aerosol/vapor-laden gases." I. J Aerosol Sci . 21:883.

Enna, S.J. and Schanker, I.S. (1972) "Absorption of drugs from the rat lung." Am J Physiol. 223:1227.

Ferron, G.A.; Karg, E. and Peter, J.E. (1993) Estimation of deposition of polydisperse hygroscopic aerosols in the human respiratory tract. J Aerosol Sci. 24:655.

Findeisen, W. (1935) "Uber das Absetzen kleiner, in der Luft suspendierter Teilchen in der menschlichen Lunge bei der" Atmung.Arch Ges Physiol. 236:367.

Freeman, B.A.; Mason, R.J.; Williams, M.C. and Crapo, J.D. (1986) "Antioxidant enzyme activity in alveolar type II cells after exposure of rats to hyperoxia." Exp Lung Res.10:203.

Ganderton, D. (1992) "The generation of respirable cloud from coarse powder aggregates,." J Biopharm Sci . 3:101.

Ganderton ,D. and Kassem, N.M. (1992) "Dry powder inhalers." Adv Pharm Sci. 6:165.

Gardiner, P.J. and Collier, H.O.J. (1980) "Specific receptors for prostaglandins in the airway." Prostaglandin. 19:819.

Gehr, P.; Bachofren, M. and Weibel, E.R. (1978) "The normal human lung: Ultrastructure and morphometric estimation of diffusion capacity." Respir Physiol . 32:121.

Gibby, E.M. and Cohen, G.M. (1984) "Conjugation of 1-naphthol by human bronchus and bronchoscopy samples." Biochem Pharmacol .33:739.

Gonda, I. (1990) "Aerosols for delivery of therapeutic and diagnostic agents to the respiratory tract." CRC Rev Ther. Drug Carrier Systems. 6:273.

Hanania, N.A.; Wittman, R.; Kesten, S. and Chapman, K.R. (1994) "Medical personnel's Knowledge of and ability to use inhaling devices." Chest. 105:111.

Hayes, M.; Taplin, G.V. and Chopra, S.K. et al. (1979) "Improved radioaerosol administration system for routine inhalation lung imaging." Radiology. 13:256.

Heyder, J. (1977a) "Gravitational deposition of aerosl particles within a system of randomly oriented tubes." J Aerosol Sci .8:289.

Heyder, J. and Rudolf, G. (1977b) "Deposition of aerosol particles in the human nose." In: Walton WH, ed. Inhaled Particles IV. Oxford: Pergamon Press. pp 107.

Heyder, J.; Gebhart, J. and Scheuch, G. (1985) "Interaction of diffusional and gravitational particle transport in aerosols." Aerosol Sci Technol .19854:315.

Hickey, A.J. (1992) In: Pharmaceutical Inhalation aerosol technology: Suµmary of coµmon Approaches to Pharmaceutical Aerosol Administration. New York: Marcel Dekker. 255.

Hickey, A.J.; Concessio N.M.; Van M.M and Platz R.M. (1994) "Factors influencing the dispersion of dry powders as aerosols." Pharm Technol . 18:58.

Hickey, A.J. and Concessio, N.M. (1994) "Aerodynamic behavior of micronized powders dispersed as aerosols." Pharm Technol . 18:88.

Hill, M. (1994) "Characteristics of an active, multiple dose inhaler." In: Byron, P.R., Dalby, R.N. and Farr, S.J. (eds.) Respiratory Drug Delivery IV. Deerfield, IL: Inter Pharm Press.

Hofmann, W.; Martonen, T.B. and Graham, R.C. (1989) "Predicted deposition of nonhygroscopic aerosols in the human lung as a function of subject age." J Aerosol Med . 2:49.

Holtzman, J.L.; Crankshaw, D.L.; Peterson, F.J. and Polnaszek, C.F. (1981) "The kinetics of the aerobic reduction of nitofurntoin by NADPH-cytochrome P-450 reductase." Mol Pharmacol . 20:669.

Horsfield, K. and Cuμming, G. (1967) "Angles of branching and diameters of branches in the human bronchial tree." Bull Math Biophys .29:207.

Inoue, K., and Yoshioka, K. (1999) "Pulmonary administration of insulin as an aerosol." Chest . 116 : 581.

Isabey, D. and Chang, H.K. (1982) "A model study of flow dynamics in human central airways." Part II: Secondary flow profiles. Respir Physiol. 49: 97.

Jager-Waldau, R.; Mehring, H. and Wiggins, J.D. (1994) "Feasibility of a low dosage dynamic powder disperser for drug delivery to the lungs." J Aerosol Med .7:205.

Kawashima, Y.; Yamamoto, H. ; Takeuchi, H. ; Fujioka, S. and Hino, T. (1999) "Pulmonary delivery of insulin with nebulized DL-lactide/glycolide copolymer (PLGA) nanospheres to prolong hypoglycemic effect." J. Controlled Release .62 : 279.

Keller, M. (1999) "Innovations and perspectives of metered dose inhalers in pulmonary drug delivery." Int. J. Pharm., 186 (1): 81-90

Kendrick, A.H.; Smith, E.C. and Denyer, J. (1995) "Nebulizers- fill volume, residual volume and matching of nebulizer to compressor." Respir Med . 89: 157.

Khanna, C.; Waldrep, J.C.; Anderson, P.M.; Weishcelbaum, R.W.; Hasz, D.E. ; Katsanis, E. and Klausner, J.S., (1997) "Nebulised interleukin II liposomes : aerosol characteristics and biodistribution." J. Pharm. Pharmacol. 49 : 960.

Kloss, M.W.; Rosen, G.M. and Rackman, E.J. (1982) "N-demethylation of cocaine to norcocaine, evidence for participation by cytochrome P450 and FAD-containing monooxygenase." Mol Pharmacol .23:482.

Kontny, M.J.; Conners, J.J. and Graham, E.T. (1994) "Moisture distribution and packaging of dry powder systems." In: Byron, P.R.., Dalby, R.N., Farr, S.J. (eds.) Respiratory Drug Delivery IV. Deerfield IL: Interpharm Press, pp. 125.

Koshkina, N.V. ; Gilbert, B.E.; Waldrep, J.C. ; Seryshev, A. and and Knight, V. (1999) "Distribution of captothecin after delivery as a liposome aerosol or following intramuscular injection in mice." Cancer Chemother. Pharmacol . 44 : i87.

Lafranconi, W.M. and Huxtable, R.J. (1984) "Hepatic metabolism and pulmonary toxicity of monocrotaline using isolated perfused liver and lung." Biochem Pharmacol . 33:2479.

Landahl, H.D. and and Black, S. (1947) "Penetration of airborne particulates through the human nose." J Ind Hyg Toxicol. 29:269.

Landahl, H.D. (1950a) "On the removal of air-borne droplets by the human respiratory tract: I. The lung", Bull Math Biophys.12:43.

Landahl, H.D. (1950b) "On the removal of airborne droplets by the human respiratory tract. II. The nasal passages". Bull Math Bniophys .12:161.

Landahl, H.D. (1964) "Schematic representation of respiratory tract" (Table 3.2). In:Hatch, T.F., Gross, P. (eds.) Pulmonary Deposition and Retention of inhaled aerosols. New York: Academic Press.

Laube, B.L.; Georgopoulos, A. and Adams, G.K., (1993) "Preliminary study of the efficacy of insulin aerosol delivered by oral inhalation in diabetic patients". JAMA . 296 : 2106.

Leflein, J.; Brown, E.; Hill, M.; Kelley, H.W.; Loffert, D.T.; Nelson, H.S. and Szeflec, S.J., (1995) "Delivery of glucocorticoids by jet nebulization: aerosol characteristics and output". J Allergy Clin Iµmunol.95:944.

LiCalsi, C.; Christensen, T.; Bennett, J.V.; Phillips, E. and Witham, C. (1999) "Dry powder inhalation as potential delivery method for vaccines". Vaccine . 17 : 1796.

Martonen T.B.; Bell, K.A.; Phalen, R.F.; Wilson, A. F. and Ho, A. (1982a) "Growth rate measurement and deposition modeling of hygroscopic aerosols in human tracheobronchial models". Ann Occup Hyg. 26:93.

Martonen, T.B. (1982b) "Analytical model of hygroscopic particle behavior in human airways". Bull Math Biol. 44:425.

Martonen, T.B. (1983a) "Deposition of inhaled particulate matter in the uppr respiratory tract, larynx, and bronchial airways: a mathematical description". J Toxicol Environ Health . 12:787.

Martonen, T.B. and Lowe, J. (1983b) "Assessment of aerosol deposition patterns in human respiratory tract casts". In: Marple, V.A., Liu ,B.Y.H., eds. Aerosols in the Mining and Industrial Work Environments. Ann Arbor Science, .151.

Martonen, T.B. and Wilson, A.F. (1983c) "The influence of hygroscopic growth upon the deposition of bronchodilator aerosols in upper human airways". J Aerosol Sci .14:208.

Martonen, T.B. (1992) "Aerodynamic size measurement of airborne fibers and health effects implications." Adv Powder Technol . 3:311.

Martonen, T.B. (1993a) "Mathematical model for the selective deposition of inhaled pharmaceuticals." J Pharm Sci . 82: 1191.

Martonen, T.B. and Katz, I.M. (1993b) "Deposition patterns of aerosolized drugs within human lungs: effect of ventilatory parameters." Pharm Res . 10:871.

Martonen, T.B.; Zhang, Z. and Lessmann, R. (1993c) Fluid dynamics of the human larynx and upper tracheobronchial airways." Aerosol Sci Technol .19:133.

Martonen T.B. and Katz I.M., (1993d) "Effects of aerosol polydispersity on deposition patterns within human lungs." J Aerosol Med. 6: 251.

Martonen, T.B. and Yang, Y. (1994a) "A mathematical model for aerosol deposition in the respiratory tract of the guinea pig." Inhal Tox .6:1.

Martonen, T.B.; Katz, I.M. (1994b) "Inter-related effects of morphology and ventilation on drug deposition patterns." J Pharm Sci . 4:11.

Martonen, T.B.; Yang, Y. and Xue, Z. (1994c) "Effects of carinal ridge shapes on lung air-streams." Aerosol Sci Tech . 21:119.

Martonen, T.B.; Yang, Y.; Xue, Z. and Zhang, Z., (1994d) "Motion of air within the human tracheobronchial tree." Partic Sci Technol .12:175.

Martonen, T.B.; Katz, I.M. and Cress, W. (1995) "Aerosol drug deposition as a function of airway disease: cystic fibrosis." Pharm Sci . 12:96.

Mather, L.E.; Woodhouse, A.; Ward, M.E.; Farr, S.J.; Rubsamen, R.A., Eltherington, L.G. (1998) "Pulmonary administration of aerosolized fentalnyl." Br. J. Clin. Pharmacol. . 46 : 37.

McBride, J.T. (1992) Architecture of the tracheobronchial tree,. In: Parent R.A. (ed.) Comparative Biology of the normal Lung, Vol. 1. Boca Raton, FL: CRC Press, pp. 49.

Melandri, C.; Tarroni, G.; Prodi, V.; De Zaiacomo, T.; Formignani, M. and Lombardi, C.C. (1983) "Deposition of charged particles in the human airways." J Aerosol Sci . 14:657.

Menkes, H.A. and Macklem, P.T. (1986) Collateral flow. In: Fishman A.P. Macklem P.T., Mead J. Geiger S.R. (eds.) Handbook of physiology, Section 3: The Respiratory System. Vol III, Mechanics of Breathing Part 1. Bethesda, M.D: American Physiological Society, pp. 337.

Mercer, T,T.; Tillery, M.I.and Chow, H.Y. (1968) "Operating cheracteristics of some compressded air nebulizers." Am Ind Hyg Assoc J .29:66.

Merkus,,P.J.F.M.; Van Essen-Zandvliet, E.E.M.; Parlevliet, E.; Borsboom, G.; Sterk, P.J.; Kerrebijn, K.F. and Qkukanjer, Ph.H., (1992) "Changes in nebulizer output over the years." Eur Respir J .5:488.

Minchin, R.F.; Barber, H.E.; Ilett, K.F. (1982) "Effect of prolonged desmethylimipramine administration on the pulmonary clearance of 5-hydroxytryptamine and b-phenylethylamine in rats." Drug Metab Dispos Biol Fate Chem .10:356.

Molinard, M.; Martin, C.A.E.; Naline, E.; Hirsch, A. and Advenier, C. (1994) "Contractile effects of bradykinin on the isolated human small bronchus." Am J Respir Crit Care Med . 149:123.

Morley, C.J.; Miller, N.; Bangham, A.D. and Davis, J.A. (1981) "Dry artificial lung surfactant and its effect on very premature babies." Lancet 356:64.

Mullins, M.E.; Michaels, L.P.; Menon, V.; Locke, B. and Ranade, M.B. (1992) "Effect of geometry on particle adhesion." Aerosol Sci Techol. 17:105.

Nerbrink, O.; Dahlback, M. and Hansson, H.C. (1994) "Why do medical nebulizers differ in their output and particle size characteristics?" J Aerosol Med, .7:259.

Newman, S.P.; Pavia, D.; Moren, F.; Sheahan, N.F. and Clark, S.W. (1981) "Deposition of pressurized aerosols in the human respiratory tract." Thorax .36:52.

Newman, S.P. and Pellow, P.G.D. (1987) "Evaluation of jet nebulizers. In: Ganderton, D.; Jones, T., (eds.) Drug Delivery to the respiratory tract. New York: Ellis Horwood, pp. 125.

Nielson, D.W.; Goerke, J. and Clements, J.A. (1981) "Alveolar subphase pH in the lungs of anesthetized rabbits." Proc Natl Acad Sci USA .78:7119.

Niven, R.W.; Ip, A.Y.; Mittelman, S.; Prestrelski, S.J. and Arakawa, T. (1995) "Some factors associated with the ultrasonic nebulizatioin of proteins." Pharm Res .12:53.

Nunn, J.F. (1993) Nunn's Applied Respiratory Physiology, 4th ed. Oxford: Butter-worth-Heinemann.

Paiva, M. (1985) Theoretical studies of gas mixing in the lung. In: Engel L.A.; Paiva. M; (eds.) Gas mixing and distribution in the lung. New York: Marcel Dekker, pp. 221.

Parthasarathy, R.; Gilbert, B. and Mehta, K. (1999) "Aerosol delivery of liposomal all-trans-retinoic acid to the lungs." Cancer Chemother. Pharmacol . 43 : 277.

Pattle, R.E. (1961) The retention of gases and particles in the human nose. In: Davies, C.N., (ed.) Inhaled particles and vapours. Oxford: Pergamon Press, pp. 301.

Pederson, S. and Steffenson, G. (1986) "Fenoterol powder inhaler techinque in children: influence of inspiratory flow rate and breath holding," Eur Respir J .68:207.

Pederson, S. (1986) "How to use a Rotahaler®." Ann Arch Dis Child. .61:11.

Pederson, S. (1994) "Clinical efficacy and safety of budesonide Turbuhaler® as compared to MDIs in children." J Aerosol Med .75:843.

Pedley, T.J.; Schroter, R.C. and Sudlow, M.F. (1979) Gas flow and mixing in the airways. In: West J.B. (ed.) Bioengineering Aspects of the Lung. New York: Marcel Dekker, .pp.163.

Persson, C.G.A. (1985) Experimental lung actions of xanthines. In: Andersson, K.E., Persson, C.G.A. (Eds.) Anti-asthma Xanthines and Adenosine. Amsterdam: Excerpta Medica, pp.61

Phelan, R.F.; Cuddihy, R.G.; Fisher, G.L.; Moss, O.R.; Schlesinger, R.B.; Swift, D.L.; Yeh, H.C. (1991) "Main features of the proposed NCRP respiratory tract model." Rad Prot Dos .38:179.

Phipps, P.R.and Gonda, I. (1990) "Droplets produced by medical nebulizers." Chest .97:1327.

Pillai. R.S.; Yeates, D.B.; Eljamal, M.; Miller, I.F. and Hickey, A.J. (1994) "Controlled release from condensation coated respirable aerosol particles." J Aerosol Sci .25:187.

Proud, D.; Macglashan, D.W.; Newball, H.H.; Schulman, E.S. and Lichtenstein, L.M. (1985) "Iμmunoglobulin E-mediated release of a kininogenase from purified human lung mast cells." Am Rev Respir Dis . 132:405.

Ribiero, L.B. and Wiren, J.E. (1990) "Comparison of Bricanyl® Turbukhaler and Berotec® dry powder inhaler." Allergy. 45:382.

Rietema, K. (1991) Theoretical derivatives of interparticle forces. In: The Dynamics of Fine Powders. New york: Elsevier, pp. 65.

Rinderknecht, J.; Shapiro, L. and Krauthaμmer, M. (1980) "Accelerated clearance of small solutes from the lungs in interstitial lung disease." Am Rev Respir Dis .121:105.

Rodrigo, G. and Rodrigo, C. (1993) "Comparison of salbutamol delilverd by nebuylizer or metered-dose inhaler with a pear-shaped spacer in acute asthma." Cur Ther Res . 54:797.

Ryan, U.S. (1986) "Pulmonary endothelium: a dynamic interface." Clin Invest Med .9:124.

Saari, S.M.; Vidgren, M.T.; Koskinen, M.O.; Turjanmaa, V.M.; Waldrep, J.C. and Nieminen, M.M. (1998) "Regional lung deposition and lung clearance of 99mTc labelled Beclomethasone-DLPC liposomes in mild and severe asthama." Chest . 113 : 1573.

SanGiovanni, M.L. (1995) (ed.) 3M reveals CFC-free inhaler for UK market,. Spray Technol Marketing. 5:26.

Scheuch, G. and Stahlhofen, W. (1988) "Particle deposition of inhaled aerosol boluses in the upper human airways." J Aerosol Med . 1: 29.

Schreier-H. (1994) "Pulmonary delivery of liposomal drugs." J. Liposome Res. 4(1): 229-238.

Schreier, H.; Gonzalez-Rothi, R.J. and Stecenko, A.A. (1993) "Pulmonary delivery of liposomes." J. Control. Rel. 24: 209-223.

Schultz, R.K.; Miller, N.C.; Smith, D.K. and Ross, D.L. (1992) "Powder aerosols with auxilliary means of dispersion." J Biopharm Sci .3:115.

Schultz, R.K.; Dupont, R.L. and Ledoux, K.A. (1994) Issues surrounding metered dose valve technology: past, present and future perspectives. In: Byron, P.R.; Dalby, R.N.; Farr, S.J (eds.) Proceedings of Respiratory Drug Delivery IV. Buffalo Grove, II: Interpharm Press, pp. 211.

Service, R.F. (1998) "New role for estrogen in cancer." Science .279:1631.

Sethi, D.K.; Norwood, D.L.; Haywood, P.A. and Prime, D. (1992) "Impact of extractable testing on MDI development programs." 3 : 63.

Sievers, R.E.; Hybertson, B.M. and Hansen, B.N. (1994) Methods and apparatus for drug delivery using supercritical solutions, US Patent # 5, 301,664, April 12, 1994.

Sleigh, M.A.; Blake, J.R. and Liron, N. (1988) "The proplulsion of mucus by cilia." Am Rev Respir Dis .137:726.

Smoluchowski, M.S. (1912) On the practical applicability of Stokes's law of resistance and modifications of it required in certain cases. Fifth International Conference of Mathematics, Cambridge, 2, 192.

(1990) "Platelet activating factor and related acetylated lipids as potent biologically active cellular mediators." Med Res Rev . 5:107.

Soumerhoff, C.P.; Caughey, G.H.; Finkbeiner, W.E.; Lazaruks, S.C.; Basbaum, C.B.and Nadel, J.A. (1989) "Mast cell chymase: a potent secretagogue for airway gland serous cells." J Iμmunol . 145:2450.

Spiro, S.G.; Biddiscombe, M.; Marriott, R.J.; Short, M.; Taylor, A.J. (1992) "Inspiratory flow rates attained by asthmatic patients though a mete red dose inhaler and a Diskhaer® inhaler." Br J Clin Res .3:115.

Stahlhofern, W.; Rudolf, G. and James, A.C. (1989) "Intercomparison of experimental regional aerosol deposition data." J Aerosol Med . 2:285.

Staniforth, J.N. (1994) The importance of electrostatic measurements in aerosol fomulation and preformulation and preformulation. In: Byron, P.R.; Dalby, R.N.; Farr, S.J. (eds.) Respiratory Drug Delivery IV. Deerfield IL: Interpharm Press, pp.303.

Staub, N.C. (1974) "Pulmonary edema." Physiol Rev .54:678.

Staub, N.C. (1991) Basic respiratory physiology. New York: Churchill Livingstone, pp. 1.

Stober, W. (1972) Dynamic shape factors of nonspherical aerosol particles. In: Mercer, T.T.; Morrow, P.E.; Stober, W. (eds.) Assessment of airborne particles. Springfield, IL: Charles C Thomas, pp. 249.

Suntres, Z.E. and Shek, P.N. (1998) "Liposomes promote pulmonary glucocorticoid delivery." J. Drug. Target. 6 : 175.

Task Group on Lung Dynamics. (1966) "Deposition and retention models for internal dosimetry of the human respiratory tract." Health Physics . 12:173.

Taulbee, D.B. and Yu, C.P. (1975) "A theory of aerosol deposition in the human respiratory tract." J Appl Physiol . 38: 77.

Taylor, R.G. (1987) In: Drug delivery to the respiratory tract, Ganderton, C.D., and Jones, T. (eds) Horwood Ellis, Chichester, England, pp. 27.

Taylor, K.M,and Farr, S.J. (1993) "Liposomes for drug delivery to the respiratory tract." Drug. Dev. Ind. Pharm. 19(1-2): 123-142.

Van Cleef, J..(1991) "Powder technology." Am Sci .79:304.

Vidgren, M.; Arpee, J.; Vidgren, P.; Hyvarinen, L.; Vaino, P.; Silvasti, M. and Tukiainen, H. (1991) "Pulmonary deposition and clinical response of 99mTc-labelled salbutamol delivered from a novel multiple dose powder inhaler." Pharm Res .11:1320.

Wang, L.Y.; Toledo-Velasquez, D.; Schwegler-Berry, D. and Ma, J.K.H., Rojanasakkul, Y., (1993) "Transport and hydrolysis of enkephalins in cultured alveolar epithelial monolayers." Pharm Res. 10:1662.

Wanger, J. (1992) Pulmonary Function Testing: A Practical Approach. Baltimore:Williams and Wilkins.

Ward, M.E.; Woodhouse, A.; Mather, L.E.; Farr, S.J.; Okikawa, J.K.; Lloyd, P.; Schuster, J.A. and Rubsamenn, R.M. (1997) "Morphine pharmacokinetics after pulmonary administration form a novel aerosol delivery system." Clin. Pharmacol. Ther. . 62 : 596.

Weibel, E.R. (1963) Morphometry of the Human Lung. Berlin: Springer-Verlag.

Weibel, E.R. (1986) Functional morphology of lung parenchyma. In: Macklem, P.T. and Mead, J. (eds) Handbook of Physiology. American Physiological Society, pp. 89.

Weibel, E.R. (1989) Lung morphometry and moderls in respiratory physiology. In: Chang, H.K. and Paiva, M. (eds.) Respiratory Physiology: An Analytical Approach. New York: Marcel Dekker, pp. 1.

West, J.B. (1990) Respiratory Physiology-The Essentials, 4th ed. Baltimore: Williams and Wilkins.

Wetterlin, K. (1988) "Tubuhaler®: a new powder inhaler for administration of drugs to the airways." Pharm Res .5:506.

White, M.V.; Slater, J.E. and Kaliner, M.A. (1987) "Histamine and asthma." Am Rev Respir Dis. 135: 1165.

Whitham, M.E.; Eagle, A.M. (1994) Alternative propellants: proprietary rights, toxicological issues land projected licensing problems. In Byron, P.R.; Dalby, R.N.; Farr, S.J. (eds.) Proceedings of Respiratory Drug Delivery IV. Buffalo Grove, IL: Interpharm Press, pp. 203.

Williams, D.E.; Hale, S.E.; Muerhoff, A.S. and Masters, B.S.S. (1985) "Rabbit lung flavin-containing monooxygenase. Purification, characterization and induction during pregnancy." Mol Pharmacol. 28:381.

Wolff, R.K. and Niven, R.W. (1994) "Generation of aerosolized drugs." J Aerosol Med. 7:89.

Yeh, H.C. and Schum, G.M. (1980) "Models of human lung airways and their application to inhaled particle deposition." Bull Math Biol .42:461.

Zeng, X.M.; Martin, G.P. and Marriot, C. (1995) "The controlled delivery of drugs to the lung." Int J Pharm. 124: 149.

Chapter 7 _____

Intraarterial and Intravascular Drug Delivery Systems

S.G. Deshpande, Amrita Bajaj, Sujata P. Sawarkar

7.1 INTRODUCTION

Novel drug delivery systems are designed with the aim of targeting the biologically active molecule to its site of action, thus avoiding a random distribution throughout the body. The second objective of the design is to control the delivery of the drug over an extended period of time (Wood, 1980).

The focus of research today has been directed to develop intravenous and intraarterial targeting and delivery systems using microspheres, nanoparticles, liposomes, microemulsions and hydrogels. The systemic infusion or local injection in the vessels ensures passive targeting of the drug. Furthermore the drug release can be controlled by diffusion through the polymer matrix and/or by erosion of the polymer (Benita et al, 1984). The rationale of using a drug delivery system to be administered through the vascular compartment of the body will be understood better with the knowledge of the anatomy of vessels.

7.1.1 Anatomy of the vasculature

The average adult has over 60,000 miles of blood vessels in the body comprising of a network of arteries, arterioles, capillaries, venules and larger veins. The major blood vessels are thick walled, muscular tubes with a smooth endothelial lining. Aorta, the largest artery, is about 2.5 cm wide whereas the smallest arterioles found just before the capillaries are about 20 μm or less in diameter. The walls of arteries and veins are made up of three layers. The outer layer called *tunica externa* or *adventitia* consists of fibrous elastic connective tissue through which run small blood vessels called *vasa vasorum*. It is through this layer that perivascular and periadventitial drug delivery systems are administered. They are applied around this coat. The middle layer, the *tunica media*, is composed of elastic filaments and muscle fibres. It is the muscle coat which gives the vessel its elasticity and contractility. The large vessels contain more elastic tissue than the smaller vessels. The tunica externa and media are much thinner in veins than in arteries. The inner layer, *tunica interna*, is also referred to as *intima membrane*. It is a thin layer of endothelial cells that are smooth and provide an ideal streamlined surface to the blood flowing-by. These cells are highly permeable. It is through these cells that nutrients and drugs reach the deeper part of the media. The characteristic features are shown schematically in Fig 7.1.

The muscle fibres and filaments facilitate the functioning of the arteries under high pressure, exerted by blood (ranging from 120 mm Hg in the aorta to 10 mm Hg in the arterioles). They also control the blood flow at a fast rate ranging from 33 cm/sec in the aorta to 0.3 mm/sec in the capillaries (Gregg & Folyey, 1993).

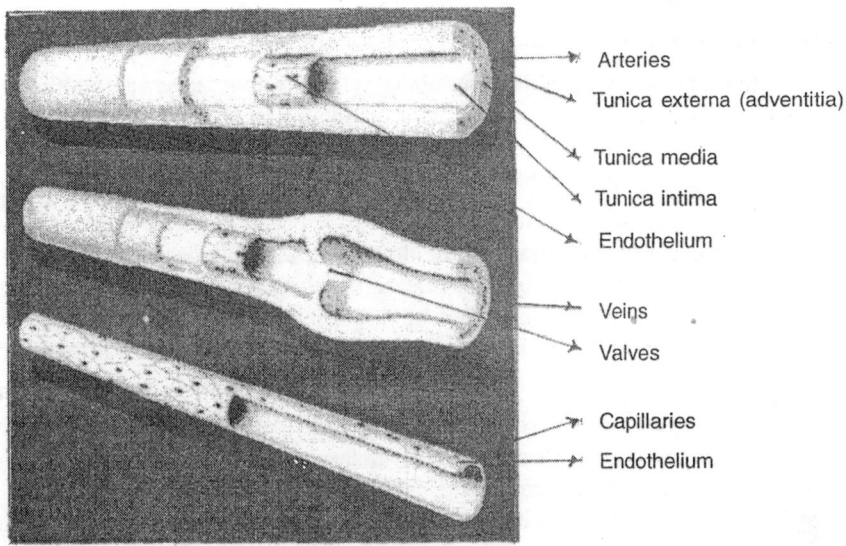

Fig 7.1 : Anatomical features of blood vessels (collected from body works version 3.0, 1993)

7.2 INTRAVASCULAR ROUTE

Intravascular routes of drug administration include either intraarterial (into arteries) or intravenous (into veins) injections (Ford, 1988). Intraarterial route involves injection of a drug directly into an artery and is used for an immediate effect in a peripheral organ, for example to improve circulation to the extremities. Drugs like peripheral vasodilators and anti-thrombotic agents are administered by this route. A drug injected into an artery terminates in a target organ. Hence, the effects are localized rather than generalized. The delivery of drug by this route for regional or systemic therapy requires the administration of drug via intraarterial infusion or injection.

7.2.1 Advantages

Several theoretical advantages have been cited in favour of this route of administration namely:

1. Increased regional drug concentration : This technique can deliver a high concentration of the particular antitumor agent to localize in the cancer region. Hence, it produces a higher response rate than the systemic route of drug administration.

2. Decreased systemic toxicity : This is due to the quick removal of the drug after the first pass through the capillary bed of the target region.

3. Enhanced activity of some drugs : When administered via the arterial route, the drug levels in the targeted tissue or organ will be significantly increased. Radio-opaque diagnostic agents are introduced by this route for roentographic studies of organs like heart, kidney, brain and to view the vascular supply to these organs.

Intraarterial route is an infrequently used method of drug administration because the technique is not simple and may require surgical procedure to reach the artery. However, almost every artery is approachable by arterial catheterization and several delivery devices have been developed for the same. Usage of this route for therapeutics encompasses organ specific cancer chemotherapy by particulate carrier therapy and chemoembolization, intraarterial infusions for thrombosis and for treatment of post angioplasty arterial restenosis.

7.2.2   Applications

When administered by intravascular route, these systems are utilized for:

1. Regional therapy via capillary filtration : When the drug carriers are administered intraarterially, particles larger than 10 mm are filtered out of the circulation largely in the capillary bed encountered after administration. By selecting the appropriate port of entry, the drug delivery system can be retained in the required organ, e.g. tumors (Daemen et. al., 1988).

2. Circulating depot : Colloidal drug particle systems introduced intraarterially can also act as circulating depots for controlled release of the drugs. These circulating particles must avoid rapid uptake by the mononuclear phagocyte system, release the drug at a required rate and be removed from the body without causing an unwanted immune response. The required particle size range for this application is reported to be 0.1-1 mm and can be utilized for indications like infections, leukemia and thrombosis (Petrak, 1993).

3. Cellular targets within vasculature: Once a particulate system that can circulate in the vascular compartment is administered, selective delivery to targets can be aimed at. Here the drug carriers are required to enter the interior of the cells, thus delivering the drug to phagocytic cells. Thus, delivery of drugs to diseased macrophages like in the case of parasitic, fungal or viral invasion, enzyme dysfunction, autoimmune diseases and gene therapy is the obvious application of this approach.

4. Cellular extravascular targets : In this application, the circulating delivery system is required to access the diseased endothelia or cross the endothelial barrier to reach cells active at an extravascular site, e.g. at the site of active rheumatoid arthritis (Weiss, 1989).

5. Chemoembolization : Chemoembolization involves the selective, temporary arterial blockage of tumor vasculature. Together with simultaneous local delivery of chemotherapeutic agents such an administration provides a synergistic effect of embolization and local chemotherapy (Fujimoto & Endoh 1985). This increases the therapeutic index of the anti-mytotic drugs that is comparatively low in systemic injection. Kato and co-workers (1980) used nondegradable microcapsules loaded with mitomycin C for the treatment of primary and secondary carcinomas of kidney, liver, bone and intrapelvic organs.

6. Diagnostic imaging : Attempts have been made to encapsulate radiocontrast agents into particulate delivery systems. Insoluble particulate contrast agents tend to produce higher contrast between normal and pathological tissue and can maintain this contrast for longer time (Seltzer, 1989).

7. Prevention of Arterial Restenosis : The proliferation of vascular smooth muscle cells is responsible for post angioplasty coronary artery restenosis. Intracoronary thrombus formation and smooth muscle cell hyperplasia are targeted for prevention of restenosis. Local intravascular site specific delivery of therapeutic agents has been used for the inhibition of smooth muscle cell proliferation. Drugs like dexamethasone,U-86983 [substituted-2-aminochromone] and tyrphostin compounds AG17 have been used in the treatment of post angioplasty restenosis (Labhasetwar et al, 1995). A few examples of carriers and drug delivery systems investigated for intravascular administration are summarised in Table 7.1.

7.3 DESIGN OF INTRAVASCULAR DRUG DELIVERY SYSTEMS

During administration of drug carriers in the vascular compartment the blood circulation plays a vital role in carrying the drug to the target tissue. The blood flow serves as the key medium for the distribution of drug delivery system through the body and as a mediator for delivering the drug to the site of action. The rate and extent to which a drug enters various tissues are influenced by the rate with which it is brought to the tissue through circulation and the ease with which the drug can leave circulation as well as regain its entry and exit from the tissue. Particulate carriers alter these rates so that a controlled drug release pharmacokinetics results. For the optimal performance of the drug its concentration, the rate of delivery to the site, the selectivity of distribution and the knowledge of the pharmacodynamics of the action, are needed to be considered in the design of an effective intravascular drug delivery system.

Table 7.1: Matrix materials utilized and potential applicationsof intravascular drug delivery systems.

Matrix material	Diameter (μm)	Intended use	Actual/Suggested Active Molecule
Ethyl cellulose	225	Chemoembolisation of cytostatics to kidney and liver	MitomycinC
Starch	40	Intraarterial administration of antitumor agents	5-Fluorouracil, BCNU, Actinomycin D
Albumin microspheres	10 - 30	Intraarterial delivery to tumors	Doxorubicin, Bleomycin, 5-Fluorouracil, Methotrexate
Ferromagnetic albumin	1-7	Dlivery to renal artery	Doxorubicin
Poly (lactide co glycolide) as nanosphere (PLGA)	300 - 400 nm	For cancer chemotherapy and post angioplasty restenosis	Dexamethasone, 5-Fluorouracil
Photopolymerized hydrogels	<50	Localized intravascular delivery of proteins	Heparin
Lipiodolized emulsion	<50	Localized treatment of hepatocellular carcinoma	Doxorubicin
Liposomes phosphatidyl - choline	25nm - 0.5 μm	Localized antifungal activity	Amphotericin B

7.3.1 Drug Carrier Systems

The drug is included in a carrier system and it is distributed to the tissues according to the properties of the carrier. The carrier seeks out the preferred site of action. Depending upon the specific indication an ideal intravascular particulate drug delivery system should facilitate following properties of drugs:

1. Retain the drug within the carrier during the transit and release the drug at the target site at the appropriate rate.

2. Prolong the drug effect due to longer circulation time as compared to free drug.

3. Increase the drug concentration at the site of action by preferential sequestering of the particles by the tissue of the site.

4. Protect the drug from metabolism and immune system recognition before it reaches targeted site. The most important requirement of a drug delivery system for the intravascular route of administration is that it should be able to avoid an uptake by the mononuclear phagocytic system. The distribution of colloidal particles after intravascular administration depends on their interfacial and physicochemical characteristics.

A detailed analysis of the surface of the human erythrocytes shows that it comprises of carbohydrates, which are a part of glycoproteins. These carbohydrates form hydration sheets at the surface. This hydration sheet is negatively charged due to the presence of sialic acid. The hydration layer shields the hydrophobic lipid cell membrane from interacting with circulating vascular components (Castoldi, 1981).

Based on this concept various attempts were made to utilize compounds containing sialic acid for modifying surface of particles and liposomes. As the hydrophobic colloids adsorb proteins on their surface, they get rapidly cleared from circulation by the mononuclear phagocytic system via the liver and the spleen. This protein adsorption can be reduced either by surface adsorption or chemical attachment of hydrated polymers at the surface of hydrophobic colloid.

The effectiveness of the hydrated polymer shell in stabilizing the particles is determined by the physicochemical properties of the polymer, the thickness of the adsorbed layer and the density of the surface coverage. The high surface density and long chain length of polyoxyethylene have been found to reduce the protein adsorption.

The surface density is predicted to have a greater effect than chain length or the steric repulsion and van der Waal's attractions. Andrade & Jeon (1991) have reported that the surface charge, surface energy, interfacial free energy and surface motion affect the blood compatibility of the polymers.

A marginally increased hemocompatibility has been reported for lipid microspheres coated with polysaccharides. However exchange between adsorbed and circulating macromolecules leads to changes in the composition of the particle surface. The lack of complete and homogeneous surface coverage leads to reversible adsorption, which is a drawback of this approach.

An alternative approach to surface modification by adsorption is to chemically attach polymers to the particle surface. However, when grafting the polymers in the presence of drugs is attempted, it is difficult to obtain uniformly covered surface due to uneven distribution of the reactive sites on the surface and the steric hindrance of already attached polymer chains.

Thus, preparation of stable surfaces saturated with suitable macromolecules is the major constraint in the development of hemocompatible particles. For surface modification it is necessary that correct chemical entities like noninteracting sugars e.g. sialic acid need to be present in a correct physical form like hydrated thick, negatively charged layer. This should be capable of screening hydrophobic interaction between circulating proteins and the drug containing particle core.

The amphiphilic block copolymers have been investigated as particles with accurately defined surface composition. These block copolymers are higher molecular weight analogues of non-ionic surfactants. They form micelles at low critical micelle concentration of approx. 10^{-8}-10^{-10} M and produce stable particles that do not interact with proteins under physiological conditions. They have long half - life of approximately 50 hr while in circulation (Petrak, 1993).

The physical nature of surface of such particles is similar to the surface of biological particles like erythrocytes. A schematic model of a micelle formed from block copolymers is depicted in Fig7.2. The core is formed from hydrophobic block and contains drug surrounded by the hydrophilic chains of the block copolymer, which extends into the aqueous environment. Thus, they prevent the interaction between the drug and the circulating proteins.

Endogenous materials such as serum albumin, glycoproteins, natural polysaccharides, polyaminoacids and synthetic materials like polystyrene are being used for this purpose. However, the particles must be nontoxic, nonimmunogenic and biodegradable even after loading the drugs.

Targetable micelles can be prepared from these functionalized micelles by linking targeting moieties including sugars and proteins. Block copolymer micelles having functional groups at each chain ends of PEG palisade have been prepared by Kataoka et al (1996). The cross-linking due to ligand exchange reaction of

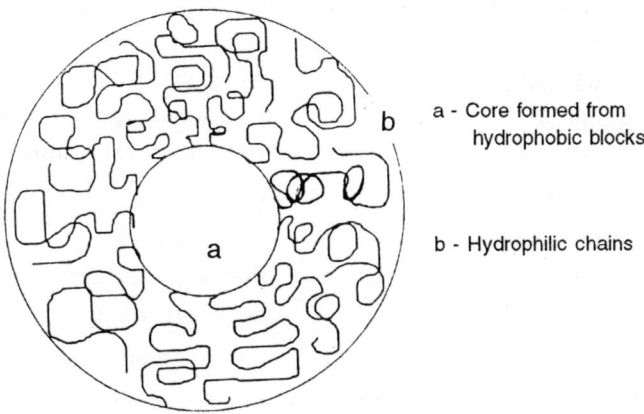

a - Core formed from
hydrophobic blocks

b - Hydrophilic chains

Fig 7.2 : Schematic model of micelle formed from block copolymers (adopted from Petrak, 1993)

cisplastin with carboxyl groups in the side chain of poly(ethyleneglycol)-poly(aspartic acid) block copolymer allows the micellization with considerably stabilized structure. Thus, stable and monodispersive, polymers approx. 30nm in diameter were prepared in aqueous media by metal complex formation. Polymeric micelles loaded with cisplastin (a platinum containing anti-tumor drug) have been developed. Micelles could also be prepared based on electrostatic interaction between a pair of oppositely charged block copolymer with PEG segments or with oligopeptides or oligonucleotides, micelle disruption was observed even in serum, suggesting a potential utility of the micelles for *in-vivo* delivery of bioactive peptides and nucleotides.

7.3.2 Particle size of carrier

In the design of site specific drug delivery systems to be administered intravascularly alteration in the size of particulate carrier and/or its site of administration leads to manipulation in targeting. The influence of particle size on the delivery of drugs is evident by the following three features related to drug administration by this route :

1   Intraarterial injection of particles 0.1-2.0 μm leads to a rapid clearance of particles from the blood stream by macrophages of the reticuloendothelial system (RES) with eventual localization of these in the Kuppfer cells of liver (Kanke et al, 1980).

2.   Particles of less than 50 nm can pass through the fenestrations of the liver endothelium and become localized after lymphatic transport in the spleen, bone marrow and tumor tissue.

3.   Intraarterial delivery of colloidal particles greater than 12 μm leads to their blockage in the first capillary bed encountered. Such blockage can lead to first order targeting to the tumor bearing organs. The second order targeting occurs due to a qualitative and quantitative difference in the capillary networks of the tumor as compared to the host organ. Hence, the drug carrier results in temporary blockage of the organ's arteries so that a co-injected drug's dwell time is extended. Its concentration gradient is maintained so as to permit greater absorption. This phenomenon forms the basis of intraarterial drug targeting. For example, the injection of microspheres greater than 15 μm into the mesenteric artery or portal vein or renal artery leads to their complete entrapment in the gut, liver or kidneys (Tomlinson et al, 1984).

7.4 DEVELOPMENT OF INTRAARTERIAL /INTRAVASCULAR DRUG DELIVERY SYSTEMS

A wide variety of polymeric drug delivery systems have been devised for protecting the active molecules and for controlling drug release in body fluids like blood and lymph. Special attention has been paid to the biodegradability and hemocompatibility of the polymer to avoid chronic toxicity especially when parenterally administered. The matrix materials investigated for use in intravascular formulations are listed below:

Starch derivatives	Collagen
Alginates	Phospholipids
Gelatin	DL-polylactic acid
Chitosan	Polyamino acid
Chylomicrons	Polyacrylamides
Lipoproteins	Polyalkyl cyanoacrylates
Albumin	Polycaprolactone
Fibrinogen	Cyclodextrins

Polylactic and polyglycolic acid are most frequently tested and used materials for intravascular administration. Lipids, although being non-polymeric, are used as constituents of vehicles for most drug delivery systems. As phospholipids and cholesterol are major structural components of biological membranes, they have also been used in variety of drug delivery devices such as microspheres, emulsions, mixed micelles and liposomes.

Biodegradable polymers such as polylactide co-glycolide, poly DL lactide and polyglycolide have been devised as delivery systems for controlled release of vaccines, cytostatics and insulin. The colloidal drug carriers such as liposomes, polyalkyl-cyanoacrylate nanoparticles facilitate transport of the potential drug from injection sites to the target sites via the vascular system because of their submicron size.

A brief discussion of several novel drug delivery systems investigated for intravascular administration is presented here:

7.4.1 Nanoparticles

These dosage forms are currently of great interest because of their colloidal nature and small size. Solid colloidal nanoparticles ranging from 1 to 1000 nm in size can be administered in fluidized form with a liquid carrier (Kreuter, 1992). This permits their usefulness in intravascular preparations. Sustained release nanoparticles have been formulated based upon the composition and surface characteristics of the specific polymers and excipients used (Tice & Tabibi, 1992).

Efficacious intraarterial administration of dexamethasone containing naonoparticles for restenosis in rat model and in a dog femoral artery model has been reported (Levy et al, 1996). The efficacy for preventing coronary artery restenosis in pigs through the use of intracoronary arterial administration of U86983 antiproliferative agents formulated into PLGA nanoparticles has been demonstrated by Labhasetwar et al (1995). Transarterial administration of nanoparticles containing anticancer agents and antibiotics is attempted in clinical studies for specific organ targeting.

Song et al (1997) have described a method to formulate and characterize nanoparticles which are compatible with therapeutic agents as well as biological macromolecules.

Preparation of nanoparticles

The method is based on the spontaneous emulsification-solvent diffusion technique. The system consists of a solvent phase for drug and polymer and an aqueous dispersion phase containing the dispersing agents. Dichloromethane or chloroform and acetone are used as the solvent for the polymer PLGA. The drug is dissolved in either phase based on its solubility. The resultant organic solution is emulsified as nanodroplets into aqueous PVA solution under stirring using a homogenizer. Then the emulsified system is stirred under reduced pressure for evaporation of the organic solvent. During evaporation of the water immiscible organic solution, the dispersed nanodroplets solidify in the aqueous solution. The entire dispersed system is filtered through a membrane filter (pore size 1mm). The nanospheres dispersed in the filtrate are then sedimented by ultracentrifugation and recovered by removing water. The schematic procedure for preparation is shown in Fig. 7.3 (Niwa et al, 1993).

The presence of acetone in the organic phase of the drug and the polymer helps to decrease the mean diameter of the spheres to submicron levels. It was found that interfacial tension between chloroform or dichloromethane phase and   aqueous phase decreased with increasing amount of acetone in equilibrium state. The acetone transfers out of the phase of higher viscosity i.e. organic phase during evaporation. The

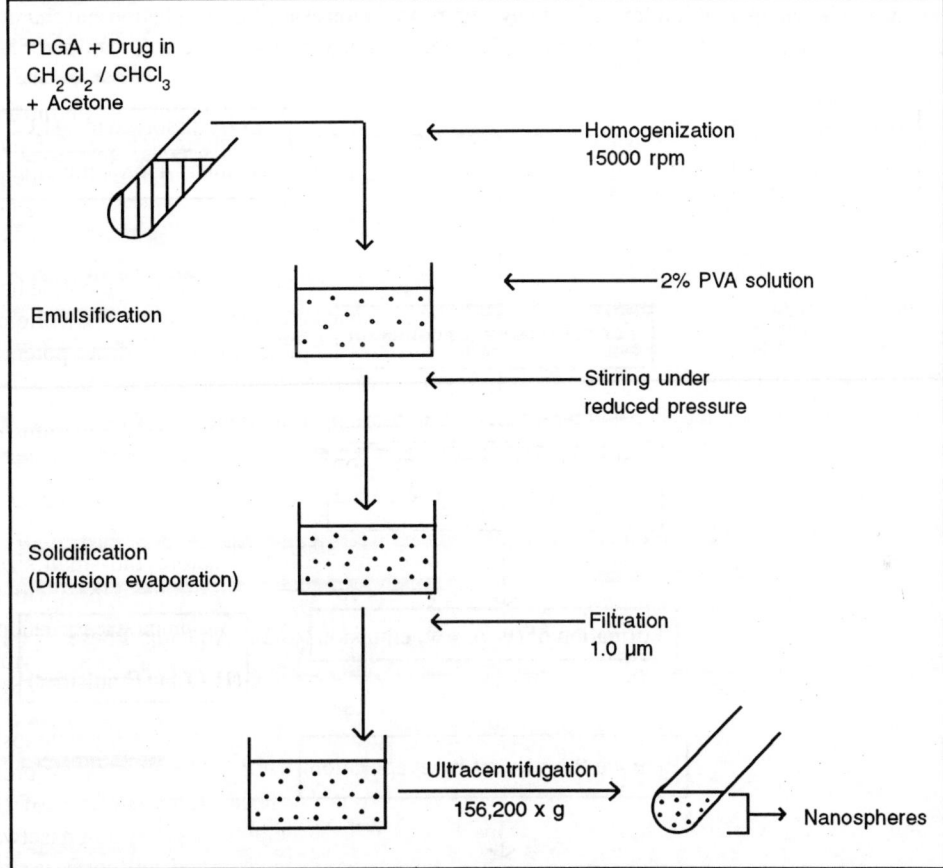

Fig 7.3 : Schematic procedure for preparation of PLGA nanospheres (Adopted from Niwa et al, 1993)

steep concentration gradient at the interface and reduction in the interfacial tension promote interfacial turbulence. This complex interfacial hydrodynamic phenomena i.e. the perturbation of the interface arising from the rapid diffusion of acetone across the interface between organic and aqueous phases spontaneously produces a much larger interfacial area. This results in formation of much smaller droplets i.e. nanospheres. Therefore this technique is called **spontaneous emulsification-solvent diffusion** method. The diffusion and evaporation of the organic solvents from the organic dispersed droplets and the counter diffusion of water into the droplets reduces the solubility of PLGA and deposits it in the droplets forming nanospheres.

Poorly water-soluble and water-soluble drugs like indomethacin, 5-fluorouracil, dexamethasone and U86983 have been loaded in PLGA nanoparticles based on these concepts.

Schematic flow chart for the preparation of bovine serum albumin (BSA) loaded particles by double emulsion-solvent evaporation method [(w1/o) / w2] is given in Fig 7.4 (Song et al, 1997).

The molecular weight of PLGA plays an important role in the incorporation of drugs. Nanoparticles made from lower molecular weight PLGA (molecular weight 58,000) showed lower BSA uptake than that from higher molecular weight PLGA (102,000). An increase in BSA entrapment was observed with increasing concentration of both PLGA and BSA solutions. It is difficult to incorporate water-soluble proteins in the nanoparticles due to the high water solubility of proteins combined with extremely small size (10nm) of nanoparticles.

During the sonication process for the second emulsification the protein tends to migrate through the nanometer sized organic droplet into the continuos aqueous phase resulting in a poor protein entrapment in the polymer matrix. The nanoparticles were sterilized by gamma radiation using ^{60}Co irradiation and characterized for the morphological and topographical properties. The mean diameters of the spherical nanoparticles were

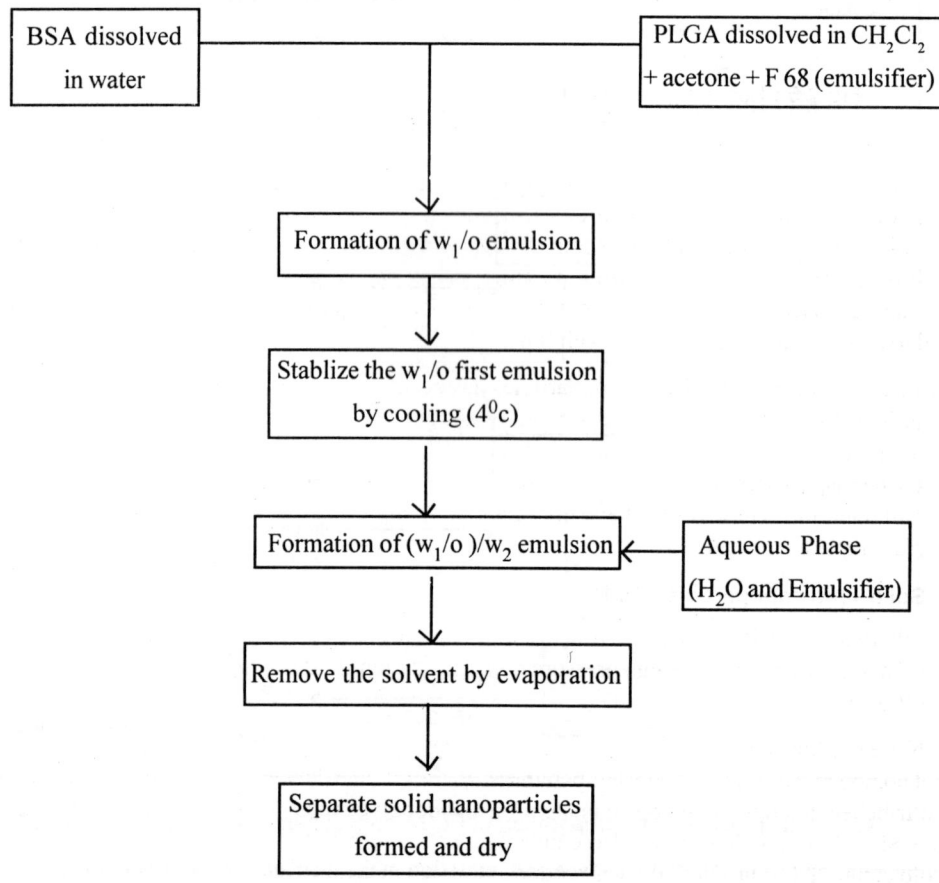

Fig 7.4 : Schematic representation of preparation of BSA loaded PLGA nanoparticles by double emulsion solvent evaporation method (adapted from Song et al, 1997)

between 100 to 300 nm. The schematic scanning electron micrograph of indomethacin nanoparticles prepared by this technique is shown in Fig 7.5.

The drug loading and release kinetics from nanoparticles have been studied. It was observed that drug released was by diffusion through the water filled channels and matrix bio-erosion. The release rate pattern of

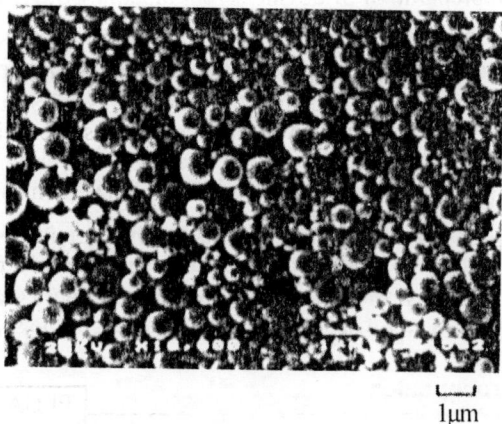

1µm

Fig 7.5 : Scanning electron microphotograph of PLGA nanospheres
loaded with indomethacin (adapted from Niwa et al 1993)

drugs could be tailored by choosing polymers with proper combination of degradation rate and molecular weight. It was possible to reduce the drug diffusion rate to moderate the initial burst release. Factors like surface cross-linking, coating and drug solubility can be modified to get the desired release pattern. In the case of solubility controlled release, the drug polymer matrix acts as a drug saturated reservoir and zero order kinetics can be observed. An erosion control system leads to a zero order release if a polymer matrix is designed to degrade in a linear manner with time.

Surface modification of PLGA nanoparticles has been investigated for design of biodegradable systems with specific release characteristics (Levy et al, 1996). Surface modification of PLGA nanoparticles with the detergent didodecyl methyl ammonium bromide (DMAB) was attempted. The surfactant improved the absorption characteristics of the surface of nanoparticles and hence significantly enhanced nanoparticle arterial wall retention. These results have important implications in terms of optimizing particle retention for coronary angioplasty restenosis.

7.4.1.1 Solid lipid nanoparticles (SLN)

SLN are alternative particulate carrier systems to polymeric nanoparticle emulsions and liposomes (Muller et al,1996). Their production using high pressure homogenization yields particles with a mean diameter between 80 nm to 100 nm.

SLN are produced by high-pressure homogenization of lipids either at elevated temperature in the melted state (hot homogenization) or at room temperature in the solid state (cold homogenization). Compritol 888 ATO (glyceroltribehenate containing approximately 15% monoglycerides) and cholesterol were used as lipids to formulate SLN. Pluronic F68 was used as emulsifier. A SLN formulation consisting of 10% Compritol 888 and 1.2% Poloxamer 188 (Pluronic F68) was produced by hot homogenization.

For drug loaded SLN, the drug was dissolved in the melted lipid prior to emulsification. Prednisolone was used as a model drug in a concentration of 1% in the lipid matrix. The entrapment efficiency of the drug was determined by measuring the concentration of the free drug in the dispersion medium.

The drug release pattern was found to be affected by the lipid matrix, concentration of emulsifier and production method. Low production temperature and low emulsifier concentration avoided burst and promoted a slow drug release pattern. Thus, SLN possess interesting features for their use as a drug carrier. Such systems being critical in physical characteristics possess a long- term stability of at least 24 months and are autoclavable at optimized conditions.

7.4.1.2 Polyalkyl cyanoacrylate nanoparticles

Polyalkyl cyanoacrylate nanoparticles have been used as carriers for the delivery of human recombinant granulocyte colony stimulating factor (rhG-CSF) (Gibaud et al., 1998). Polyalkylcyanoacrylate nanoparticles have been prepared by anionic polymerization or nanoprecipitation.

Isobutylcyanoacrylate (IBCA) and isohexylcyanoacrylate (IHCA) were used as monomers to prepare the polymers, polyisobutyl cyanoacrylate (PBCA) and polyisohexyl cyanoacrylate (PHCA).

By anionic polymerization it was possible to associate more than 66% of rhG - CSF with nanoparticles when the glycoprotein was added at the end of polymerization process. The rhG-CSF was mainly adsorbed on the surface of the nanoparticles and most of the colony stimulating activity was conserved. The in-vitro release of rhG-CSF from polyhexylcyanoacrylate nanoparticles was found to be progressive for 8 hr.

7.4.2 Microspheres and microcapsules

Microspheres have been investigated for intravenous and intraarterial targeting and delivery systems. Microspheres and microcapsules have been injected in the vessels to ensure the passive targeting of drugs. The drug release is controlled by diffusion through the polymer matrix and/or by erosion of the polymer. The role of microspheres and microcapsules depends on their size and site of injection.

Microparticles of diameters smaller than 2 mm can be injected in an intravenous, intraarterial and intraperitoneal manner in order to target the RES. I.V. injection of microspheres of size from 3 to 12 μm is intended to block the capillaries of lungs, liver and spleen.

Vessels can be hyperselectively embolized with drug loaded particulate materials of more than 10μm. Microspheres and microcapsules are used as particulate agents for the embolization of tumors and arteriovenous malformations. In these delivery systems microspheres or microcapsules have a two fold action as embolic agents and drug carriers. Microspheres of 100 to 300 μm size are the most appropriate embolic agents. They reach the intralesional precapillary arteries and cause reduction of blood flow.

Drugs can be incorporated in these particulate systems by two methods:

1) The polymer can either surround a core of drug (encapsulation type), or

2) The drug can be dissolved or homogeneously dispersed in the polymer (matrix device-microsphere type).

Microcapsules are similar in many respects to microspheres but they consist of small spheres that have an outer layer or membrane enclosing a core material that can be the drug itself. Microcapsules are generally large compared to the microspheres.

Polymers that are most commonly used in these formulations are ethylcellulose, cetyl alcohol, PLA polymers, PLGA copolymers, carnauba wax and proteins viz. serum albumin and gelatin. Table 7.2. Sums up the main characteristics of these materials and drugs loaded in them (Flandroy et al, 1993)

The kinetics of drug release from the microparticles and the biodegradation rate of the drug carrier are of major importance since they determine the amount of drug released per unit of time, accordingly the bioavailability of the drug and its effect.

A summary of different types of microspheres/miccrocapsules investigated for intravascular administration is as follows:

Table 7.2 : Characteristics of polymers used in microspheres
(adapted from Flandroy et al, 1993)

Polymer	Mean size (μm)	Degradation status	Drug	Kinetics of drug release
Ethyl cellulose	200-300	Non-degradable	Cisplatin, Mitomycin	Burst effect
PLGA	100-200	Degradable (days-months.)	Cisplatin, Adriamycin	Sustained release
Albumin	7-80	Degradable (few days)	Mitomycin, Adriamycin	Burst effect
Gelatin	45-50	Degradable (few days)	Adriamycin	Burst effect
Cetylalcohol	300	Degradable (20 days)	BCNU	Burst effect
Wax	125-800	Non- degradable	5FU	First order release
Chitosan Chitin	150-200	Degradable	Cisplatin	Sustained release

7.4.2.1 Albumin microspheres

Albumin microspheres are biodegradable and allow incorporation and sustained release of variety of drugs. Hence they have been clinically inve..tigated for the intraarterial delivery of chemotherapeutic agents.

Albumin microspheres are prepared by high-speed ultrasonic emulsion and suspension technology. The particle solidification is achieved by heat or chemical cross-linking as represented in schematic chart given in Fig 7. 6 (Gupta et al, 1986). Following hydration, these particles swell 50 to 100% of their size with concurrent slow matrix erosion.

An early work compared the efficacy of 3.3% w/w 5-FU loaded albumin microspheres with the delivery of an equivalent dose of drug solution. It was observed that tumor growth rate over 20 days after the microspheric drug delivery was one third of that when the drug was administered as solution. Similar results were obtained on using epirubicin loaded albumin microspheres (Leucuta et al, 1988). Apart from albumin, proteins like caesin and gelatin can also be used to formulate microspheres. Caesin microspheres are prepared by emulsification followed by polymer cross-linking with glutaraldehyde.

7.4.2.2 Polylactide (PLA)/ Polylactide - co-glycolide (PLGA) microspheres

Polylactide(PLA) and Poly (lactide-co-glycolide) microspheres are prepared by emulsion solvent evaporation process. In order to make microspheres that would degrade in required time, combination of two poly DL-lactide samples of different molecular weights in different ratio can be used. This is because high molecular weight polymers yield microspheres of high mechanical strength whereas low molecular weight polymers decrease the lifetime of the particles.

A solution of two polymers in dichloromethane is dispersed in an aqueous phase and microdroplets are then solidified by the slow evaporation of the organic solvent. This technique is convenient to control the size distribution of the microspheres. Extensive research has been carried out on the use of PLA/PLGA microspheres as drug carriers.

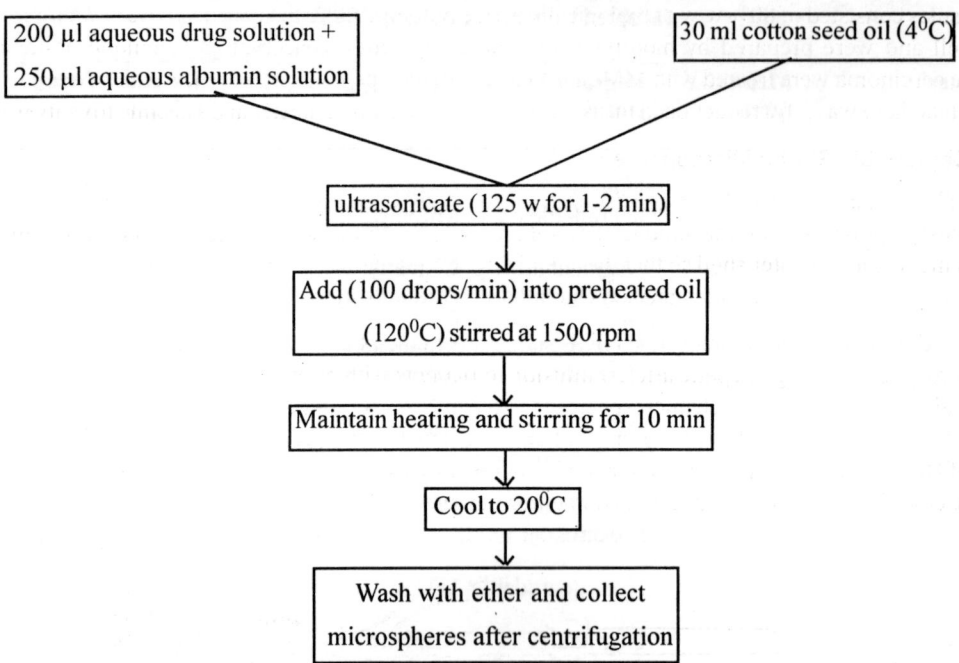

Fig 7.6 : Schematic representation of steps involved in the preparation of albumin
microspheres by heat denaturation (adapted from Gupta et al, 1986)

Ichihara et al (1989) loaded PLA microspheres with mitomycinC and performed clinical studies on two groups of patients, one being treated by chemoembolization and another by systemic chemotherapy, which formed the control group. It was observed that the cumulative survival rate for 59 patients with unressectable hepatocellular carcinoma was 54.3% for one year. For the control group, the cumulative survival rate was 11.6% for 6 months and zero percent after one year.

Sah et al (1995) prepared biodegradable PLA/PLGA microcapsules for controlled release of model proteins viz. BSA, transferrin and trypsin by w/o/w emulsion solvent evaporation method. The influence of microcapsule formation on degradability and permeability to proteins was studied. It was demonstrated that the degree of water uptake and their susceptibility to hydrolysis affected the *in-vitro* release of proteins.

Microcapsules provided continuous release profiles of proteins rather than polyphasic or pulsatile kinetics. Therefore the microcapsules providing controlled release of antigen can be an effective alternative to multiple injections of antigen and have a potential use as vaccine adjuvants.

PLA/PLGA polymers have also been used to encapsulate L-thrombin, a potent coagulation factor to be used in combination with antimitotic agent to increase the efficiency of chemoembolisation. The gelatin microspheres were produced as a chemoembolization material to deliver anticancer drug and L-thrombin was microencapsulated in PLA microcapsules (Ruiz et al., 1989) by coacervation. PLA/PLGA polymer solutions in dichloromethane were coacervated by slow addition of silicone oil to yield microcapsules.

7.4.2.3 Ethylcellulose microcapsules

Selective intraarterial infusion of the ethylcellulose microcapsules of mitomycinC exerts its potential therapeutic effect through both infarction and prolonged local drug activity.

Kato et al (1981) treated tumors with elthylcellulose microcapsules loaded with mitomycinC. MMC microcapsules consisted of 80% w/w of biologically active mitomycinC as the core and 20% w/w ethylcellulose as the shell and were prepared by modifying the phase separation coacervation technique. Patients with metastatic carcinoma were treated with MMC- microcapsules via percutaneous arterial catheterization. It was observed that there was 30% reduction in measurable maximum tumor diameter and systemic toxicity was mild.

7.4.2.4 Degradable Starch Microspheres

The degradable starch microspheres consist of specially formulated cross-linked spheres produced by traditional emulsion polymerization technique. The spheres are 40 ± 5 mm in diameter and the degree of cross -linkage is highest in the outer shell so that the spherical shape is maintained until the final stage of disintegration. The spheres are stable in dry state and can be stored at room temperature.

Dakhil & William, (1982) administered BCNU (1,3, -bis 2 chloroethyl - 1-nitrosourea) mixed with degradable starch microspheres through hepatic arterial infusion to patients with primary and metastatic cancer. This co-administration of degradable starch microspheres resulted into temporary blockage of the arterial block through the liver. Such occlusion at the arteriolor capillary bed enhances regional uptake and decreases systemic toxicity of BCNU. As the spheres are degraded by serum amylase, rapid blood circulation is reestablished 15 min. after embolization and is found to become normal after 30 min. A schematic representation of starch microspheres induced arteriolor capillary occlusion and drug egress from blood column is shown in Fig 7.7.

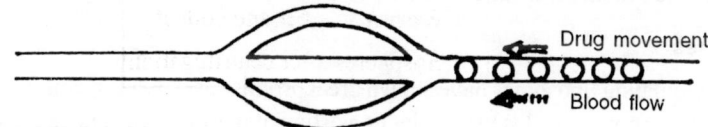

Large solid spheres in blocked blood column

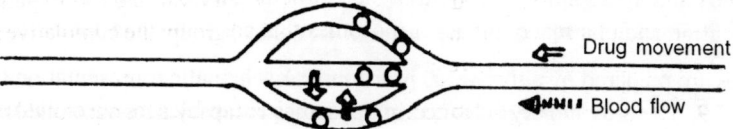

Restriction of blood flow in capillary bed with small spheres

Fig 7.7 : Schematic representation of starch microspheres induced arteriolar capillary occlusion and drug egress from blocked blood coloumn (adapted from Dakhil et al, 1982)

7.4.2.5 Magnetic nanoparticles/microspheres

The incorporation of magnetic Fe_3O_4 particles of size of 10-20 nm in diameter into albumin, poly (isobutyl) cyanoacrylate and chitosan nanoparticles enables the preparation of magnetically responsive particles. By placing a magnet in close vicinity of organs or extremities, it is possible to increase the concentration of the magnetic particles and hence of particle bound drug in the kidneys, lungs or hind limbs . (Ibrahim et al, 1983).

Drugs bound to these particles are then released at the target site leading to higher concentration at this site and lower concentration in other parts of the body, in comparison to the intravascular injection of solution of the same drug.

Widder & Senyui (1980) used a rat tail Yoshida tumor model as the target site. Magnetically responsive albumin microspheres were injected and a magnet with a field strength of 0.55T was placed at this site. Transmission microscopy revealed that microspheres are endocytosed by endothelial cells as early as 10 min. after infusion. By 30 min. microspheres were seen in tumor cells and within 24 hr., they were endocytosed by the tumor cells and resided there for 12 hr. Similar results were obtained for 1-7 mm sized doxorubicin albumin microspheres in lung metastasis tumor by placing a magnet of strength 0.6T at each side of the rat close to the lungs. Doxorubicin concentration of magnetic microspheres was increased to about 10-fold in comparison to free drug and about 1.3-fold in comparison to plain doxorubicin microspheres. The mean survival time of these animals increased by 44% with doxorubicin magnetic particles and by 29% in free drug (Papisov et al, 1987).

However it should be noted that the localization of the target site in the tail and the use of small animals (like mice and rats) enabled the use of a relatively small magnetic field. In a larger three-dimensional patient body, it will not be possible to focus the magnetic field exclusively on a restricted target area in the interior of the body. Unless the particles are injected into the tissues or organs within the magnetic field or into a location where blood flow reaches the magnetic field area immediately after injection, they will come into contact with the RES which would remove them from circulation before they could pass through the magnetic field. The use of magnetic field requires the knowledge of the exact position of the tumor or target site. Undetected metastases cannot be treated by this method. Nevertheless the use of magnetic particles is an interesting approach that is worth studying when rapid removal of the particles by the RES can be prevented by other methods.

7.4.3 Liposomes

Targeted long circulating liposomes have shown great promise as a tissue specific drug carrier for intravascular administration. Liposomes are closed vesicles consisting of one or more concentric spheres of lipid bilayers or lamellae enclosing an equal number of aqeous compartments. Liposomes range in size from 25 nm to as much as 10 mm and hence can be administered intravascularly.

The potential advantages that liposomes offer as intravascular delivery vehicles are (1) they can incorporate both hydrophobic and hydrophilic drugs within their structure, and (2) their surface can be modified to alter their biodistrubution and pharmacokinetics. Liposomes that are stable can act as slow release drug depots.

Liposomes are prepared by a three-step procedure. A schematic representation of liposome preparation is given in Fig 7.8. The drug moiety is loaded in liposomes either by passive or active loading process.

Liposomes are more than an inert vehicle in that they can also alter drug distribution based on their size, chemical composition, nature and surface charge. They are made from naturally occuring phospholipids such as phosphatidyl choline, cholestrol as well as synthetic phospholipids such as phosphatidyl inositol.

When liposomes become associated with the cell plasma membrane they can modify the cell membrane phospholipid composition. During phagocytosis these changes may alter enzymes and carriers in the cell membrane resulting in the liposomal lipids becoming an active participant in the therapeutic manoeuvre.

Depending on their construction, liposomes can be made to release entrapped drugs at increased temperature. This increases the potential for regional therapy because parts of body can be made hyperthermic by various techniques.

A number of anti-cancer drugs and anti-microbiologic agents are trapped in liposomes viz. cytosine, arabinoside, methotrexate, doxorubicin, dactinomycin, amphotericinB (Arnold et al, 1986).

It has been observed that the pH of the tumor cells is reduced. Hence liposomes have been made that will release their contents much more effectively at pH 5-6 than at pH 7.2 with the intention of specific release of drugs only in tumors.

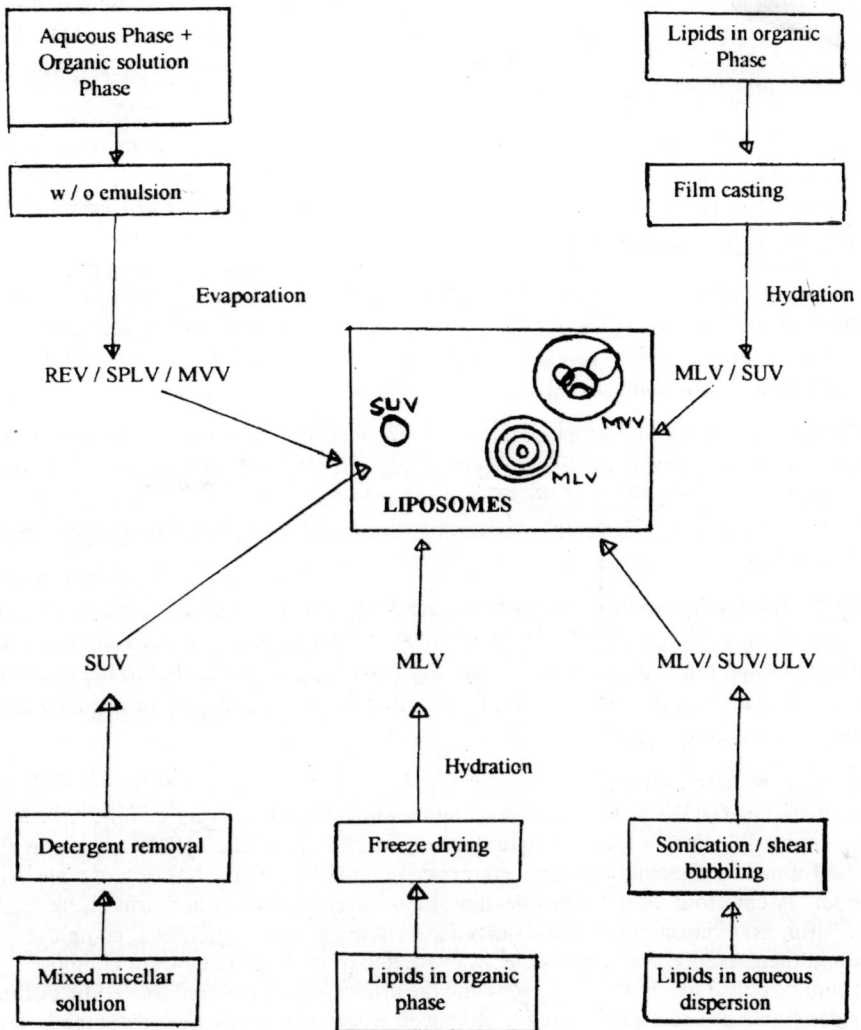

ULV, SLV, MLV, SPLV, MVV and REV represent uni, small, multi, stable pluri lamellar, multi vesicular and reverse phase evaporation vesicles respectively.

Fig 7.8 : Schematic diagram for preparation of liposomes (adapted from Crommelin, 1994)

A large number of investigators demonstrated in preclinical studies that liposomes modulated the biodistribution of doxorubicin resulting in a significant reduction of dose limiting toxicity (Rahman & White, 1985). Gel state liposomes released their contents following uptake by liver macrophages, which served as a reservoir for prolonged release of doxorubicin into the circulation (Crommelin et al, 1983). Hence the therapeutic index of the drug increased. Recently it has been reported that amphotericinB encapsulated in liposomes was substantially less toxic than free amphotericinB in mice model. Attaining comparable antifungal efficacy, former was found to be upto ten times less toxic than the free drug in the form of conventional deoxycholate solubilized formulation (Crommelin, 1994).

Conventional liposomes comprised of only phosphatidylcholine and cholesterol for colloidal systems. Surface characteristics play a crucial role after they are intravascularly administered. Hence the development of sterically stabilized long circulating liposomes represented a milestone in the search for liposomes that can bypass mononuclear phagocytic system. This stabilization is achieved by incorporation of natural hydrophilic components viz. gangliosides (GM1), phosphatidyl inositol essentially mimicking the outer surface of red blood cells or of synthetic hydrophilic polymers especially PEG.

However recent studies indicate that for PEG-PE stabilized liposomes, steric hindrance was introduced by the PEG. This can block the recognition of the surface attached targeting ligand and hence binding activity of liposomes at target site is reduced (Huang et al, 1995). This problem has been resolved by either,

(i)   using PEG of moderate chain length, or

(ii)   introducing a long spacer by attaching the targeting ligand to the distal end of PEG-PE coated liposome. The important limitation to be taken into account, considering the use of liposomes as drug carriers is their inability or limited ability to extravasate and to reach target sites in the extravascular space and nonvascular tissues (Torchillin, 1995).

However there exist many important targets within the vascular system itself, such as blood cells, vessel wall components and pathological structures exposed into circulation (thrombi, atherosclerotic lesions and malignancies). Furthermore, targeting of certain extravascular sites (eg. subendothelial layer, smooth muscle cells, tumor cells) after vascular disruption is possible in case of atherosclerotic lesions, acute myocardial infarction and neoplasia.

Drugs in cyclodextrins in liposomes : Water-insoluble drugs that cannot be effectively incorporated into the bilayers of liposomes or are incompatible can be administered in the form of water-soluble cyclodextrin complexes via liposomes and reach target tissues. This approach appears preferable to the use of cyclodextrins alone, for drug adminstration in terms of drug localization in the tissues and may reduce the problems of cyclodextrin toxicity including drug displacement by other molecules.

Mc Cormack & Gregoriades (1995) prepared cyclodextrin complexes with model drugs dehydroepiandrosterone (DHEA), dexamethasone and retinol. The drugs were complexed with ^{14}C labelled HPbCD and entrapped in liposomes by dehydration-rehydration procedure (DRV Liposomes). The *in-vivo* studies were performed by injecting liposome entrapped complexes into the tail vein of male Wistar rats used as animal model. Twenty four hours after injection, blood plasma, tissues and urine were analysed for [14]C (HPbCD) and [3]H(drugs) radioactivity. It was observed that entrapment of drug/HPbCD complexes into liposomes was efficient and their retention in the vesicles was greater when liposomes were composed of distearoyl phosphatidyl choline only. Quantitative drug loss into the urine after injection of free HPbCD, drug complexes reduced considerably and tissue uptake greatly enhanced when complexes were entrapped into liposomes.

7.4.4 Microemulsions

Microemulsions are thermodynamically stable emulsions having small droplet size of less than 140 nm. Microemulsions of phospholipids have been prepared by prolonged sonication and microfluidization of the components.

Soyabean oil microemulsions can be prepared by adding polyoxyethylene hydrogenated castor oil (HCO 60) as surfactant. HCO surfactants were found to be most suitable emulsifiers in stabilizing emulsions containing lipiodol oily phase. Low concentrations of emulsifier HCO 60 (1%) have been reported to give stable emulsions with longer sustained release characteristics. A ready to inject lipiodol based emulsion containing a water - soluble cytotoxic drug, doxorubicin has been developed by Jeong et al (1998).

Lipiodol has three functions in the emulsion systems. It acts as a contrast medium for visualizing the tumors. Secondly, it slows the arterial circulation as an embolic agent, thereby effectively blocks the blood supply feeding hepatocellular carcinoma. Third, it shows a preferential uptake into tumor tissue and hence can be used as a vehicle for the targeted delivery of cytotoxic or radiotherapeutic drugs. Lipiodolized emulsion as a carrier for anticancer drugs has been proved successful in targeted chemotherapy.

Kurihara et al (1995) formulated a highly lipophilic antitumor agent RS-1541 (130- palmitoyl rhizoxin) as HCO60 emulsion for intravascular injection. The lipolysis of such emulsions is evaluated by lipoprotein lipase and these emulsions were less susceptible to lipolysis as compared to conventional lecithin emulsified emulsions. Lecithin emulsions were rapidly taken up by liver leading to low blood levels, HCO 60 emulsions in contrast showed less uptake by RES, long circulation time in the blood and high distribution of antitumor agent into the tumor tissues.

7.4.5 Photopolymerised hydrogels

Interfacial photopolymerised hydrogels provide an effective means of local delivery of proteins and offer biological materials to the vessel wall. Controlled amounts of hydrogels can be placed on the luminal surface for intravascular delivery or they can be applied around the tunica externa to allow periadventitial drug delivery.

The hydrogel is a three dimensional network that allows restricted cell permeation. Small molecular weight species such as oxygen, glucose, aminoacids can diffuse through it freely whereas permeability to protein depends upon their molecular weight.

The hydrogel barrier is impermeable to macromolecules hence it may be used for the controlled release of macromolecular drugs. The drug is entrapped in the 3D meshwork of the gel and as the meshwork loosens by degradation the drug is slowly released.

A method for the application of very thin (< 50 μm) hydrogel films to the inner surface of blood vessel by interfacial photopolymerization has been described by West & Hubbell (1995).

The hydrogel precursor consists of three subunits: a central PEG domain (M.W. 8,000, biocompatible), flanked by lactyl groups (biodegradable) and terminated by two acrylic groups (photo cross-linkable). A central PEG chain is copolymerised at each end with five average lactic acid units and further capped at each end with reactive acrylate.

In this process a nontoxic photoinitiator is adsorbed to the luminal surface of the vessel. The vessel is then filled with the hydrogel precursor and illuminated, resulting in the formation of a gel at the vessel surface.

Philbrook et al (1995) have described the method for incorporating heparin into hydrogel by interfacial polymerization. The arterial segment was filled with eosin Y (20 ppm) and the excess of eosin was flushed through the lavage. Following this macromer application, triethanolamine (e donor) is applied. Illumination with visible light (480-514nm) initiates photopolymerization whereby the hydrogel grows from the tissue surface where eosin-macromer interface is formed. The cross section of a rat carotid artery where an interfacial hydrogel coating has been applied to the endoluminal surface is shown in Fig 7. 9. Bulk photopolymerization can be evaluated *in-vitro* as well as by *in-vivo* methods using isolated arterial segments from rat.

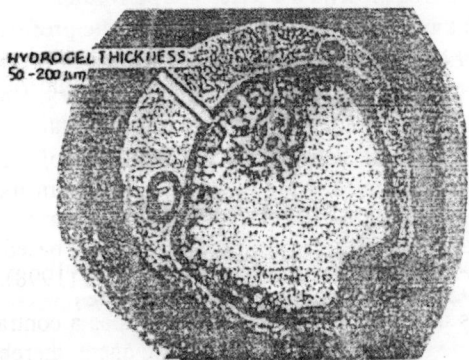

Fig 7.9 : Cross section of a rat carotid artery where an interfacial hydrogel coating has been applied to the endoluminal surface (adapted from Philbrook et al, 1995)

7.4.5. 1 Assessment of formation and degradation kinetics of the hydrogel

The formation and degradation kinetics of interfacially photopolymerized hydrogels was assessed in rat carotid arteries. Fluorescent microspheres (1 μm) were added to the hydrogel precursor formulation to aid in visualization. To evaluate polymerization kinetics, illumination times were varied and the thickness of the hydrogel was measured. The hydrogel thickness was found to increase with increasing illumination time. This can be used as an effective means to control thickness of intravascular hydrogel. To assess degradation, illumination time was held constant and duration of *in-vivo* exposure to blood flow was varied. It was concluded that it is possible to design hydrogels with desired degradation kinetics by changing the length and composition of the degradable polymer.

7.4.5.2 *In-vitro* release kinetics

In-vitro release kinetics was studied by dissolving proteins of molecular weights ranging from 6,000 to 150,000 Da in aliquots of the precursor solution and then converting the solution to hydrogel by bulk photopoiymerization. The hydrogel samples were incubated with buffered saline solution. The samples were withdrawn at frequent intervals and the buffer was changed to approximate sink conditions and the release was quantified by a suitable assay. The average release rate for 0-80 % release was computed for each protein. A linear relationship between the release rate and protein molecular weight was observed. For proteins of molecular weight approx. 80,000 Da and less, release appeared to be controlled by diffusion without polymer degradation, whereas the proteins of molecular weight 150,000 Da were released by degradation of the hydrogel.

7.4.5.3 In-vivo drug delivery studies

The potential to locally deliver a protein from a hydrogel to the arterial segment and affect a change in the healing response of an injured vessel can be assessed in a rat carotid arterial balloon injury model. Arterial injury is induced in male rats after which a hydrogel containing platelet derived growth factor, PDGF is applied periadventitially via bulk photopolymerization. Rats are euthenized and the carotid arteries subjected to histological analysis. The thickness of intimal layer is measured and compared with the control. It has been observed that protein can be delivered from photopolymerized hydrogel while retaining its biological activity and the released protein is able to permeate the vessel wall to act on its target.

7.4.5.4 The arterial uptake

The ability to deliver heparin from heparin loaded biodegradable hydrogel coating on the endoluminal surface of carotid arteries of rats formed by *in-situ* photopolymerization has been evaluated by Philbrook and coworkers (1995). During the study blood and urine samples were taken to evaluate biodistribution and elimination rates of heparin. A qualitative analysis of drug present in arteries was performed by audioradiography. Blood levels of heparin from hydrogel showed a two compartment elimination rate profile, where faster elimination was observed in the beginning and later constant rate of elimination followed over a period of time. Persistent site-specific delivery of heparin to vessel wall was assessed for over 48 hours. The hydrogel was able to sustain high concentration of the drug in locally treated vessel tissue. These results indicate the feasibility of using hydrogel deposited endovascularly as a platform for the local delivery of drugs to blood vessel wall. Low levels of therapeutic agents can be delivered using this technology with the added benefit of decreased systemic levels with minimum exposures to sensitive organs.

Pluronic gels : Pluronic gel solutions have been used for periadventitial application of antisense c-myb oligonucleotides (Simons et al, 1992). Pluronic gels are soluble at cold temperature (4°C) and form a gel at body temperature.

The antisense oligonucleotide have been added to pluronic solutions at the concentration of 1 mg/ml stored at 4°C. Immediately after balloon angioplasty, 200 ml of solution is applied to the carotid artery from which the adventitia has been stripped. On contact with tissues at 37°C the solution gels, generating a translucent layer that envelops the vessel.

The suppression of smooth muscle cell accumulation by antisense oligo-nucleotide incorporated in pluronic gel has been investigated *in-vivo* in rat carotid artery model. Morphological examination revealed that minimum intimal accumulation occured with antisense oligonucleotide in pluronic gels as compared to control groups.

7.4.6 Polymeric matrices

The polymer based drug delivery systems provide a means of controlling local drug levels in an efficient manner and more effective means of examining the effects of various compounds in the control of smooth muscle cell proliferation following vascular inujury.

Ethylene vinyl acetate [EVA] polymer has been used to form drug containing matrices. EVA polymer based drug delivery system has been implanted perivascularly to injured artery. The polymer-matrices are prepared by dissolving drug and EVA in dichloromethane. The solution is then poured in glass petri dishes. Dried and cast polymeric matrix is cut into rectangular pieces. Various drugs that are incorporated in EVA matrices and implanted perivascularly are tyrphostin compounds, colchicine and heparin (Golomb et al, 1995).

Silicon polymer matrices : Silicon polymer is a non-degradable polymer that has been used because of its high biocompatibility and hydrophobicity linked to excellent sustained release properties. Local periadventitial delivery of dexamethasone using silicon polymer matrix has been studied to inhibit proliferation after balloon injury in the rat carotid model (Villa & Guzman, 1994). The agent, as dry powder (90 - 120 mm) is incorporated by levigating it with prevulcanized silicon rubber and then exposing it to vacuum. Drug-polymer matrices are cast into thin slabs in aluminium moulds under pressure and vulcanizing. The surfaces of slab matrices are scaled using silicone polymer to allow unidirectional drug release.

7.4.7 Perivascular drug delivery systems

A periadventitial polymeric drug delivery system is one strategy for obtaining and maintaining high tissue levels of drugs at the site of vascular injury. The periadventitial (around the outer core of the artery) polymer systems can be impregnated with different drugs and have been implanted perivascularly i.e. around the periphery of blood vessel. Drug clearance and arterial uptake after local perivascular delivery to the rat carotid artery have been studied (Fishbein et al, 1996).

Attempt was made to characterise how drug released into the perivascular space enters the arterial wall and how it is cleared from the local environment. It was observed that drugs could enter the artery either from the adventitial aspect or from the lumen after absorption by the extraarterial capillaries. Almost all the drug released into the perivascular space is cleared through the extravascular capillaries. Virtually all the deposited drug diffuses directly from the perivascular space. This local drug release leads directly to increased local drug concentration within the arterial walls.

Controlled release polymeric matrices, as mentioned earlier, have been devised for perivascular administration using ethylene vinyl acetate polymers, silicone polymers or pluronic gels.

Polymeric matrices containing 0.1% colchicine were implanted perivascularly in rats following balloon catheter injury. The polymers were retrieved 1,7,14 and 21 days post implantation and the amount retained in the matrices was determined. Pieces of arteries treated with the perivascular implants were harvested and blood samples were withdrawn at the above time points, the amount of colchicine was determined in the serum. The rate and extent of colchicine transport across rat carotid artery were studied.

A good correlation was found between the amount of drug released and $T_{1/2}$ for various drug loads and matrix thickness. Matrices with the rate limiting membranes released drug at a constant rate. It was possible to design the implants with specific geometric size and delivery rate, large surface area matrices could cover a larger infused area of vessel. Adjustment of thickness of the matrix and drug load was possible to get the desired delivery amount and rate.

One has to consider the diameter of the artery in design of such matrices since all the local effect is sought. The diffusion experiments reveal that the drug is sufficiently permeated across bovine arteries. The calf artery is much thicker than rat. Therefore the rate - limiting step in the controlled delivery of drug from perivascular matrices is the release rate of the drug from the implanted matrices rather than the diffusion through the artery.

Thus by using a polymeric based drug delivery system implanted perivascularly to the injured artery the continued therapeutic effect of the drug on the developed neointima could be evaluated while avoiding systemic adverse effects due to the relatively low systemic levels of the locally released drug (Mishaly et al, 1997). The local perivascular delivery of specific growth factors and their inhibitors as well as therapeutic agents permits the evaluation of novel agents and represents a practical solution for examining longitudinal *in-vitro* drug effects.

7.4.8   Endovascular drug delivery

Local drug delivery for the treatment of vascular diseases is being utilized recently. Anatomic targeting involves approaches delivering high drug concentrations at specific sites (Markou et al, 1998).

Anatomic targeting intends to provide local drug delivery directly into the injured vessel wall with minimal systemic exposure. Antithrombotic drugs have been introduced directly into the vascular tissues by perforated balloon angioplasty catheterization but the residence time of drug in the vessel wall is typically short (approximately one hour).

The recently developed methods of iontophoresis or of coating of balloons with drug releasing hydrogels tend to produce short-term effects. As an alternative, a new local delivery approach has been developed. In concept, an antithrombotic drug is infused around the circumference of the vessel and adjacent to the wall. The drug remains close to the wall achieving high concentration just distal to the infusion site. As the infusate enters the blood stream along the vessel, its radial velocity should be low compared to the centre stream flow so as to produce minimal flow disruption. As the drug propagates downstream under fluid convection forces, it remains adjacent to the wall in a boundary layer. This concept has been evaluated in-vivo and in-vitro. Its major advantages include:

(1)   Higher drug concentration levels than could be achieved by intravenous infusion.

(2)   Use of agents which might be toxic systemically, expensive or less available.

(3)   Avoidance of bleeding complications and side effects.

(4)   Reduced total drug requirements and hence reduced cost of therapy.

(5)   Longer periods of drug administration for controlled release of drug in vessel.

To demonstrate the efficiency of this technique, its capacity to inhibit thrombosis was evaluated in a baboon thrombosis model (Chen & Hanson, 1995). The catheter was inserted into a femoral arteriovenous shunt (blood flow rate 100ml/min) and placed proximal to a segment of highly thrombogenic Dacron vascular graft. Integrelin (an inhibitor of platelet glycoprotein IIB / IIIA, dose 1mg) and hirudin (an antithrombin. dose 100mg /ml/ min) were used to inhibit thrombin formation. Experimental flow visualization studies indicated that high concentrations of infused drugs retained near the vessel wall. Platelet deposition on the Dacron graft surface was reduced by 82-97 % (Integrelin) and 68-92 % (hirudin) over 1-2 hr. of blood exposure. The local antithrombic effects produced were found to be 200 fold and 30 fold more efficient than systemic administration of the same agents. A schematic diagram of an endovascular drug delivery system is included in Fig 7.10.

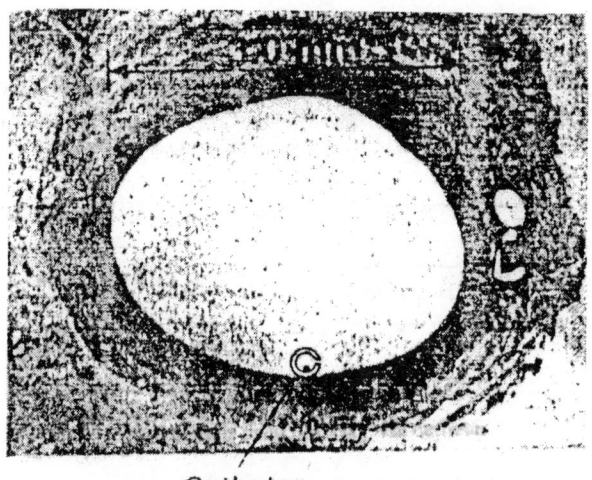

Catheter

Fig 7.10 : Schematic diagram of endovascular drug delivery (adapted from Markou et al 1998)

Vascular grafts :Vascular grafts are microporous fibrillar structures that can be implanted in the vessels. The microporous graft exhibits a mesh like arrangement of the polyurethane fabricated by a simultaneous spraying phase inversion technique.

Improving small diameter grafts is the focus of vascular research. An implanted graft is analogous to a native vessel deprived of its endothelium and sustained modification of the graft may be required for satisfactory endothelial growth. In a simple way we can emulate the native environment of arteries by providing factors to control growth via controlled release microspheres in grafts.

A technique has been developed for the inclusion of PLA microsphere in polyurethane vascular grafts (Krietz & Webber, 1995). Cardiothane-51, a medical grade polyether urethane polymer that is safe in humans was used. One or more drugs can be loaded into microspheres to deliver the drugs to the immediate environment. This inclusion technique was developed primarily to assist vascular graft healing, tissue matrix regeneration and cell substrate attachment.

7.4.5 Pharmacokinetic considerations

A pharmacokinetic model based on the physiology of the mammalian circulation is shown in Fig 7.11. This method is used to study the behaviour and characteristics of intraarterial infusion. The drug is given by either intravenous or intraarterial infusion into the body and is assumed to be eliminated by all the organs and tissues. The mechanisms of drug elimination are excretion, metabolism by liver or by hydrolysis in the body fluids.

Pharmacokinetic analysis outlining the crucial elements and potential drug exposure increases with intraarterial drug infusions has been carried out (Ensminger & Gyres, 1984).

To quantitate the delivery advantage to the target site, the ratio of regional exposure after regional arterial infusion is compared to that after venous infusion at the same dose rate.

The advantage of increased drug delivery resulting from arterial infusion is determined by factors which influence the time integrals of the arterial drug levels obtained by arterial versus venous infusion respectively.

It is demonstrated that the regional drug exposure advantage (Rd) for agents with linear pharmacokinetics is related to the rate of drug elimination in the rest of the body and the blood perfusion rate into the target region by the formula:

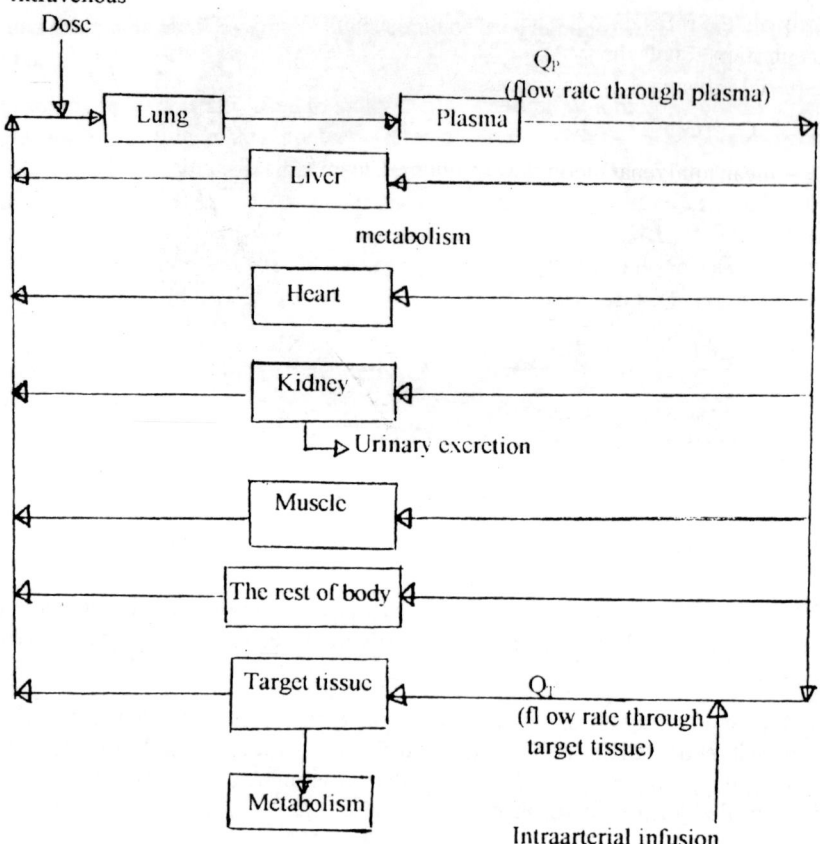

Fig 7.11 : Pharmacokinetic model for intraarterial and intravenous infusion systems

$$\text{Advantage } (R_d) = 1 + CL_{app} \times Q_T \qquad (1)$$

Where Capp is the total body drug clearance from the rest of the body, excluding the tumor (target) region and Q_T is the blood flow through the regional artery being infused. Intraarterial infusion will reduce drug delivery and availability to the rest of the body by:

$$R_d = 1 - E_T \qquad (2)$$

Where E_T = extraction ratio of the drug by the target region. Combining the advantage gained through the total body clearance relative to regional blood flow plus that gained by regional extraction, the general equation defining the regional advantage of intraarterial infusion is:

$$\text{Regional advantage; } R_d = 1 + \frac{CL_{TB}}{Q_T(1 - E_T)}$$

Where CL_{TB} = total body drug clearance and Q_T and E_T are as mentioned above. Hence regional selectivity is a direct function of a drug's total body clearance. Thus agents with high total body clearance are essential for maximum regional - effect for intraarterial chemotherapy.

Blood Clearance CL (ml/min) is calculated by:

$$CL = \text{inf.}/C_T$$

Where inf. equals the infusion rate and C_T is the concentration at steady state in the renal artery. This renal artery concentration equals the systemic arterial concentration (C_s) in the case of systemic infusion. In the case of intraarterial infusion C_T is calculated by:

$$C_T = C_S + \text{inf} / Q_T$$

Where Q_T = mean total renal blood flow (ml/min). Clearance is also calculated from urinary excretion,

$$C_L = U/C_T$$

Where U = urinary excretion rate (mg/min). The extraction ratio is calculated by the formula:

$$E_T = U/C_T Q_T.$$

The advantages of intraarterial over systemic drug delivery were calculated, using formula for local advantage:

$$\frac{C_T \text{ ia}}{C_T \text{iv}} = 1 + \frac{CLs}{Q_T}$$

Where $C_T$ia = target artery concentration during local and $C_T$iv = Target artery concentration during systemic drug delivery of the same dose. The CLs is defined as the total body clearance of the drug minus the clearance of the drug by the target organ. For systemic advantage:

$$\frac{C_s \text{ ia}}{C_s \text{ iv}} = 1 - E_T$$

Where C_s ia equals the systemic concentration during local and $C_s$iv equals the systemic concentration during systemic drug delivery of the same dose.

The relevant pharmacokinetic parameters and estimates of the improved regional hepatic exposure with hepatic arterial drug infusion for a number of drugs are presented in Table 7.3 (Chen & Gross, 1980).

Table 7.3: Pharmacokinetic properties of drugs used for hepatic arterial infusion.

Drug	T ½(min)	CL_{TB} lit / min	E_H exposure of hepatic arterial infusion	Estimated increased
FU	10	2-5	0.80	50-100
FUDR	<10	5-15	0.69-0.92	100-400
BCNU	<5	2.5		7-13
Mitomycin	£10	0.6	0.07-0.18	3-5

Most of the drugs used in hepatic arterial chemotherapy have short plasma half - lives and high total body clearances. The two most commonly utilized drugs FU and FUDR have half - lives of < 10 min. with high total body clearance plus extensive hepatic extraction (E_H). Calculations based on direct blood level determinations indicate as much as a 100 fold advantage for FU and 400 fold advantage for FUDR of hepatic arterial over intravenous infusion resulting in the generation of an improved hepatic drug exposure. Significantly (i.e. > 2 fold) increased exposure with hepatic arterial infusion is seen for a number of other agents, including methotrexate, mitomycin, cisplatin etc. These principles assumed that the rate coefficients of drug lost remained constant over the complete range of drug concentration and throughout the time period involved.

Pharmacokinetic advantages of local drug delivery by intraarterial infusion are observed if either the target organ has a high extraction ratio for the drug or the systemic clearance of the drug is high with respect to the blood flow through the organ.

Deviations from theoretical predictions are expected because of saturation kinetics. It has been reported by Daemen et al (1986) that a homogeneous flow distribution can cause localised saturation kinetics in the target organ. Since renal size and vascularization could be a function of genetic line, care should be taken in selecting experimental models. Disposition of ^{51}Cr EDTA and ^{125}I OIH following the constant rate of infusion either intravenously or intraarterially into the right or left kidney of the Wistar Kyoto rat was investigated. Both the compounds were eliminated by the kidney, the former by glomerular filtration and latter by glomerular filtration as well as tubular excretion. This study supported the target organ directed drug delivery but also revealed pitfalls i.e. nonlinearity in pharmacokinetics. The clearance and extraction of both substances by the right kidney were independent of the route of administration. In steady state the advantage of intrarenal over systemic delivery was limited because of the relative high blood flow of the kidney. Only a small reduction (30%) in systemic concentration was achieved by ^{51}CrEDTA infusion.

One of the methods for decreasing hepatic arterial blood flow is the use of microparticles or microspheres. At sufficiently high doses using biodegradable starch microspheres (40 μm diameter), hepatic arterial blood flow could be totally blocked in about 25 % of patients. By 30 min. after hepatic arterial injection the starch microspheres are completely lysed by serum amylase and flow resumes through the hepatic arterial tree, as ascertained by contrast angiograms. In the remaining 75% of patients hepatic arterial flow was found to decrease by 80% and arterial venous shunting occurred. The use of hepatic arterial starch microspheres is an additional method to deliver more drug to tumor within the liver.

Three varieties of microspheres have been used clinically, two for drug delivery and one for radiotherapy. Ethyl cellulose microspheres which are 225±55 μm in diameter and contain 80% by weight of biologically active mitomycin have undergone extensive testing. Preclinical investigation in dogs indicate that drug release occurs over hours and that there is approximately a 60% reduction in circulating systemic mitomycin when the drug is encapsulated in microspheres and administered intraarterially. Because of the increased drug delivery to the liver and to the hepatic tumor, systemic drug exposure was reduced.

Improved regional selectivity of hepatic arterial BCNU with degradable starch microspheres was investigated (Dakhil et al, 1982). The ratio of the value of AUC with BCNU plus microspheres over the value of AUC with BCNU alone was 0.08 indicating much lower systemic concentrations.

In addition to being pharmacokinetically rational, a second element in the evaluation of appropriateness of a drug for intraarterial chemotherapy is the dose response curve for that given drug in the tumor type in question.

By arterial infusion one exposes the tumor to more drug than is otherwise possible. And if tumor is sensitive to given drug then the exposure with intravenous chemotherapy may be sufficient to kill entire sensitive cell population. But if tumor is absolutely resistant to drug, then by increasing the exposure 100 fold with hepatic arterial infusion of some drugs, may not produce response. If an agent has marginal activity when given intravenously in a tumor then hepatic arterial infusion may be profitable. FU or FUDR both have definite marginal activity in colorectal cancer, hence marked increase in exposure by hepatic arterial infusion of FU or FUDR is of benefit than the use of another agent cytarabine which has no activity in the disease.

When the dose response for an agent is sufficiently steep and the pharmacokinetics appropriate, it should be possible to generate cytotoxic drug levels in the hepatic arterial tree with lower nontoxic systemic levels. The dose limiting toxicity should be regional (liver) rather than systemic (bone marrow). This is possible with FU despite its 50-80% hepatic extraction, where a constant hepatic arterial infusion of 1000 mg/m^2/day produces same steady state systemic level as 300 mg/m^2/day given intravenously.

A third consideration in successful intraarterial chemotherapy is knowledge of drug's schedule dependency. Schedule dependency is based on the biochemical and cytokinetic actions of the agent. In alkylating agents bolus injection for short term peak exposure may produce maximal damage to the nucleic acid of cells. Lower drug level with constant infusion allows rate-limited repair to occur and prevent lethality.

The drug schedule dictates type of delivery system necessary. Short infusion or bolus may be given by injection or by temporary pump attachment. Prolonged controlled infusion will require catheterization and pumping.

7.6 INTRAARTERIAL CATHETER INFUSION DRUG DELIVERY SYSTEMS

As intraarterial drug administration involves direct injection or infusion of drug into the artery supplying the blood to target organ, location of drug delivery site becomes important.

The drug must be delivered directly into the tumor blood supply in a reliable and reproducible manner. Several catheters and infusion pumps have been devised for the purpose. Pattern of distribution of the agents injected intrarterially is dependent on the flow rate of the infusion.

When percutaneous angiographic catheters are used, tips of the catheters tend to move about leading to unpredictable flow distribution changes. Nucleide angiography has been used to guide the catheter placement and to ascertain complete drug flow distribution with continuous hepatic arterial infusion using percutaneous angiographic catheter surgically placed. Progressive hepatic arterial thrombosis occurs at a high rate and gradually decreased blood flow and ultimately occlusion occurs. Hence a catheter system free of thrombosis and movement which reliably infuses the target region is a pre-requisite for maximal response with minimal toxicity.

7.6.1 Catheters

Catheter systems are used for local delivery of intravascular drugs at the desired site. Soft silastic catheters are placed surgically in a manner to minimise turbulence in blood flow.

1. **Porous balloon catheters :** The balloon catheters are developed to administer drugs with high pressure, forcing delivery into the arterial wall through the pore. One of the catheters has a diameter of 3 mm and length of 25 mm. It is perforated by a laser beam, creating 12 pores, each with an average diameter of 75 mm.

    In another design, 35 perforations are arranged radially around the circumference and along the length of the balloon catheter. The catheters can tolerate hydraulic pressure from 6-10 atm., for both to inflate the balloon and to produce outward flow through the pores (Gonchior & Clemens, 1995)

    Porous balloon with mechanical expansion PB/ME is another type that permits mechanical expansion before infusion of drug. This catheter is porous reservoir balloon with 50 holes that are 75 mm in diameter and covers a graded cure cage. A rotation knob allows the operator to enlarge the mechanical cage and expand the balloon against the vascular wall without infusing the agent. After mechanical inflation is done, direct infusion of the agent is attained, under infusion pressure of 6 atm. Schematic diagram of a balloon catheter is given in Fig. 12.

2. **Needle Injection Catheter :** It contains six circumferential needles that can be extended and used to inject the drug into the vessel wall and adventitia. This device is made up of flexible polyethylene with a central lumen for a guide wire and six outer needles of 250 mm of positioned symmetrically. When the catheter is placed in the vessel lumen, the needles are advanced by a mechanism at the external end of the catheter, thus extending the needles proximally so that they fan out to encompass a diameter of 5.5 mm. The needles are shaped such that there is a cover at the end so that they can penetrate laterally into the media

or perivascular area. It has been suggested that adventitia plays an important role in the vessel response to catheter induced injury and the drug delivery into the adventitia creates a depot, which may provide a method of prolonged therapeutic action. It is important that local drug delivery devices do not in themselves cause injury and tissue hyperplasia or infection. Antimicrobial bonded catheters have also been developed (Yang et al, 1998).

3.   **Micro Catheters :** A very sophisticated and powerful catheter system is a minute sized catheter made up of shafts of variable thickness with a very flexible and supple distal extremity. It's external diameter is 1.5 to 2.7 F (1F = 1/3 mm). A gold or platinum ring is inserted in the tip that increases the opacity under fluoroscopy. The microcatheters are equipped with stearable micro-guide wire for torque advancement and thus to reach upto the sixth division branches of arteries. Intravascular navigation using such devices makes regions accessible that were thought to be out of reach a few years ago (e.g. brain carotid artery).

The distal aperture of microcatheters are narrow and only liquids or particles of diameter upto 350mm can be injected. Colloidal spherical particles of diameter 200-300 mm can pass when correctly dispersed and sufficiently diluted. Flow of non-spherical particles of similar size is difficult to control.

4.   **Helical Catheter :** Such catheters are devised for local endovascular drug delivery (Markou et al, 1998). The catheter is placed adjacent to the vessel wall proximal to the treatment site (e.g. vascular lesion or thrombus). The catheter is made from a polyethylene tubing with an outer diameter of 0.356 mm and internal diameter of 0.203 mm. The end of the catheter is in the form of helix, which comes in contact with the vessel wall. A number of small holes are laser drilled in the coils of the catheter (25 mm in diameter) through which drug is infused. This allows for drug infusion to lie in slowly moving layers of blood adjacent to the wall i.e. within the blood fluid 'boundary layer. The catheter profile can be optimised to minimise flow disturbances created by the catheter geometry. Fig 7.12 illustrates the concept of the helical catheter for endovascular local drug delivery.

The catheter systems require infusion pumps to generate pressure for the delivery of the drugs. Intraarterial drug infusions have been limited by the type of pumping systems involved. Following problems have been reported:

1.   Pumps worn externally by patients are inconvenient because of their bulkiness and are a major hindrance to normal daily activities.

2.   The pumps and the external catheter connections are sites for the interruption of the infusion path leading to the bleeding, catheter thrombosis or infection.

3.   Delivery catheters may induce problems due to clotting, breaking, kinking, leaking, dislodgment, embolism, fever, septicemia or hemorrhage.

4.   The technique is inconvenient for outpatients and hospital staff necessitating the use of portable infusion pumps and percutaneous infusion catheters, with their inherent restriction on patient's activities.

5.   There is a need for a team of supportive personnel to maintain a prolonged outpatient infusion and the clumsiness and unreliability of the infusion systems have limited their widespread applicability.

Hence a totally implanted drug delivery pump has been developed to overcome many of the problems noted with intravascular administration.

Totally implanted drug delivery pump system for hepatic arterial chemotherapy : A small flexible silastic catheter of 0.92 inch in diameter is implanted to infuse the entire liver arterial vasculature (Buchwald & Grage, 1980).The catheter is attached to a subcutaneously placed model 400 Infusaid pump Fig 7.12. This pump has a side port with an auxillary septum. There is delivery mechanism for continuous infusion through the pump.

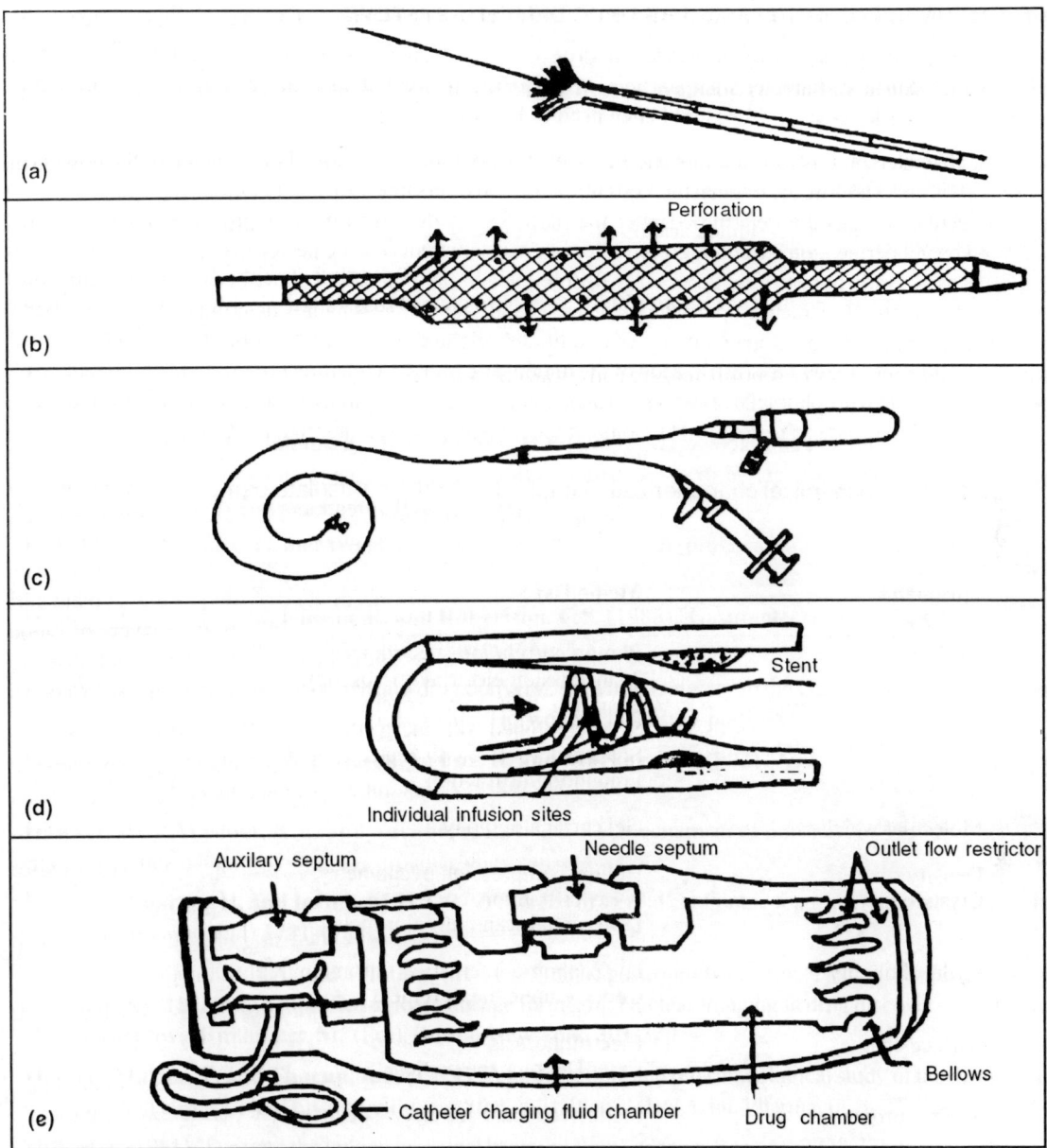

(a)

Perforation

(b)

(c)

Stent

(d)

Individual infusion sites

Auxilary septum   Needle septum   Outlet flow restrictor

Bellows

(e)   Catheter charging fluid chamber   Drug chamber

Fig 7.12 : Different catheters and pumps used for intravascular drug delivery

The disk shaped pump is separated into two chambers. The inner drug chamber contains the solution to be infused, the outer charging chamber contains a fluorocarbon liquid in equilibrium with its vapour phase. This vapour pressure produces the power source exerting pressure on the bellows and forces the infusate through a flow - regulating element. Each pump has a 50ml volume and a set rate (3-6 ml/day) and requires refill every 8-16 days. Pump refills and side port injections are performed by percutaneous injection.

A superselective one shot intraarterial method for treating inoperable cancer of the liver has been investigated. Selective one shot administration is a simple procedure, one can insert a catheter percutaneously via femoral artery into the celiac or hepatic artery and is able to obtain the antitumor effect.

7.7 EVALUATION OF INTRAVASCULAR DRUG DELIVERY SYSTEMS

Physicochemical evaluation of intravascular drug delivery systems is critical to assess their design and performance. Surface characteristics, particle size, density, crystallinity, surface charge and hydrophobicity affect the release kinetics of drugs and hence need to be evaluated.

For characterization of surface morphology, a high- resolution microscope like scanning probe microscope is used. SEM and TEM are the optimal methods that allow most versatile sizing and morphology characterization. The molecular weights are determined after the particles are dissolved in an appropriate solvent and then analyzed by gel permeation chromatography. Density measurements can be performed by helium pycnometry and by density gradient centrifugation. X-ray diffraction and thermoanalytical methods like DSC are used to evaluate the structural characteristics of the particles. The surface charge is mainly determined by electrophoretic mobility, using laser Doppler anemometry or amplitude weighted phase structuration. Hydrophobicity of the molecule influences the *in-vivo* distribution of the moiety after intravascular injections. Two major methods for determination of hydrophobicity exist viz. water contact angle measurement and hydrophobic interaction chromatography (Carstensen et al, 1991). Some of these methods are summarized in Table 7.4.

Table 4: Physicochemical characterization methods of drug particulate carriers for intravascular administration (Kreuter, 1994).

Parameter	Method (s)
Particle size	Photon correlation spectrometry Transmission electron microscopy Scanning electron microscopy SEM combined with energy dispersive X-ray spectrometry Scanned probe microscopes Fraunhofer diffraction
Molecular weight	Gel chromatography
Density Crystallinity	Helium compression pycnometry X-ray diffraction Differential scanning calorimetry
Hydrophobicity	Hydrophobic interaction chromatography Contact angle measurement
Surface charge	Electrophoresis Laser Doppler anemometry
Surface properties	Static secondary ion mass spectrometry

7.7.1 Drug loading analysis

Drugs may be loaded onto the carriers either by solid dispersion, adsorption or chemical binding. The adsorption isotherm of the drug is an important criterion for determining the type of binding and the binding capacity of the carrier. Drug content is determined by noting the bathochromic shift or the quenching of the fluorescence caused by that amount of drug that is bound to the particles. Colloidal nature of the drug carrier can cause problems in the drug content determination. Separation or extraction of the drug by ultracentrifugation or ultrafiltration is a prerequisite to the drug content determination.

7.7.2   Degradation pathways (DP) for intravascular drug delivery systems

DP is an indicator of the release mechanism of the drug. Hence most drug delivery systems are evaluated for their degradation pathway. The degradation of poly (alkyl cyanoacrylates) is studied most extensively. One pathway of degradation is by erosion of the polymer backbone by formation of formaldehyde. The second pathway is cleavage of the ester via formation of a soluble polymer acid. Other types of drug carrier systems may degrade by hydrolysis, e.g. polylactic acid microspheres.

7.7.3 Drug release kinetics

Drug release may occur by desorption of surface bound drug or by diffusion through the nanoparticle matrix or the nanocapsule polymer wall material may erode by a combined erosion-diffusion process. The release mechanism, the diffusion coefficient and the biodegradation rate are the main factors governing the drug release rate. The release kinetics of drugs from carriers are strongly influenced by the biological environment. Nanoparticles may be coated by plasma - proteins that poses an additional diffusion barrier and may lead to a retardation of the release.

Following methods have been used for the determination of the *in vitro* release kinetics.

i)   Side-by-side diffusion cells with artificial or biological membrane

ii)   Dialysis bag diffusion technique

iii)   Reverse dialysis sac technique

iv)   Ultracentrifugation

v)   Ultrafiltration

vi)   Centrifugal ultrafiltration technique.

7.7.4   Bioacceptability and Toxicity

Drug carriers distribute very rapidly into the phagocytic cells of the RES, especially the liver, mainly the Kupffer cells. The poly (cyanoacrylate) nanoparticles possess a slight but definite toxicity toward a number of cells including fibroblasts, hepatocytes, endothelial cells, macrophages, osteogenic sarcomas, round cell sarcomas etc. The toxicity decreases with increasing side chain ester length with the exception of the methyl ester, which is less toxic than the ethyl ester. Partly degraded nanoparticles were more toxic than undegraded. In addition to cell toxicity the mutagenicity of the drug delivery system can also be tested using Ames test.

7.7.5   Body distribution of Intravascular drug carriers

Intravascularly injected colloidal drug carriers are mostly taken up by the reticuloendothelial organs like liver (60 - 90 % of the injected dose), spleen (2 - 10 %), lungs (3 - 10 %) and a low amount (< 1 %) into the bone marrow. To maximize the local effect of the drug at the desired site the uptake by these organs needs to be minimized. A number of models have been developed to study the arterial uptake and the extent of organ distribution of the drug.

7.7.6   Ex-vivo model for nanoparticle uptake by artery

The schematic diagram of the arterial perfusion system used for the ex- vivo evaluation of nanoparticle uptake by the artery is given in Fig 7.13 (Song et al, 1997).

The apparatus consists of a pressure- gauged syringe connected to a piece of artery (e.g. canine carotid artery) about 2.0 cm. in length. The base of the arterial piece is connected to a container via a three - way stopcock.

The artery is inflated with 250 ml of saline at 1 atm. pressure for one minute to induce an injury before infusion of the nanoparticle suspension that is contained in the pressurized syringe. The nanoparticle suspension

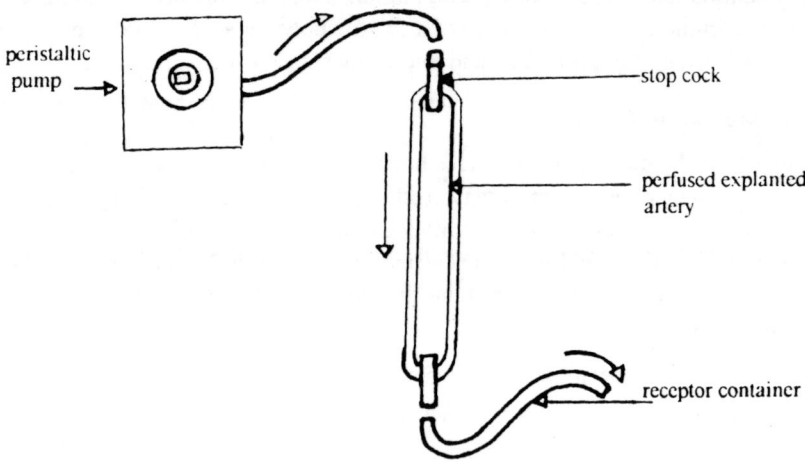

Fig 7.13 : Schematic representation of the arterial perfusion system used for the ex vivo evaluation of arterial uptake (adapted from Song et al, 1997)

is allowed to remain in the arterial channel for about 30 sec at 37°C under 1.0 atm. pressure with the system closed by the stopcock. At the end of the test period, the pressure in arterial channel is released by emptying it through the bottom opening. Then, the arterial segment is flushed with lactated Ringer's perfusion solution (at room temp.) for 30 sec. at 1 ml/min. flow rate using a peristaltic pump. At the end of the experiment, the artery is frozen and later analyzed for drug content.

7.7.7 Quantification of drug amount in artery

The arterial tissue samples are finely cut into small pieces and transferred to homogenization tubes. Drug is extracted from the tissue samples by mixed organic solvents in suitable proportions. The tissue is ground at spin speed of about 3000 - 3500 rpm using Teflon paddle driven lab-mixer for 15 min. at 37°C in a water bath. The procedure is repeated to ensure complete extraction of drug. The cumulative extract is centrifuged at 1000 rpm to remove particulate matter. The supernatant is evaporated to dryness under vacuum at 50°C. It is then quantified by HPLC for drug content.

Following extraction, the arterial tissue is lyophilized and its dry weight is recorded. The drug uptake by artery is calculated by relating the measured drug amount in the artery to the level of drug loading in the drug delivery system. The drug retention in the artery is expressed as mg/10 mg of dry weight of arterial tissue.

7.7.8 Animal model to check optimum microparticle size suitable for chemoembolization

A preliminary animal model has been developed for estimating the extent of chemoembolization caused by the biodegradable microparticles. It is possible to analyze the tissue distribution and tumor localization using the animal model employing a lipophilic marker molecule e.g. Fluorescence-dilaurate (FDL) (Bastian et al, 1995).

7.7.9 Tumor model

Single tumor nodules are induced in Sprague-Dawley (female) rats by injecting Novikoff hepatoma cells under the central liver lobe. Seven days after tumor inoculation the mean tumor diameter is noted and then laparotomy is performed in the anaesthetized animal (Fig 7.14).

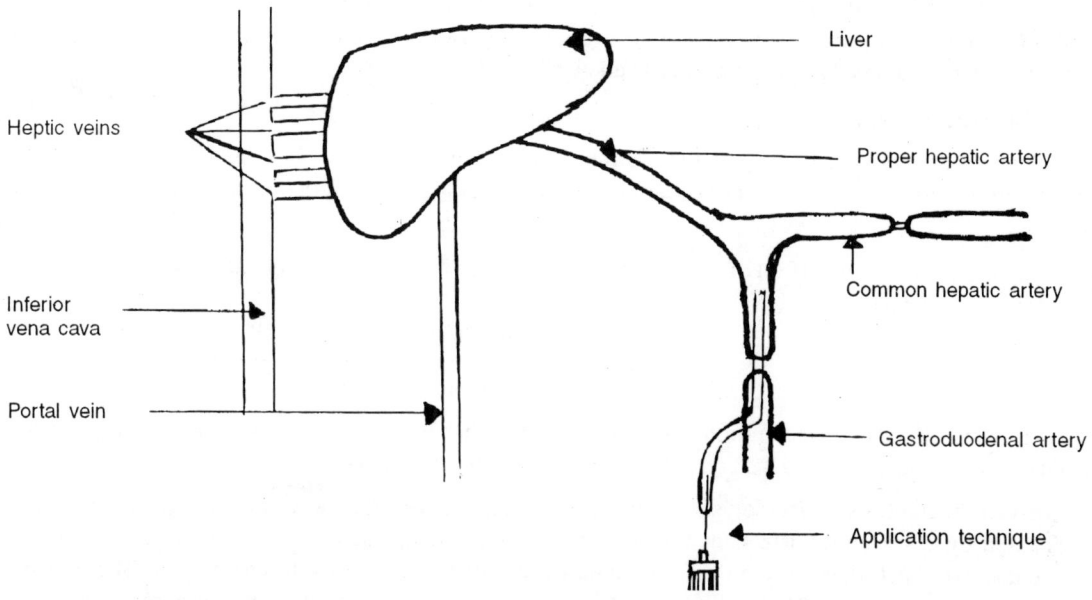

Fig 7.14 : Schematic representation for evaluation of optimum particle size for hepatic embolization
(adapted from Bastian et al, 1995)

The microparticle suspension is injected through the gastroduodenal artery in a total volume of 1 ml over a period of 5 min. During the injection the common hepatic artery is clamped to prevent retrograde embolization. At the end of the treatment, the animals are sacrificed, liver tumors are dissected to separate material from the tumor centre and border.

Other organs like spleen and lungs are also dissected to check for the distribution of drug particles. Frozen sections are prepared from liver and tumor tissues. They are screened under a fluorescence microscope and the density of the particle is evaluated.

The tumor tissue is homogenized in water and FDL is extracted with methylene chloride. The *extraction ratio* as the means of the deposition of particles in the tumor is evaluated as follows (Bastion et al, 1995):

$$ER_{T/L} = C_T/C_L$$

Where, $ER_{T/L}$ describes the ratio of the detected particle concentration in tumor (C_T) and in the liver tissue(C_L).

The extraction ratio indicates the particle concentration in tumor and normal liver tissue. Using this rat model it has been reported that 40 mm diameter microparticles are most suitable for liver tumor embolization. They accumulate in the border of the tumor and block further back flow. Furthermore, they are rarely detected in other organs, whereas smaller particles are deposited in the lung and spleen. This leads to less side effects of the drug during chemoembolization therapy.

7.7.10 Screening for administration related problems associated with intravascular drug delivery

The intravascular route is the most rapid and the most bioavailable method of getting a drug into the systemic circulation. However, this route is prone to many problems that are independent of the formulation as well as those related to the drug delivery. The major adverse effects of intravascular administration that result from the formulation are haemolysis, precipitation, phlebitis and pain. Hence, any intravascular drug delivery system designed may be evaluated for their absence (Yalkowsky et al,1998).

7.7.11 In - vivo studies

Of the various animal models for screening formulations in animals, rabbit ear vein is the most convenient, reliable, inexpensive and readily accessible as compared to the veins of other commonly used laboratory animals.

Effective concentration (EC) of a drug is its concentration in the injected vein at the site of the injection at the time of the injection.

$$EC = \frac{\text{Formulation concentration x injection rate}}{\text{blood flow rate}}$$

It is the effective concentration that determines whether the formulation will produce precipitation, toxicity to red blood cells, or to the cells of the inner wall of the blood vessel or vein.

a) **In-vivo haemolysis :** Haemolysis is a function of solution toxicity and vehicle composition. It can be caused by cosolvents, surfactants and sometimes by the drug itself. The red blood cells that are in contact with a sufficiently high concentration of formulation are prone to haemolysis. The maximum tolerable concentration that will not produce haemolysis is dependent upon the composition of the formulation.

Haemolysis can be measured *in-vivo* by analysis of either blood or urine at some time after an intravenous injection. Because intravascular haemolysis increases the concentration of circulating haemoglobin in the blood, the blood level of haemoglobin is a fair indicator of haemolysis.

b) **In - vivo precipitation :** A number of injectable drugs must be administered in concentrations greater than their aqueous solubility. There will be less precipitation from a very rapid injection than from a slow or moderate rate injection. It is possible to physically test for precipitation *in-vivo* by excising the injected ear vein and examining it under polarized light.

c) **In-vivo phlebitis :** Many factors have been reported to cause phlebitis, particulate matter being the most clearly documented. Infusion solutions containing negligible amounts of particles can also produce phlebitis upon prolonged administration.

For evaluation of phlebitis the formulation is injected in the marginal ear vein of rabbit and the same vein on the other ear is used as a control. Rating scales are used to quantify phlebitis. Visual evaluation of phlebitis is assessed using vein-colour change, region of edema or erythema or inflammation over the entire ear. However, visual evaluation is somewhat subjective and arbitrary although simple and convenient.

Less subjective and more quantitative *in-vivo* techniques of measuring phlebitis have been developed by White & Yalkowsky (1991). A specified amount of formulation is injected at a specified rate onto the marginal ear vein of a rabbit. The injected and uninjected ears are monitored for the temperature fluctuations for upto 24 hr after injection (Fig 7.15).

A thermal imaging camera or simple thermo-couples that are placed at a point, 3cm downstream from the point of injection site, are used to measure the increase in temperature of the injected ear vein with respect to control. Both veins are compared visually and by thermal means for about 4 hours. A temperature difference of about 2°C indicates severe phlebitis and a difference of less than 0.5°C suggests no phlebitis. The relationship between an increase in the temperature difference and phlebitis can be confirmed by histological evaluation of both veins after 24 hr.

In-vivo pain : Pain is a primary symptom of cell damage such as phlebitis, local burning, itching, stinging, aching. It may be caused after intravascular administration. Hence, the intravascular systems are evaluated using animal models for absence of such symptoms. A novel method has been developed for measuring

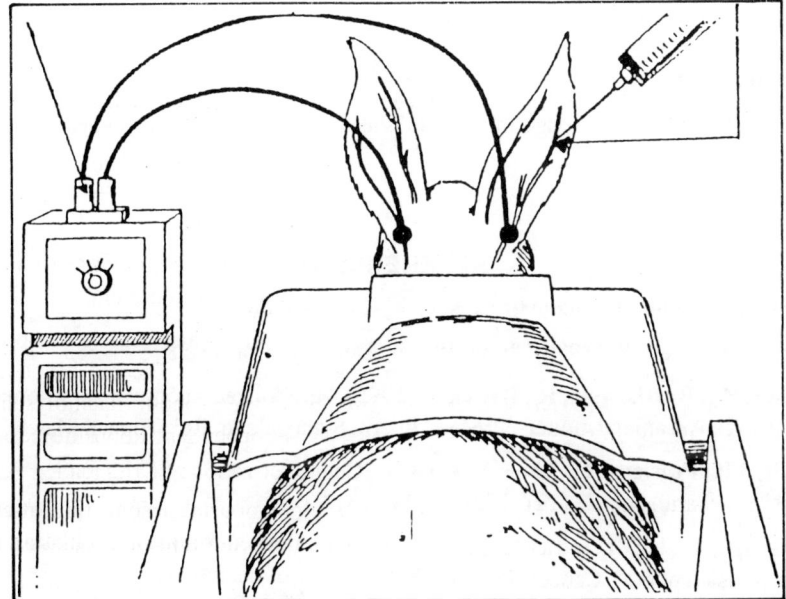

Fig 7.15 : Schematic diagram of experimental setup for screening of intravascular drug delivery system for haemolysis, phlebitis and pain (adapted from White & Yalkowsky, 1991).

intravascular pain. Rats were restrained and connected to strain gauges. The struggling during and following an intravascular injection is taken as a measure of the pain produced by the injection (Yalkowsky et al, 1998).

Serum levels of phosphokinase could also be measured. Phosphokinase is an enzyme produced and released by cells in response to damage and can be used as an indicator of pain on injection. This method is a more quantitative and less subjective method of evaluating pain.

Such extensive evaluation of the physicochemical and biological characteristics by *in-vivo* and *in-vitro* models would enable the design and development of a safe and effective intravascular drug delivery system.

7.8 SCOPE

As per the principles of targeting an effective intravascular device should be so designed that the drug delivery system is supplied to the first level (organ), the particulate carriers at the second level (lesion) and the drugs should be released in situ (third level). Based upon this concept, intravascular drug delivery systems have been designed with nanoparticles, microspheres, liposomes and hydrogels as carriers for the drugs to be administered into the vascular bed for local or systemic action.

Using this type of intelligent drug delivery system, the agent or drug is directly delivered to the site of injury. Intravascular administration is a mode of localized drug delivery in which the therapeutic agent is directly infused into the arterial intima i.e. intraluminally, using various types of catheters.

An alternate approach for maintaining the tissue level of drugs at the site of vascular injury is periadventitial polymeric drug delivery system. Nanoparticles and photopolymerized hydrogels have been administered intravascularly for the retention into the vascular bed of artery thereby providing sustained release of drugs. Colloidal drug carriers for intravascular administration represent a potentially powerful means of local administration of therapeutic agents including pharmaceutical proteins and nucleic acids to the arterial wall. Site selective drug delivery is the main reason for administering colloidal drug delivery systems into the vascular compartment of the body.

7.9 ACKNOWLEDGMENT

The authors appreciate and acknowledge the valuable assitances of Ashwini Pande and Savindu K. in the compilation of this work.

REFERENCES

Andrade, J.D.; Jeon, S.I. (1991) J. Colloid Interf. Sci.,142(1) : 159 -166.

Arnold, I. Freeman.; Mayhew; E. (1986) "Targeted Drug Delivery",Cancer, 58 : 573- 583.

Bastian, P.; Kohler, H.;, Bartkowski, R.; Kissel, T. (1995), "Embolization of liver carcinoma optimization of microparticle size in an animal model", Proceed Intern. Symp. Contr. Rel. Bioact. Mater. 22 : 422 - 423.

Benita, S.; Benoit, J.P.; Puisieux, F.; Thies, C. (1984); "Characterization of Drug loaded Poly (d,l - lactide) microspheres" , J. Pharm. Sci., 73 (12) : 1721 - 1724.

Buchwald, H.; Grage, T. (1980) "Intraarterial infusion chemotherapy for hepatic carcinoma using a totally implanatable infusion pump", Cancer, 45 : 866 - 869.

Carstensen, H.; Muller, B.W.; Muller, R.H. (1991) "Adsorption of ethoxylated surfactants onb nanoparticles; I. Characterization of hydrophobic interaction chromatography", Int. J. Pharm.,67 :   29 - 31.

Castoldi, G.L. (1981) "Erythrocyte" in Zucker Franklin D. et al. ed, " Atlas of Blood Cells" Lea and Febiger, Philadelphia.

Chen, C. and Hanson, S.R. (1995) "Boundary layer infusion of heparin prevents thrombosis and reduces neointimal hyperplasia in venous polytetrafluoroethylene graft" J. Vasc. Surg., 22 : 237 - 247.

Chen, H.S.G. and Gross, J.F. (1980) "Intraarterial infusion of anticancer drug", Cancer treatment reports, 64, (1) : 31 - 40.

Crommelin, D.J.A. (1994) "Liposomes" in Kreuter J. ed . "Colloidal Drug Delivery Systems", Drug and Pharmaceutical Sciences Vol 66, Marcel Dekker Inc., New York , pg . 87 - 88, 149 - 150.

Crommelin, D.J.A.; Slaats, N. and Bloois, L.V. (1983) "Preparation and Characterization of doxorubicin con-taining liposomes; influence of liposomes charge" , Int. J. Pharm., 16 : 79 - 92.

Daemen M. J. A. P.; Vervoort H.J.M.; Peter and Thijssen H.H.W. (1988) Pharmacokinetic evaluation of local drug delivery, the intratesticular and intrarenal administration of acenocoumarol in the rat, J. Pharm. Pharmacol, 40, pg. 283-285.

Daemen, M.J.A.; Essen, H.V. and Smits J.F.M. (1986) "Target organ directed drug delivery; evaluation of renal infusion of Chromium 51 - ethylene diamine tetraacetate and Sodium o-(125 I) iodohippurate in   the Wistar Kyoto rat", J. Pharm. Sci. , 75(12) : 1137 - 1138.

Dakhil, S. and William, E. (1982) "Improved regional selectivity of hepatic arterial BCNU with degradable microspheres", Cancer, 50 : 631 - 635.

Ensminger, W.D.; Gyres, J.W. (1984) "Regional cancer chemotherapy", Cancer treatment reports, 68, (1) : 101 - 113.

Fishbein, I.; Banai, S.; Levitzki, A.; Moscovitz, D.; Gertz, S.D.; Gazit, A. and Golomb, G. (1996) "Perivascular and intraluminal delivery system of a tyrphostin for treatment of restenosis", Proceed. Intern. Symp. Contr. Rel. Bioact. Mater. 23 :17 - 18.

Flandroy M.J.; Grandfils C. and Jerome R.J. (1993) "Clinical application of microspheres in embolization and chemoembolization", in Rolland A., ed., "Pharmaceutical Particulate Carriers", Drugs and Pharmaceutical Sciences, Vol 61, Marcel Dekker inc. New York pg.331.

Ford J.L. (1988) "Parenteral Products" in Aulton M.E. (ed) "Pharmaceutics; The Science of Dosage Form design" Churchill Livingstone, pg 360.

Fujimoto S. and Endoh F. (1985) "Natural history of hepatocellular carcinoma and prognosis in relation to treatment", Cancer, 56, pg. 2404 - 2410.

Gibaud S. G.; Rousseau C.; Weingarten C.; Favier R.; Douay L. and Andreux J.P. (1998) "Polyalky cyanoacrylate nanoparticles as carriers for granulocyte colony stimulating factor (G - CSF)", J. Cont. Rel. 52 pg. 131 - 139.

Golomb G.; Fishbein I.; Banai I.; Moscovitz D. and Banai S. (1995) "Inhibition of restenosis in a rat model by perivascular delivery of a Tyrphostin compound" Proceed. Intern. Symp. Contr. Rel. Bioact. Mater. 22, pg.151 - 152.

Gonchior P. and Clemens P. (1995) "Comparison of local intravascular drug delivery system", Am. Heart J., 130, pg. 1174 - 1181.

Gregg G. and Folyey B. (1993) Body Woks, Version 3; Mythos Software, Encyclopedia on CD. Rom.

Gupta P. K.; Hung C.T.; Huang L. T.; Lam F. C. and Perrier D.G. (1986) " Albumin Microsphere Part 3, Synthesis and Characterization of microsphere containing adriamycin and magnetite", Int. J. Pharm. 33 pg 137- 143.

Huang L.; Leen R. J.; Atsuhide M. and Maruyama K. (1995) "Target for liposomes within the vascular system", Proceed. Intern. Symp. Cont. Rel. Bioact. Mat, 22, pg. 36- 37.

Ibrahim A.; Rolland C.; Couvreur P. and Speiser P. (1983) " New magnetic drug carrier", J. Pharm. Pharmacol. , 35, pg 59 -61.

Ichihara T.; Sakamoto, K.; Mori K. and Akagi M. (1989) "Transcatheter arterial chemoembolization therapy for hepatocellular carcinoma using polylactic acid miocrospheres" Cancer Research, 49, pg. 4357 - 62.

Jeong S.Y.; Yi S.W.; Yong H.K.; Kwon I.C.; Chung J.W.; Park J.H. and Choi Y.W. (1998) "Stable lipiodolized emulsions for hepatoma targeting and treatment by transcatheter arterial chemoembolization" J. Cont. Rel., 50, pg. 135 - 143.

Kanke M.; Simmons G. H.; Weiss D.L.; Bivins B. A. and Deluca P. P. (1980) "Clearance of 141Ce labelled microspheres from blood and distibution in specific organs following I.V. and intraarterial admn. In beagle dogs", J. Pharm. Sci. 69, pg. 755 - 756.

Kataoka K.; Yokoyama M.; Sakurai Y.; Suwa S.; Yokoyama H. and Okaro T. (1996) "Introduction of cisplatin into polymeric micelle", J. Cont. Rel. 39, pg. 351 - 356.

Kato J.; Mori H.; Kumagai I.; and Nemoto R. (1980) Sustained release properties of mcroencapsulated MitomycinC with ethyl cellulose infused into renal artery of the dog kidney, Cancer, 46, pg 14 -21.

Kato T.; Nemoto R.; Mori H. and Kumagai I. (1981) "Arterial chemoembolization with Mitomycin C microcapsules in the treatment of primary carcinoma of kidney, liver, bone and intrapelvic organs" Cancer 48, pg 674 - 680.

Kreitz M.R. and Webber W.L., (1995) "Incorporation of Polymer microspheres in porous polyurethane vascular grafts" Proceed. Intern. Symp. Cont. Rel. Bioact. Mater.,22,(1995), pg. 79.

Kreuter J. (1992), "Nanoparticles preparation and applications" in Danbrow M. ed., "Microcapsules and Nanospheres in Medicine and Pharmacy", CRC press Boca Raton, F. L. pg. 125 - 128.

Kreuter J., (1994), "Nanoparticles"in Kreuter J. ed. "Colloidal drug delivery systems" , Drugs and Pharmaceutical Sciences,Marcel Dekker Inc. Vol. 66, pg.248 - 249.

Kurihara A.; Yamashita Y.; Mizota A.; Yasino A.; Sasagawa K.; Kobayashi T. and Hiraoka M. (1995) "Lipid emulsions for parenteral drug delivery of antitumor lipophilic agent", Proceed. Intern. Symp. Contr. Rel. Bioact. Mater. 22, pg.402 - 403.

Labhasetwar V.; Song. C.; Humphrey W.R.; Shebusk R.J. and Levy R.J. (1995) "Nanoparticles for site specific delivery of U86983 in restenosis in pig coronary arteries", Proceed. Intern. Symp. Cont. Rel. Bioact. Mater. 22, pg 182 - 183.

Leucuta S. E., Risca R., Daicoviciu D., and Portutiu D.,(1988), "Albumin microspheres as a drug delivery system for epirubicin : pharmaceutical,pharmacokinetic and biological aspects", Int. J. Pharm., 41, pg. 213-217.

Levy R. J.; Song C. X.; Labhasetwar V.;Davis J. and Underwood T. (1996) "The effect of Nanoparticle surface modification on arterial retention post angioplasty in a dog femoral artery model" Proceed. Intern. Symp. Cont. Rel. Bioact. Mat. 23 , pg 393 - 394.

Markou C. P.; Brown J. E.; Pursley M.D. and Hanson S. R. (1998) "Boundary Layer drug delivery using a helical catheter", J. Contr. Rel., 53, pg. 281 - 288.

Mc Cormack B. and Gregoriades G. (1995) "Drugs in Cyclodextrin in Liposomes ; Evaluation of the concept in vivo"; Proceed. Intern. Symp. Contr. Rel. Bioact. Mater. 22, pg. 190 - 191.

Mishaly D.; Fishbein I.; Dorit M. and Golomb G. (1997) "Site specific of colchicine in rat carotid artery model of restenosis", J. Contr. Rel., 45, pg 65 - 73.

Muller R. H.; Mehnert W.; Freitas C. and Muhlen A. Z. (1996) "Solid lipid nanoparticles for intravenous drug delivery", Proceed. Intern. Symp. Cont. Rel. Bioact. Mat. 23, pg. 184 - 185.

Niwa T.; Hino T.; Takeuchi H.; Kumou N. and Kawashima Y. (1993) "Preparation of biodegradable nanospheres of water soluble and insoluble drugs", J. Cont. Rel. 25, pg. 89 - 98.

Papisov M.I.; Sanelyev V.Y.; Sergienko V. B. and Torchilin V.P. (1987) "In vivo kinetics of radiolabelled manetic drug carriers", Int. J. Pharm. 40, pg. 201 - 205.

Petrak K. (1993) "Design and properties of particulate carriers for intravascular administration" in Rolland ed. "Pharmaceutical Particulate Carriers", Drugs and Pharmaceutical Sciences, Vol. 61, Marcel Dekker Inc. New York, pg. 277-278, 280-282.

Philbrook M.; Weselcouch E.; Roth L.; Lovich M.; Gallant M.; Edelman E. and Leavitt R. (1995) "Local sustained delivery of heparin via in situ photopolymerized biodegradable hydrogel", Proceed. Intern. Symp. Contr. Rel. Bioact. Mater. 22, pg.19- 20.

Rahman A and White (1985) "Pharmacological toxicological and therapeutic evaluation in mice of doxorubicin liposomes, Cancer Research, 45, pg. 796 - 803.

Ruiz J.M.; Tissier B. and Benoit J.P. (1989) "Microencapsulation of Peptide; Study of phase seperation of poly (D,L lactic acid - co - glycolic acid) copolymer 50/50 by silicon oil", Int. J. Pharm. 49, pg. 69- 74.

Sah. H.; Chien Y. W. and Toddywala R. (1995) "Continuous release of proteins from biodegradable microcapsules and in vivo evaluation of their potential as a vaccine", J. Cont. Rel., 35, pg. 137 -144.

Seltzer S.E. (1989), "The role of liposomes in diagnostic imaging", Radiology 171, pg. 19 - 21.

Simons M.; Elazer R. and Edelman. (1992) "Antisense C mylo oligonucleotides inhibit intimal arterial smooth muscle cell accumulation in vivo", Nature ; 359, pg. 67 - 70.

Song C. X.; Labhasetwar V.; Murphy H. and Levy R.J. (1997) "Formulation and characterization of biodegradable nanoparticles for intravascular local drug delivery", J. Cont. Rel. 43, pg. 197 - 212.

Tice T. R. and Tabibi S.E. (1992) "Parenteral drug delivery , injectables", in Kydonieus ed., "Treatise on Controlled Drug Delivery", Marcel Dekker Inc., New York pg. 3 19 - 326.

Tomlinson E.; Burger J.; Mcvie I. and Hoefnager K. (1984); "Albumin microspheres for intraarterial drug targeting", in Anderson J. M. et al , ed., "Recent Advances in Drug Delivery Systems" , Plenum Press, New York pg 199 - 208.

Torchillin V.P. (1995) "Targets for Liposomes within the vascular system", Proceed. Intern. Symp. Contr. Rel. Bioact. Mater. 22, pg. 190 - 191.

Villa A. E. and Guzman (1994) "Local delivery of dexamethasone for prevention of neointimal proliferation in a rat model on balloon angioplasty", J. Clin. Invest. , 93, pg. 1243 - 1249.

Weiss M.M. (1989) " Corticosteroids in Rheumatoid Arthritis", Sem. Arth. Rheum. 19 (1), 9 - 21.

West J. L. and Hubbell J. (1995) "Localized intravascular protein delivery from photopolymerized hydrogels", Proceed. Intern. Symp. Contr. Rel. Bioact. Mater. 22 pg.17-18.

White M. and Yalkowsky S.H., (1991) "Studies in Phlebitis (III) , Evaluation of diazepam and phenytoin", Pharm. Res. 8, pg. 1340 - 1341.

Widder K. J. and Senyui (1980) "In vitro release of biologically active adriamycin by magnetic responsive microspheres", Cancer Research, 40 , 3512 - 3514.

Wood D.A. (1980) "Biodegradable Drug Delivery Systems", Int. J. Pharm., 7, 1980, 1-18.

Yalkowsky S.H.;Kryzaniak J. F. and Ward G. H. (1998) "Formulation related problems associated with intravenous drug delivery", J. Pharm. Sci. , 87, pg. 787 - 796.

Yang S.M. and Hasaniya N. (1998) "Impact of antimicrobial bonded catheters on the incidence of catheter related infection", Crit. Care Med., Vol. 26, 1, Suppl. A140.

Chapter 8

Implantable Therapeutic Systems

R.S.R. Murthy

8.1 INTRODUCTION

Lafarge pioneered the concept of implantable therapeutic systems for long term and continuous drug administeration in 1861 with the development of subcutaneously implantable drug pellet. The technique was then improved and solid pellets containing crystalline hormones were prepared to mimic the steady and continuous secretion of hormones from the gland (Deanesly & Parkes, 1936, 1937; Ballard & Nelson, 1975) However, the chronic use of implantable pellets for human care declined over the years and at present there are a few steroid pellets available. Subcutaneous drug administration by pellet implantation is known to have several drawbacks particularly irregular drug release profile.

8.2 HISTORICAL DEVELOPMENT

Accidental discovery of controlled drug permeation characteristics of silicon elastomers paved the way for the bio-medical applications of polymers in designing implantable therapeutic systems. Potential bio-medical applications of silicon elastomers were studied by fabricating a very small capsule shaped implant containing thyroid hormone powder which released the hormone steadily for a long time when tested in-vitro. Similar results were obtained with isoproterenol, digitoxin, EDTA etc. when encapsulated in silicon capsules (Folkman & Long, 1964, 1964a). Power (1965) reported the use of silicon capsules containing Pyrimethamine to protect chicks from malaria. Use of silicon implants in veterinary medicine for contraception received much attention with the findings by Dzink and Cook. The slow release progesterone over one year period from silicon capsules were lately extended to the controlled release device for long term contraceptive activity.

8.3 MECHANISM OF DRUG RELEASE FROM IMPLANTS

The ideal system for drug release should approach zero order kinetics. The device should be biocompatible, non-toxic, non-mutagenic, non-immunogenic, and non-carcinogenic. In general, implants should possess a high drug to polymer ratio. It should have good mechanical strength, be free of drug leakage, be easily sterilizable and be easy and inexpensive to manufacture. The rate of drug release can be regulated by the shape and size of the implants, as well as by selecting suitable polymer or polymer blend for fabrication. The mechanism of drug release from the implants can be classified as described below.

8.3.1 Diffusion controlled release

Fundamentally solute diffusion through polymer membrane or from the polymer matrix is related to Fickian and non-Fickian diffusion. These equations with appropriate boundary conditions constitute the initial model that can be applied to various drug release polymer systems.

8.3.2   Mathematical modeling of diffusion process

The process of drug release from a polymeric drug delivery system can be described in most cases by Fickian diffusion. Some exceptions include the swellable release system. The equations describing Fickian diffusion are solved to provide the following information:

(a) Determination of the release rate dM_t/dt and the normalized quantity of the drug M_t/M_∞ released in the surrounding medium

(b) Analysis of drug concentration profile in the polymer during release generally in terms of normalized concentration of drug c_i/c_{io} as a function of dimensionless depth or position x/δ for various dimensionless times $Dim.t/\delta^2$.

(c) Determination of the concentration profile of a countercurrently diffusing penetrant for expressing drug diffusion coefficient Dim as a function of structural changes in the polymer.

Fick's law: For three-dimensional diffusion in a binary system standard notation reported by Bird et al (1960) is generally used:

$$J_i^* = - cD_{im}.\nabla x_i. \tag{1}$$

where J_i^* is the molar flux of the diffusing component (solute) with respect to the molar average velocity, Vxi is the mole fraction of the solute and D_{im} is the solute diffusion coefficient in the polymer.

In most cases of controlled release systems, Fickian diffusion occurs through thin films or membranes where the diffusion may be considered one-dimensional. Therefore, under the assumptions of ideal thermodynamic systems concentration independent diffusion coefficients, and one-dimensional diffusion, we can write:

$$J_i^* = - D_{im}.dc_i/dx. \tag{2}$$

where $c_i = x_i c$. Integration of this equation between the interfacial concentrations c_{i1} and c_{i2} of a membrane or a polymer film of thickness d, under the assumption of constant flux, gives

$$J_i^* = D_{im}(c_{i1} - c_{i2})/ \delta. \tag{3}$$

Since experimental determination of the interfacial concentrations of drug i. is rather cumbersome, the concentration in bulk solution can be used, if expressed by means of a thermodynamic partition coefficient K, which is defined as

$$K = c_{i1}/c_{i2} = \text{concentration of drug at interface/ concentration of drug in bulk.}$$

Then the equation for flux is written as,

$$J_i^* = \{D_{im}.K / \delta\}(c_{i2} - c_{i1}) \tag{4}$$

Where the term $Dim.K / d$ represents the drug permeability coefficient, P_{im}. However, in circumstances especially when the thickness of the sample is unknown, the permeability is defined as, $P_{im} = D_{im}.K$

Although drug diffusion through most of the polymeric devices is described by Fickian diffusion, recently there has been considerable interest in the development of "swellable controlled" delivery systems (Langer, 1980). Drug release kinetics from this system does not follow Fickian diffusion but anomalous diffusion is observed (Reinhart et.al, 1981; Good, 1976; Korsmeyer & Peppas, 1981, 1983) as a result of relaxation of the macromolecular chains. Relaxational effect are the result of polymer transition from the glossy to the rubbery state due to water (or solvent) swelling. The mode of transport of the solvent is described usually by case-II transport as per the equation,

$$Dc_s/dt = d/dx \{D (c_s) dc_s/dx - v'c_s\} \tag{5}$$

where v' is the velocity of the moving front separating the glassy from the rubbery state. As a result of this transition, the diffusion coefficient of the drug D_m may increase by three or four orders of magnitude as diffusion proceeds from the glassy to the rubbery state.

8.4 DIFFUSION CONTROLLED SYSTEMS

8.4.1 Reservoir (membrane) systems

In reservoir or membrane release system, the drug is enclosed in relatively large quantities in a permeable synthetic membrane and is placed in contact with a fluid at constant temperature. After an initial period of transient diffusion, steady state is established and diffusive release rates can be easily determined.

Here, two interesting cases of mathematical modeling are distinguished. According to Baker & Lonsdale's (1974) classification they are devices with (i) constant activity, and (ii) non-constant drug activity sources.

8.4.1.1 Constant activity sources: Constant activity reservoir type devices include systems where the drug activity is maintained constant throughout prolonged use. Modeling of these devices in done by applying Fick's'law in the integrated form expressing the flux Ji* in terms of the actual release rate dMt/dt, as under.

$$J_i^* = D_{im} K/\delta \, (c_{i2} - c_{i1}) \tag{6}$$

The integrated form of the above equation be written as

$$dM_t/dt = D_{im}.K.A/\delta \, (c_{i2} - c_{i1}) \tag{7}$$

where, A is the effective membrane area for diffusion of the drug. This equation is applicable to thin film geometry with thickness δ. The total amount of drug released as a function of time can be determined by simple integration of the above equation.

$$M_t = \{D_{im} K A (c_{i2} - c_{i1})/\delta\} t = K_1.t \tag{8}$$

The above equation is modified depending on the geometry of the delivery system. Hence, for cylindrical devices with internal and external radii ri and re respectively, the equation is

$$dM_t/dt = \{D_{im} K A / \ln(r_e/r_i)\} \, (c_{i2} - c_{i1}) \quad \text{or,} \tag{9}$$

$$M_t = \{D_{im} K A \, (c_{i2} - c_{i1})/\ln(r_e/r_i)\} \, t = K_2.t \tag{10}$$

Similarly the total amount of released drug from a spherical reservoir device is expressed by the equation,

$$M_t = [4\pi D_{im}.K \, (c_{i2} - c_{i1})] \, t / [(r_e - r_i)/r_e.r_i] = K_3.t \tag{11}$$

In all three cases the amount of drug released M_t is proportional to the release time t, which is generally called "zero order release behavior" and is highly desirable as such device can provide drug for long periods of time at constant rates.

8.4.1.2 Non constant Activity source

Modeling of non-constant activity reservoir system is important for devices where the drug is available in solution, below the solubility limit. Some of these models may also be applied to the late release stage of a constant activity reservoir system, where most of the drug has been depleted, and drug activity cannot be kept constant. For these systems, Baker & Lonsdale (1974) have formulated a model as under:

$$dM_t/dt = \{D_{im} KA/\delta\} \, (c_{i2} - c_{i1}) \tag{12}$$

Or, $\quad dM_t/dt = \{Dim \, KA/\delta\} \, (M_{t2}/V_2 - M_{t1}/V_1) \tag{13}$

Since the total amount of drug $M_\infty = M_{t2} + M_{t1}$, and at the initiation (t=0) all the drug is in the device,

$$M_{t1} = M_\infty$$

$$DM_{t1}/dt = \{M_\infty Dim\, K\, A/V_1\, \delta\}\, \exp\{(-D_{im}\, K\, A_t/\delta)\, (1/V_1 + 1/V_2)\} \qquad (14)$$

Consequently, drug release behaviour for non-constant activity device is first order.

8.4.2 Matrix (Monolithic) systems.

Matrix (monolithic) devices usually contain drug or bioactive agents incorporated either as a solution or as a dispersion in the polymer phase. They are prepared in many geometric shapes depending on the place of implantation.

8.4.2.1 Systems with dissolved drug

In this system the drug is dissolved in the polymer below its solubility limit either by preparing a drug-polymer solution, casting in a desirable geometric form and evaporating the solvent, or soaking the polymer in a drug solution.

For plane sheet matrix of thickness δ, with initial drug concentration $c_{i.o}$, and surface concentration c_i, with negligible edge effect, release profile may be explained by the equation

$$dci/dt = D_{im}\, (d^2ci/dx^2) \qquad (15)$$

Above equation on integration gives (Crank, 1975)

$$M_t/M_\infty = 1 - \sum_{N=0}^{\infty} \frac{8}{(2n+1)^2\, \pi^2} \exp[\{-Dim(2n+1)^2\pi^2 t\}/\delta^2] \qquad (16)$$

At long times, the first term of the summation of this expression is dominant (n=0), and this equation can be simplified as follows:

$$M_t/M_\infty = 1 - \frac{8}{\pi^2} \exp[\{-D_{im}\pi^2 t\}/\delta^2] \text{ for } M_t/M_\infty > 0.6 \qquad (17)$$

Similar modeling can be applied for the prediction of dissolved drug release from cylindrical matrix (Crank, 1975) systems of radius r with initial loaded drug concentration of cio and surface concentration ci. The amount of drug released follows the equation,

$$M_t/M_\infty = 1 - \sum_{N=1}^{\infty} \frac{4}{r^2\, \alpha^2 n} \exp(-D_{im}\, \alpha^2_n\, t) \qquad (18)$$

where an are the positive roots of the Bessel function of the first kind of order zero. These roots are tabulated in standard reference (Crank, 1975).

For spherical matrices under the same boundary conditions, the total quantity of drug released is calculated by the equation;

$$M_t/M_\infty = 1 - \frac{6}{\pi^2} \sum_{N=1}^{\infty} \frac{1}{n^2} \exp.[\{-D_{im}n^2\pi^2 t\}/r^2] \qquad (19)$$

For long times, the first term of the summation of the above equation is the dominant one and hence we can write as:

$$M_t/M_\infty = 1 - \frac{6}{\pi^2} \exp.[\{-D_{im}\pi^2 t\}/r^2] \qquad (20)$$

Release rates dM_t/dt can be calculated by simply differentiating the equations.

8.4.2.2 Systems with dispersed drug

When the matrix system consists of a drug dispersed in the polymer at a concentration c_{io} that is greater than the drug solubility c_{is}, the previously developed models do not apply. In this case, the well known pseudo-steady state approximation model is used (Higuchi, 1961). This model adopts the following assumptions:

1. Drug is uniformly dispersed in the matrix

2. Particle size is much smaller in comparison to the polymer film thickness

3. Diffusent concentration at the interface c_{is}, is always zero.

4. No polymer volume change.

5. Boundary effect is negligible

Integrating Fick's first law over the polymer film layer thickness x*, which contains only dissolved drug:

$$dM_t / dt = D_{im} A \{(c_{is}-0) /x^*\} \qquad (21)$$

A mass balance over the dispersed drug area can also be written as

$$dM_t = \{ c_{io} -(c_{is})/2)\}dx^* \qquad (22)$$

Solving the above equations for the value of x* and substituting the value in the previous equation and further integrating over time, we get,

$$M_t = A[D_{im}.c_{is} (2c_{io} -c_{is})t]^{1/2} \qquad (23)$$

The release rate is expressed by the equation:

$$dM_t /dt = A/2 [D_{im}.c_{is}(2c_{io} -c_{is})^{1/2}.t^{-1/2} \qquad (24)$$

This model predicts a square root of time dependence for the drug released in a well-stirred infinite medium This model has been extended to cylindrical and spherical matrices as under:
For cylindrical matrix,the fraction of drug released is expressed as,

$$M_t/M_\infty +[1- M_t/M_\infty][\ln (1- M_t/M_\infty)] = (4D_{im}/r^2)(c_{is}/c_{io})t \qquad (25)$$

For spherical matrix, the fraction drug released is expressed as,

$$M_t/M_\infty -3/2[1-(1-M_t/M_\infty)^{2/3}] = -(3 D_{im}/r^2)(c_{is}/c_{io})t \qquad (26)$$

8.4.3.3 Diffusion in porous systems

Although considerable experimental work has been reported on the release of drugs through porous polymeric materials (Langer, 1980), mathematical modeling is still at a rather primitive stage. For diffusion of drug through a porous polymer with initial concentration c_{io} above the drug solubility c_{is}. The model developed by Higuchi, 1963) has wide acceptance today which incorporates the void fraction and tortousity t of the polymeric system in the diffusion coefficient D_{eff}. The model is based on a pseudo steady-state approximation and the total amount of released drug can be calculated as

$$M_t = A [D_{eff} C_{is}(2c_{io} - \varepsilon.c_{is}) t]^{1/2} \qquad (27)$$

where

$$D_{eff} = D_{iw} (\varepsilon / t)$$

Where D_{iw} is the solute diffusion coefficient in water. However these models fail to predict the unique release behaviour observed in controlled release monolithic devices for the sustained release of macromolecules. It has been shown that in these systems solute diffusion occurs almost exclusively through large interconnecting channels at almost zero-order release rates (Langer et al., 1980). Another model developed by Swan & Peppas (1981) treats the release of drugs from porous systems as dissolution and diffusion controlled phenomenon.

8.4.3.4 Swelling controlled systems

Numerous pharmaceutical formulations are prepared by incorporating drug in a polymer matrix in a dissolved or dispersed phase. In most of these formulations the matrix undergoes considerable swelling when placed in contact with thermodynamically compatible liquid (water for hydrophilic and organic solvents for other polymers). As a result a considerable increase in drug diffusion occurs through the relaxing gel-like phase.

Preliminary modeling of drug release from swellable hydrophilic matrices was reported by Lapidus & Lordi (1968). Using a pseudo-steady state approximation equation, no.27 was used to understand the release of drugs with limited water solubility and equation 28 for completely dissolved drug.

$$M_t/M_\infty = 2\,[D_{im}/\Pi\delta^2]^{1/2} \tag{28}$$

8.4.3.5 Chemically controlled systems

Chemically controlled systems include bioerodible and pendent-group polymer matrices. These drug delivery systems are becoming very popular because of their special characteristics, such as complete bio-degradation of the polymer and release rates controlled by the geometric shape of the device (Heller, 1980).

8.4.3.5.1 Polymer dissolution and bio-erodible systems

Polymer dissolution process depends on geometric shape of the materials and therefore surface kinetics and the expected functional expression of the dissolution rate is important to consider. Expressions developed by Cooney (1971; 1972) for polymer dissolution of cylindrical, spherical and other devices; and expressions derived by Hopfenberg (1976) for drug release from slab, cylinder and sphere; determine the erosion rate dM_t/dt described in terms of an erosion constant K_e and the continuously changing available area for bio-degradation A_e:

$$DM_t/dt \;=\; K_e.A_e \tag{29}$$

Solution for this equation for various geometries gives

$$M_t/M_\infty = 1 - [\,1 - (K_e t/c_{io}l)\,]_n \tag{30}$$

Here n=1 for a plane sheet of thickness $\delta = 2l$, n=2 for a cylinder of radius r=1 and n=3 for a sphere of radius r = l.

8.4.3.5.2 Pendent chain system

Modeling of pendent chain delivery system is not based on diffusion equation, but rather on the kinetics of the reaction that leads to the removal of the pendent chain. Harris et al (1976) and Ringsdorf (1978) have proposed kinetic models for some specific systems.

In conclusion, modeling of drug release from or through controlled delivery polymeric systems has been achieved based predominantly on the steady state and transient description of drug diffusion by use of Fick's law. Drug release from reservoir (membrane) and matrix (monolithic) devices is straight forward and so release rate and the total amount of the released drug may be predicted for devices of varying geometry also. Areas where more accurate mathematical description is presently needed include drug release from swellable and porous material. With the advent of co-delivery polymeric systems, new models will need to be developed for interacting and non-interacting multicomponent diffusion through polymers.

8.5 DEVELOPMENT OF IMPLANTABLE THERAPEUTIC SYSTEMS

Historically, the subcutaneous implantation of drug pellets is known to be the first medical approach aiming to achieve prolonged and continuous administration of drugs. This first generation of implantable therapeutic systems was produced by simple compression of drug crystals either alone or in combination with small quantity of pharmaceutical adjuvant into tiny cylinder-shaped pellets that can be implanted readily in to a subcutaneous tissue. Over the years, a number of approaches have been developed to achieve the controlled administration of biologically active agents via implantation or insertion in the tissue. The approaches are outlined as follows:

A. Diffusion controlled systems

1. Membrane permeation-controlled systems containing

    a. Non porous membranes

    b. Microporous membranes

    c. Semipermeable membranes

2 Matrix diffusion controlled systems containing

    a. Lipophilic polymers

    b. Hydrophilic swellable polymers

    c. Porous polymers

3 Microreservoir dissolution controlled systems containing

    a. Hydrophilic reservoir/ Lipophilic matrix

    b. Lipophilic reservoir/ Hydrophilic matrix

B. Activation controlled systems

    1. Osmotic pressure activated

    2. Vapor pressure activated

    3. Magnetically activated

    4. Ultrasound activated

    5. Hydrolysis activated

8.5.1 Types of devices based on route of administration

In spite of the fact that the therapeutic systems are classified in the categories mentioned above based on the mechanism of drug release, it is difficult to fabricate devices based on any one mechanism. Most of the devices work on the combination of two or more mechanisms and so the systems discussed in this chapter are dealt based on the routes of administration as under.

    1. Subcutaneous implants

    2. Intra-ocular implants/ inserts

    3. Intra-vaginal inserts

    4. Intra-uterine implants/ inserts

8.5.1.1 Subcutaneous implants

Subcutaneous tissue is basically a sheet of areolar tissue lying directly underneath the skin (dermal tissue). It is rich in fat but poor in nerve network and hemoperfusion. Therefore, subcutaneous tissue is an ideal location for implantation and prolonged drug administration because of it's ready access, slow drug absorption, and low reactivity to the insertion of foreign materials. In addition, drug delivery systems for the subcutaneous implantation offer one unique advantage of retrieval whenever medical or personnel reasons dictate such a need.

Most of the approaches listed above can be adopted to fabricate the systems for controlled release of

Table 8.1 : Fabrication and evaluation of reservior devices.

Coating material	Drugs	Method of preparation	Results and comments
Polyethylene glycol/ Cellulose (Salicylic acid, Tripelennamine (Caffeine)	—	Film Casted on Teflon Coated Plates	The release rate profile showed a square root of time dependence. Release rate was independent of film thickness and proportional to the drug concentration in pure ethyl cellulose films.
Hydroxy propyl cellulose/polyvinyl acetate (Pentobarbital, Methapyrilene)	—	Film casted on Teflon coated plates	Drug release followed a diffusion controlled model
Gelatin-Sodium sulphate (Clofibrate)	—	Microcapsules by simple coacervation	Thinner walled microcapsules showed release rate $\sqrt{t}$ model while thicker walled one showed zero order kinetics.
Ethyl cellulose Caffeine	—	Fims prepared using Gardner's ultra applicator	Films demonstrated timed release rate of diffusion controlled mechanism.
2-Hydroxy methacrylate, diethylene glycol dimethacrylate, trimethacrylate glycidyl methacrylate and hydroxy-ethyl acrylate.	Potassium chloride	Micro spheres prepared by cold precipitation followed by irradiation polymerization	Drug release was found dependent on the monomer and the precipitating medium.
Dimethylpolysiloxane	Butamben	Sheets of 0.127 mm was prepared	Sustained release fo the durg was observed
Polymers and waxes	Potassium chloride	Polymer coating by spray coating, was coating by melting and dispersion.	Gelatin-gum Arabic vates offered effective controlled release of the Coacervation in case of drug gelatin-gum Arabic system.
Gelatin	Clofibrate	Spherical dropet prepared by a capillary jet method was coated by simple coacervation	Following initial burst, the release followed zero order kinetics until nearly 90% of the drug wsa released.
Silicon tubing	Megestrol Acetate Anti- inflammatory Drugs	Suspension of the drug was filled in the tubing and sealed on both ends.	The effectiveness produced was approximately 10 times that of orally administered implant at a daily dose of 2.85 mg/day produced more anti-arthritic effect than the 10 mg/day of phenyl butazone by subcutaneous injection.

biologically active agents via subcutaneous implantation. Polymers of both non-biodegradable and biode-gradable types are used depending on the requirement. The methods used to develop reservoir devices include (a) press coating or air suspension coating technique to coat the drug particles/drug reservoir using water insoluble polymeric materials, (b) prepared by filling drug reservoir in silicone tubing of a suitable wall thickness and then sealing both the ends securely, and (c) preparing films containing drug and polymer by placing the solution on Teflon coated surface and allowing the solvent to evaporate to form film. Some examples of these devices reported in the literature are given in Table 8.1.

Even though diffusion controlled delivery systems are appropriate for constant drug release from implants the matrix systems are more popular due to simplicity of fabrication and commercialization.

In this system solid drug is dispersed in an insoluble matrix. The rate of drug release is dependent on the rate of drug diffusion but not on the rate of dissolution. However, in such a system, zero order release is not commonly achieved in-vivo. The three major types of matrix diffusion control devices generally fabricated are insoluble plastic, fatty, are hydrophilic matrices. Insoluble plastic matrices are designed as swallowable tablets or implants. The drug present within the pores and channels of the polymeric matrix would be released very quickly (dose dumping) in vivo which could be dangerous for drugs with a narrow therapeutic index. This problem is particularly seen in case of chewable tablets of insoluble drug dispersed in a polymeric matrix. This problem could be overcome to some extent by dissolving the drug in the polymer itself. A representative type of such a formulation is given in Fig 8.1.

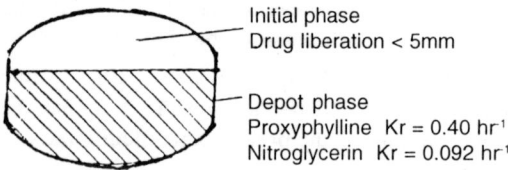

Initial phase
Drug liberation < 5mm

Depot phase
Proxyphylline $Kr = 0.40 \text{ hr}^{-1}$
Nitroglycerin $Kr = 0.092 \text{ hr}^{-1}$

Structure of depot phase

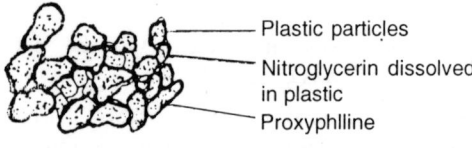

Plastic particles

Nitroglycerin dissolved in plastic

Proxyphlline

Drug release from depot phase

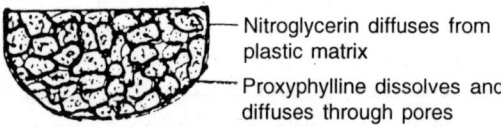

Nitroglycerin diffuses from plastic matrix

Proxyphylline dissolves and diffuses through pores

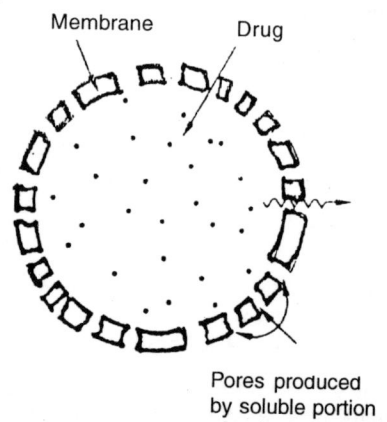

Membrane   Drug

Pores produced by soluble portion of polymer membrane

Fig 8.1: Diagramatic structure of matrix type controlled release depot formulations

Fig 8.2 : Diagramatic representation of diffusion control drug release from a coated system

Fatty matrices generally consist of waxes and are prepared by dispersing the drug and excipients in molten wax. This mixture is then congealed, granulated and compressed in to cores and may be coated. Hydrophilic matrices are prepared using non-digestible hydrophilic gums like hydroxypropyl methylcellulose or sodium carboxy methyl cellulose. The drug is mixed with a hydrophilic gum and then compressed in to tablets. Such a tablet when exposed to body fluid, rapid initial drug release occurs, but hydration and gelation of gums at the tablet interface result in the formation of a viscous gel barrier which retards further drug release (Fig 8.2). Generally in this system drug release follows Higuchi's diffusion controlled model. Some examples of the matrix devices fabricated as implants are given in Table 8.2.

Table 8.2 : Fabrication and evaluation of matrix type implants.

Matrix material (Drugs)	Fabrication procedure	Results and comments
Hydrated methyl cellulose (Chlorpheniramine maleate)	Drug in ether mixed with the polymer was granulated with ethanol and compressed	Drug release appeared to follow Higuchi's model
Carnauba wax and stearyl Alcohol (Tripelenamine HCl)	Drug and surfactants were blended with molten wax mixture congealed, granulated and compressed	Water soluble surfactants increased alcohol dissolution rate, probably by creating more channels.
Carbopol (Mepyramine maleate)	Aqueous dispersion of the drug stirred with aqueous dispresion of Carbopol 934. Gummy product obtained was dried and ground to 200-500 mm particles.	Release profile was found linear with time in the initial 5 hrs during in-vitro dissolution study.
Silicon elastomer (Morphine sulphate)	Drug mixed with simethicone fluid and polydimethyl siloxane Elastomer and moulded to cylinder and polymerised.	Release was slow but increased by the addition of water soluble carrier. Release mechanism by pores through matrix secondary to the swelling.
Methyl acrylate and methyl methacrylate. (Sod. pentobarbital Ephedrine HCl Dextrometharphan HBr)	Drug-polymer mixture was compressed	Drug release followed square root of time dependence.
Glyceryl tristearate (Sulfaethylthiadiazole)	Drug dispersed in molten wax was dispersed in hot water containing dispersant. Particles was separated and air-dried.	Drug release by diffusion and partially by disintegration.
Polyvinyl chloride Polyethylene Halogenated fluorocarbon (Sod. salicylate)	Drug plastic mixture was compressed and embedded in wax to expose only one surface of the compact.	Drug release profile followed Higuchi's model.
Ethylene glyco methacrylate (Norgestomet)	Drug dissolved in the alcohol solution of the polymer and then polymerised by adding ethylene dimethacrylate as cross linking agent.	Steady release rate for 16 dyas observed when tested in-vivo by subdermal implantation.
Silicone elastomer (Estradiol)	By coating drug polymer dispersion around a rigid silicone rod by extrusion.	Steady release rate for 200-400 days following sub cutaneous implantation behind ear of steer.
Silicone elastomer and silicone tubing (Norgestomet)	Dispersion of the drug in an aqueous solution of PEG 400 mixed with a viscous mixture of silicone elastomer and extruded into silicone tubing, polymerised and cut into cylinders.	A constant zero order release profile was achieved

One of the patented subcutaneous implant device for contraception is Syncro-Mate-B Implant, which is fabricated by dissolving norgestomet crystals in an alcoholic solution of ethylene glycomethacrylate (Hydron S) and then polymerizing the drug polymer mixture by the addition of a cross-linking agent, such as ethylene dimethacrylate, and an oxidizing catalyst to form a cylinder shaped insoluble Hydron implant (Chien, 1978). Another subdermal implant device for contraception is 'Compudose Implant' which is fabricated by dispersing micronised estradiol crystals in a viscous mixture of silicone elastomer and catalyst and then coating the estradiol- polymer dispersion around a rigid silicone rod by extrusion technique to form a cylinder shaped implant. The device was tested in steers for 200-400 days to release a controlled quantity of estradiol for growth promotion.

8.5.1.2 Intra uterine devices

The invention of an intrauterine plastic spiral by Margulies and a plastic loop by Lippes opened up the modern era of IUD development (Tiatze & Levit, 1962). A 'T'shaped polyethylene device was later developed by Tatum (1970) which significantly reduced IUD related side effects such as pain, bleeding and expulsion. However, its good uterine tolerance property was recognized after the development of IUDs containing contraceptive agents like copper (Copper T) and progestins. This development initiated new era of research in the field of medicated IUDs.

8.5.1.2.1 Development of medicated intrauterine devices

The effectiveness of conventional IUDs in preventing pregnancy depends primarily on their mechanical effect on the endometrial surface and so they are designed to contact greater areas of the endometrial surface. Hence the larger size IUDs were designed but they suffer from the disadvantage of irritation, provoke bleeding, cramping and expulsion leading to undesirable responses after the insertion of IUDs.

The controlled release of anti-fertility agents from IUDs was conceived in 1968 by Zipper et al (1968) who prepared copper bearing IUDs for easy tolerance and suitable size control. Antifibrinolytic agents such as amino caproic acid and tranexamic acid were also tried to suppress incidences of bleeding and pain.

8.5.1.2.2 Design of IUDs

A logical consideration for designing the IUDs is that the device should conform to the endometrial cavity with regard to its anatomical and functional characteristics. When the uterine cavity is empty, the endometrial surface is separated by only a thin layer of mucus and other secretions. The volume and shape of the endometrial cavity depend on the contractile state of the myometrium as a result of the summation of myometrial forces. The average dimensions of the endometrial cavity at several levels have been computed schematically in the Fig 8.3 .

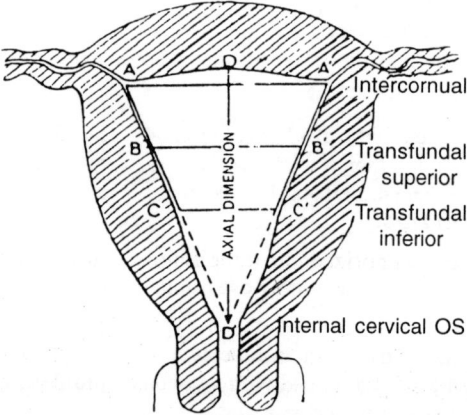

Fig 8.3 : Endometrial dimentions . A-A' = 30.3 ± 4.3 mm; B-B' = 22.5 ± 5.2 mm; C-C' = 38.5 ± 4.3 mm
D-D' = 38.5 ± 5.3 mm; AA'-BB' = 10 mm; and bb'-cc' = 10mm

As myometrial fibers contract, the uterine wall thickens and shortens, and in response the endometrial cavity becomes smaller in all dimensions. As the contraction increases, the lateral walls of the cavity approximate one another, and the cavity assumes the shape of the capital letter 'T'. Apparently, the intrauterine device in the shape of a 'T' can easily conform to the shape and size of the endometrial cavity, causing minimal myometrial distention and endometrial compression..

8.5.1.2.3 Hormone releasing IUDs

Doyle & Clewe (1968) first initiated use of hormone releasing IUDs with the objective of enhancing the intrauterine retention of a silicone device in animals. Initially, progesterone containing silicone capsules were affixed to modified Lippes loops which on short term studies demonstrated induction of histological changes in the endometrium, which otherwise could not be brought about by the oral administration of progesterone. Further development has resulted in the evolution of a 'T' shaped progesterone-releasing IUDs in which the drug containing silicone capsule forms an integral part of the vertical arm of the device. New version of the progesterone releasing IUDs, consisting of a medicated core with progesterone suspended as microcrystals in a silicone medical fluid, which is then encapsulated in a rate-limiting barrier of an ethylene/vinyl acetate copolymer. Here also the progesterone releasing compartment forms an integral part of the vertical arm of the 'T' shaped IUD. By varying the characteristics of the polymer, it becomes possible to deliver the progesterone at constant rate. The basic design of such IUD system is given in Fig 8.4.

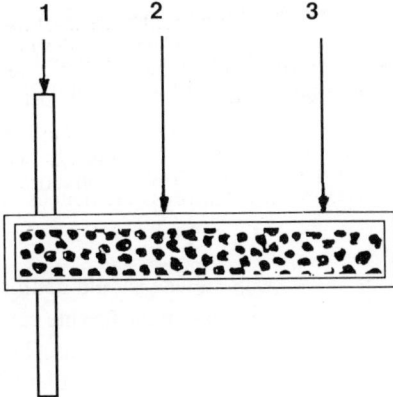

Fig 8.4 : Diagramatic sketch of Intra Uterine Devices (IUD): (1) Permeable tbe wall ;
(2) Drug crystals suspended in viscous base ; (3) Transverse bar to avoid expulsion

The major advantage of the IUDs delivering progesterone is negligible localization of the drug in non-target tissues. This property is attributed to the ability of the endometrium to metabolize progesterone as it traverses the endometrial layers, therefore deep layers of the endometrium would not be subjected to the action of the intrauterinally administered progesterone and would continue to respond to the endogenously secreted ovarian hormones with cyclic changes and normal desquamation.

8.5.1.2.4 New developments of interest in IUDs.

Intrauterine drug delivery systems may be categorized into three major groups considering the current research and developments.

(a) Encapsulated drug delivery : This type consists of a polymeric membrane which both encapsulates and controls the release of the therapeutic agents. They may be single component or multiple component systems. In the single component system, drug in the pure solid form is present in a capsule fabricated from biocompatible polymeric material notably silicon elastomer and polyethylene polymer. For improving biocompatibility, tensile strength and elastic modulus copolymers of polydimethyl siloxane with polycarbonate or polyurethane are used. In multiple component systems a liquid medium saturated with excess drug particles is enclosed in a rate controlling polymeric membrane generally made up of ethylene/vinyl acetate copolymer. A zero-order release rate is maintained until the encapsulated drug solution becomes unsaturated. The duration of medication can be adjusted by incorporating an approximate amount of drug into the solution system (Baker and Lansdale, 1974)

(b) Drug-dispersing matrix device : This type of the device is prepared by homogeneously dispersing the drug particles in a cross-linked polymeric matrix. They may be retrievable or biodegradable devices. Retrievable devices are fabricated from silicone elastomers by pre-mixing solid drug powder with semisolid silicone elastomer before vulcanization at room or low temperature (Chien et al, 1976. It can also be fabricated from polyethylene by dry mixing the drug powder with low density polyethylene particles before melt extrusion . The rate of drug release from this device is not constant but time-dependent. The amount of drug release is linearly proportional to $t_{1/2}$ (Chien et. al,1976). In case of bio-degradable devices, both the drug and a bio-degradable polymer like poly(lactic/glycolic acid) are dissolved in a common solvent and then melt pressed at an elevated temperature. The rate of drug release from this type of drug delivery system is a combination of polymer bio-degradation and drug diffusion.

(c) Composite drug delivery devices : This type of drug delivery system is a hybrid of encapsulated drug delivery device with drug dispersing matrix device. Here the core, which is a matrix, is coated with the rate controlling membrane. By this technique, desired release rate can be achieved for most drugs, especially when a highly drug-permeable membrane, such as silicone elastomer, is used on a porous support.

8.5.1.3 Intravaginal Controlled Drug Release Devices

It has been known for several decades that various pharmacologically active agents, such as steroids, may be absorbed effectively through the vaginal mucosa. Using of vagina as the root of administration for contraceptive steroids has several advantages, the most practical of which is that self-insertion and removal are possible. It also provides continuous administration of an effective dose level, thus insuring better patient compliance. It can also prevent the possibility of systemic toxicity or inefficient biological activity resulting from the alternately surging and ebbing plasma drug levels that occur with the intermittent use of oral dosage form. The advantage of intravaginal Medroxy progesterone acetate (MPA) over the conventional oral administration is illustrated in the Fig 8.5.

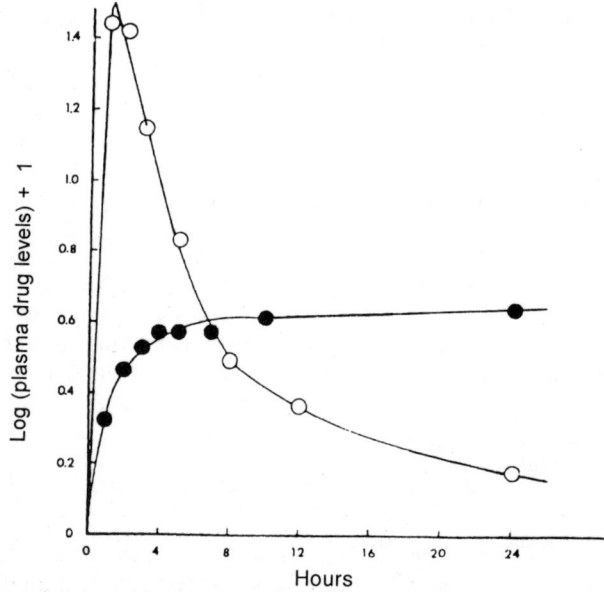

Fig 8.5 : Comparitive plasma profiles of Medroxy progesterone acetate(MPA) in five women following oral administration of 10 mg MPA in tablets(o) and Intravaginal administration of 100 mg MPA in a vaginal ring(l)

Another advantage of the intravaginal route of administration is its ability to avoid 'first pass metabolism'. The perennial venous plexus, which drains the vaginal tissue and rectum, flows in to the pudentum vein and ultimately into the vena cava, which circumnavigates the liver in first pass. Thus the vaginal route may be of great value with drugs like progesterone and estradiol, which are poorly available when taken orally because they are extensively metabolized by the liver (Flynn et al, 1976). In addition, the intravaginal route can also be beneficial to drugs such as prostaglandin that cause GI irritation.

8.5.1.3.1 Bio-pharmaceutics of Intravaginal controlled drug release devices

Intravaginal absorption of a therapeutically active agent from a controlled release device should be visualized as a consecutive process of several definable steps. For the drug dispersing vaginal ring, the steps consist of the dissolution of the finely divided, well dispersed drug particles into the surrounding polymer structure; diffusion through the polymer matrix to the device surface; partition into and then diffusion across the vaginal secretion fluid; uptake by and then penetration through the vaginal epithelium; and finally, transport and distribution of the drug molecules by circulating blood and/or lymph to a target tissue.

Assuming that the finally divided drug particles are homogeneously dispersed throughout the polymer matrix, the dissolution of the drug in the polymer phase is not a rate limiting step. A sharp interface is maintained between the drug dispersion zone and the drug depletion zone, which recedes continuously into the core of the device with time. It is also assumed that the drug has a finite solubility C_p in the polymer phase and the total drug content per unit volume A, including the undissolved solid particles, is much greater than C_p. Under these conditions, the rate of intravaginal release of a drug species from the matrix type medicated vaginal ring is defined as

$$\frac{dQ}{dt} = \frac{D_p\, C_p\, A}{\{[\, D_p\, K_s\, (\, 1/P_{aq} + 1/P_m)]^2 + 4D_p\, C_p\, At\}^{1/2}}$$

where,

D_p = diffusivity of the drug in the polymer matrix

K_s = interfacial partition co-efficient

P_{aq} = permeability co-efficient across the aqueous diffusion layer

P_m = permeability co-efficient across the vaginal membrane

In the beginning when the drug depletion zone is very narrow the rate-limiting step is either the hydrodynamic diffusion layer or the vaginal wall. In such circumstances, the equation is reduced to:

$$\frac{dQ}{dt} = \frac{C_p\, P_{aq}\, P_m}{K_s\, (\, P_{aq} + P_m)}$$

This indicates that a zero order drug release profile results.

As the residence of the device prolongs, drug depletion zone increases and the release predominantly follows matrix diffusion process as depicted in the following equation:

$$dQ/dt = 1/2\{\, D_p.C_p.A/t\}^{1/2} \quad or, \quad Q/t^{1/2} = (2.A.C_p.D_p)^{1/2}$$

8.5.1.3.2 Fabrication of intravaginal devices

Intravaginal devices are fabricated using drug (generally contraceptive steroid) dispersed in a viscous mixture of silicone elastomer and catalyst and then extruding the drug-polymer dispersion into a mould to form a donut shaped ring as shown in Fig 8.6. It is designed for insertion into the vagina and positioned around the cervix.

This type of device is not completely free from problems. It causes breakthrough bleeding and requires cyclic insertion for 21 days with removal for remaining 7 days to minimize the problem.

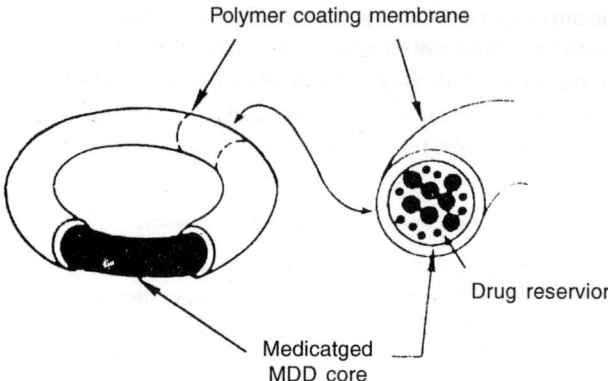

Fig 8.6 : Diagramatic sketch of Intravaginal insert along with it's transverse section.

A new generation of vaginal rings to facilitate this multicycle contraception has been developed in which the drug dispersing polymer matrix was coated with a nonmedicated polymeric coating to minimize the initial drug concentration spike frequently observed in the first treatment cycle. A schematic diagram of the device is given in Fig 8.6.

8.5.1.4 Intra-ocular implants

Most ocular treatment call for the topical administration of drugs to the tissues around the ocular cavity. Several types of ophthalmic delivery systems are commercially available. Most prescribed dosage form is the eye drop solutions, which are easy to use even though they suffer from inherent disadvantage of immediate dilution and drug loss through the naso-lacrimal drainage. Hence bio-availability following intraocular administration of drops may hardly be 1.2 % to the aqueous humor and therefore demands suitable intra ocular delivery system to increase bio-availability to a substantial level.

8.5.1.4.1 Bio-pharmaceutics of ocular drug administration

Topical administration of ophthalmic active drugs to the eye is the most prescribed route of administration for the treatment of various eye disorders. Unfortunately, drugs administered to the eye as conventional dosage-form like eye drops shows very low bioavailability. For example, pilocarpine administered in glaucoma as eye drops is available only 2-3% to the aqueous humor. Many factors affect the intra-ocular bioavailability of topically applied ophthalmic active drugs: (1) continual inflow and outflow of lacrimal fluid, (2) efficient naso-lacrimal drainage, (3) interaction of drugs with the proteins of the lacrimal fluid, and (4) productive and nonproductive absorption of the drug into various ocular tissues notably cornea and conjunctiva. Taking pilocarpine as an example, following instillation of a pilocarpine eyedrop dose (50 to 70 μl) into the pre-corneal area of the eye, greater part of the drug solution (80% of the drug dose) is drained away within 5 minutes by the naso-lacrimal drainage system until the solution volume returns to the normal resident tear volume of 7.5 μl (Chrai et al, 1973). The remaining drug gets diluted with the tears and the concentration declines and so the uptake by the corneal and conjunctival tissue. This results into biphasic decline of the drug concentration in the precorneal area; initial rapid decline due to the nasolacrimal drainage followed by slow decline due to corneal/ conjunctival absorption.

The pre-corneal disposition of pilocarpine eye drop solution by various routes was observed to follow a first order kinetic pattern. Naso-lacrimal drainage being the major route of disposition, the volume of the eye drop instilled into the pre-corneal area of the eye influences greatly the intra-ocular bioavailability.

So far as the trans-corneal permeation of drugs is concerned the prevailing theories include, all or in part, the following hypothesis.: (1) existence of a permeation barrier in the lipophilic corneal epithelium, (2) rapid uptake and transport of pilocarpine by the cornea, (3) release of pilocarpine from the cornea to the anterior chamber is controlled, (4) existence of pilocarpine depot somewhere in the cornea. The extent of permeability of the corneal epithelial barrier varies with the solubility character of the permeating molecule. The barrier being lipophillic, shows higher permeability to lipid soluble drugs. The sequences of transcorneal permeation of pilocarpine following its instillation in the cul-de-sac can be outlined as in the following scheme:

Tear flow

$\downarrow q_T$

Precorneal drug pool $\xrightarrow{K_a}$ Epithelial surface $\xrightarrow{K_{aE}}$ Corneal epithelium $\xrightarrow{K_{eE}}$ Stroma endothelium

$\downarrow K_{nl}$ $\searrow K_c$ $\downarrow K_{em}$ K_{aS} $K_{eS} \downarrow K_{aAH}$

Nasolacrimal $\qquad$ Conjunctiva $\qquad$ Metabolism $\qquad$ Aqueous humor

Drainage system $\qquad\qquad\qquad\qquad\qquad\qquad\qquad\qquad\qquad$ $\downarrow K_{eAH}$

$\qquad\qquad\qquad\qquad\qquad\qquad\qquad\qquad\qquad\qquad\qquad\qquad\qquad$ Elimination

where

q_T = normal tear fluid production rate (0.66 µl / min)

K_{nl} = composite first order elimination rate constant of naso lacrimal drainage

K_c = apparent rate constant for conjunctival uptake of drug

K_a = apparent rate constant for epithelial uptake of drug

K_{aE} = apparent absorption rate constant into epithelium

K_{eE} = apparent elimination rate constant from epithelium

K_{aS} = apparent absorption rate constant into stroma-endothelium

K_{eS} = apparent elimination rate constant from stroma-endothelium

K_{aAH} = apparent absorption rate constant into aqueous humor

K_{eAH} = apparent elimination rate constant from aqueous humor

K_{em} = apparent metabolism rate constant from epithelium

By considering the eye as consisting of two major compartments, the precorneal area and the aqueous humor, rate profile for the disappearance of the drug from the pre-corneal compartment is mathematically expressed as,

$$\frac{dC_T}{dt} = \frac{-q_T C_T - (K_p S_c / h_c)(C_T - C_{AH})}{v_D e^{-K_{nl}t} + V_o}$$

and the rate profile for the appearance of pilocarpine in the aqueous humor compartment is defined by

$$\frac{dC_{AH}}{dt} = \frac{K_p S_c}{V_{AH} h_c}(C_T - C_{AH}) - K_{eAH}\frac{C_{AH}}{V_{AH}}$$

where,

C_T = drug concentration in the tear fluid

K_p = specific transcorneal permeability rate ($3.675 \times 10\text{-}4$ µl / ml cm^{-1} min^{-1})

S_c = surface area of the cornea (2cm^2)

H_c = thickness of the cornea (0.035)

C_{AH} = drug conc. In the aqueous humor

V_D = drop size of the drug solution instilled

K_{nl} = $(0.25 + 0.0113\ V_d)\ min^{-1}$

V_0 = normal resident tear volume (7.5 µl)

V_{AH} = volume of the aqueous humor

V_{pc} = volume of the drug pool in the precorneal area after instillation of the drug dose.

The pilocarpine concentration in the aqueous humor can be increased by multiple instillation (Himmelstein, et al, 1978). By multiple instillations of one drop dose every 30 minutes for 5 doses, the pilocarpine concentration profile in the aqueous humor compartment was significantly increased and prolonged as compared to the single instillation. Hence it is evident that controlled slow release implants could increase the bio-availability in a significant way.

8.5.1.4.2 Controlled release ocular devices

The controlled release ocular devices are flexible, oval inserts which consist of a medicated core reservoir prepared out of a hydrogel type of materials. Based on the mechanism of release and types of constructions, the device may be essentially three types.

(a) Diffusion controlled ocular devices

These consists of a medicated core prepared out of a hydrogel polymer like alginates, sandwiched between two sheets of transparent, lipophilic, rate controlling polymer like ethylene / vinyl acetate copolymer membrane designed to the required geometry suitable for insertion in to the cul-de-sac as given in Fig 8.7.

When the device is placed in the cul-de-sac , the drug molecule penetrate through the rate controlling membranes at zero order rate process as defined by the following mathematical expression

$$dQ/dt = D_p\ K_m\ (C_R - C_T)\ /\ \delta_m$$

Where dQ/dt is the release rate of drug from a unit surface area of the device, D_p is the diffusivity of the drug in the polymer membrane, Km is the partition co-efficient of the drug towards the membrane, δ_m is the thickness of the device (0.3 mm) and $(C_R - C_T)$ is the difference in the drug concentration. Between the drug reservoir and

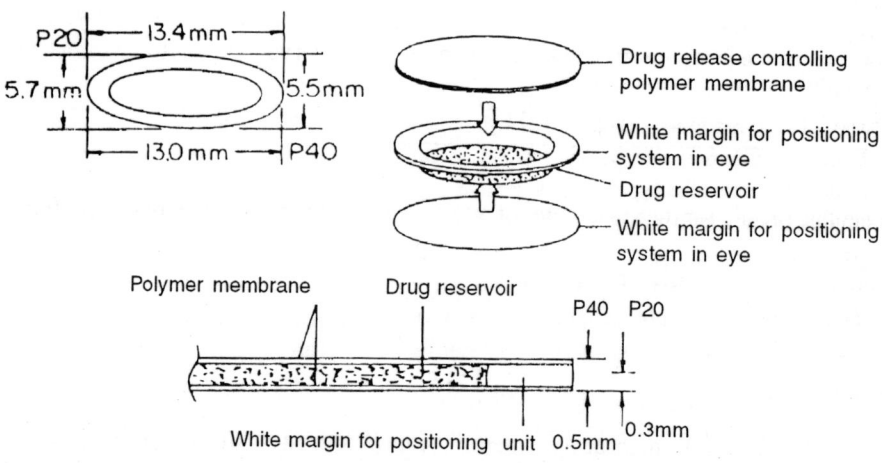

Fig 8.7 : Schematic diagram of an Ocusert controlled release drug delivery device.

in the tear fluid. If an infinite sink condition is maintained in the ocular cavity, that is $C_R \gg C_T$, then equation is reduced to

$$dQ/dt = D_p \, K_m \, C_s \, / \, \delta_m$$

By maintaining the drug concentration constant in the reservoir, the release rate of the drug could follow the first order kinetics. A range of release rate can be achieved by changing the composition and thickness of the polymer membrane

A typical in-vivo release rate profile of pilocarpine from the ocusert Pilo-20 is illustrated in the Fig 8.8. During the first hours, the system releases pilocarpine at a rate, which is three times higher than the programmed rate, i.e, 20μg per hour. The programmed release rate is then achieved in approximately six hours and is maintained for seven days. The system administers a total of less than 70% of the pilocarpine loading dose to the eye at the end of seven days medication (Mikkelson et al, 1973).

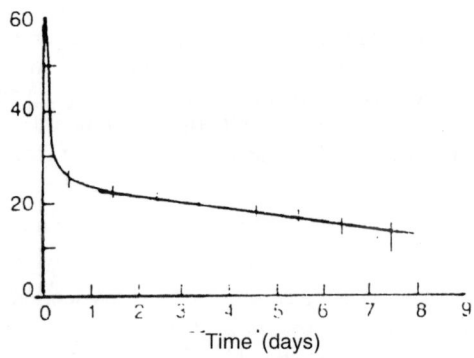

Fig 8.8 : In-vitro release pattern of pilocarpine from Ocusert pilo-20 system.

Incorporating the additives during the membrane preparation can also modify the membrane permeability of pilocarpine across the rate controlling ethylene/vinyl acetate co-polymer membrane. For example, di-(2-ethylhexyl)-phthalate is added into the membrane of ocusert Pilo-40 to enhance the rate of membrane permeation of pilocarpine (Mikkelson, et al, 1973). Similarly, ocular inserts of this type have been reported for various other ophthalmic medications like carbonic anhydrase inhibitor, epinephrine, anesthetics, anti-biotics, anti-inflammatory steroids etc.

(b) Hydrophilic matrix type ocular devices (contact lens type)

This type of device is a matrix prepared out of hydrogel polymers, which are generally used to fabricate contact lenses. Even, contact lens can be used to deliver drug at a predetermined rate by the selection of a suitable polymer composition. This type of device substantially prolongs the drug/eye contact time and thus increases bioavailability. Some of the polymers that could be used for preparing the device are 2-hydroxy ethyl methacrylate, vinylpyrrolidone acrylic co-polymer etc. When contact lenses are used as device, the lens is presoaked in the drug solution for sufficient time for equilibration and is then inserted just like a contact lens. The potential bio-medical application of hydrophilic contact lenses has been extended to the intra-ocular controlled administration of antibiotics, antiglacoma drugs, anti-inflammatory steroids etc.

(c) Erodible devices

This type of device is fabricated from bioerodible or bio-degradable polymers of hydrogel or non-hydrogel type. The mechanism of drug release in these systems is dependent on rate of erosion or rate of degradation. Several erodible types of ocuserts have been prepared using polymers like carboxymethyl cellulose, polyvinyl alcohol, collagen etc. containing drugs like pilocarpine, gentamycin etc in the form of discs and wafers.

Erodible ocular inserts containing hydrophobic polycarboxylic acids have been reported by Heller & Baker (1974) . Some of the products of this type are also marketed recently. They are: (i) Lacrisert, a cylindrical shaped device made up of hydroxypropyl cellulose for the treatment of dry eyes in conjunction with artificial tear drops, (ii) Soluble ocular drug inserts (SODI), a small oval shaped wafer containing anti-glaucoma drugs fabricated out of acrylamide, N-vinyl pyrrolidone and ethyl acrylate (ABE) system. The device is inserted in the cul-de-sac after soaking for 10-15 minutes, which release drug for a long time. Generally it replaces 4 to 12 drops instillation. (iii) Ocular therapeutic system or minidisc, is a miniature contact lens with a diameter of 4 to 5 mm made of silicone based prepolymer: a-w-bis(4-methylacryloxy)-butyl poly dimethyl siloxane. Dissolution studies reported claim the extended release of the entrapped drug for more than 170 hours from this device. (iv) Corneal collagen shield, prepared by molding collagen mixed with the drug into a contact lens configuration is dehydrated and sterilized by gamma radiation and packed. The device on insertion releases the drug as the polymer dissolves slowly in the tear fluid. Large number of devices containing drugs in the category of antibiotics, steroids have been reported (Bloomfield, 1978).

(d) Implantable Silicone Devices

Silicone rubber device was developed for the local delivery of an anti-neoplastic drug to the intraocular site and has been tested in animal model. The system is composed of two sheets of silicone rubber glued to the edge with silicone adhesive to form a baloon like sac through which a silicone tubing (0.3 mm dia) is inserted as showed in Fig 8.10. The device was tested by implantation into the episcleral tissue of rabbit. The rate of drug release through such a device can be expressed by a simple steady-state expression

$$\frac{1}{A}\frac{dx_t}{dt} = \frac{D_K}{h}d_C$$

where dx_t/dt represents the rate of release, A is the cross-sectional area of diffusion, D is the apparent diffusivity of the permeating species across the silicone membrane, K is the apparent partition coefficient between the water and the polymer phase and dC is the concentration gradient across the membrane.

Such silicone devices have significant potential for local controlled delivery of antibacterial, anticancer and antiviral drugs to the anterior chamber of the eye.

(e) Implantable Infusion Devices

Patients suffering from dry-eye require frequent instillation of artificial tear preparations. A continuous infusion device containing these solutions was developed by Refojo et al (1978) and has been tested successfully in

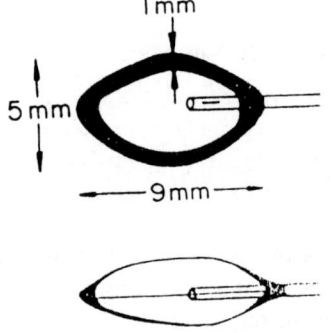

Fig 8.9 : Schematic diagram of an expandable silicone implant type ocular insert.

mongrel dogs model. In this device, the canalicular system is intubsted with fenestrated silastic tubing, which is subcutaneously tunneled and then attached to a miniaturized and computerized pumping device, which is capable of pumping a pre-determined volume of the solution continuously.

Another intraocular drug delivery pumping device is the Infusaid, wherein the energy for pumping is met by an expanding fluid like a fluorocarbon in gas-liquid equilibrium at body temperature (Infusaid Corp. user manual). The device was tested by implantation in the lumbar region of a rabbit, which delivered drug continuously for six weeks to the rabbit eye through a tube implanted into the superior conjunctival fornix.

(f) Future directions

An unusually high number of aggravated ocular conditions due to over treatment by repeated instillation have been seen as a result of mechanical injury and sensitivity reactions. This is particularly the case with antiviral therapy, which demands instillations every hour. Besides being cytotoxic, these agents have both mutagenic and oncogenic potential. Therefore, such treatment modalities should be intervened with controlled release devices to minimize the toxic potential and to enhance therapeutic potential.

Iontophoretic devices have been utilized for evaluating herpes simplex infection and reactivation as well as epinephrine distribution and concentration in full thickness corneas and in trigeminal ganglia of rabbits (Dunkel & Paron, 1987). Iontophoretic delivery of sulfa drugs in pyocyaneous infections has been reported to be 3 to 12 times greater in the cornea and 3 to 15 times greater in the aqueous humor than that resulting from diffusion alone (Von Sallmann, 1942).

Although controlled release devices could be more useful in the management of many ophthalmic conditions, they are not very much popular because such devices have to be put in place and taken out from under the eyelid periodically. Moreover the device can move around in the precorneal space resulting in discomfort and visual disturbances. Proper design of the device particularly with respect to size and shape using polymers that are compatible and preferably degradable in the tear fluid would solve most of the problems and can bring about a significant change in the use of ocular drug delivery systems.

8.5.1.5 Dental implants

Dental diseases are recognized as a major health problem throughout the world. Pain, discomfort and cosmetic considerations are the factors that demonstrate the severity of the problems associated with the dental diseases today. Most of the dental diseases need therapeutic agent to concentrate at a specific part of the dental structure and therefore targeting drugs to the specific area minimizes superfluous distribution of the drug to other body organs. Sustained release drug delivery systems in the form of dental implants offer many advantages to achieve this objective. They are (i) implants could be homed in periodontal pockets where actually drug release is required, (ii) secreting saliva offers an environment suitable for release of the drug, (iii) in most of the cases the device could be retrieved and re-inserted without the intervention of the expert.

Several suggestions for designing sustained release of fluoride in tablet form have been reviewed in the literature (Mishima, 1965). Intraoral device is one of the types of sustained delivery of fluoride which is prepared using dental cement for intracoronal restoration (Holly, 1973). Fluoride, as stannous fluoride (SnF_2), was incorporated into different dental cements: polycarboxylate, zinc oxide and zinc oxide phosphate. In vitro experiments have shown that 70% of SnF_2 incorporated into polycarboxylate released a greater amount of fluoride than other formulations.

A different device for locally controlled release of fluoride was designed to be attached onto the tooth's surface using copolymer hydrogel HEMA and MMA. The device was designed to release 0.02 to 1.0 mg of fluoride per day during a period of 30 to 180 days.

A sustained release device composed of ethyl cellulose, polyethylene glycol, and chlorhexidine as an active agent was applied as a coat to a removable partial acrylic denture (Jirschfeld et al, 1984) . Low plaque index was observed during the 12 days of the trial.

One of the clinical features of periodontal disease is the formation of a periodontal pocket, which is a pathologically deepened sulcus. In a normal sulcus, the gap between the gingiva and the tooth is normally between 1 to 3mm deep. However, during periodontitis, the depth of the pockets usually exceeds 5mm generally associated with a dramatic change of the microflora.

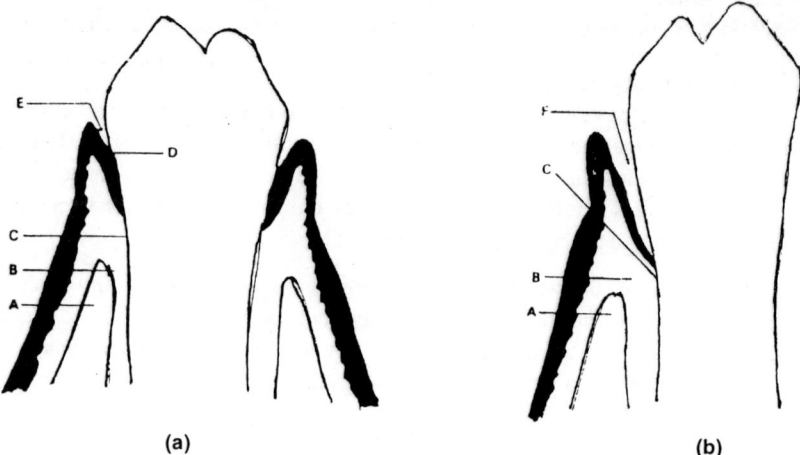

Fig 8.10: .(a) Healthy periodontum and (b) periodontal pocket : Legend; A = alveolar bone, B = periodontal ligament, C = cementum, D = cementum-enamel junction, E = sulcus, and F = periodontal pocket.

The number of Gram-negative bacteria can increase to 70% of the total flora, most of it being anaerobic rods. This condition is generally associated with inflammation and thus treatment with antibiotic and anti - inflammatory agent is warranted. Growing attention has been given to topical and local drug delivery system for treating periodontal diseases. One type of a slab form for treatment of periodontal disease is an ethylcellulose film (Friedman & Golomb, 1982) containing chlorhexidine which released the drug over a period of 205 days when tested in-vitro. Similar film containing metronidazole (30%) was prepared containing polyethylene glycol, which released 90% of the drug in vivo in 24 hours. Dental implantation strips containing chlorhexidine in several matrix materials like acrylic polymers, HPMC etc. have also been reported (Addy et al, 1982).

8.5.2 Activation controlled system

Several implantable pumps for the sustained delivery of drugs have been developed utilizing activated systems to mechanically push the medication into body at a controlled rate. Among many such systems the following category of products have received much attention and some of them have also undergone commercialization.

　　Osmotic pressure driven devices

　　Vapor pressure driven devices

　　Mechanical pumps involving peristaltic and solenoid pumping device

　　Magnetically activated systems

　　Ultrasound activated implant devices

Among these systems osmotic pressure device has been studied at length and has been commercially developed for controlled delivery of Insulin.

8.5.2.1 Osmotic pumps

These have been dealt with in a separate chapter.

8.5.2.2 Vapor pressure activated infusion pumps

In this mode of controlled drug delivery, the drug reservoir, in a solution formulation, is contained inside an infusate chamber, which is physically separated from the vapor pressure chamber by a freely movable bellow(Fig 8.11. The vapor chamber contains a vaporizable fluid, e.g. fluorocarbon, which vaporizes at body temperature and creates a vapor pressure. Under the vapor pressure created, the bellows move upwards and forces

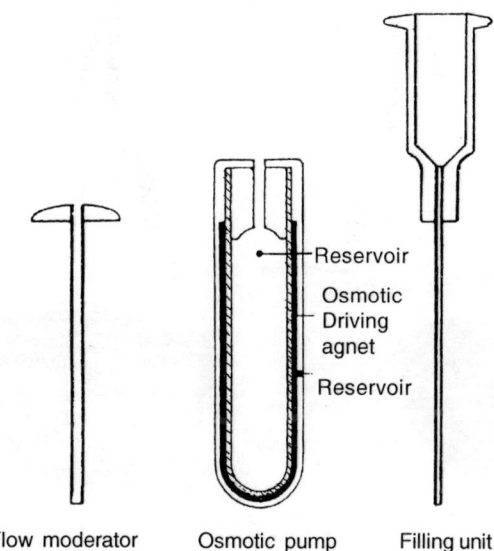

Flow moderator   Osmotic pump   Filling unit

Fig 8.11 : Cross-sectional view of a vapor pressure-activated drug delivery system, (1) flow regulator, (2) silicone polymer coating, (3) bellows, (4) fluorocarbon chamber, (5) infusate chamber, (6) fluorocarbon fluid filling tube, (7) filter, (8) inlet septum, (9) needle stop.

the drug solution in the infusate chamber to release, through a series of flow regulators and delivery cannula, into the blood circulation at a constant flow rate (Chien, 1982; Blackshear et al, 1979) as defined by the formula,

$$dQ/dt = \frac{3.1416 \, d^2 \, \Delta p}{128 \, \mu l}$$

Where d and l are the inner diameter and the length of the delivery canula; dp is the pressure difference between the vapor pressure in the vapor chamber and the pressure at the implantation site; and μ is the viscosity of the drug solution. The viscosity of the infusate could be adjusted by the addition of a calculated quantity of a water-soluble, high molecular weight polymer, such as dextran. A range of dextran concentration from 0 to 4% provides a wide latitude of flow rate changes with the pump in situ (1.95 to 0.6 ml per hour). The FC-88 used as propellant in the pump has an effective vapor pressure of approximately 8 lb/ sq.in. at 37^0C (Blackshear et al, 1972).

A typical example is the development of Infusaid, an implantable infusion pump, for the constant infusion of heparin for anti coagulation therapy (Blackshear et al, 1975), of insulin for antidiabetic medication (Blackshear et al, 1979) and of morphine for patients suffering from the intensive pain of terminal cancer.

8.5.2.3 Magnetically activated drug delivery

Macromolecular drugs, such as peptides, have been known to release only at a relatively low rate from a polymeric drug delivery device. This could be achieved by incorporating the therapeutic agent in a magnetism-triggering mechanism into a polymeric drug delivery device. The device is fabricated by positioning a donut shaped magnet at the center of a biocompatible polymer matrix which contains a homogenous dispersion of a macro molecular drug at a rather high drug : polymer ratio, to form a hemispheric magnetic pellet. The pellet is then coated with a polymer like ethylene-vinyl acetate copolymer or silicone elastomer, on all sides, except the cavity at the center of the flat surface, to permit the release of the macromolecular drug under pressure. Under the vapor pressure created, the bellows move through the cavity. The hemispheric magnetic delivery device

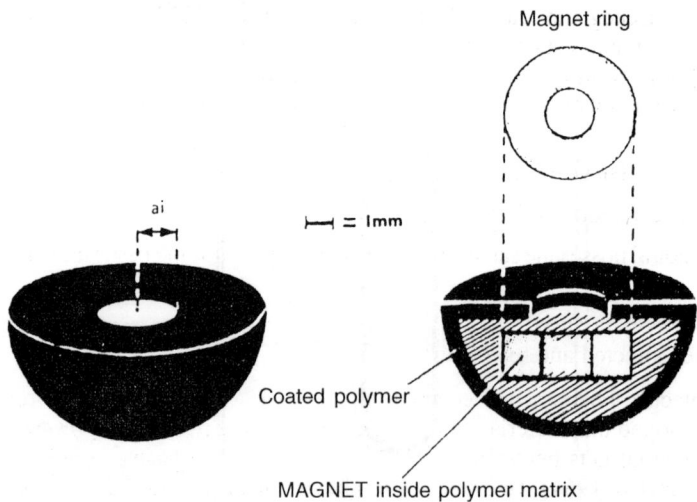

Fig 8.12 : Diagrammatic illustration of a magnetism-activated drug delivery device of hemispherical type.

can release macromolecular drug at a controlled basal rate, by diffusion process, under non-triggering condition or release the same drug at a much higher rate under the activation from an external magnetic field.

8.5.2.4 Ultrasound activated drug delivery

It was recently discovered (Kost et al, 1984) that ultrasonic waves can also be utilized, as an energy source, to facilitate the release of drug at a higher rate from polymeric drug delivery device containing a bio-erodible polymer matrix, e.g., poly{bis (p-carboxyphenoxy) alkane anhydride}. The potential application of ultrasonic wave for the modulation of drug release is still undergoing evolution.

8.6 MEDICAL ASPECTS OF IMPLANTATION

The environment of the living tissue, in which the device is implanted, determines the release rate of the drug. Animal tissue contains approximately 70% body fluid consisting in two major compartments: intracellular fluid and extracellular fluid. The extracellular fluid bathing all tissues is further subdivided into interstitial and intravascular (which includes plasma and lymph) fluid. The interstitial fluid, which the implants mostly encounter on the site of implantation, contains the electrolytes. Oxygen is freely available and is readily replaced by complex biochemical processes and homeostatic controls (Bloch et al, 1972). At cellular level, the pH value may be lower than the pH of 7.4 measured in extracellular fluid. Many enzymes, which are capable of oxidation, reduction or hydrolysis, are present in the environment of living tissues.

8.6.1 Reaction of host to implant

Inflammation is the defensive reaction of the living body to any irritant, whether physical, chemical, or bacterial. The acute phase of the inflammatory reaction leads to the formation of an exudate and fibrinous network at the affected site. Vascular and lymphatic systems are activated resulting into the accumulation of leukocytes and mast cells which along with red blood cells permeates the capillaries to the affected site. The presence of a surgically implanted device calls for major adoption by the host tissues unless the device is absorbable. The non-absorbable polymer device may remain as an incompletely covered foreign body with a barrier of connective tissue forming between it and the surface epithelium. Absorption and permeation of drugs may be effectively blocked (Coutinho et al, 1970; Benegiano et al, 1973; Benegiano & Ermini, 1972). Successful implantation may also be jeopardized by the immune response from the lymphatic system. In this process of disruption and liquefaction the tissue may become antigenic, resulting in the rejection of the implant. In addition, the leaching out of any additives from the implant may also cause toxic reactions. These reactions may be minimized by the following measures :

(1) the polymer device should have minimum surface area,

(2) the device should have smooth surface finish,

(3) ideally the implant should posses the same structural characteristics as the tissue in which it is embedded, and

(4) as far as possible the polymer used should be flexible as, a rigid plastic material inserted into a soft tissue often becomes infected and rejected.

Many a times the electric phenomena occurring at the interface could lead to thrombus formation (Mirkovitch, 1963). It was hoped that material with a high negative zeta potential might resist this tendency. However, this negetive potential gets neutralized on contact with blood, plasma, albumin, fibrinogen and gamma globulin (Mirkovitch et al, 1964). To prevent thrombosis, the device should be smooth and in contact only with an area of high velocity (Bloch et al, 1972).

Silicone capsules were found to show least degree of reactions among synthetic polymeric implants particularly when implanted in the subcutaneous or intra-peritonial space (Folkman & Long Jr, 1964). More often it is observed that the additives added in the fabrication of the device cause more damage than the basic polymeric material. For example a 2% phenolic anti-oxidant, if used , caused a marked inflammatory reaction while the same could be minimized by using a 2% amine anti-oxidant (Bloch et al, 1972).

8.6.2   Reactions of implant to host

No polymer is totally impermeable to the body fluids. Even highly lipophilic polymers like silicone elastomers absorb fat-soluble substances of the blood like cholesterol and steroids (Folkman et al, 1969). Most important in the clinical use of polymeric devices are the effects of tissue enzymes and free radicals as well as hydrolysis caused by the absorption of body fluids. Changes in physical property of the devices seen often may be due to environmental stress or as a result of chemical change. Carbon-carbon bond cleavage may account for the loss of tensile strength in hydrophobic polymers (Oppenheimer, 1955).

In conclusion, an ideal implantable therapeutic system should be biostable, biocompatible with minimal tissue-implant interactions, non-toxic, noncarcinogenic, retrievable and should release the drug at a constant, programmed rate for a pre-determined duration of medication.

8.7 CONCLUSION

The concept of implant delivery system though conceived long back was commercialized only after the use of bio-compatible polymers were developed. Understandings on the mechanism of drug diffusion made the fabrication of controlled release and long term release drug formulation more scientific and dependable. Implants with diffusion controlled delivery systems were mainly used for subcutaneous and intradermal delivery of many drugs for extended duration of action. Out of these, polymer-based matrix delivery systems have become popular, particularly for drugs like naltrexone and other anti-abuse drugs. Activation controlled systems were designed based on the principle of osmotic pressure, vapor pressure, magnetically activated, ultrasound etc. Out of these, osmotic pressure activated implant device was developed for commercial utilization for the controlled delivery of insulin. In addition, many insert devices like intra-vaginal, intra-uterine and intra-ocular were developed using non-biodegradable but diffusible polymers. To overcome the disadvantages of retrieval of ghost implants after complete drug release, bio-degradable polymers were used for developing devices for implantation in the deep areas of the body. Extra-corporal devices using conventional and programmable techniques for infusion of drugs at constant rate over a long time were also developed. Application of medicated implant devices for dental therapeutics is the recent development which has immense commercial potential in treating dental infections, particularly of anaerobic organisms.

Inspite of these investigations development of an ideal and bio-compatible polymer free from toxic and allergic manifestations is yet to be brought about. However, with the available polymers, a reasonably good implant device with minimal tissue interactions, non-toxic, non-carcinogenic could be developed commercially.

REFERENCES

Addy, M.; Rawie, L.; Handley, R. N.; Newman, H. and Coventry, J. F. (1982) "In vitro studies into the use of denture base and soft line materials as carriers of drug in mouth." J. Periodontol., 53: 693.

Baker, R. W. and Lansdale, H. K. (1974) "Controlled release: Mechanisms and rates." In A. C. Tanquarry and Lacey, R. E. (eds), "Controlled Release of Biologically Active Agents", Plenum Press, Newyork,

Ballard, B.E. and.Nelson, E. (1975) "Prolonged action Pharmaceuticals". In : Remington's Pharmaceutical Sciences." 15th ed. (A. Osol et al.,Eds.), Mack, Easton, PA Chap. 91.

Benegiano, G. and Ermini, M. (1972) Continuos steroid treatment by sub-dermal polysiloxane implants.,

Acta. Eur. Fertil. 3: 119.

Benegiano, G.; Ermini, M.; Carenza, L. and Rolfini, G. (1973) "Studies on sustained contraceptive effect with subcutaneous poly-dimethyl siloxane implants 1. Diffusion of megestrol acetate in humans." Acta Endocrinol. 73 : 335.

Bird, R. B.; Stewart, W.E. and Lightfoot, E. N. (1960) "Transport phenomenon." Wiley, New York .

Blackshear, P. J.; Dorman, F. D.; Blackshear, P. L.(Jr.); Varco, R. L. and Buchwald, H. (1972) "The design and initial testing of an implantable infusion pump." Surg. Obstet. Gynacol. , 134 : 51.

Blackshear, P. J.; Rohde, T. D.; Varco, R. L. and Buchwald, H. (1975) "One year of continuos heparanization in the dog using a totally implantable infusion pump." Surg. Gynecol. Obstet. 141:176.

Blackshear, P. J.; Rohde, T. D.; Grotling, J. D.; Dorman, F. D.; Perkins, P. R.; Varco, R. L. and Buchwald H. (1979) "Control of blood glucose in experimental diabetics by means of a totally implantable insulin infusion device." Diabetes, 28: 634.

Bloch, B. and Hastings, G. W. (1972) In; Thomas(Ed), "Plastics materials in Surgery", 2nd ed., Springfield, IL, Chapter. VI.

Bloomfield, S. E.; Miyata, T.; Dunn, M. W.; Bueser, N.; Stenzel, K. H. and Rubin, A. I. (1978) "Soluble gentamycin ophthalmic insert as drug delivery system." Arch. Ophthalmol, 96: 885.

Chien, Y. W. (1978) In: "Sustained and controlled drug del. System", Marcel Dekker, Inc, N.Y, 1978. Ch.4

Chien, Y. W. (1982) "Implantable controlled release drug delivery systems." In; Novel drug delivery Systems: Fundamental, developmental concepts, and Biomedical assessments, Marcel Dekker, Inc., New york, Chap. 7.

Chien, Y. W.; Lambert, H. J. and Rozrek, L. F. (1976) In; ACS symposium series, No. 33 on "Controlled release polymeric formulations", (Paul, D. R., and Harris, F. W., Eds.), American Chemical Society, Washington, D. C., p. 72.

Chrai, S. S.; Patton, T. F.; Mehta A. and Robinson, J. R. (1973) "Lachrymal and instilled fluid dynamics in rabbit eyes." J. Pharm. Sci. , 62: 1112.

Cooney, D. O. (1971) "Slow dissolution of implanted beads of spherical particles as a method for prolonged release medication." AIChE J. 17: 754.

Cooney ,D. O. (1972) "Effect of geometry on the dissolution of the Pharmaceutical tablets and other solids: Surface detachment kinetics controlling." AIChE J. 18: 446.

Coutinho, E. M.; Ferreira, D. A. M.; Prates, H. and Kincl, F. A. (1970) "Excretion of (6 -14 C) megestrol acetate (6-Me-17-Acetoxy-pregna-4,6-diene-3,20-dine) - release from subcutaneous silastic implants in women." J. Reprod. Fertil. 23: 345.

Crank, J. (1975) The Mathematics of Diffusion, Clarendon Press, Oxford.

Deanesly, R. and Parkes, A.S. (1936) "Comparative activity of compounds of the androsterone-testorterone" Series, Biochem. J. 30: 291

Deanesly , R. and Parkes, A.S. (1937) "Factors influencing the effectiveness of administered hormones, Proc.Roy. Soc. (London) S.B. 124: 279.

Doyle, L. L., and Cleve, T. (1968) "Preliminary studies on the effect of hormone releasing intrauterine devices." Am. J. Ostet. Gynecol.. , 101: 564.

Dunkel, E. C. and Paron Langston, D. (1987) "HSV induced reactivation : Contribution of epinephrine after corneal intophoresis." Curr. Eye. Res., 6 (1): 75-86.

Eckenhoff, B.; Theeuwes, F. and Urquhart. (1981) "Osmotically driven pumps for rate controlled delivery of solutions and viscous suspensions." J. Pharm. Technol., 5: 35.

Flynn, G. L.; Hormone, N. F. H.; Hwang, S.; Owada, E.; Molokhla, A.; Behl, C. R.; Higuchi, W. I.; Yotsuyanagi, T.; Shah Y. and Park , J. In; Paul, D. R. and Harris, F. W. (1976) (Eds.) "Controlled release polymeric formulations." Am. Chem. Society, Washington, D.C., p. 87.

Folkman, J. and Long, D.M. jr. (1964) "The use of silicon rubber as a carrier for prolonged release therapy." J. Surg. Res. 4: 139-142

Folkman ,J. and Long, D.M. jr. (1964b) "Drug pace makers in the treatment of Heart block." Ann. NY Acad. Sci. 8: 857

Folkman, J. , Reiling, W. and Williams,G. (1969) "Chronic analgesia by silicone rubber diffusion." Surgery 66: 194.

Friedman, M. and Golomb, G. (1982) "New sustained release dosageform of chlorhexidine for dental use I Development and kinetics of release." J. Periodon. Res., 17: 323.

Good, W. R. (1976) "Diffusion of water-soluble drugs from initially dry hydrogels. In Kostelnik,R. (ed), Polymeric delivery systems." Gordon and Breach, NewYork.

Harris, F. W., Aulabaugh, A. E., Case, R. D., Dykes, M. K. and Feld W. A. (1976) "Polymer containing pendent Herbicide substituents." In; Paul, D. R. and Harris, F. W. (eds), controlled release of polymeric ormulations, ACS Symposium Series, Vol 33, American Chemical Society, Washington D. C. , p. 222.

Heller. J. (1980) "Controlled release of biologically active compounds from bioerodible Polymers." Biomaterials, 1: 51.

Heller, J., Baker, R. W. (1974) "Bio-erodible devices." U.S.Patent # 3811144.

Higuchi, T. (1961) "Rate of release of medicaments from ointment bases containing drugs in suspension." J. Pharm. Sci. 50: 874.

Higuchi, T. (1963) "Mechanism of sustained-action medication." J. Pharm. Sci. 52: 1145.

Himmelstein, K. J., Guvenir, I., and Patton, T. F. (1978) "Preliminary pharmacokinetic model of pilocarpine uptake I distribution in eye., J. Pharm. Sci. , 67: 603.

Holly, F. J. (1973) "Formation and rapture of tear film." Int. Ophthalmol. Clin. , 13: 73.

Hopfenberg, H. B. (1976) "Controlled release from Erodible Slabs, Cylinders and Spheres." In; Paul, D. R. and Harris, F.W (eds) Controlled release polymeric formulations, ACS Symposium Series, Vol 33, American Chemical Society , Washington D. C. p.26.

Jirschfeld, Z., Friedman, M., Golomb, G. and Ben-Yacoov, D. (1984) "EDTA enhancement of strontium uptake by intact human enamel." J. Oral Rehabil., 11: 477

Korsmeyer, R. W. and Peppas, N. A. (1981) "Effect of morphology of the hydrophilic polymeric matrices on the diffusion and release of water-soluble drugs." J. Membr. Sci., 9: 211.

Korsmeyer,R. W. and Peppas, N. A. (1983) "Swelling controlled delivery systems for Pharmaceutical Applications: Macromolecular and modeling considerations." In Mansdorf, S. Z. and Roseman, T. J. (ed), Controlled release delivery systems, Marcel Dekker, Newyork, 1983, p. 77.

Kost, J., Leong, K. W. and Langer, R. (1984) "Ultrasonic controlled polymeric delivery sysems." In; Meyers, W. E. and Dunn, R. L.(Eds.), Proceedings of 11th International symposium on "Controlled release of Bioactive materials" The controlled release society, Inc. , Lincolnshire, IL, p. 84.

Langer, R. (1980) Polymeric delivery systems for controlled drug release." Chem. Engg. Commun. 6: 1

Langer, R., Rhine, W, Hsieh, D. and Bawa, R. (1980) "Polymers for the sustained release of macromolecules. In Baker, R (ed) Controlled Release of Bioactive Materials, Academic Press, Newyork, p. 83.

Lapidus, H. and Lordi. H.N. G. (1968) "Drug release from compressed hydrophilic matrices." J. Pharm. Sci. 57: 1292.

Mikkelson, T. J., Chrai S. S., and Robinson, J. R. (1973) "Competitive inhibition of drug- protein interaction in eye fluids and tears., J. Pharm. Sci. , 62: 1942.

Mirkovitch, V. (1963) "Bioelastic phenomena, thrombosis and plastic : A review of current knowledge." Cleveland Clin. Q. 30: 241.

Mirkovitch, V., Beck, R. E. and Andres, P. G. (1964) "The zeta potential and blood compatibility characteristics of some selected solids." J. Surg. Res. 4: 395.

Mishell, D. R. Moore, Jr,. D. E. Roy. S. Brenner, P. F. and Page, M. A. (1978) "Clinical performance and Endocrine profile with contraceptive vaginal rings containing a combination of estradiol and d-norgestrol. Am. J. Obstet. Gynacol.,130: 55.

Mishima, S. (1965) "Some physiological aspects of the pre-corneal tear films." Arch. Ophthalmol., 73: 233

Oppenheimer, B. S. (1955) "Further studies of polymers as carcinogenic agents in animals." Cancer Res. 15: 333.

Powers, K. G. (1965) "The use of silicon rubber implants for the sustained release of anti-malarial and Antischistosomal agents." J Parasitology 51: 53.

Refojo, M. F., Liu, H. S., Leong, F. L., and Sidebottom, D. (1978) "Release of nitrosourea derivative for refillable silicone rubber implants for the treatment of intra-ocular malignancies." J. Bioengineer.,2: 437.

Reinhart, C. T., Korsmeyer, R. W. and Peppas. N. A. (1981) "Macromolecular network structure and its effect on drug and protein diffusion." Internatl. J. Pharm. Technol, 2: 9.

Ringsdor, H. (1978) "Synthetic Polymeric Drugs." In: Kostelnik, R. J.. (ed). Polymeric Delivery Systems, Gordon and Breach, New york, p. 197.

Swan, E. A. and Peppas, N. A. (1981) "Drug release kinetics from hydrophobic porous monolithic devices." Proc. Symp. Controlled Rel. Bioact. Mater. 8, (1981) 18.

Tatum, H.J. (1970) "Fertility control and acceptability in women of contraceptive steroids released in microquantities from subcutaneous silastic capsules." U. S. Patent, # 3,533,406 (October 13, 1970).

Theeuwes F. and Yum, S. I. (1976) "Principles of the design and operation of generic osmotic pumps for the delivery of semisolid or liquid drug formulations." Ann. Biomed. Eng., 4: 343.

Theeuwes F. and Eckenhoff, B. (1980) "Controlled release of bioactive materials.:" (R.Baker, ed.). Academic Press, New york, p.61.

Tiatze, C. and Levit, S. (1962) "Intauterine contraception devices, International congress series." No. 54, Excerpta Medica , Amsterdam.

Von Sallmann, L. (1942) "Sulfadiazine iontophoresis in pyocyaneus infection of rabbit cornea." Am. J. Ophthalmol., 25: 1292

Zipper, J. A., Medel, M. and Prager, R. (1968) In: Abstracts of the 6th world congress on fertility and sterility, Tel Aviv, Israel, May 20-27, P. 154.

Chapter 9

Oral Delivery of Proteins and Peptides : Biochemical Considerations

Girish K. Jain

9.1 INTRODUCTION

Peptides or polypeptides are low and/or high molecular weight biopolymers, which yield two or more amino acids on hydro-lysis. Peptides and polypeptides are important constituents of proteins. Proteins are the principle components of the protoplasm of cells and are high molecular weight compounds consisting of alpha-amino acids connected together by peptide linkages. Twenty different aminoacids are commonly found in various pro-teins of biological importance. Each protein has a unique genetically defined amino acid sequence which determines its specific configuration and function. These proteins serve as enzymes, structural elements, hormones, or immunoglobulins, and are involved in metabolic processes, cell growth, immunogenic defence mechanisms, and other biological activities (Hey & John, 1978; Dence, 1980; Matthews, 1975; Walker & Isselbacher, 1974).

Peptides, polypeptides, or proteins are, therefore, an important class of biological substances which are not only the essential nutrients of human body, but some of the polypeptide hormones, e.g., insulin, are used in treating various diseases resulting from hormonal deficiency (Klostermeyer & Humble, 1966). These type of compounds are known for their proteolytic instability as well as for their limited potential to cross membranes (Lee, 1988) and therefore oral delivery of peptide and protein drugs necessitates that a sizable fraction of the adminstered dose reaches the systemic circulation.

The former general belief that all peptide and proteins are entirely decomposed in gastrointestinal (GI) tract before absorption occurs, has turned out to be a misconception (GI tractler, 1964). Today several lines of evidence sug-gest that peptide and proteins are capable of traversing through the intestinal epithelium in intact form, however with yet unpre-dictable and often insufficient bioavailability due to severe presystemic degradation in GI tract. It is known today that small amounts of intact peptides and proteins can enter the circulation under normal circumstances (Gardner, 1984; Gardner, 1991, Gebert, 1991). Indica-tion for absorption of some peptides and proteins derive from the detection of antibodies to various food proteins in the circula-tion of humans (Bazim et al 1973; Cunningham, 1987; Paganelli, & Lewinsky 1980). Additional evidence is provided by direct determination of orally administered proteins such as ovalbumin in blood (Husby et al, 1987; Jacobasson et al, 1986) and by isolated tissue experiments in which the passage of intact oligopeptides and of high molecular weight fragments of protein across isolated animal jejunum has been demonstrated (Takaori et al, 1986; Warshaw et al, 1974; Heyman et al, 1982). In case of peptides the beliefs that, the significant amount of undegraded compound can enter the circula-tion in intact form and exert profound effect, is relatively new but gaining acceptance (Webb et al, 1992; Gardner et al, 1991). In other words the delivery of pep-tides, proteins and other macromolecules to human beings and animals, in intact forms, has become increasingly important to medical community.

232

Numerous studies have been carried out to investigate enzyme inhibition, transport, and hydrolysis of peptides and proteins across the epithelia of the GI tract and plasma membranes of animal and vegetable cells (Hey & John, 1978; Walker & Jasselbacher, 1974; CIBA Foundation Symposium, 1977). The development of drug delivery systems for oral administration of peptide and protein drugs involve systematic case by case study on proteolytic degradation mechanism, kinetics, segmental differ-ences in degradation rate and intestinal permeability. A variety of techniques such as incubation with pancreatic enzymes, mucosal homogenates, brush border membrane residues, intestinal rings and perfusion experiments may be utilised to determine the above mentioned parameters. LHRH agonists for example buser-elin and immunoactive thymopoitin fragments are example of the compounds readily degraded by pancreatic trypsin, chymotrypsin and carboxypeptidases where as metkephamide, a pentapeptide has been shown to completely resist proteases of pancreatic origin (Langyuth et al, 1977). Investigations on degradation of several enkephalin analogs catalysed by brush border membrane demonstrate the versatility of the enzyme system involved in the degradation and also the saturabil-ity of the degradation reaction rate (Langyuth et al, 1977). The later findings suggest that at higher peptide doses the fraction absorbed may be expected to increase due to saturability of the degradation process. For proteolytically labile compounds, appropriate means to stabilise the molecule within the GI tract are mandatory in order to improve the absorption of intact molecule. These may involve the stabilisation of the molecule itself, for example by insert-ing unnatural D-amino acids in the molecule, N-methylation of peptide bond or cyclization. On the other hand co-administration of protease inhibitors may significantly enhance the bioavailability of proteolytically labile peptide (Langyuth et al, 1977).

The extensive biochemical and physiological studies may help in understanding the phenomenon of absorption, distribution, metabolism, and elimination of peptide and protein drugs, which in turn may accelerate the overall development of appropriate dosage form(s) for the delivery of therapeutically and nutrition-ally important peptide/protein drugs.

Since the inception of genetic engineering, the peptides and proteins produced commercially may be comparatively cheaper and easier to obtain than those, which are derived from natural sourc-es. From pharmaceutical viewpoint, it is important to develop a viable dosage form, which would allow the efficient delivery of peptides or proteins to the site of disorder. A number of such pharmaceutical dosage forms are being used either to treat a disease (e.g., cyclosporins and insulin) or to provide nutrients (e.g., protein hydrolysate) to the human body. Aspartane, a dipeptide, is also being used as a sugar supplement (Ovais & Chein, 1995).

Peptide and protein drugs are often administered parenteral-ly. Recent investigations have demonstrated the feasibility of non-parenteral routes of administration including ocular, oral, buccal, nasal, transdermal, rectal, and vaginal. For peptide and protein drugs, which are used for long term therapy, the oral route is still considered, by many pharmaceutical scientists, as the ideal route of administration. However, it is recognized that the nasal, transdermal, rectal, and vaginal routes are also viable for the delivery of drugs for systemic effect.

Therefore, new research programms should be introduced with an aim to develop dosage form(s) for the effective adminis-tration of such drugs through nonparenteral routes.

The oral administration of peptide and protein drugs faces two formidable problems. The first is the protection against the hazard of digestion in stomach and small intestine. 2nd is absorption from the GI tract in the absence of a carrier system for peptide of more than three amino acid residues. It is a difficult premise upon which such macromolecules can be delivered across the GI tract in a reliable manner to provide therapeutic concentra-tions in the systemic circulation or at the site of action.

The oral administration of peptide and protein drugs, which may be identified as antigens by the body, is likely to be more susceptible to the immunological or antibody response in compari-son to nonpeptide drugs. The antigen-antibody reaction in the GI tract may result in the breakdown of peptide drugs and, therefore, minimize the overall systemic bioavailability of such drugs. It is recognized however, that the normal GI tract is permeable to macro-molecules in sufficient amounts to be antigenically or biologi-cally active. These observations are based on the fact that a number of local and systemic diseases are caused by gastrointestinal abosrption of toxic quantities of bacteria, endotoxin, antigens, and hydrolytic enzymes (Walker & Jasselbacher, 1974; Ganong, 1977; Spiro, 1983). Therefore, the presence and the likely interference of immunoglobulins in the uptake and the transport of peptide drugs in the GI tract (Walker & Jasselbacher) should also be consid-ered druing the formulation of oral dosage form(s).

An understanding of the mechanism of the peptide hydrolysis and absorption in the GI tract is a prerequisite for the development of a commercially feasible delivery system for peptide and pro-tein drugs. During process development of such a system for the oral delivery of peptide and protein drugs, the following param-eters must be considered:

☞   Protection of peptides / proteins from the hydrolytic enzymes in GI tract.

☞   Enhancement of mucosal transport of the peptides / pro-teins.

☞   Mode of release, controlled release or instant release, since a controlled release form of the drug in some thera-peutic indications may be desirable.

☞   The ability of peptide/protein drug and their formulations to penetrate the GI tract.

☞   The ability of protease inhibitors to specifically prevent proteolytic breakdown of peptide and protein drug and not of other toxic or antigenic substrates.

The study with peptide and non peptide drugs have already demon-strated the capability of the intestine to perform several phase I and II metabolic reactions that can lead to considerable presys-temic elimination of therapeutic agents e.g. cyclosporin A and calcium channel antagonists (oxidation by cytochrome P_{450}), pivampicillin (hydrolysis by esterases), salicylazosulphapyridine (azoreduction) and estrogen and morphine (glucuronidation). Intraluminal metabolism may take place by pepsin secreted by gastric cells and by trypsin, chymotrypsin and elastase secreted by pancreatic cells. Brush border enzymes like carboxypeptidases can also act upon oligopeptides having 2-6 amino acid residues. The cytosolic fraction of enterocytes can also convert peptides to their constituent aminoacids primarily on account of the peptidases present therein.

The peptide and protein molecules which escape intraluminal and brush border hydrolysis can enter mucosal cells by a carrier mediated process, which can be followed by intracellular hydrolysis to constituent aminoacids.

The large size and the polar nature coupled with high diffu-sional resistance of the gastrointestinal mucosa to these mol-ecules make their transport difficult. Even if these compounds are taken up intact, there is the very likely possibility that these macromolecules will undergo storage or metabolism within the enterocytic cells without being transferred to the systemic circulation. However if this barrier is overcome, the compounds can still be metabolised by the liver and/or excreted into the bile.

Considering that one of the physiological functions of the GI tract is to digest ingested proteins, until abosrbable tri and dipeptides and amino acids remain, the problem of metabolism of peptides and proteins by digestive enzymes is a difficult one to solve. The potential sites of presystemic metabolism are the intestinal lumen, brush border, cytosol of the epithelial cells (enterocytes), and the liver (Davis, 1986). Various luminal, brush border, intestinal cytosolic, and liver enzymes could be involved in the presystemic metabolism, as shown by the examples in Table 9.1 which includes a list of enzymes, selected bioactive peptides, their proteolytic sites and general protease inhibitors. This list is meant to serve only as a general illustration of how bonds in a few selected peptides are cleaved by these enzymes and what types of inhibitors could be used to inhibit the enzyme activity. It is not intended to be comprehensive in its scope. The liver is the primary site of xenobiotic metabolism, yet the intestinal enterocytes are qualitatively similar in enzymic activity and are capable of performing many of the same enzymatic reactions (Chandler & Varandani, 1972). The metabolism by cytosolic enzymes can generally be studied with intestinal homogenates. These activities vary along the length of the intestinal tract. The relative contributions of the liver and intestinal mucosa to presystemic drug elimination can be evaluat-ed by comparing portal and oral bioavailabilities.

This chapter will describe the various enzymatic barriers to peptide and protein drug delivery including the brush border region. The present article will attempt to focus on metabolic fate of this class of compounds as they pass through GI tract following oral delivery and the enzymes they will encounter along that path. The chapter will also describe the role of enzyme inhibi-tors in enhancing peptide protein uptake via oral route of admin-istration. Conclusions and suggestios relative to circumventing enzyme barriers and enhancing oral bioavailability of peptide and protein drugs will also be discussed.

9.2   BARRIERS TO ORAL DELIVERY OF PROTEINS AND PEPTIDES

9.2.1 Enzymatic barriers to protein delivery

By structure the GI tract is highly efficient in preventing the absorption of intact polypeptides and proteins. Orally adminis-tered peptide and protein drugs can be metabolised by a number of peptidases at one or more sites before reaching the systemic circulation as schematically shown in Fig 9.1. To better under-stand the role of the enzymatic barrier in peptide and protein absorption, it is necessary to have information on the types and distribution of proteases, their substrate specificities, and the probablity of the contact with a peptide or protein. On this basis the proteases may be classified into five families:

(a)   Aspartic Proteases

(d)   Serinyl Proteases

(b)   Cystein Proteases

(e)   Threonine Proteases

(c)   Metallo Protease

These proteases are essentially hydrolases and rarely show absolute specificity in their action. Newly isolated proteases can be classified by their responses to general inhibitors, which are specific for each family of proteases. It is widely believed that all enzymes in each family cleave the peptide bond using the same basic mechanism and the same or similar catalytic residues (Table 9.1). As more proteases are isolated and characterised it is becoming clear that there are subgroups or subfamilies within each family of enzymes. For example, both the chymotrypsin/tryp-sin subfamily and the subtilisin subfamily of serine proteases have evolved separately although they both cleave the peptide bonds using the same chemical mechanism. At present there are some enzymes which can not fit into any of the five families of proteases since they have no sequence homology with other known proteases, a good example being the multicatalytic protease which has multiple subunits and atleast four different proteolytic activities. As these new enzymes are characterised mechanistically, it is likely that most will be members of new sub families within the five classes or families of proteases and will operate by the same general mechanism of peptide bond cleavage. However, there still remains the possibility that an entirely new mechan-ism of peptide bond hydrolysis is discovered in times to come.

On account of the ubiquitous nature of proteases there are multiple sites where such degradations may occur. A typical example is that of the metabolism of insulin by glu-tathione transhydrogenase in various tissues (Lee, 1988). Conse-quently, peptides and proteins need to be protected against degradation at more than one site for them to reach their target site intact. In a given protein or peptide, there may be more than one degradation site along the structure. Each locus may be mediated by a certain peptidase, as seen in the case of hydro-lysis of substance P (Llet et al, 1990). Often a suitable modifica-tion of one linkage to circumvent one protease may make the rest of the molecule vulnerable to other proteases. Moreover, all the proteases capable

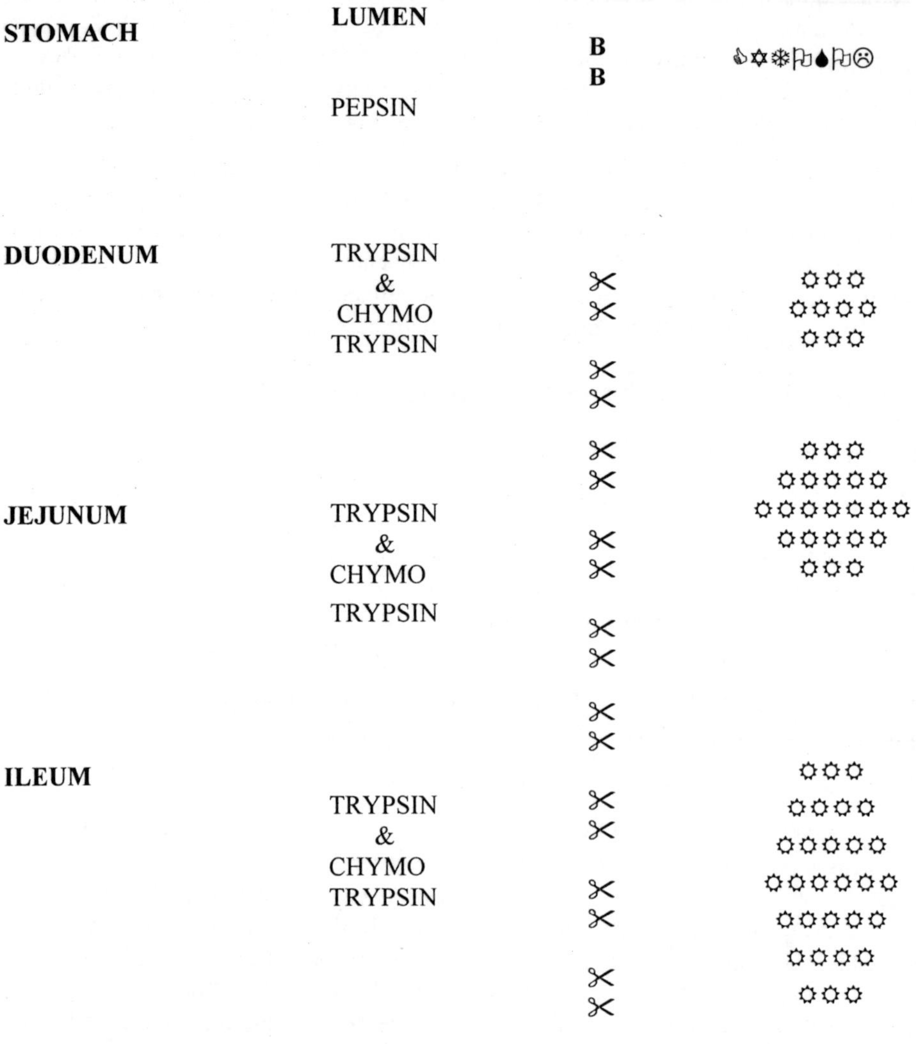

	LUMEN		
STOMACH		B B	♦✿❄🏠♦🏠⊗
	PEPSIN		
DUODENUM	TRYPSIN & CHYMO TRYPSIN	✂ ✂ ✂ ✂	✿✿✿ ✿✿✿✿ ✿✿✿
JEJUNUM	TRYPSIN & CHYMO TRYPSIN	✂ ✂ ✂ ✂ ✂ ✂	✿✿✿ ✿✿✿✿✿ ✿✿✿✿✿✿✿ ✿✿✿✿✿ ✿✿✿
ILEUM	TRYPSIN & CHYMO TRYPSIN	✂ ✂ ✂ ✂ ✂ ✂	✿✿✿ ✿✿✿✿ ✿✿✿✿✿ ✿✿✿✿✿✿ ✿✿✿✿✿ ✿✿✿✿ ✿✿✿

Fig 9.1: Potential sites of degradation of orally administered protein and peptide drugs by proteases of different sections of GI tract

BB: Brush Border

✂✿: Proteases of Brush Border and Cytosol origin

of degrading a peptide or protein are usually present at an anatomical site. Additionally transport, being the rate-limiting barrier to a number of peptide drugs, complete absorption of enzymatically stable peptide and proteins will also be an exception rather than rule.

Many proteases are involved in various human diseases and these enzymes are the targets for the development of protease inhibi-tors as new therapeutic agents. Within the serine protease family, potential target enzymes include neutrophil elastase, which is involved in pulmonary emphysema; thrombin, which is essential in platelet dependent thrombus formation; and dipeptidyl peptidase IV and granzymes, both of which are involved in immune defense. Within the metalloprotease family, potential target enzymes include angiotensin

Table 9.1 : Peptideases and their characteristics

Enzymes	Active Site	Specificity	Peptide/Protein	Bonds hydrolysed
Exopeptidases: **.....NH₂Terminus**				
Aminopeptidase N (EC 3.4.11.2)	Zn^{++}	■-□-□- (many)	Enkephalin (Met) Oxytocin Vasopressin Desmopressin	Tyr^1-Gly^2 Cys^1-Tyr^2 Cys^1-Tyr^2 Cys^1-Tyr^2
Aminopeptidase A (EC 3.4.11.7)	Ca^{++}	■-□-□- (Asp, Glu)	Angiotensin-I Angiotensin-II	Asp^1-Arg^2 Asp^1-Arg^2
Aminopeptidase P (EC 3.4.11.9)	Zn^{++}	□-■-□- (Pro)	Bradykinin TRH	Arg^1-Pro^2 His^2-Pro^3
Aminopeptidase W (EC 3.4.11.--)	Zn^{++}	□-■-□- (Trp)	RO-23-7014	Gly^3-Trp^4
Dipeptidyl peptidase (EC3.4.14.5)	Serine	□-■-□- (Pro, Ala)	Substance P (deaminated) β-Casomorphin	Pro^2-Lys^3; Pro^4-Gln^5 Pro^2-Phe^3; Pro^4-Gly^5; Pro^6-Ile^7
γ-Glutamyl Transpeptidase (EC 2.3.2.2)	Zn^{++}	■-□-□- (γ-Glu)	TRH	$γ$-Glu^1-His^2

Table 9.1 continued

Table 9.1 continued

Enzymes	Active Site	Specificity	Peptide/Protein	Bonds hydrolysed
Exopeptidases: **...COOH Terminus**				
Angiotensin Converting Enzyme (EC 3.4.15.1)	Zn^{++}	-□-□-■-■ (Many)	Angiotensin I Substance P (deaminated)	Phe^8-His^9; Phe^8-Gly^9 Gly^9-Leu^{10}
Carboxypeptidase P (EC 3.4.17.-)	Zn^{++}	-□-□-■-□ (Pro, Ala, Gly)	Angiotensin II	Pro^7-Phe^8
Carboxypeptidase M (EC 3.4.17.12)	Zn^{++}	-□-□-□-■ (Lys, Arg)	Bradykinin	Phe^8-Arg^9
γ-Glutamyl carboxypeptidases (3.4.13.19)	Zn^{++}	-■-■-■-■ $(γ\text{-}Glu)_n$	Gastrin I Big Gastrin	$-(γ\text{-}Glu)_n$-Glu^{27} $-(γ\text{-}Glu)_n$-Glu^{27}
.....Dipeptidases				
Microsomal Dipeptidase (EC 3.4.13.19)		■-■ (Many)		Gly-D-Phe
Gly-Leu Peptidase		■-□ (Neutral)		Gly-Leu
Zn Stable Peptidases		■-□ (Asp,Met)		Asp-Lys

Table 9.1 continued

Enzymes	Active Site	Specificity	Peptide/Protein	Bonds hydrolysed
Endopeptidases				
Enteropeptidase (3.4.21.9)	Zn^{+-}	-□-■-□- Pentapeptide $(Asp)_4$-Lys	Trypsinogen	Asp-Lys
Endopeptidase (EC 3.4.24.11)	Zn^{--}	-□-□-■-□- (Hydrophobic)	Insulin B Chain	Tyr^{16}-Leu^{17}
			Oxytocin	Pro^7-Leu^8
			Neurotensin	Pro^{10}-Tyr^{11}-Ile^{12}
			GnRH	His^2-Trp^3 ; Gly^6-Leu^7
			CCK-8	Gly^4-Trp^5 ; Asp^7-Phe^8
			Gastrin	Gly^{13}-Trp^{14} ; Asp^{16}-Phe^{17}
			Enkephalin (Met)	Gly^3-Phe^4
			Angiotensin II	Tyr^4-Ile^5
			Bradykinin	Gly^4-Phe^5 ; $Pro^7 Phe^8$
			Substance P	Gln^6-Phe^7 ; $Phe^7 Phe^8$; Gly^9-Leu^{10}
			α-Atrial Natriuretic Factor (human)	Cys^7-Phe^8 ; Ser^{25}-Phe^{26}
			Somatostatin	Asn^5-Phe^6 ; Phe^6-Phe^7 ; Thr^{10}-Phe^{11}
			Vaso Intestinal Peptide	Thr^7-Asp^8 ; Ser^{25}-Ile^{26}

Enzymes	Active Site	Specificity	Peptide/Protein	Bonds hydrolysed
Endopeptidase (EC 3.4.24.18)	Zn^{++}	-□-■-□-□- Aromatic/ Hydrophobic	Angiotensin I CCK-8 Bradykinin Substance P GnRH Melanotropin Serpin/α-1 Antitrypsin EBV Transformed human B cell line BC-5	Tyr^4-Ile^5 Met^3-Gly^4 Gly^4-Phe^5; Phe^5-Ser^6 Gln^6-Phe^7-Gly^8 Tyr^5-Gly^6-Leu^7 Phe^7-Arg^8 Asp^{12}-Thr^{13}·; Asp^6-Ala^7 Glu^{298}-Ser^{299} Ser^{155}-Ser^{156}

DFP : Diisopropylfluorophosphate

TRH : Thyrotropin Releasing Hormone

GEMSA : Guanidinoethylmercaptosuccininc acid

MGTA : DL-2- Mercaptomethyl-3-guanidinoethyl thiopropanoic acid

CPAB : N-[1(R,S)-Carboxy-2-phenylethyl]-Phe-p-aminobenzoate

Source : Data adapted from : Kenny et al, 1987; Kenny & Stephenson, 1987; Erdos & Skidgel, 1990; Turner et al, 1987; McDonald & Barret, 1986; Tobey et al, 1988l Guan et al, 1985; Gros et al, 1991; Harbeck & Mentlein, 1991; Simmons & Orawski, 1992; Heymann Mentlein, 1978; Skidgel et al, 1984; Drapeau et al, 1991; Metsas et al, 1983; Turner, 1987; Metsas et al, 1984; Katayama et al, 1991; Stephenson & Kenny, 1988; Morita et al, 1983; Erickson et al, 1992; Yoshioka et al, 1988; Thorsett & Wyvrett, 1987; Rahfeld et al, 1991; Cushman & Ondetti, 1980; Nagae et al, 1992; Deddish et al, 1989; Chipkin, 1986; Ferrariolo et al, 1993) converting enzyme, which is involved in hypertension; stromolysine which is implicated in inflammatory disorders such as rheumatoid arthritis; Pseudomonas aeruginosa elastase which is involved inlung infections particularly in cystic fibrosis. Within the aspartic protease family, potential target enzymes include renin, which is involved in hypertension and the HIV protease. Within the cystein protease family poten-tial target enzymes include cathepsin B, which is involved in tumors; and calpain which is involved in brain destruction during stroke and related diseases.

9.2.2 Mechanistic aspects of enzymatic barrier

9.2.2.1 Catalytic mechanism of peptisases

The structures of several members of all five classes of proteases have been determined by X-ray crystallography. In general catalytic site lies in the cleft on the surface of the enzyme molecule. The substrate polypeptide chain binds to the active site cleft with the scissile peptide bond adjacent to the catalytic residues. There are special subsites on the either side of the catalytic site, which will interact with the individual amino acid chains of the polypeptide. The aminoacid residues of the substrate are designated P_1, P_2, P_1', P_2' and the correspond-ing subsites of the enzyme are termed S_1, S_2, S_1' and S_2, S_1 and S_2 subsites are on the carbonyl side of the scissile peptide bond towards the N-terminus of the substrate and the S_1' and S_2' subsites are numbered away from the scissile bond towards the C-Terminus of the substrate (Schecter & Berger, 1967). The active site residues, representative examples and general inhibitors for each family of proteases are given in Table 9.2.

9.2.2.2 Aspartic proteases

Aspartic proteases mainly include Pepsin, Renin, Cathepsin D, Cathepsin E and HIV protease. These are all restricted in their actions either by pH or intolerance to the medium, which some times serve in a protective manner. The aspartic proteases contain two active site aspartic acid residues Asp-32 and Asp-215 in pepsinogen numbering (Tang et al, 1973). A general acid-base mechanism has been proposed in which water attacks the carbonyl of the scissile peptide bond with the active site carboxylate mediating the appropriate proton transfer to form a tetrahedral intermediate (Fruton, 1976).

Aspartic protease inhibitors include mainly reversible inhibitors including competitive and transition state inhibitors, activation sequence peptides, pepstatins and pepstatins analogs. One of the pepstatin analogs Pepstatin A is a potent inhibitor of pepsin. Many statin containing peptides have been described as potent inhibitors of renin and HIV proteases (Boger, 1983). Recent investigations have revealed that hydroxymethyl carbonyl isosteres, DMP-850, DMP-851, cyclic ureas, pyran-2-ones, nonapeptide mimetics, JG-365, nelfinavir, indinavir, saquinavir, ritonavir, A-77003, A-80967, KN-1-272 and CGP-61755 are excellent inhibitors of HIV proteases (Kiso et al, 1999; Bing et al, 1999;Sorvillo et al, 1999; Zhang et al, 2000; Sloand et al, 1999; Rodgers et al, 1998; Prasad et al, 1999; Friedler et al, 1999; Patick et al, 1998; Veronese et al, 2000; Ren & Lien, 1998; Hoegl et al, 1999).

9.2.2.3 Cystein proteases

Cystein proteases mainly include Calpains, Cathepsins B, H, I, L, S, M, N T, Interleukin Converting Enzyme, Papain and Pro-line endopeptidases. These proteases contain a catalytic cystein sulfhydryl group and a histidine imidazole group at the active site of the enzyme. The sulfhydryl group of cystein can be alky-lated by a variety of reagents such as N-ethyl maleimide, iodoa-cetate and p-chloro mercuric benzoate. The sulfhydryl group attacks the amide or ester carbonyl group of a substrate to form a thioester covalent intermediate with the release of the first product. Then the acyl group of thioester is transferred to a water molecule to release the carboxylic acid portion of the substrate and regenerates the active enzyme. The attack of water molecule on the thioester in the acylation step is catalysed by the imidazole group of histidine. This imidazole group can act as a proton donor or acceptor in the catalytic process.

Cystein protease inhibitors have been reviewed earlier (Rich, 1986; Dermuth, 1990) and mainly include

Table 9.2 : Protease classification , their active site residues, representative examples and inhibitors.

Proteases	Active Site Residue	Representative Example	Inhibitors
Aspartic	Asp-32, Asp-215	Pepsin, Renin, Cathepsin-D, Cathepsin-E, HIV Protease	Statin Derivatives (Pepstatin, Pepstatin-A, Chymostatin etc.), Competitive and Transition State Analogs, Activation Sequence Peptides, Hydroxy methyl carbonyl isostere, DMP-850, DMP 851, Cyclic ureas, Pyran-2-ones, Nonapeptidic mimetics, JG-365, Nelfinavir, Indinavir, Saquinavir, Ritonavir, A-77003, A-80987, KN-1-272, CGP-61755
Cysteinyl	Cys-25, His-159	Cathepsins-B,H,I,L,M,N,S andT Calpains, Papain, Proline Endopeptidase, Interleukin Converting Enzyme	Peptidyl chloromethyl ketones, Peptidyl diazomethyl ketones, Peptidyl fluromethyl ketones, Peptidyl epoxides, Peptidyl alde- hydes, Peptidyl -α-ketoesters, Peptidyl- O-acyloxy hydroxamates, Peptidyl acyloxy methyl ketones, Nethyl maleimide, Iodo-acetate, Antipain, p-Chloromercuric benzo-ate, Chymostatin, CA-074, CA-074 Me, E-64, E-64-c, E-64-d, α-Aminoaziridine-2,3-di-carboxylic acid, Peptidyl vinyl sulphones, Peptidyl acyloxy vinyl esters, Cystatin-C
Metallo	Zn^{++},His and Glu	Peptidyl dipeptidase-A Endopeptidase 24.11 Endopeptidase 24.15 Aminopeptidase M Carboxypeptidase A Stromolysin, Gelatinase A, Gelatinase B, Collagenase Angiotensin Converting Enzyme Thermolysin	Zinc Specific Chelating Agents (e.g. 1,10-Phenanthroline), N-Carboxy alkyl peptides, Thiol containing peptides, Peptide ketones, Peptide hydroxamic acids, Phosphoinidates, Phosphoramidon, Diprotin, Thiorphan, Actinonin, Captopril, Lisinopril, Enalapril, DFP and CPABetc, Fasidotrilat, Ramiprilat, Kininogen, Amlodipine, Neprilysin, SQ 28603, Aminophosphinic derivatives, Mercaptoacetyl based fused heterocyclic dipeptides
Serinyl	His-57, Asp-102, Ser-195	Thrombin, Trypsin, Chymotrypsin, Elastase (PPE, HNE), Kallikrein, Cathepsin A, G, R, Tissue Plasminogen Activator, Dipeptidyl peptidase III, Dipeptidyl peptidase IV Tripeptidyl peptidase	Reversible Inhibitor (Simple Substrate Analogs, Transition State Analogs), Irreversible Inhibitors (Alkylating agents which react with active site histidine, Acylating agents which react with active site serine), Suicide Inhibitors (Mechanism based inhibitors), BCH-2763, Monocyclic lactams, Boronic acid derivatives, Cyanopyrrolidides, Diaryl phosphonates, Fluostatin, TMC-2A TMC-2B, TMC-2C , TSL-225 , N-Peptidyl-O-hydroxyl amines.

irreversible inhibitors including peptidyl chloromethyl ketones (Drenth et al, Shaw, 1981), peptidyl diazomethyl ketones (Green & Shaw, 1981; Shaw, 1983), peptidyl fluromethyl ketones (Rasnick, 1985; Rauber et al, 1986; Angliker et al, 1987), peptidyl epoxides (Barret et al, 1982), peptidyl acyloxymethyl ketones (Smith et al, 1988) and peptidyl O-acylhydroxamates (Smith et al, 1988b; Bromme et al, 1989). Reversible cystein proteinase inhibitors include peptidyl al-dehydes57, 58 peptidyl-a-ketoesters (Angelastro et al, 1990; Hu & Abeles, 1990), peptidyl vinyl sulphones and peptidyl acyloxy vinyl esters (Billson et al, 1998). Other potent inhibitors include a-amino acid aziridine-2, 3-dicarboxylic acids (Schirmeister, 1999), cystatin C (Nycander et al, 1998) and E-64 derivatives (Billson et al, 1998; Matsumoto et al, 1999).

9.2.2.4 Metallo proteases

Metalloproteases mainly include Peptidyl dipeptase-A, Endo-peptidases, Aminopeptidase-M, Carboxypeptidaes-A, Stromolysine, Gelatinase-A, B, and Collagenase. The native enzyme contains a zinc atom with four ligands (two histidine residues, a glutamic acid residue and a water molecule) arranged in a tetrahedral geometry (Kester & Mathews, 1977). The substrate binds to the active site with scissile carbonyl group coordinating to the native enzyme. The zinc polarises the scissile peptide carbonyl group and an adjacent glutamic acid residue acts as a general base, catalysing the addition of water to the substrate. Usually the primary recognition between the enzyme and the substrate is the interaction of the P_1'side chain with S_1' subsite. However other residues in the substrate can also interact with extended substrate-binding sites of the protease.

General inhibitors of metalloproteases are zinc specific chelating agents such as 1,10-phenanthroline while specific inhibitors are compounds, which lack scissile peptide bond and instead have a functional group, which is capable of chelating with zinc at the active site of the enzyme. These inhibitors include N-carboxyalkyl peptides (Maycock et al, 1981), thiol containing peptides, peptide carboxylic acids (Grey et al, 1981), peptide hydroxamic acids (Delaisse et al, 1985; Odake et al, 1990), pep-tide ketones (Wallace et al, 1986), phosphoimidates (Mookhtiar et al, 1987; Powers & Harper, 1986), fasidotrilat (Marie et al, 1988), ramiprilat (Zhang et al, 1999; Massien et al, 1999; Kitamura et al, 2000), kininogen ramiprilat (Zhang et al, 1999; Massien et al, 1999; Kitamura et al, 2000), amlodipine ramiprilat (Zhang et al, 1999; Massien et al, 1999; Kitamura et al, 2000), neprilysin (Gurbanov et al, 1999), SQ-28607 (Gurbanov et al, 1999), aminophosphinic acid derivatives (Chen et al, 1998; Vincent et al, 1997), mercaptoacetyl based fused heterocyclic dipeptides (Robl et al, 1997) and sulphonimidamides (Cathers & Schloss, 1999). Recent studies on comparative evaluation have shown that ACE inhibitors can effectively protect symptomatic radiation pneumonitis in human subjects (Wang et al , 2000).

9.2.2.5 Serine proteases

Serinyl proteases can be devided mainly into three major groups, Tryptases (Trypsin like), Chymases (Chymotrypsin like) and Elastases (mainly Neutrophil Elastases). Other serine pro-teases include Thrombin, Kallikrein, Cathespin A, G, & R and Tissue Plasminogen Activators, Dipeptidyl peptidase III (Akiyama et al 1998), Dipeptidyl peptidase IV (Wilmouth et al, 1999) and Tripeptidyl peptidase (Tomkinson, 2000; Tomkinson, 1999; Otlewski et al, 1999). Catalytic residues of serine proteases including Ser-195, His-57 and Asp-102 (chymotrypsin numbering system) are referred to as the catalytic triad. The catalytic residues form hydrogen bonds and hydrolyse peptide bond by a specific mechan-ism, in which the reactive γ-OH group of ser-195 attacks the carbonyl group of the scissile amide bond of the substrate to form a tetrahedral intermediate. It is stabilised by hydrogen bonding to the backbone NH-groups of gly-193 and ser-195 of the enzyme, which form the oxy anion hole. Decomposition of tetrahe-dral adducts result in the release of the amino function (kraut, 1977).

Trypsin like enzymes cleave substrates with positively charged residues such as Arg, Lys at the P_1 site due to interac-tion with Asp-189 in the S_1 pocket of this group of enzymes. Chymotrypsin and Elastase like enzymes preferably cleave sub-strates with aromatic or large hydrophobic and small aliphatic residues at P_1 respectively. General serine inhibitors include DipF, DMSF and DC1. They react with the active site ser-95 and form inactivated enzyme derivatives.

Serine protease inhibitors (Powers & Harper, 1986) are mainly reversible and irreversible inhibitors. Major class of compounds include simple substrate analogues, transition state analogues, alkylating agents which react with active site histidine, acylating agents which react with serine forming acyl enzymes and mechanism based suicide inhibitors.

Recent studies have demonstrated that BCH-2763 (Finkle et al, 1998), monocyclic lactams (Wilmouth et al, 1999; kahne et al, 1999), peptidyl boronic acid derivatives (Tomkinson, 2000; Augustyn, 1999; Shimazawa, 1999), cyanopyrrolidides (Tomkinson, 2000; Augustyn, 1999; Shimazawa, 1999), N-phenyl phthalimides (Tomkinson, 2000; Augustyn, 1999; Shimazawa, 1999), TMC-2A/B/C (Yamada et al, 1998), TSL-225 (Yamada et al, 1998), N-peptidyl-O-hydroxyl amines (Lin et al, 1998; Tanaka et al, 1998) and fluostatins A/B (Akiyama et al, 1998) are excellent inhibitors of serine proteases.

9.2.6 Threonine proteases

It is an entirely new sub class of protease. It mainly includes proteasomes which are basically multi catalytic endopeptidases complex (EC 3.4.99.46) of non-lysosomal origin and are located in the nucleus and cytoplasm of all eukaryotic cells (Gardner et al, 2000). These enzymes play key role in the catabolism of proteins within the cellular environment. Proteasomes are the first member of threonine sub class of enzymes. These are large multi sub units proteases with distinct catalytic sites and are known to have an unusual catalytic mechanism in which N-terminal threonine residue of a-subunit is the catalytic nucleophile. The proton donor or acceptor role in the catalysis may be performed either by a conserved lysine residue (Lys-33 in Thermoplasma proteasome) or a water molecule bonded to (a-amino group of the N-terminal threonine. The proteinases can cleave peptide bonds on the carboxyl side of basic, hydrophobic and acidic amino acid residues. These activities have been termed trypsin-like, chymotrypsin-like and peptidylglutamylpeptide hydrolase activities respectively.

Specific inhibitors of proteasomes include lactocystin, peptidyl aldehydes, peptidyl vinyl sulphones, di and tri peptidyl boronic acid derivatives and other transition state analouges (Gardner et al, 2000).

9.2.3 Physicochemical properties of peptides / proteins

Peptides and proteins present a unique problem for their delivery across the intenstinal mucosa. High molecular weight coupled with their unique molecular properties (e.g. hydrogen bonding leading to low thermodynamic activity and thus low escaping tendency from aqueous phase) makes the task more difficult. A peptide or protein may demonstrate aggregation and exhibit con-formational changes (unfolding and denaturation) which in turn may have a direct bearing on the biological response. A typical example is that of Immunoglobulin G, which has two flexible do-mains (Fab 2 regions) and is believed to be responsible for antigen binding and which because of conformational changes leads to immunogenic responses. Self-association involving H-bonds and hydrophobic interactions can also lead to decreased solubility of the peptides and thus reduced availability. Finally, aggregation and polymerisation of the molecule may also lower their potential for oral delivery.

There appears to be a strong interplay of penetration and proteolytic barriers in the abosrption of macromolecules across the gut. Macromolecules, like polyethlene glycols (PEGs) have been utilized to study permeability across the intestine (Donovan et al , 1990). Since these PEGs traverse the intestinal mucosa by a mechanism different from that of proteins, they may not be good markers for assessing membrane permeability of proteins. The transient increase in permeability to macromolecules may be attributed to an interaction of several factors:

➔ Enhanced endocytosis of macromolecules,

➔ Increased membrane fluidity, and

➔ Decreased intestinal proteolysis.

Proteolysis is not a dominant factor limiting macromolecu-lar antibody absorption at a young age (Telemo et al, 1987). The more extensive absorption of immunoglobulin G (IgG) in spite of its molecular size is attributed to the involvement of its specific receptor in its uptake.

9.3 PROTEIN ABSORPTION AND METABOLISM:

9.3.1 PHYSIOLOGICAL IMPORTANCE OF PEPTIDE ABSORPTION:

The intestinal assimilation of dietary protein occurs pri-marily through breakdown followed by dipeptide, tripeptide and amino acid absorption. Serval studies have indicated that the products of protein digestion accumulate in the gut lumen (Hare, 1990; Bond & Beynon, 1987; Adibi, 1971). Further clinical studies on patients with hereditary deficiencies in amino acid transport also tend to support this hypothesis (Adibi & Mercer, 1973).

Patients with Cystinuria and Hartnup Syndrome have a greatly reduced capacity for absorption of basic and neutral amino acids, respectively. The dipeptide absorption however was normal when studied in these patients indicating that protein nutrition can be maintained with an adequate number of amino acid dipeptide carrier systems. Therefore the peptide absorption can become largely responsible for dietary protein assimilation (Asatoor et al, 1971; Asatoor et at, 1970).

Amongst the important parameters that influence the peptide absorption are the maximal number of amino acid residues, the length of the amino acid side chain and the stereoisomerism of the side chain. Di- and triglycines are not hydrolyzed at all in human jejunal fluid, where as tetra to hexaglycines are hydro-lyzed, though there seems to be no statastically significant difference in the hydrolytic rates of the last three peptides. Similarly, di and triglycides are stable in the luminal fluid, whereas their leucine counterparts are hydrolyzed luminally. In humans and monkeys there exists one dipeptide uptake system with an extremely broad specificity (Silk et al, 1975). Intestinal mucosal uptake of oligopeptides is limited to di and tripeptides only. This uptake is mediated by a specific carrier system which shows preference for peptides with bulky side chains and L-stereoisomer amino acid residues at both the N and C terminals.

The peptide that does not possess the molecular features for interaction with the carrier system probably gets absorbed across the intestine by simple diffusion. Those peptides that exceed a molecular weight of 1 KD cannot utilise this aqueous pore pathway and are probably absorbed across the intestinal wall by endocytosis. However, the fate of such peptides, after receptor mediated endocytosis, is post-internalization degradation by the lysosomes (Blay & Brown, 1985).

9.3.2 Peptide metabolism by luminal, enterocytic and lysosomal proteinases

The metabolism of peptide and protein drugs by the intralu-minal enzymes, namely gastric, pancreatic and intestinal proteas-es, followed by enterocytic and hepatic lysosomal enzymes will be addressed in the following segments in an orderly fashion.

9.3.2.1 Gastric enzymes

Digestion is intiated in the stomach upon oral administra-tion of peptides and proteins in the gastric juice by family of aspartic proteinases called pepsins, which are most active at pH 2-3 but become inactive at a pH above 5. However, pepsins rarely degrade peptides or proteins to their constituent amino acids.

Hydrolysis of b-casein by gastric proteases has been studied by comparing the activity of bovine chymosin and pepsin A (Guillou et al, 1991). The cleavage patterns revealed that only six of the peptide bonds were hydrolyzed by chymosin and seven others by pepsin. The results indicated that the preferential splitting occurred at the Leu-X, Ser-X, and Trp-X bonds by chymosin and Leu-X, Met-X and Thr-X by pepsin A. However the above information does not promote an adequate understanding of the way peptides are degraded when all the peptidases act together in concert. To illustrate this point Fig 9.2 shows what can happen during the concerted hydrolysis of bradykinin and substance-P because in the small intestine, the process of concerted hydrolysis is particularly important in cases of peptides containing proline as one of the amino acid residue. Important dietary proteins such as collagen, gliadin and a-casein contain relatively high amounts of this amino acid.

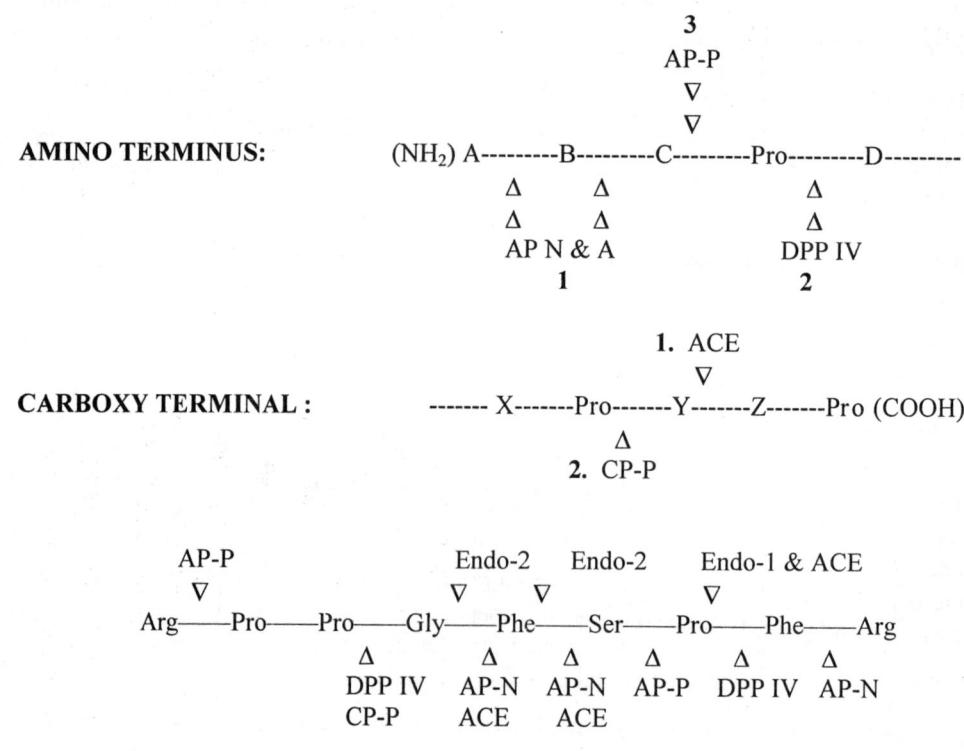

BRADYKININ

SUBSTANCE – P

Fig 9.2 : Typical examples of concerted hydrolysis of peptide bonds by brush border enzymes

∇...	Potential initial sites of hydrolysis	∇...	Secondary sites of hydrolysis
ACE	Angiotensin Converting Enzyme	**AP-N**	Aminopeptidase-N
AP-P	Aminopeptidase-P	**CPP-P**	Carboxypeptidase-P
DPP IV	Dipeptidyl peptidase IV	**Endo-1**	Endopeptidase-24.11
Endo-2	Endopeptidase-24.18		

Pepsin has been known to exist in a variety of molecular forms in vivo, which have been studied in pre-term and post-term infants (Adamson, 1988). The levels of total enzyme activity and gastric acidi-ty were lower in the pre-term infants when compared to post-term infants. Differential development of the enzymes and the isoenzymes may have an important bearing on the subsequent pancreatic hydrolysis and may provide a basis for evaluating the gastric capacity for peptide hydrolysis and nutritional management.

9.3.2.2 Pancreatic enzymes

The pancreas is a storage site for most of the exo and endopeptidases, notably Elastases, Aminopeptidases (Dipeptidyl Aminopeptidase IV), Chymotrypsin, Trypsin and Carboxypeptidase-A. Aminopeptidases, carboxypeptidases and dipeptidases belong to the exopeptidase class because these enzymes hydrolyse peptides sequentially from either the N- or C-terminal. -The combined activity of pancreatic proteases against dietary proteins is quite remarkable. However, their activity towards small peptides is very much restricted and much of the luminal fluid acitivity against small peptides is derived from either the brush border or the cytoplasm of the enterocyte. Functional alterations have also been observed in cases of ure-mia. In case of acute uremia the levels of intestinal peptidases have been found to be elevated, especially aminopeptidases and jejunal peptidases (Magnusson et al, 1991).

Carboxypeptidase A is a fully characterized exopeptidase. The two requirements of the substrates for this enzyme are:

(i) A free terminal carboxyl group and

(ii) A C-terminal amino acid bearing a branched aliphatic or aromatic group.

The three endopeptidases work in concert to cleave almost all of the internal peptide linkages in most peptides and pro-teins. a-Chymotrypsin prefers to cleave peptide bonds near hydro-phobic amino acids (e.g.leucine, methionine, tryptophan and tyrosine). Trypsin on the other hand preferentially cleaves peptide bonds near basic amino acids such as arginine and lysine. Elastase complements the other two proteases by cleaving peptide bonds of amino acids bearing smaller, unbranched, nonaromatic side chains. All three proteases have optimum pH of about 8.

Unlike porcine and rat pancreatic elastase, oxidised alpha-1-proteinase inhibitors can inhibit human pan-creatic elastase. Such an inhibitor has been shown to be effective in diminishing the elastolytic activiy of elastase, thus preventing the degradation of blood vessels during acute hemorrhagic pan-creatitis (Donohue et al, 1988). Pancreatic proteases may also play an important role in the control of brush-border disaccharidase activities (Padres et al, 1992). The possible role of pancreatic proteases in the turnover of intes-tinal brush border proteins has also been suggested (McNamare et al, 1981). The sur-face of intestinal absorptive cells is being constantly renewed, and certain surface enzymes are in part removed from the membrane by the action of pancreatic proteases, denoting again an import-ant physiological role for elastase.

The role of bile in the regulation of intestinal proteolytic activity in rats has been investigated. The diversion of bile and pancreatic juice from the intestine causes an increase in pan-creatic enzyme secretion. Bile duct obstruction results in a three times increase in pancreatic juice chymotrypsin activities but causes a large decrease in intestinal mucosal trypsin, chymo-trypsin, and total proteolytic activities. These results in-dicate that an interruption in bile flow causes an accelerated rate of degradation of pancreatic proteolytic enzymes. However, it also induces pancreatic proteolytic secretion in response to decreased intestinal proteolytic activity (Alpers nad Tedesco, 1975). Chronic diversion of bile pancreatic juice exerts hypergrowth of pancreas and hyperse-cretion of proteases in the fasting state. However, it also imparts less sensitivity of pancreatic enzyme secretion to die-tary feeding 9 Green and Nasset, 1977).

The role of cholecystokinin (CCK) has been implicated in the putative feedback mechanism between intraduodenal pancreatic proteases and pancreatic enzyme secretion. Rosewicz et al (Rosewicz et al, 1990) studied the effects of CCK on gene expression of endocrine pan-creatic hormones. CCK at physiological postprandial plasma con-centrations stimulates pancreatic protease gene expression but has no effect on gene expression of endocrine pancreatic hor-mones. The effects of pH and fasting on the pancreatic serine protease levels and on the extent of oral absorption in dogs and humans have been examined (Sinko,1992). Chymotrypsin levels in fasted dogs are ten times higher than in humans. Since pharmacokinetic stud-ies and preclinical screening of peptidic candidates in animals and humans are routinely performed during the fasted state, this finding has significance in the correlation of bioavailability results between dogs and humans (Sinko, 1992).

The pancreatic proteases have been extensively investigated due to the fact that they tend to inactivate one of the most widely studied model peptdie drugs, insulin. Relevant literature in this area has been summarized in which some recent findings from various groups have been incorporated.

The proper management of Type I diabetes (and some Type II) requires daily subcutaneous insulin injections. The inconvenience and poor patient acceptance have prompted extensive investigation of alternative and nonparenteral insulin delivery pathways, such as rectal, enteral, nasal, and even transdermal routes of administration. Although other delivery modes may improve diabetic therapy, the oral route is still regarded as the most acceptable one. For this reason, intense investigations of oral insulin delivery have been persued such as the incorporatiion of enhancers, use of enteric coating, targeting insulin release to certain regions of the intestine, and the use of protease inhibitors.

To design a better and an effective oral delivery system for insulin, several factors limiting the intestinal insulin uptake need to be fully explored and variables defined. Such variables include the intrinsic permeability difference along the intestinal lumen, the enzymatic barrier difference in the GI tract, and the effects of additives on intestinal permeability and insulin transport characteristics. Early in vitro everted gut sac experiments using different segments of the rat intestine revealed that a signifi-cant permeability difference exists for insulin (Schilling and Mitra, 1990). The duodenum showed little or no absorption, while the jejunum and the ileum absorbed low but significantly greater amounts of insulin. No significant insulin metabolism was observed during flux measure-ments, but in tissue homogenates significant metabolism was observed. Insulin uptake across the intestinal mucosa appears to be by passive transport only. This evidence tends to suggest that the oral delivery of insulin may be viable by selective release of insulin in the mid-jejunum to ileum segments, thereby exposing insulin to the optimal region of absorption. In situ closed intestinal loop studies also indicated bioavailability differences for insulin solution delivered to different regions of the rat intestine (Schilling and Mitra, 1992). With addition of sodium glycocholate and linoleic acid, absorption in the duodenum and medial and distal jejunum was increased eight, three and two fold respectively.

The enzymatic inactivation of insulin by luminal and brush border enzymes is well known. Schilling and Mitra (Schilling and Mitra, 1991) conducted in vitro degradation studies of insulin by trypsin and a-chymotrypsin and suggested that the apparent Km values (Michaelis constant) for the two enzymes were nearly the same, whereas the apparent V_{max} (limiting velocity) of chymotrysin was found to be 8.6 times higher than trypsin. Their results indicate that α-chymotrypsin possesses much stronger proteolytic activity against insulin than trypsin. Initially, a-chymotrypsin attacks insulin at the carboxyl side of B_{26}-Tyr and A19 Tyr residue, and then at the B16 Tyr, B_{25}-Phe, and A14-Tyr sites. The extensive deactivation of insulin by α-chymo-tropsin makes any structural modification of insulin for improved stability in the intestinal tract unattractive.

Since insulin molecules aggregate in aqueous solution, forming dimers, hexamers and large aggregates, the influence of insulin dissociation on enzymatic cleavage has been a matter of intense study. Liu et al (Liu et al,1991) reported that the rate constant for a-chymotrypsin mediated insulin degradation was accelerated in the presence of ethylenediamine tetracetic acid disodium salt (EDTA), a zinc che-lating agent. Complexation of zinc by EDTA essentially disso-ciates insulin hexamers to dimers in a concentration dependent manner thereby exposing more insulin cleaving sites to the enzyme. A study using a naturally occuring bile salt, sodium gly-cocholate, indicates that this bile salt is also capable of completely dissociating insulin oligomers (Li et al, 1992). Interestingly enough, this adjuvant however, does not appear to inhibit the activity of chymotrypsin to any sginficant extent. An inhibiting effect of bile salts on nasal aminopeptidases has been reported in the literature. Recently, (Shao et al, 1993) extended this study further to evaluate the differential effects of anionic, cationic, and nonionic surfactants on the a-chymotryptic degradation and enteral absorption of insulin oligomers. The re-sults suggest that these surfactants exert their action on insu-lin dissociation and enzymatic degradation in a quite different manner. Anionic surfactants such as sodium lauryl sulfate effi-ciently dissociates insulin oligomers and denatures a-chymotryp-sin at concentrations above its critical micellar concentration. Cationic surfactants like hexadecyltrimethylammonium bromide (CTAB) interacts with negatively charged insulin molecules at lower CTAB concentration, while completely solubilizing insulin at higher concentrations. CTAB solubilization of insulin tends to retard its a- chymotrypsin degradation probably by repelling the positively charged enzyme molecules away from substrate. Nonionic surfactants such as Tween 80 failed to exert any effect on insulin degradation. Anionic surfactants may serve as better insulin absorption enhancers than other types of surfactants due to their ability to dissociate insulin oligomers thus producing smaller diffusing species, and also due to their ability to retard the presystemic degradation of insulin by luminal proteases.

9.3.2.3 Intestinal proteases

Most of the intestinal mucosal proteases are of the brush border variety. When considering absorption from the intestine, it must be empahsized that it is the regional protease distribution that causes wide variability in peptide absorption. In addition to the anatomical differences that exist in the various segments there is also the pH differential. It has also been shown that uremia and similar disorders lead to an increase in activities of intestinal proteases, mainly aminopeptidases. A significant increase in aminopeptidase N activity and a positive correlation between aminopeptidase N activity and serum urea has been observed in uremic rats. However, the disaccharidase activity remains unaltered. These observations are also compat-ible with different regulation mechanism for the brush border peptidases and disaccharidases.

9.3.3   Other metabolic factors

9.3.3.1 Peptide hydrolases along small intestinal mucosa

The distribution of peptide hydrolase activity between brush border membrane and cytosol varies considerably with species. Peptide hydrolases show dual location in the cells along the intestinal tract, i.e. brush border membrane and cytosol, and it is often difficult to evaluate the exact proportion of activity in each location. The intestinal mucosa is the most likely source of luminal oligopeptide hydrolase activity. It is well known that the

Table 9.3 : Protease classification, their active site residues, repersentative examples and inhibitors

Peptide	Brush Border %	Cytosol %
Tetra peptides: Phe-Gly-Gly-Phe	95	5
Tri peptides : Tyr-Tyr-Tyr	87	13
Leu-Leu-Leu	81	19
Tyr-Gly-Gly	64	36
Phe-Gly-Gly	50	50
Leu-Gly-Gly	33	67
Di peptides : Tyr-Gly	55	45
Phe-Gly	42	58
Tyr-Tyr	36	64
Leu-Leu	25	75
Leu-Gly	14	86

enzymes associated with the cytosol and brush border fractions of the intestinal mucosa are capable of hydro-lysing oligopeptides (Table 9.3) (Leonard et al, 1976; Fujita et al, 1972; Peters, 1973; Silk et al, 1975; Kim et al, 1972). The peptide hydrolases bound to the intestinal brush borders are distinct from those in the cytosol (Kim et al, 1974). It has also been established that the jejunal luminal peptide hydrolase activity originates from the cytosol fraction of the mucosal cells (Heizer et al, 1972; Parson, 1972). A major biological role for intestinal cytosolic peptide hydrolases may be the catabolism of intracellular proteins (Nicholson and Peters,1978). Therefore, the quantitative significance of luminal peptidases, in the digestion of exogenous proteins, must be determined by comparing luminal and total cellular enzymic activity.

9.3.3.2 Distribution of peptide hydrolases

Studies on the subcellular distribution of peptide hydrola-ses have shown peptidase activities in both the soluble and brush border fractions of the small intestinal mucosa (Silk et al, 1975), the former consitituting about 85% and the latter 10-15% of the total activ-ity. The subcellular distribution studies of peptidase activities in the normal human jejunum against glycine and leucine homopeptides have indicated variability in the activities of these enzymes along the intestinal mucosa (Parson, 1972). Leucine and glycine aminopeptidases exhibit variation in the cytosolic distribution and the bioactivity also varies markedly with the chain length of the substrate.

Zymogram studies of peptide hydrolases of cytosolic frac-tions have yielded multiple bands indicating multiple zones of enzymic activity. Such zymogram patterns of the brush border membrane fractions however are quite different from those of the soluble fraction indicating that the enzymes from the two sources may be different (Silk et al, 1975).

Attempts have been made to determine, indirectly, the func-tional localization of peptidase activity in intact intestinal mucosa. The results and the interpretation of those studies have often been conflicting (Nicholson and Peters, 1978; Newy and Smith, 1960; Peters et al, 1969). In vitro studies where the rate of uptake of peptides and their constituent amino acids on intestinal segments have been compared, have suggested that hydrolysis precedes transport (Matthews et al, 1969; Fern et al, 1969). The relevance of these studies to the in vivo situation is not clear as the peptidases are rapidly released from the mucosa into the incubation medium (Kushak and Ugollev, 1966).

The regional, cellular and subcellular distribution patterns of the aminopeptidases have also been found to be variable (Table 9.4). The cytosolic fraction of the intestinal enterocyte contains aminopeptidases, which are distinct from the membrane bound varieties (Josefsson and Sjostrom, 1966). Moreover, cytosolic aminopeptidases appear to be closely related to the brush border membrane peptidases, which tend to point towards the involvement of these enzymes in the assembly of the final surface membrane amino peptidases (Miura et al, 1983).

Table 9.4 Dipeptdase activity in homogenates of biopsied specimens from various regions of human gastro intestinal tract

Region	Infant*	Adult
Stomach	13.6 ± 8.3	57.1 ± 36.0
Proximal duodenum	11.5 ± 7.4	39.8 ± 18.7
Jejunum	26.3 ± 5.4	111.4 ± 13.7
Ileum	41.8 ± 9.2	211.6 ± 11.6
Colon	9.5 ± 3.7	44.5 ± 10.6

*1 Week old child

9.3.3.3 Lysosomal proteolytic pathways

Lysosomes are responsible for degrading exogenous and endog-enous proteins. Exogenous proteins enter the cells by endocyto-sis and are degraded within endosomes or rerouted to the lysosome for degradation (Maze and Gray, 1980; Das and Radhakrishnan, 1975). This process is referred to as heteropha-gy. Little doubt exists as to the role played by lysosomes in the breakdown of intracellular proteins in certain situations (nutritional depravation and pathological states). However, aside from cathepsins, little is known about other lysosomal proteases and their mecahnism (Diment et al, 1988; Glaumann and Ballard, 1986; Mayer and Doherty, 1986). Degradation of endogenous proteins by lysosomal pathways is referred to as autophagy and these proteins enter the lysosomes by four distinct processes: macroautophagy, microautophagy, crinophagy and transport mediated by the 73kDa heat-shock cognate protein (hsc 73).

Macroautophagy involves sequesteraion of a portion of cytoplasm by a preexisting intracellular membrane to form an autopha-gic vacuole. Nascent autophagic vacuoles mature in a stepwise manner, first acquiring lysosomal membranes and becoming acidi-fied, followed by acquisition by lysosomal hydrolases and degra-dation of the vacuoular contents. Macroautophagy appears to modulate overall intracellular protein levels rather than to specifically regulate the levels of certain proteins, as seen in states of amino acid depravation. Microautophagy is a pathway for basal protein degradation defined biochemically under condi-tions where macroautophagy is suppressed. Microautophagic strucutre arise during in vitro incubation of lysosomes isolated from livers of starved rats. Crinophagy is the fusion of secretory granules with lysosomes, resulting in digestion of the granule contents. Crinophagy can be induced in the liver by drugs that block secretion, and under normal conditions occurs mainly in the endocrine glands. Crinophagy appears to be an efficient mechanism for preventing an overabudance of intracellular hormone when its extracellular secretion is low.

Proteins sequestered by a non selective bulk process within the lysosomes turn over with an apparent half -life of about 8 minutes and this rapid lysosomal proteolysis is initiated by endopeptidases, in particular by the cathepsins D and L. While there is still inadequate information about catheptic enzymes it appears that cathepsins D, E and L are the major endopeptidases, especially in the reticuloendothelial system (RES). Cathepsins, which show mainly exopeptidase activity include cathepsin A, B, C and H and they may in turn attack the carboxy or amino terminus of proteins. Cathepsin H is most probably the only lysosomal amino-peptidase in a number of cell types (Mortimore and Poso, 1984). Cathepsin B has been reported to have some endopeptidase activity in that it activates trypsinogen to trypsin under acid pH (Bohley and Seglen, 1992).

Lipoproteins and cholesterol levels, in the circulating blood, play an important role in heart disorders. High levels of high density lipoproteins (HDL) is associated with decreased risk of heart disease whereas increased levels of low density liporoteins (LDL) aid in atherosclerosis. Native LDLs are degraded by the proteases of the lysosomal extract but they are not sensitive to cathepsin D. This degradation reaction was most rapid at pH 4 and 4.5 (Greenbaum et al, 1959). Administration of compounds like thyroxine and chloroquine tend to increase proteolysis. Chloroquine increased the number of autophagic vacuoles in the rat pancreas, leading to enhanced proteolytic lysosomal enzyme activities, especially acid phosphatase and cathepsin B activi-ties (Skrzydlewski and worowsky, 1978).

The degradation of metallothionein has been observed to be greater in the rat liver homogenates than in cytosol and predomi-nates under acidic pH. The role of lysosomal proteases in degra-dation of metallothionein is now well established (Yucel et al, 1991). This degradation could be inhibited by leupeptin, a known blocker of the lysosomal proteases, cathepsin B and L. However, another independent study revealed that injections of leupeptin not only increased the activity of cathepsin A and D but also produced moderate increases in the activities of cathepsins B and L (Choudhuri et al, 1992). The results, therefore, suggest that the lysosomal proteinase may be involved in the activation of some aldolases. Furthermore, the role of lysosomal proteinases in the modification of other cyto-solic enzymes has also been revealed.

A new cathepsin has been isolated from rat liver and has been shown to be a lysosomal protease. This particular cathepsin inactivates glucose-6-phosphate dehydrogenase and also differs from cathepsin B in that it scarcely hydrolyses N-substituted derivatives of arginine (Katunuma et al, 1982).

Usually, all cathepsins are stable and are optimally active under acidic pH conditions. It has been a long held belief that cathepsins are virtually inactive under neutral and basic pH conditions. Nevertheless cathepsin E has a proteolytic activity and also has cleavage specificity towards the B chain of oxidized insulin at physiological pH (Towatari et al, 1978). In an attempt to correlate alcohol consumption to the activity of cathepsins and thus to hepatic lysosomal protease activity, metabolism experiments conducted after acute ehtanol administration revealed that alterations in hepatic protein catabolism following ethanol administration was not related to the changes in the activities of cathepsins contradicting prevous report(Athauda et al, 1991).

Thus, the initial events in the breakdown of proteins may occur outside the lysosome, but the final stages are inherently intralysosomal. Despite the fact that the route taken by a given protein may be different and vary with the hormonal status, environmental conditions and nutritional status, the underlying pathway for final degradation is purely lysosomal.

9.3.3.4 Cytosolic proteolytic pathways

Proteolytic pathways in cells are highly regulated. In contrast to the lysosomal enzymes, any protease activity free in the normal cytosol must be under rigid control. Since the pro-tein hydrolysis is a thermodynamically favoured reaction, the enzymes participating in such cytosolic degradation must be more than simple catalysts for the hydrolytic process. Changing the susceptibility of individual substrates may block protein degradation but the cells are able to modulate the activity of other pathways, such as the ubiquitin dependent pathway or the calcium dependent pathway.

Ubiquitin, a highly conserved 76-amino-acid polypeptide serves as a marker for proteins to be attacked. It is found free or covalently conjugated to a variety of protein targets within all eukaryotic cells (Hershko, 1988;Rechsteiner, 1988). Ubiquitin is covalently attached to certain proteins in a stable form that may alter protein's con-formation or aid in its assembly into macromolecular struc-tures (Rechsteiner, 1988). Covalent links between substrate proteins and ubiquitin are thought to commit proteins to degradation. Ubquitin-mediated protein degradation involves a series of intermediary reactions starting with an ATP-requiring ubiquitin activation step. The ubiquitin moieties are attached to ε-amino groups of the lysine residues on the fated protein. Proteins so marked are then, digested by specific cytosolic enzymes. Remarkably ATP is needed for both the protein activation and the protein cleavage steps.

Molecular determinants within proteins determine their susceptibility to ubiquitin conjugation (Ciechanover and Schwartz 1989). Hershko and Ciechano-ver (1982) have proposed that ubiquitin binding acts as a signal for attack by proteinases specific for ubiquitin-protein conjugates. This regulation is interesting at a basic biochemical level. Protein and peptide pharmaceuticals can be engineered so that they are not susceptible to degradation during synthesis. In addition, they can be modified to be substrates for a specific proteolytic pathway or not to be substrates if they naturally are, so as to control their half-lives in the cell. Caution needs to be excercised in the fabrication of peptide and protein delivery systems so as not to potentially "mark" the protein pharmaceutical for rapid hydrolytic degradation.

In addition, two calcium-dependent neutral proteases have been isolated from eukaryotic cells(Murachi et al., 1989; Mellgren et al., 1989). Calpain I reqires micromolar concentration of calcium while calpain II requires millimolar concentrations of calcium. Calpains degrade a limited number of proteins in vitro(Wang et al (1989), mainly cytoskeletal or membrane proteins. The degree to which calpains contribute to overall proteolysis is not yet clear.

9.3.3.5 First pass metabolism

The liver is a potential site for removal of macromolecules like peptides and proteins following oral delivery. Being well perfused and composed of several cell types, including hepato-cytes, Kuppfer and endothelial cells, the liver is an important organ for protein metabolism. These cell types have receptors for different proteins, which enable them to recognize and internalize proteins and peptide drugs.

The transendothelial passage of proteins and peptide drugs depends upon the physicochemical properties of the drug and also the capillaries. Uptake of peptides and proteins from plasma by hepatocytes occurs by two distinct, yet not entirely separable processes: receptor-mediated endocytosis and non-selective pino-cytosis.

In receptor-mediated endocytosis plasma derived proteins become internalized post-binding by hepatocyte receptor proteins located within the plasma membrane. Receptor mediated endocytosis is operative in hepatocytes for several proteins, including insulin, glucagon, growth hormone, and intestinal and pancreatic peptides, and metallo and hemoproteins (Jones et al., 1982).

Receptor-mediated endocytosis starts with plasma-derived proteins becoming internalized following specific recognition and binding by hepatocyte receptor proteins. These receptors are typically integral membrane glycoproteins(Jones et al, 1979). The receptors can be of "functional" and clearance types, and therefore clearance of a protein can be accentuated if a protein binds to both. The liver contains both these receptors and so there is a fast turnover of proteins(Sugiyama and Hanano, 1989). In the indirect shuttle pathway of polypeptide internalization by hepatocytes, the ligand-receptors complexes proceed through coated vesicles to the endocytic compartment(Stahl and Scwartz, 1986). This process regulates the receptors-ligand binding affinity and also enables the receptor protein to recycle efficiently. The receptor-mediated endocytosis process is both of high capacity because of receptor recycling and of a high affini-ty due to the highly specific recognition.

Proteins and peptide drugs may gain access to the cytoplasm of hepatocytes by another process known as nonselective pinocyto-sis (Kaplan,1981). The amount of proteins internalised by this process is only a small fraction of the total proteins. Albumin, some pancreatic proteins as well as glycoproteins are examples of proteins removed from plasma by hepatocytes by a non-receptor-mediated process.

It is, therefore, necessary to determine the peripheral sites of degradation and the cellular mechanism involved in regulating catabolism or processing of an administered protein since they may contribute to the design of molecules possessing desirable kinetic and/or pharmacological properties.

9.4   METABOLISM OF SELECTED PEPTIDE DRUGS:

9.4.1 Insulin

Insulin one of the most widely studied peptide drugs is variably absorbed in diabetics. Degradation of insulin occurs following uptake into cells by receptor mediated endocytosis. Two principal enzymes have been implicated in the degradation of insulin, namely, glutathione insulin transhydrogenase and insulin-degrading enzyme. Though the relative roles of these two enzymes is still controversial, it is generally accepted that the former enzyme cleaves insulin at the disulfide bridges(Varandani, 1972), whereas the later breaks it at the Tyr16-Leu17 bond in the B chain of insulin (Duckworth et al 1979). Another widely held belief is that the insulin degrading enzyme initiates the degradation resulting in three peptide chains held together by disufide bonds. This molecule is further degraded by non-specific proteases(Varandani et al, 1972). There is an abundance of reports on the binding and subsequent degradation of insulin by skeletal muscle preparation and liver homogenates. All of these studies point towards mainly to these two enzyme systems.

9.4.2 Substance P

This 11 amino acid peptide is found mainly in the central nervous system (CNS) as well as in the GI tract. The action of this peptide is terminated by proteases at the end of a synapse, though the enzymes have not been identified. It has been proposed that membrane bound proteases are involved in the degradation, mainly metallo endopeptidases(Endo et al., 1985). The role of angiotensin converting enzyme has been implicated, though only in the CNS(Hooper and Turner., 1987). This particular enzyme also cleaves the Phe8-Gly9 bond of amidated substance P releasing the C-terminal tripeptide, followed by removal of the successive dipeptides.

9.4.3 Thyrotropin releasing hormone (TRH)

This hypothalamic regulatory hormone which stimulates release of thyrotropin, prolactin, and growth hormone from the pituitary, has a pyroglutamyl residue at its amino terminus and an ami-dated carboxyl terminus, and is thus stable towards classical exopeptidases. However, the hormone is potentially susceptible to attack by aminopeptidases, primarily, pyroglutamyl aminopepti-dase (Griffiths and Kelly, 1979; Hersh and McKelvy,1979;Prasad and Peterkosfky, 1976; Krider et al, 1981;Griffiths et al, 1980). This enzyme has been found in the rat colon and other intestinal tissues. Also further degradation of the pep-tide occurs by deamidation of the terminal amide and this reaction is assisted by prolyl endopeptidase, an enzyme found exten-sively in the liver, pancreas, ileum, lung and skeletal muscle of rats. Studies with some analogs of TRH have shown that they are resistant to degradation by gastrointestinal and liver enzymes (Morier et al, 1981).

9.4.4 Vasopressin

Arginine vasopressin (AVP) is a neurohypophysial nonapeptide hormone with antidiuretic effect on the kidney (Gibbs, 1986). Vasopressin is stable in normal plasma in vitro though, it has been shown to be extensively degraded in the proximal renal tubule (Carone et al, 1974). In vivo there is rapid endocytotic uptake of the intact peptide followed by lysosomal degradation in the proximal tubule. Several analogs with significant antidiuretic activity have been synthesized and tested (Vavra et al,1974 ;Sawyer et al, 1974; Rado et al, 1976). The enhanced activity of these analogs upon oral administration has been attributed to their resistance to proteolytic degradation before and after absorption and improved membrane permeation.

9.5 APPROACHES TO CIRCUMVENTING THE METABOLIC BARRIER

In GI tract, enzymatic barrier efficiently digests proteins to a mixture of amino acids and small quantities of peptides consisting of 2-6 amino acid residues. The poor oral availability of peptides and proteins has prompted the examina-tion of various other non-invasive pathways, including the nasal (Mosses et al, 1983; Nagai et al,1984), pulmonary (Yoshida et al,1979), rectal (Ichikawa et al,1980; Nishita et al,1985), ocular (Stratford et al 1988; Yamamoto et al, 1989), buccal (Ishida et al,1983), and vaginal routes (Okada et al, 1983), as alternatives sites for administering peptide and protein drugs. However even with these routes the enzymatic barrier is substantial.

The approaches to circumventing the protease action should be based entirely upon the principal site of degradation of the peptide drug: intracellular, luminal, or the brush border. The approaches may include:

1. Chemical modification of the peptide or protein sturucture

2. Co-administration of protease inhibi-tors, and surfactants

3. Formulation approaches to minimize the contact of the peptide or protein with proteases or selection of delivery site with less enzyme distribution.

9.5.1 Chemical modifications of peptide/protein drug

Proteins are quite labile due to the susceptibility of the peptide backbone to proteolytic degradation, as well as their large molecular size and complex secondary, tertiary, and sometimes even quaternary structures. Prodrugs of peptides have been prepared and tested in vitro. Approaches to reducing proteolysis have included amongst others chemical modification of the peptide backbone, and N- and C-terminal modification or blocking (Samamen, 1985). Bioreversible N-hydroxyalkylation of the peptide bond to bring about protection against carboxypeptidases or other proteolytic enzymes has been one of these approaches. Additional structural modifications include subsititution of nondisulfide-bonded cysteine residues with nonsulfur containing amino acids (Mark et al, 1986) and chemical replacement of labile methionine residues with nonoxidizable analogs such as norleucine.

A classical approach to circumventing enzymatic degradation and increasing plasma half life of peptides has been the covalent attachment of polyethylene glycol (PEG) to amino groups (Chen et al, 1982; Abuchowsky et al, 1977; Davis et al, 1981). PEG modification of other nonenzyme proteins have also been reported (Kater et al, 1987; Ajisaka, 1980). Some of the other modifications utilised to reduce peptide degradation include carbonyl reduction, D-amino acid substitution, olefin substitution, N-terminal to C-terminal cyclisation, dehydro amino acid substitution, retro-inversion modification, and thiomethylene modification amongst other strategies (Davis et al, 1981). Some of the other modifications employed to minimise proteolytic degradation of peptides mainly include the following strategies:

➔ Olefinic substitution, for example: substitution or reduction of amide bond. For the angiotensin converting enzyme inhibitor benzoyl-Phe-Gly-Pro and for the human immunodeficiency virus protease inhibitors, replacement of CONH- group by -COCH$_2$- enhanced the inhibitor activity (Wyvratt, 1985).

➔ Analogoues with C- and N-termini, for example: acylation or alkylation of N-terminus or alteration of the C-terminus by reduction or amide formation (Roemer and Pless, 1979).

➔ Introducing conformation constraints by steric or stereochemical means, for example: by using unnatural or D-amino acids or N-methyl amino acids (Roemer and Pless, 1979; Humphrey and Ringrose,1986).

➔ Co-valent constraints, i.e. the use of cyclic amino acids, bridged dipeptides, cyclic peptides, or N- to C-terminal cyclisation (Wyvratt, 1985; Brewster and Waltham,1981).

➔ Dehydro amino acid substitution(Wyvratt, 1985).

➔ Retro-inversion modification, i.e. the direction of the peptide backbone is reversed and the chirality of each amino acid is inverted. This approach is limited if the amide linkages are important in the interaction with a target receptor (Brewster and Waltham,1981).

➔ Thiomethylene modification (Brewster and Waltham,1981).

Modifying the amino acid composition to afford stability against proteases has led to enhanced peptide absorption as shown in the case of Tyr-D-Ala-Gly-L-Phe-D-Leu (DADLE), a leucine enkephalin analog and metenkephamid (Su et al,1985). Certain nonapeptides e.g. 1-deamino-8-D-arginine vasopressin and 1-deamino-2-tyrosin (O-ethyl)-oxytocin) were shown to be orally effective in con-scious dogs and human volunteers, probably because of higher permeability and thus reduced contact time with proteases Vilhardt and Bie, 1983). The development of S-GnRH-A, a nonapeptide with D-Arg6 has exhibited higher order of fish spawning activity than parent salmon gonadotrophin releasing hormone (Kundu and Jain, 1996). Another significant example is the development of GHRP-6, a growth promoting hexapeptide which has shown remarkably better growth promoting response and wound healing potential than the parent molecule (Kundu and jain, 1996; Kundu et al, 1988). Table 9.5 gives the structure and clinical utility of some stable and biologically active peptide analogs from natural peptide leads.

Table 9.5 : Some stable peptide analouges of high medicinal value designed from natural peptide leads

Peptide	Primary Structure	Known Therapeutic Application
Melanotan	Ac-Ser-Tyr-Ser-**Nle**-Glu-His-D-Phe-Arg-Trp-Gly-Lys-Pro-Val-NH₂	Potential use as a stimulant of skin pigmentation
Ebiratide	**Met(O₂)**-Glu-His-Phe-D-Lys-Trp-NH-(CH₂)₄-NH₂	Treatment of CNS Disorders
Metkephamide	Tyr-D-Ala-Gly-Phe-MeMet-NH₂	Potential Analgesic
Busereline	Glu-His-Trp-Ser-Tyr-D-Ser-(ᵗBu)-Leu-Arg-Pro-NH-Et	Treatment Prostate Cancer and Endometriosis
GHRP-6	His-D-Trp-Ala-Trp-D-Phe-Lys-NH₂	Growth Hormone secretagogue
HOE-140	D-Arg- Lys-Arg-**Hyp-Thi**-Ser-D-Tic-**Oic**-Arg	Treatment of Pain, Inflammation, Rhinitis and Asthma
MDL-28050	**Suc**-Tyr-Glu-Pro-Pro-Glu-Glu-Tyr-Ala-**Cha**-Gln	Anticoagulant : Thrombin Antagonist
L-365209	Cyclo(Pro-D-Phe-Ile-D-**Dhp-Dhp**-D-MePhe)	Uterine relaxant; Oxytocin Antagonist
RX-77368	Glu-His-**Dmp**-NH₂	Potential use for CNS disorders
A-75998	Ac-D-**Nal**-D-**Phe(p-Cl)**-D-Pal-Ser-MeTyr-D-Lys-(**Nic**)-Leu-Lys-(Isp)-Pro-D-Ala-NH₂	Treatment of Prostate Cancer and Endometriosis Treatment of Acromegaly and Carcinoid Syndrome
Sandostatin	Phe-Cys-Phe-D-Trp-Lys-Thr-Cys-**Thr-ol**	Treatment of Diabetes insipidus Artificial Sweetener, Glucose mimetic
Desmopressin Aspartane	**Mpa**-Tyr-Phe-Cln-Asn-Cys-Pro-D-Arg-Gly-NH₂ Asp-Phe-OMe	

[**Nle**: norleucine]; [**Met(O₂)**: methionine sulphone]; [**Hyp**: 4-hydroxy proline]; [**Thi**: thienylalanine]; [**Oic**: octahydroindole-2-carboxylic acid]; [**Suc**: succinyl]; [**Cha**: cyclohexyl alanine]; [**Dhp**: dehydropiperazyl]; [**Dmp**: β,β-dimethylpro]; [**Nal**: 3-(2-naphthyl)Ala]; [**Phe(p-Cl)**: p-Chloro-Phe]; [**Pal**: (3-pyridyl)-Ala]; [**Nic**: nicotinyl [**Isp**: isopropyl]; [**Thr-ol**: threoninol]; [**Mpa**: 3-mercaptopropionic acid] ; **Source**: Collected from Fauchere & Thurieau, 1986; Ward, 1991 Fauchere, 1986; Eberley, 1991; Hider & Baelow, 1991; Sawyer et al, 1994; Olson et al, 1993; Wiley & Rich, 1993.

9.5.2   Co-administration of protease inhibitors

A major step towards enhanced oral peptide and protein delivery can be achieved by circumventing the enzymatic barriers that limit the amount of these compounds from reaching the target site. Proteases are essentially hydrolases, which rarely show absolute specificity in their action. The in vivo kinetics and specificity of proteases are likely to be different from those in vitro (Hanley, 1983). The aspartic proteases, i.e., renin, cathepsin D and pepsin are all restricted in their action either by pH or intolerance to the medium which sometimes serve in a protective manner. Inactivation of the protease may also occur in the neutral-alkaline environment of the duodenum in GI tract as seen in the denaturation of pepsin. Peptidases, in vivo may be kept in check by excess of proteinase inhibitors such as α-1-antitrypsin, α-2-antiplasmin, and α-2-macroglobulin (Travis and Savesen, 1983). Relative distribu-tion, and hence the proteinase/inhibitor concentration ratio, may vary considerably in body fluids, particularly in the splenic microenvironment where the concentration of macrophages is high. Thus, the results from an in vitro model to assess the specificity of preoteases need to be analysed with caution. Such an in vitro method does not allow direct in vivo extrapolation since the peptides and proteins may be degraded by peptidases acting together in concert. One also needs to excercise caution in using appropriate experimental conditions while performing in vitro studies so as not to denature, inactivate, or potentiate the proteases.

Various protease inhibitors have been examined with respect to their ability to suppress proteolytic activity. This approach has met with mixed results. Positive results have been observed in the oral absorption of tetragastrin (Jennewein et al,1974), insulin (Kidron et al, 1982), arginine, vasopressin (Saffran et al, 1988) and a nonapeptide renin inhibitor (Takaori et al, 1986). The inhibi-tors used include bacitracin (a non-specific protease inhibitor), phosphoramidon (a metalloprotease inhibitor), p-hydroxy-mercuribenzoate (a cysteine protease inhibitor), aprotinin, diisopropyl flurophosphate (serine proteinase inhibitors), bestatin, puromycin, and α-aminobornic acid derivatives (aminopeptidase inhibitors). Sodium glycocholate, a penetration enhancer, has been shown to inhibit leucine aminopeptidase activity and protect insulin from proteolysis (Hirari et al, 1981). Calcitonin absorption through small and large intestine has been remarkably increased by use of protease inhibitors in the formulation (Tozaki et al, 1998). Also ligating the pancreatic duct to exclude the pancreatic juices from the small intestine can cause a 12-fold increase in absorpition of pentagastrin from the duodenum of rats (Jennewein et al, 1974).

9.5.3 Formulation approach

A third strategy to circumvent the enzymatic barrier is the formulation approach and studies have been carried out using insulin as a model peptide. The delivery systems have been designed to (a) protect insulin from coming in contact with proteases, primarily in the lumen, and (b) release the protein only upon reaching a favourable area for absorption.

Several formulations tested include emulsions(Kidron et al, 1982; Saffran et al, 1988), liposomes (Takaori et al, 1986 ; Hirari et al, 1981), nanoparticles (Oppenheim et al, 1982), and soft gelatin coated cap-sules (Touitou and Rubinstein, 1986). An azo polymer, which is stable along the GI tract but decomposes at the ileocecal junction to release insulin, has been tried to deliver insulin upon oral administration (Saffran et al, 1986). Novel bioadhesive drug carrier matrix systems (Bernkop-Schnurch and Pasta; 1998) and chitosan-EDTA-protease inhibitor conjugates (Bernkop-Schnurch and Scerbe-Saiko; 1998) have also been used to deliver many other biologically active peptide and protein molecules through oral route by shielding them from enzymatic attack.

9.6 CONCLUDING REMARKS

Systemic avaiibility of many peptide and proteins following oral administration has been extremely low (0.1-2%) rendering this mode of drug administration unsuitable for such macromolec-ules. As described here, several luminal, pancreatic, cytosolic and lysosomal proteases can severely limit the systemic absorption of these compounds. This enzymatic barrier sets an upper limit to the percent of dose of a peptide or protein drug that can be orally absorbed. The design of better peptide drugs and protease inhibitors will become possible once we have a better understanding of the type, properties and distribution of proteases at a given mucosal site. Knowledge of the rate and extent of various metabolite formations and an examination of the sequential steps in a metabolite scheme might aid in the design of peptidase resistant prodrugs, analogues and peptidomimetics. Formulation approaches can also be utilized to protect the compound from luminal proteases either by coating, site directed release, and/or inclusion of specific protease inhibitors. The synthetic and site directed mutagenesis approach to peptide structure alteration coupled with the rapid development of the newer generation of non-toxic permeation enhancers and site specific bioadhesive polymers may make the oral delivery of peptide and protein drugs commercially feasible in the near future.

REFERENCES

Abuchowski, A.; McCoy, J.R.; Van Es, T.; Palczuk, N.C. and Davis, F.F. (1977) J. Biol. Chem. 252,, 3582-3586.

AC Moses, A.C.; Gordon, G.S.; Carey, M.C. and Flier, J.S. (1983) Diabetes, 32, b 1040-1047.

Adamson, I.; Esangbedo, A.;Okolo A.A. and Omene, J.A. (1988) Biol. Neonate, 53, 267-273.

Adibi, S.A. (1971) J. Clin. Invest., 50, 2266-2275.

Adibi, S.A. and Mercer, D.W. (1973) J. Clin. Invest., 52, 1586-1594.

Ajisaka, K. and Iwashita, Y. (1980) Biochim. Biophys. Res. Commun., 97, 1076-1080.

Akiyama, T.;S Harada, S.; Kojima, F.; Takahashi, Y.; Imada, C.; Okami, Y.; Muraoka,Y.; Aoyagi, T. and Takeuchi, T. (1998) J Antibiot (Tokyo), 51:6 553-9.

Alpers, D.H. and Tedesco, F.J. (1975) Biochim. Biophys. Acta., 401, 28-40.

AM Asatoor, A.M.; Cheng, B.; Edwards, K.D.G.; Lant, A.F.; Matthews, D.M.; Milne, M.D.; Navab, F. and Richards, A.J. (1970) Gut, 11, 380-387.

Angelastro, M.R.; Mehdi, S.; Burkhart, J.P.; Pest ,N.P. and Bey, P. (1990) J. Med. Chem., 33, 11-13.

Angliker, H.; Wickstrom, P.; Rauber, P. and Shaw, E. (1987) Biochem. J., 241, 871-875.

Asatoor, A.M.; Crouchman, M.R.; Harrison, A.R.; Light, F.W.; Lough-ridge,L.W.; Milne, M.D. and Richards, A.J. (1971) J. Clin. Sci., 41, 23-33.

Athauda, S.B.; Takahashi, T.; Inoue, H.; Ichinose,M. and Taka-hashi, K. (1991) FEBS Lett., 292, 53-56.

Augustyns, K.; Bal, G.; Thonus, G.; Belyaev, A.; Zhang, X.M.; Bollaert, W.; Lambeir, A.M.; Durinx, C.; Goossens, F. and Haemers, A. (1999) Curr Med Chem., 6:4 311-27.

Baici, A. and Gyger-Marazzi, M. (1982) Eur. J. Biochem., 129, 33-41.

Barret, A.J.; Kembhavi, A.A.; Brown, M.A.; Kirschke, H.; Knight, C.G.; Tamai, M. and Hanada, K. (1982) Biochem. J., 201.

Bazim, H.; Andre, C. and Heremans, J.F. (1973) Ann. Immunol. Inst. Pasteur, Paris, 1246, 253-272.

Bernkop-Schnürch, A. and Scerbe-Saiko, A. (1998) Pharm Res., 15:2 263-9

Bernkop-Schnürch, A. and Pasta, M. (1998) J Pharm Sci., 87:4 430-4

Billson, J.; Clark, J.; Conway, S.P.; Hart, T.; Johnson, T.; Langston, S.P.; Ramjee, M.; Quibell, M.and Scott,R.K. (1998) Bioorg. Med. Chem. Lett. May 5 8:9 993-8

Bing, E.G.; Kilbourne, A.M.; Brooks, R.A.; Lazarus, E.F. and Senak, M. (1999) J Acquir Immune Defic Syndr Hum Retrovirol, 20:5 474-80.

Blay, J. and Brown,K.D. (1985) Biochem. J., 225, 85-94.

Boger, J. (1983) In: Peptides: Structure - Function, Proc. 8th Am. Pept. Symp., VJ Hruby and DH Rich (Eds), Pierce Chem Co., Rockford, IL, p-569-579.

Bohley, P. and Seglen, P.O. (1992) Experentia, 48, 151-157.

Bond, J.S. and Beynon, R.J. (1987) In: Proteolysis and Physiological Regulation (H. Baum ed), Pergamon Press, Oxford, pp. 173-285, 1987.

Brewster, D. and Waltham, K. (1981) Biochem. Pharmacol., 30, 619.

Brömme, A.; Schierhorn, A.; Kirsch, H.; Wiederanders, B.; Barth, A.; Fittkau, S. and Dermuth, H.U. (1989) Biochem. J., 263, 861-866.

Carone, F.A.; Christensen, E.J.; G Flouret, G. (1987) Am. J. Physiol., 253, F1120-F1127, 1987.

Cathers, B.E and Schloss, J.V. (1999) Bioorg. Med. Chem. Lett., 9:11 1527-32.

Chandler, M.M and Varandani, P.T. (1972) Biochem. Biophys. Acta., 286, 136-140.

Chen, H.; Noble, F.; Coric, P.; Fournie-Zaluski, M.C.; Roques, B.P. (1998) Proc. Natl. Acad. Sci. U S A, 95:20 12028-33.

Chen, R.H.L.; Abuchowski, A.;van Es, T.; Palczuk, N.C. and Davis, F.F. (1982) Biochim, Biophys Acta., 660, 293-296.

Chipkin, R.E. (1986) Drugs Future, 11, 593-606.

Choudhuri, S.; McKim, J.M. and Klassen, C.D. (1992) Toxicol. Appl. Pharma-col., 115, 64-71.

Choudry, Y. and Kenny, A.J. (1991) Biochem. J., 280, 57-60.

Chung, Y.C.; Kim, Y.S.; Shadchehr, A.; Garrido, A.; MacGregor, I.L.; and Sleisenger,M.H. (1979) Gastroen-terology, 76, 1415-1421.

CIBA Foundation symposium, Peptide Transport and Hydrolysis, Elsevier/North-Holland, New York 1977.

Ciechanover, A. and Schwartz, A.L.(1989) Trends Biochem. Sci., 14, 483-488.

Cunningham-Rundles, C. (1987) Failure of antigen exclusion In: J. Brostoff and SJ Challacombe (Edn). Food Allergy and Intol-erance, Tindall, London, p 223-236.

Cushman, D.W. and Ondetti, M.A. (1980) In: Progress in Medicinal Chemis-try, GP Ellis, GB West (Eds), Elsevier- North Holland Bio-medical: Amsterdam, The Netherlands, p 41-104.

Das, M. and Radhakrishnan, A.N. (1975) Biochem. J., 146, 133-139.

Davis, S.; Abuchowski, A.; Park, Y.K. and Davis, F.F. (1981) Clin. Exp. Immunol., 46, 649-653.

Davis, S.S. (1986) In : Delivery Systems for Peptide Drugs, Plenum Press, New York, p 1.

Deddish, P.A.; Skidgel, R.A. and Erdös, E.G. (1989) Biochem. J., 261, 289-291.

Delaisse, J.M.; Eeckhout, Y.; Sear, C.; Galloway, A.; McCullah, K. and Vaes, G. (1985) Biochem. Biophys. Res. Commun., 133, 483-490, 1985.

Dence, J.E. (1980) In: Steroids and peptide: Selected chemical As-pects for biology, Biochemistry and Medi-cine John Wiley and Sons, New York, Chapter 4.

Dermuth, H.U. (1990) J. Enzyme Inhibition, 3, 249-278.

Diment, S.; Leech, M.S. and Stahl, P.D. (1988) J. Biol., 263, 6901-6907.

Donohue Jr., T.M. Drey M.L.and Zetterman, R.K. (1988) Alcohol-Alcohol, 23, 265-270.

Donovan, M.D.; Flynn, G.L. and Amidon, G.L. (1990) Pharm. Res., 7, 863-868.

Drapeau, G.; Chow, A. and Ward, P.E. (1991) 12, 631-638.

Drenth, J.; Kalk, K.H. and Swen, H.M. (1976) Biochem., 15, 3731-3738.

Duckworth, W.C.; Stentz, F.B.; Heinemann, M. and Kitabachi, A.E. (1979) Proc. Natl. Acad. Sci., USA, 76, 635-639.

Eberley, A.N. (1991) Chimia, 45, 145-53.

Endo, S.; Yokosawa, H. and Ishii, S. (1985) Biochim. Biophys. Res. Commun., 129, 684-700.

Erdös, E.G. and Skidgel, R.A. (1990) Kidney Int. 38, 524-527.

Ericksom, R.H.; Suzuki, Y.; Sedlmeyer, A. and Kim, Y.S. (1992) J. Biol. Chem., 267, 21623-21629.

Fauchere, J.L. (1986) In: Advances in Drug Research; B Testa (Ed), Academic: London, Vol 15, 29-69.

Fauchere, J.L. and Thurieau, C. (1992) Adv. Drug. Res., 23, 128-159.

Fern, E.B.; Hider, R.C. and London, D.R. (1969) Biochem J., 111, 30-33.

Ferrariolo, R.L.; Mohler, M.A. and Gloff, C.A. (Eds) (1993) In: Protein Pharma-cokinetics and Metabolism: Pharmaceutical Biotechnology Sereis, Plenum, New York.

Finkle, C.D.; St. Pierre, A.; Leblond, L.; Deschenes, I.; DiMaio, J.; Winocour. P.D. (1998) Thromb Haemost 79:2 431-8.

Friedler, A.; Blumenzweig, I.; Baraz, L.; Steinitz, M.; Kotler, M. and Gilon, C. (1999) J Mol Biol., 287:1 93-101.

Fruton, J.S. (1976) Adv. Enzymol. 44, 1-36.

Fujita, M.; Parsons, D.S. and Wojnarowska, F. (1972) J.Physiol., London, 227, 377-394.

Ganong, W.F. (1977) Review of Medical Physiology, 8th Ed., Lange Medical Publication, Los Altos, California.

Gardner, M.I.G. (1984) Biol. Rev. Biol. Proc. Cambridge Phil. Soc., 59, 289-331.

Gardner, M.I.G. (1987) Adv. Bio. Sci., 65, 99-106.

Gardner, M.L.G.; Illingworth, K.M.; Kelleher, J. and wood, D. (1991) J. Physiol., 439, 411-422.

Gardner, R.C.; Assinder, S.J.; Christie, G.; Mason, G.G.; Markwell, R.; Wadsworth, H.; McLaughlin, M.; King, R.; Chabot-Fletcher, M.C.; Breton, J.J.; Allsop, D. and Rivett, A.J. (2000) Biochem J., 1 346 Pt 2: 447-54

Gebert, G. (1991) Algemin Medizin, 19, 125-131.

Gibbs, D.M. (1986) Psychoneuroendocrinology, 11, 131-140.

GI tractler, C. (1964) In: Protein Digestion and Absorption in Nonrumin-ants; Mammalian Protein Metabolism Vol 1, Academic Press, New York, p-35-69.

Glaumann, H. and Ballard, F.J. (1986) In: Lysosomes: Their role in protein breakdown, Acad. Press, New York.

Green, G.and Nasset, E.S. (1977) Am. J. Dig, Dis., 22, 437-444.

Green, G.D.J. and Shaw, E. (1981) J. Biol. Chem., 256, 1923-1928.

Greenbaum, L.M.; Hirshkowitz, A. and Shoichet, I. (1959) J. Biol. Chem., 234, 2885-2887.

Grey, R.D.; Saneii,H.H.; and Spatolla, A.F. (1981) Biochem. Biophys. Res. Commun., 101, 1251-1258, 1981.

Griffiths, E.C. and Kelly, J.A. (1979) Mol. Cell. Endocrinol., 14, 3-17.

Griffiths, E.C.; Kelly, J.A.; White, N. and Jeffcoate, S.L. (1980) Acta. Endocrinol., 93, 385-391.

Gros, C.; Giros, B. and Schwartz, J.C. (1985) Biochemistry, 24, 2179.

Guan, D.D.; Yoshioka, M.; Erickson, R.; Heizer, W. and Kim, Y.S. (1988) Am. J. Physiol., 255, G212-G220.

Guicherit, O.R.; Gooszen, H.G.; Jansen, J.B.; Van-der-Burg M.P. and Lamers, C.B. (1990) Digestion, 47, 226-31.

Guillou, H.; Miranda, G. and Pelissier, J.P. (1991)Int. J. Pept. Protein Res., 37, 494-501.

Gurbanov, K.; Shuranyi, E.; Kaballa, A.; Fudim, E.; Blumberg, S. and Winaver, J (1999) Gen Pharmacol Sep 33:3 277-81.

Hanley, M.R. (1983) In: Degradation of Endogenous Opiods: Its rele-vance in Human Pathology and Therapy, Raven Press, New York, p 129.

Hara, H. and Kiriyama, S. (1991) Proc. Soc. Exp. Biol. Med., 198, 732-736, 1991.

Harbeck, H.T. and Mentlein, R. (1991) Eur. J. Biochem., 198, 451-458.

Hare, J.F. (1990) Biochem. Biophys. Acta., 1031, 71-90.

Heizer, W.D.; Kerley, R.L. and Isselbacher, K.J. (1972) Biochim. Biophys. Acta., 264, 450-461.

Hersh, L.B. and McKelvy J.F. (1979) Brain Res., 168, 553-564.

Hershko, A. (1988) J. Biol. Chem., 263, 15237-15240.

Hershko, A. and Ciechanover, A.(1982) Annu. Rev. Biochem., 51, 335-364.

Hey, D.H and John, D.I. (1978) In: Aminoacids, Peptides and related compounds, in organic chemistry, Vol 6 Chapters 1 to 3 and 5, University Park Press, Baltimore.

Heyman, M.; Ducroc, R.; Desjeux, J.F. and Morgaat, J.L. (1982) Am. J. physi-ol., 242 G 558-G 564.

Heymann, E. and Mentlein, R. (1978) FEBS Lett., 91, 360-364.

Hider, R.C. and Barlow, D. (Eds), (1991) Polypeptide and Protein Drugs- Production, Characterization and Formulation; Ellis Horwood, Chichester, England.

Hirai, S.; Yashiki, T. and Mima, H. (1981) Int. J. Pharm., 9, 173-184.

Hoegl, L.; Korting, H.C. and Klebe, G. (1999) Pharmazie, 54:5 319-29

Hooper, N.M. and Turner, A.J. (1987) Biochem. J., 241, 625-633.

Hu, L.Y. and RH Abeles, R.H. (1990) Arch. Biochem. Biophys., 281, 271-274.

Humphrey, M. and Ringrose, P.S. (1986) Drug Metab. Rev., 17, 283-310.

Husby, S.: Foged, N.: Host, A. and Swehag, S.E. (1987) Gut, 28, 1062-1072.

Ichikawa, K.; Ohata, I.; Mitomi, M.; Kawamura, S.; Maeno, H. and Kawata, H. (1980) J. Pharm. Pharmacol., 32, 314-318.

Ilett, K.F.; Tee, L.B.G.; Reeves, P.T.; Minchin, R.F. (1990) Pharmacol. Therap., 46, 67-93.

Ishida, M.; Machida, Y.; Nambu, N. and Nagai, T. (1981) Chem. Pharm. Bull., 29, 810-816.

Jacobasson, I.: Lindberg, T.: Lothe, L.; Axelson, I. and Bene-diktsson, B. (1986) Gut, 27, 1029-1034.

Jennewein, H.M.; Waldeck, F. and Konz, W. (1974) Arzneim. Forsch., 24, 1225-1228.

Jones, A.L.; Vierling, J.M.; Steer,C.J. and Recihen, J. (1979) In: Progress in Liver Diseases, Vol. 6 (H. Popper and F. Schaffner, Eds), Grune and Stratton, New York, p 43-80.

Jones,A.L.; Renston, R.H. and Burwen, S.T. (1982) In: Progress in Liver Diseases, Vol. 7, Grune and Stratton, New York, p 51-69.

Josefsson, L. and Sjostrom, H. (1966) Acta Physiol. Scand., 67, 27-31.

Kahne, T.; Lendeckel, U.; Wrenger, S.;Neubert, K.; Ansorge, S. and Reinhold, D. (1999) Int. J. Mol. Med., 4:1, 3-15.

Kaplan, J. (1981) Science, 212, 14-20.

Katayama, M.; Nadel, J.A.; Bunnet, N.W.; Di Maria, G.V.; Haxhiu, M. and Borson, D.B. (1991) 12, 563-567.

Katre, N.V.; Knauf, M.J and Laird, W.F. (1987) Proc. Natl. Acad. Sci., USA, 84, 1487-1492.

Katunuma, N.; Kominami, E.; Hashida, S. and Wakamatsu, N. (1982) Adv. Enzyme Regul., 20, 337-350.

Kenny, A.J. and Stephenson, S.L. (1988) FEBS Lett., 232, 1-8.

Kenny, A.J.;Stephenson, S. and Turner, A.J. (1987) In: Mammalian Ectoen-zymes, Elsevier Science Publishers B.V., Amsterdam, Nether-lands, 169-210.

Kester W.R.and Mathews, B.W. (1977) Biochem., 16, 2506-2516, 1977.

Kidron, M.; Bar, O.J.; Berry, E.M. and Ziv, E. (1982) Life Sci., 31, 2837-2841.

Kim, Y.S.; Sleisenger, M.H. and Kim, Y.W. (1974) Biochim. Biophys. Acta., 380, 283-296,.

Kim, Y.S.; Birtwhistle, W. and Kim, Y.W. (1972) J.Clin. Invest., 51, 1419-1430.

Kiso, Y.; Matsumoto, H.; Mizumoto, S.; Kimura, T.; Fujiwara, Y. and Akaji, K. (1999) Biopolymers, 51:1 59-68.

Kitamura, K.; Akahori, K.; Yano, H.; Iwao, K.and Oka, T. (2000) Naunyn Schmiedebergs Arch Pharmacol., 361:3 273-8.

Klostermeyer, H. and Humble, R.E. (1966) Agnew. Chem. Intern., Ed. 5, 807.

Kraut, J. (1977) Ann. Rev. Biochem., 46, 331-358.

Kreider, M.S.; Winodur, A. and Krieger, N.R. (1981) Neur. Endocrin. Lett., 3, 115-118, 1981.

Kundu, B. and Jain, G.K. (1996) Indian Patent Application No. 296/DEL/96.

Kundu, B.; Singh, G.; Jain, G.K.; Shukla, A.; Srivastava, N. and Patnaik, G.K. (1988) Protein and Peptide Lett., 5, 83.

Kundu, B.; Singh, G.; Tripathi, A.; Jain, G.K. and Raghubir, R. (1998) Indian Patent Application No. 747/DEL/98.

Kushak, R.I. and Ugolev, Dokl. A.M. (1966) Biol. Sci., 168, 411-413.

Langyuth, P.; Bohner, V.; Heizmann, J.; Merkle, H.P.; Wolffram, S.; Amidon, G.L. and Yamashita, S. (1997) J. Controll. Rel., 46, 39-57.

Lee, V.H. (1988) CRC Crit. Rev. Ther. Drug carrier Syst., 5, 69-97.

Lee, V.H. (1988) CRC Critical Reviews in Therpeautic Drug Carrier Systems, 5, 69-97.

Leonard, J.V.; Marrs, T.C.; Addison, J.M.; Burston, D.; Clegg, K.M.; Lloyd, J.K.; Matthews, D.M. and Seekins, J.W. (1976) Pediatr. Res., 10, 246-249.

Li, Y.; Z Shao Z. and Mitra, A.K. (1992) Pharm. Res., 9, 864-869.

Lin, J.; Toscano, P.J. and Welch, J.T. (1998) Proc Natl Acad Sci U S A., 95:24 14020-4

Liu, F.Y.; Kildsig D.O. and Mitra, A.K. (1991) Pharm. Res., 8, 925-929.

Magnusson, M.; Sjostrom, H.;Noren, O.; Asp, N.G. and Denneberg, T. (1991) Nephron., 58, 456-460.

Marie, C.; Mossiat, C.; Lecomte, J.M.;J Bralet, J. (1998) Pharmacology 1998 Jun 56:6 291-6.

Mark, D.; Lin, L. and Su, S. (1986) US Patent "Human Recobinant Cysteine Depleted Interferon-b Muteins", Nos 4,518,584, 1985, and 4,588,585.

Massien, C.; Azizi, M.; Guyene,T.T.; Vesterqvist, O.; Mangold, B.and Ménard, J. (1999) Clin Pharmacol Ther Apr 65:4 448-59.

Matsumoto, K.M.;K Mizoue, K.;K Kitamura, K.;WC Tse,W.C.; CP Huber, C.P.; Ishida,T. (1999) Biopolymers 51:1 99-107.

Matthews, D.M. (1975) Physiol. Res. 55, 537.

Matthews, D.M.; Lis, M.T.; Cheng, B. and Crampton, R.F. (1969) Clin. Sci., 37, 751-754.

Maycock, A.L.; DeSousa, D.M.; Payne, L.G.;TenBroeke, J.; Wu, M.T.; and Patchett, A.A. (1981) Biochem. Biophys. Res. Commun., 102, 963-969.

Mayer, R.J. and Doherty, F. (1986) FEBS Lett., 198, 181-193.

Maze, M. and Gray, G.M. (1980) Biochem., 19, 2351-2358, 1980.

McDonald, J.K. and Barret, A.J. (1986) In: Mammalian Proteases. A Glos-sary and Bibliography Vol. 2: Endopeptidases; Academics, London.

McNamara, D. ; Teitelbaum, J. and Potier, M. (1981) Biomedicine, 35, 122-124.

Mellgren, R.L.; Renno, W.M. and Lane, R.D. (1989) Cell Biol. Rev., 20, 139-159.

Metsas, R.; Fulcher, I.S.; Kenny, A.J. and Turner, A.J. (1983) Proc, Natl. Acad. Sci. USA, 80, 311-3115.

Metsas, R.; Kenny, A.J. and Turner, A.J. (1984) Biochem. J., 223, 433-440.

Miura, S.; Song, I.S.; Morita, A.; Erickson, R. and Kim, Y. S. (1983) Biochim. Biophys. Acta., 66-75.

Mookhtiar, K.A.; Marlowe, C.K.; Bartlett, P.A. and Van Wart, H.E. (1987) Biochem., 26, 1962-1965.

Moore W.M. and Spilburg, C.L. (1986) Biochem., 25, 5189-5195.

Morier, E.H.; Han, K.K.; Patsouris, L.; Mareau, O. and Rips, R. (1981) Int. J. Peptide Protein Res., 18, 113-515, 1981.

Morita, A.; Chung, Y.C.; Freeman, J.J.; Erickson, R.H.; Sleisenger, M.H. and Kim, Y. S. (1983) Clin. Invest.72, 610-616.

Mortimore, G.E. and Poso, A.R. (1984) Fed. Proc., 34, 1289-1294.

Murachi, T.; Takano, E.; Maki, M.; Adachi, Y. and Hatanaka, M. (1989) Biochem. Soc. Symp., 55, 13-28.

Nagae, A.; Deddish, P.A.; Becker, R.P.; Anderson, C.H.; Abe, M.; Tan, F.; Skidgel, A. and Erdös, E.G. (1992) J. Neurochem., 59, 2201-2212.

Nagai, T.; Nishimoto, Y.; Nambu, N.; Suzuki, Y. and Sekine, K. (1984) J. Controlled Resease, 1, 15-22.

Newy, H. and Smyth, D.H. (1960) J. Physiol., London, 152, 367-371.

Nicholson, J.A. and Peters, T. J. (1978) Clin. Sci. Mol. Med., 54, 205-207.

Nishita, T.;Okamura,Y.; Kamada, A.; Higuchi, T.; Yagi, T. and Shichiri, M. (1985) J. Pharm. Pharmacol., 37, 22-26.

Nycander, M.; Estrada, S.; Mort, J.S.; Abrahamson, M.I (1998) BjörkFEBS Lett Jan 23 422:1 61-4

Odake, S.; Okayama, T.; Obata, M.; Morikawa, T.; Hattori, S.; Hori, H. and Y Nagai, (1990) Chem. Pharm. Bull., 38, 1007-1011.

Okada, H.; Yamazaki, I.; Yashiki, T. and Mima, H. (1983) J. Pharm. Sci., 72, 75-78.

Olson, G.L.; Bolin, D.R.; Bonner, M.P.; Bos, M.; Cook, M.; Fry, D.C.; Graves, B.J.; Hatada, M.;Hill, D.E.; Kahn, M.; Madison, V.S.; Rusiecki, V.K.; Sarubu, R.; Sepinwall, J.; Vincent, G.P. and Voss, M.E. (1993) J. Med. Chem., 36, 3039-3049.

Oppenheim, R.C.; Stewart, N.F.; Gordon, L. and Patel, H.M. (1982) Drug Dev. Ind. Pharm., 8, 531-546.

Otlewski, J.; Krowarsch, D. and Apostoluk, W. (1999) Acta Biochim Pol., 46:3 531-65.

Padres, M.; Rabaud M.and Bieth, J.G. (1992) Biochim. Biophys. Acta., 1118, 174-178.

Paganelli, R. and Levinsky, R.J. (1980) J. Immunol. Methods, 37, 333-341.

Parson, D.S. (1972) In: Transport Across the Intestine, Church Hill, London, p. 253-278.

Patick, A.K.; Duran, M.; Cao, Y.; Shugarts, D.; Keller, M.R.; Mazabel, E.; Knowles, M.; Chapman, S.; Kuritzkes, D.R. and Markowitz, M. (1998) Antimicrob Agents Chemother., 42:10 2637-44.

Peters, T.J. (1973) Clin. Sci. Mol. Med., 45, 803-816.

Peters, T.J.; Modha, K.and MacMahon, M.T. (1969) Gut, 10, 1055-1058.

Powers, J.C. and Harper, J.W. (1986) In: Proteinase Inhibitors (Barett, A.J. and Salvensen,G. Eds) Elsevier: Amsterdam, New York, Oxford, p-219-298.

Powers, J.C. and Harper, J.W. (1986) In: Proteinase Inhibitors (AJ Barett and G Salvensen Eds) Elsevier: Amsterdam, New York, Oxford, p-55-152.

Prasad, C. and Peterkosfky, A. (1976) J. Biol. Chem., 251, 3229-3234.

Prasad, J.V.; Boyer, F.E.; Domagala, J.M.; Ellsworth, E.L.; Gajda, C.; Hamilton, H.W.; Hagen, S.E.; Markoski, L.J.; Steinbaugh, B.A.; Tait, B.D.; Humblet, C.; Lunney, E.A.; Pavlovsky, A.; Rubin, J.R.; Ferguson, D.; Graham, N.; Holler, T.; Hupe, D.; Nouhan, C.;Tummino, P.J.; Urumov, A.; Zeikus, E.; Zeikus, G.; Gracheck, S.J. and Erickson, J.W. (1999) Bioorg Med Chem., 7:12,775-800.

Publishers B.V., Amsterdam, Nether-lands, 211-248.

Rado, J.P.; J Marosi, J.; Szende, L.; Borbely, L.; Tako, J. and Fisch-er, J. (1976) J. int. Clin. Pharmacol., 13, 199-209.

Rahfeld, J.; Schierhorn, M.; Hartrodt, B.; Neubert, K. and Heins. (1991) J. Biochim. Biophys. Acta, 1076, 314-316.

Rasnick, D. (1985) Anal. Biochem., 149, 461-465.

Rauber, P.; Angliker, H.; Walker, B. and Shaw, E. (1986) Biochem. J., 239, 633-640.

Rechsteiner, M. (Eds) (1988) In: Ubiquitin, Plenum Press, New York.

Ren, S. and Lien, E.J. (1998) Prog Drug Res., 51: 1-31

Rich, D.H. (1986) In: Proteinase Inhibitors (AJ Barret, A.J.; Salven-sen,G. Eds), Elsevier: Amsterdam, NY, Oxford, 153-178.

Robl, J.A.; Sun, C.Q.; Stevenson, J.; Ryono, D.E.; Simpkins, L.M.; Cimarusti, M.P.; Dejneka, T.; Slusarchyk,W.A.; Chao, S.; Stratton, L.; Misra,R.N.;Bednarz,M.S.; Asaad, M.M.; Cheung, H.S.; Abboa-Offei, B.E.; Smith, P.L.; Mathers, P.D.; Fox, M.; Schaeffer, T.R.; Seymour, A.A.and Trippodo, N.C. (1997) J Med Chem., 40:11 1570-7.

Rodgers, J.D.; Lam, P.Y.; Johnson, B.L.; Wang, H.; Li, R.; Ru, Y.; Ko, S.S.; Seitz, S.P.; Trainor, G.L.; Anderson, P.S.; Klabe, R.M.; Bacheler, L.T.; Cordova, B.; Garber, S.; Reid, C.; Wright, M.R.; Chang, C.H. and Erickson-Viitanen, S. (1998) Chem Biol., 5:10 597-608.

Roemer, D. and Pless, J. (1979) Life Sci., 24, 621.

Rosewicz, S.; Riecken E.O. and Logsdon, C.D. (1990) Digestion, 46, 390-395.

Saffran, M.; Bedra, C.; Kumar, G.S. and Neckers, D.C. (1988) J. Pharm. Sci., 77, 33-38.

Saffran, M.; Kumar, G.S.;Savariar, C.; Burnham, J.C.; Williams, F. and Neckers, D.C. (1986) Science, 233, 1081-1084.

Samamen, J.M. (1985) In: Polymeric Material in Medication, Plenum Press, New York, p 227.

Sawyer, T.K.; Cody, W.L.; Leonard, D.M. and Hadley, M.E. (1994) In : Encyclopedia of Molecular Biology; RA Meyers (Ed), VCH, New York.

Sawyer, W.H.; Acosta, M. and Manning, M. (1974) Endocrinology, 95, 140-145.

Schecter, I. and Berger, A. (1967) Biochem. Biophys. Res. Commun., 27, 157-162.

Schilling, R.J. and Mitra, A.K. (1992) Pharm. Res., 9, 1003-1009.

Schilling, R.J. and Mitra, A.K. (1990) Int. J. Pharm., 62, 53-64.

Schilling, R.J. and Mitra, A.K. (1991) Pharm. Res., 8, 721-727.

Schirmeister, T. (1999) J. Med. Chem. Feb 25 42:4 560-72

Shao, Z.; Krishnamoorthy, R.; Chermak. T. and Mitra, A.K. (1993) Pharm. Res., 10, 243-251.

Shaw, E. (1980) In: Design of Irreversible Inhibitors: Enzyme In-hibitors as Drugs, (M Sandler, Ed), p 25-43.

Shaw, E.; Wikstrom, P. and Ruscica, J. (1983) Arch. Biochem. Biophys., 222, 424-429.

Shimazawa, R.; Takayama, H.; Kato, F.; Kato, M. and Hashimoto, Y. (1999) Bioorg Med Chem Lett., 9:4 559-62.

Siddiqui, Ovais and Chien, W.Y. (1995) CRC Critical Reviews in Therapeu-tic Drug Carrier Systems, 3 (3), 195-208.

Silk, D.B.A.; Perret, D. and Clark, M.L. (1975) Clin. Sci. Mol. Med., 49, 523-526.

Silk, D.B.A.; Perret, D.and Clark, M.L. (1975) Gastroenterology, 68, 1426-1432.

Simmons, W.H. and Orawski, A.T. (1992) J. Biol. Chem., 267, 4897-4903.

Sinko, P.J. (1992) Pharm. Res., 9, 320-325.

Skidgel, R.A.; Defendini, R. and Erdös, E.G. (1987) In: Neuropeptides and Their Peptidases, AJ Turner (Ed), Ellis Horwood, Chichester, England, p 165-182.

Skidgel, R.A.; Engelbrecht, S.; Johnson, A.R. and Erdös, E.G. (1984) Pep-tides, 5, 769-776.

Skrzydlewski, Z. and Worowski, K. (1978) Acta. Biol Acad. Sci. Hun-gary, 29, 19-22.

Sloand, E.M.; Kumar, P.N.; Kim, S.; Chaudhuri, A.; Weichold, F.F. and Young, N.S. (1999) Blood, 94:3 1021-7.

Smith, R.A.; Coles, P.J.; Spencer, R.W.; Copp, L.J.; Jones, C.S. and Krantz, A. (1988) Biochem. Biophys. Res. Commun., 155, 1201-1206.

Smith, R.A.; Copp, L.J.; Coles, P.J.; Pauls, H.W.; Robinson, V.J.; Spencer, R.W.; Heard, S.B. and Krantz, A. (1988) J. Am. Chem. Soc., 110, 4429-4431.

Smith, R.A.; Copp,L.J.; Donnelly, S.L.; Spencer, R.W. and Krantz, A. (1988) Biochem., 27, 6568-6573.

Sorvillo, P,; Kerndt, S. O.; Castillon, M.; Carruth, A. and Contreras, R. (1999) AIDS Care, 11:2 147-55.

Spiro, H.M. (1983) Clinical Gastroenterology, 3rd Ed., Macmillan, New York, p 467 and 587.

Stahl, P. and Schwartz, A.L. (1986) J. Clin. Invest., 77, 657-662, 1986.

Steizt, T.A. and Shulman, R.G. (1982) Ann. Rev. Biophys. Bioeng., 11, 419-444.

Stephenson, S.L. and Kenny, A.J. (1987) Biochem. J., 241, 237-247.

Stephenson, S.L. and Kenny, A.J. (1988) Biochem. J., 255, 45-51.

Stratford, R.E.; Carson, L.W.; Dodda-Kashi, S. and Lee, V.H.L. (1988) J. Pharm. Sci., 838-842.

Su, K.S.E.; Campanale, K.M.; Mendelsohn, L.G.; Kerchner, G.A. and Gries, C.L. (1985) J. Pharm. Sci., 74, 394-398.

Sugiyama, Y. and Hanano, M. (1989) Pharm. Res., 6, 192-202.

Takaori, K.; Burton, J. and Donowitz, M. (1986) Biochim. Biophys. Res. Commun., 137, 682-687.

Takaori, K.; Burton, J. and Donowitz, M. (1986) Bioochem. Biophys. Res. Commun., 137, 682-687.

Tanaka, S.; Murakami, T.;Nonaka, N.; Ohnuki, T.; Yamada, M. and SuGI tracta, T. (1998) Immunopharmacology 40:1 21-6

Tang, J.; Sepulveda, P.; Masciniszyn, J.; Chen, K.C.S.; Huang, W.Y.; Too, N.; Lin, D. and Lanier, J.P. (1973) Proc. Natl. Acad. Sci., USA, 70, 3437-3439.

Telemo, E.; Westrom, B.R.; Ekstrom G.and Karlsson, B.W. (1987) Biol. Neonate, 52, 141-148.

Thorsett, E.D. and Wyvratt, N.J. (1987) In: Neuropeptides and Their Peptidases, AJ Turner (Ed.) Ellis Horwood, Chichester, England, p 229-292.

Tobey, N.; Heizer, W.; Yeh, R.; Huang, T.I. and Hoffner, C. (1988) Gastroen-terology, 88, 913-926.

Tomkinson, B. (1999) Trends Biochem Sci., 24:9 355-9.

Tomkinson, B. (2000) Arch Biochem Biophys., 376:2 275-80.

Touitou, E. and Rubinstein, A. (1986) Int. J. Pharm., 30, 95-99.

Towatari, T.; Tanaka, K.; Yoshikawa,D. and Katunuma, N. (1978) J. Bio-chem., Tokyo, 84, 659-672

Tozaki, H.; Odoriba, T.; Iseki, T.; Taniguchi, T.; Fujita, T.; Murakami, M.; Muranishi, S. and Yamamoto, A. (1998) J Pharm Pharmacol.,50:8 913-20

Travis, J. and Savesen, G.S. (1983) Ann. Rev. Biochem., 52, 655-709.

Turner, A.J. (1987) In: Neuropeptides and Their Peptidases, AJ Turner (Ed.) Ellis Horwood, Chichester, England, p 183-201.

Turner, A.J.; Hooper, N.M. and Kenny, A.J. (1987) In: Mammalian Ectoen-zymes, Elsevier Science

Varandani, P.T. ( ) Biochim. Biophys. Acta., 286, 126-135, 197Varandani, P.T.; Shroyer, L.A. and Naf, M.A. (1972) Proc. Natl. Acad. Sci. USA, 69, 1681-1684.

Vavra,I.; Machova, A. and I Krejci, I. (1974) J. Pharmacol. Exp. Ther., 188, 241-247.

Veronese, L.; Rautaureau, J.; Sadler, B.M.;Gillotin, C.; Petite, J.P.; Pillegand, B.; Delvaux, M.; Masliah, C.; Fosse, S.; Lou, Y. and Stein, D.S. (2000) Antimicrob Agents Chemother.,44:4 821-6

Vilhardt, H. and Bie, P. (1983) Eur. J. Pharmacol., 93, 201-205.

Vincent, B.; Jiracek, J.; Noble, F.; Loog, M.; Roques, B.; Dive, V.; Vincent, J.P.and Checler, F. (1997) Br J. Pharmacol., 121:4 705-10.

Walker, W.A. and Isselbacher, K.J. (1974) Gastroenterology, 67, 53.

Wallace, D.A.; Bates, S.R.E.; Walker, B.; Kay, G.; White, J.; Guth-rie, D.J.S.; Blumson,N.L. and DT Elmore, D.T. (1986) Biochem. J., 239, 797-799.

Wang, L.W.; Fu, X.L; Clough, R.; Sibley, G.; Fan, M.; Bentel, LB Marks, L.B. and Anscher, M.S. (2000) Radiat Res., 53:4 405-410.

Wang, K.K.W.; Villalobo, A. and Roufogalis, B.D. (1989) Biochem., 262, 693-706.

Ward, D.J. (1991) In: Peptide Pharmaceuticals-Approaches to the Design of Novel Drugs; Open University, Buckingham, England.

Warshaw, A.L.; Walker, W.A. and Isselbacher, K.J. (1974) Gastroenterology, 66, 987-992.

Webb, K.E.; Matthews, J.C. and Di Rienzo, D.B. (1992) J. Animal Sci., 70, 3248-3247.

Wiley, R.A.; Rich, D.H. (1993) Med. Res. Rev., 13, 327-384.

Wilmouth, R.C.; Kassamally, S.; Westwood, N.J. Sheppard, R.J. Claridge, T.D. Aplin, R.T. Wright, P.A.; Pritchard G.J.,and Schofield C.J. (1999) Biochemistry, 38:25 7989-98.

Wyvratt, M.J. and Patchett, A.A. (1985) Med. Res. Rev., 5, 483.

Yamada, M.; Okagaki, C.; Higashijima, T.; Tanaka, S.; Ohnuki, T. and SuGI tracta, T. (1998) Bioorg Med Chem Lett., 8:12 1537-40

Yamamoto, A.; Luo, A.M.; Dodda-Kashi, S. and Lee, V.H.L. (1989) J. Pharmacol. Exp. Ther., 249, 249-255.

Yoshida, H.; Okumura, K.; Hori, R.; I Anmo, I. and Yamaguchi, H. (1979) J. Pharm. Sci., 68, 670-671.

Yoshioka, M.; Erickson, M.H. and Kim, Y. S. (1998) J. Clin. Invest., 81, 1090-1095.

Yucel, L.T.; Jansson, H. and Glaumann, H. (1991) Virchows. Arch. Cell. Pathol., 61, 141-145.

Zhang, W.; Gorset, C.B.; Washington, T.F.; Blaschke, D.L.; Kroetz, K.M. and Giacomini (2000) Drug Metab Dispos., 28:3 329-34.

Zhang, X.; Recchia, F.A.; Bernstein, R. Xu, X.; Nasjletti, A. and Hintze, T.H. (1999) J Pharmacol Exp Ther 1999 Feb 288:2 742-51.

Chapter 10

Prodrug Based Novel Approaches in Drug Delivery

Alok Namdeo, N. K. Jain

10.1 INTRODUCTION

The drugs, mostly organic, elicit the pharmacologic response by interacting with receptors at the site of action, and any factor that limits the optimum access to this site is considered barrier in its usefulness, which may range from formulation problems to in-vivo limitations. As shown in Fig 10.1, the barriers can be overcome by chemically linking promoiety to form prodrug which undergoes biotransformation to release the parent drug

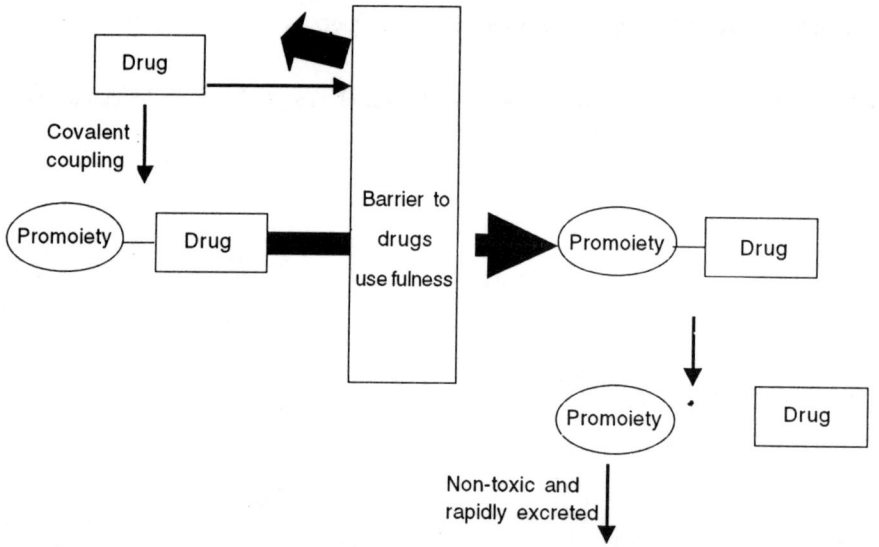

Fig 10.1: Concept of Prodrug

once the barrier is circumvented. The term 'prodrug' was introduced by Albert (1957) to describe compounds which undergo biotransformation prior to exhibiting their pharmacologic effect. The use of the term has since been expanded to include compounds, which undergo chemical as well as hydrolytic transformation (Kupchean et al, 1965). Intensive research on prodrug can be realized from a search through chemical abstract service since 1987 for 8 years, which revealed 4000-6000 papers and 500-1000 patents concerning those directly and indirectly related to prodrugs and their clinical applications (Stella, 1996). The research on prodrug should be multidisciplinary involving medicinal chemist to synthesize appropriate modifications; biologist/biochemist to observe activity and reversion mechanism; and formulation and development scientist to relate structure with delivery/formulation of prodrugs. The concept of prodrug in general has been reviewed earlier (Sinkula & Yalkowski, 1975: Sharma, 1986), therefore the chapter confines to the recent novel prodrug approaches in the successful development of novel drug delivery formulations and in drug targeting.

10.2 PRODRUGS IN NOVEL DRUG DELIVERY SYSTEMS

The novel systems of drug delivery offer a means of improving the therapeutic effectiveness of incorporated drugs by providing sustained, controlled delivery and/or targeting the drug to desired site. The effectiveness of system depends upon the entrapment efficiency, which is governed by physicochemical properties of drugs, therefore prodrugs have been widely investigated and utilized successfully to transiently modify the properties of drugs in a manner to improve the drug loading. The prodrugs must be hydrolysed in the body to release the active drug. For this reason, most of the prodrugs designed are esters, amides etc. involving -OH, -COOH, $-NH_2$ free groups of drug to covalently couple with promoieties. These are hydrolysed easily by esterases and amidases present in the body. The rate of hydrolysis can also be predictably modulated by using different promoieties or using spacers, to accrue the sustained delivery.

The low incorporation in novel drug delivery systems is generally observed for polar hydrophilic drugs. The simplest strategy therefore appears to prepare the lipophilic prodrugs by covalent attachment with long chain alkyl carboxylic acids. The lipidic prodrug can be encapsulated in the carrier system or drug can be linked to carrier system or lipidic prodrug itself may acquire mesomorphic character assembling in delivery system. These strategies are discussed below in detail.

10.2.1 Prodrug incorporated delivery systems

The colloidal system of drug delivery provides sustained and controlled delivery by releasing the encapsulated drug while in circulation or after encapture by cells; the targeting is achieved when the system carries the drug to desired site after administration. Therefore, it is imperative that delivery system must incorporate maximum quantity of drug for optimum efficacy and cost effectiveness. Comparison of encapsulation efficiency of a drug in system with therapeutic dose will indicate their usefulness. When a large amount of carrier is required for the encapsulation of a low dose of drug, then the system is neither administerable nor economic. Furthermore, if the encapsulation efficiency is very low, removal of free drug is necessary both from the therapeutic (to avoid undesirable effects) and commercial (to reduce cost) points of view. Therefore, ideal system will have nearly 100% encapsulation efficiency. The encapsulation depends upon the physicochemical properties which can be suitably modified by linking appropriate promoiety, obtaining prodrug that will be suitably formulated into delivery system as described below.

10.2.1.1 Prodrugs in liposomes

Liposomes, widely reported drug carriers, are vesicles consisting of stacked lipid bilayers with intervening sheets of water. The drug is incorporated into aqueous compartment or lipid bilayer structure or associate with polar head groups of the bilayer depending upon their hydrophilicity/lipophilicity. The less hydrophobic drugs exhibit low entrapment efficiency (EE) and making them more hydrophobic by derivatization with various fatty acids has been the most encouraging approach to improve the EE. The triamcinolone 21- palmitate (prodrug) showed 85% EE compared to 5% EE of triamcinolone acetonide (Goundalkar & Mezei, 1984). Shaw et al (1976) prepared various fatty acid derivatives of hydrocortisone and found that hydrocortisone-21-palmitate had maximum encapsulation efficiency in multilamellar vesicles. The 6-mercaptopurine is another drug showing very low (about 1.5%) EE due to non-interaction with bilayers and low solubility in water. Taneja et al (2000) linked it to glyceryl monostearate and EE was found to have improved upto 98%. Liposomal encapsulation of palmitoyl-L-asparaginase resulted in prolongation of blood half-life (from 2.8 hr to longer than 23.7 hr), abrogation of acute toxicity and preservation of antitumour activity as compared to free drug (Jorge et al, 1994).

5-Fluorouridine (FUR), is an effective anticancer agent but with severe side effects. Encapsulation in liposomes of this water soluble drug showed low (26%) encapsulation efficiency (EE) and rapid leakage during storage (>50% in 12 days) (Crossaso et al, 1997). Therefore lipophilic prodrugs were encapsulated and EE was improved to 45% and 95% for 5'-succinyl-FUR and 5'-palmitoyl-5-FUR respectively. The palmitoyl prodrug showed no evident sign of drug release for three months of storage; no appreciable change in vesicle size and no drug precipitation or liposome aggregation, thereby predicting long chain aliphatic chain as better promoiety because of better anchoring of palmitoyl prodrug intercalated between phospholipid bilayer. The REV liposomes (prepared by reverse phase evaporation method) bearing 5'palmitoyl-5-FUR were coupled with thiolated monoclonal antibody AR-3 obtaining immunoliposomes which showed best antitumor activity on HT-29 cells than liposomes or 5-FUR (Crossasso et al, 1997). Ozaki et al (1989) have reported higher activity of intraperitoneally administered 5' and 3',5'-long chain acyl derivatives of 5'-Fluoro-2'-deoxyuridine (dFUR) which was attributed to slow release leading to higher and more persistent level of drug in the organism; this is because 5-dFUR is active as antitumor only after phosphorylation of its 5'-hydroxyl group, the fatty acid chain must therefore be first removed via hydrolysis by aspecific esterases to make it cytotoxic. The investigation of intracellular degradation of dipalmitoyl ester of 5-FUdR incorporated in egg PC lipsomes showed intracellular drug depot, from which drug is slowly released (Van et al, 1990; Kawaguchi et al, 1985).

versluis et al (1998) incorporated lipophilic daunorubicin derivative in liposomes anchored with apolipoprotein E (apo-E). These showed 20- to 50- fold greater effectiveness than liposomes lacking apo-E. The affinity of apo-E liposomes for LDL receptor on B16 cells was 15 fold higher than that of LDL (0.77 Vs 11.5 nM respectively) indicating LDL- receptor mediated higher tumor uptake.

10.2.1.2 Prodrug in niosomes

Niosomes are vesicles of non-ionic surfactant which are cheap and chemically stable compared to costly and instable phospholipids. Uchegbu & Duncan (1997) encapsulated PK1, an N-(2-hydroxypropyl) methacrylamide (HPMA) copolymer doxorubicin conjugate in niosomes for sustained release. The PK1 has shown 4-fold increase in the maximum tolerated dose (relative to doxorubicin) and antitumor activity under phase I clinical trial (Vasey et al, 1996). This is due to enhanced penetration and retention effect of tumour tissues (Matsumura & Maeda, 1986). However, this preferential uptake is accompanied by rapid renal excretion of most of the remaining conjugate (Seymour et al, 1990; Pimm et al, 1996) because of low molecular weight of HPMA while increasing the mol. wt. of HPMA is not practicable due to non-biodegradable nature of the polymer backbone. The encapsulation of PK1 in niosomal formulation composed of Span 60, cholesterol and Solulan C24 showed maximum entrpment of 49%, good storage stability and doxorubicin was liberated slowly during incubation of these PK1-niosomes with a mixture of lysosomal enzymes in-vitro. The vesicles of hexadecyl diglycerol ether $(C_{16}G_2)$ showed higher (61%) EE as well did not induce RBC lysis. The PK1-$C_{16}G_2$ niosomes were mainly taken up by liver and spleen following in-vivo administration, after 24 hr 25% and 3% of dose administered was present as free doxorubicin in these organs respectively (Uchegbu & Duncan, 1997).

10.2.1.3 Prodrug in lipoproteins

Lipoproteins are endogenous transporter of lipids in the circulation, they are non-immunogenic and escape recognition by RES. Their structural artificial mimics are NeoHDL particles consisting of apolar triglyceride core surrounded by phospholipid monolayer in which specific apoproteins, extracted from natural LDL, are embedded (Schouten et al, 1993). Since the qpoproteins on the particles are essential for he LDL recognition, drugs should preferably be into the lipid moiety, but most of the drugs are not sufficiently lipophilic, therefore lipophilic prodrug have been investigated. Bijsterbosch et al (1994) prepared dioleoyl derivative of iododeoxyuridine (IDU-Ol$_2$) to incorporate into NeoHDL finding similar properties as native HDL. After intravenous administration hepatic association of the prodrug was higher supposedly due to physiological HDL-specific processing. Lactosylation to IDU- Ol$_2$ loaded ^{125}I Neo-HDL (contains galactose residues) rapidly cleared from plasma and approximately 75% of injected amount was recovered in liver at 10 min., enabling effective treatment of diseases like hepatitis B. Monard et al (1993) also achieved higher incorporation of linolenate prodrug of ametantrone and mitoxantrone into LDL compared to free drug.

10.2.1.4 Prodrugs in emulsions

The oil-in-water (o/w) emulsions are useful in sustained drug delivery, passive targeting to macrophages (Singh & Revin, 1986) and in active targeting by ligand attachment (Iwamoto et al, 1991). The formulation of etoposide (VP-16) and teniposide (VM-26), the podophyllotoxin derivatives, could not be developed because drugs are poorly soluble in a lipid emulsion with cholesteryl ester as oil component (Halbert et al, 1984). For this, Lundberg (1994) esterified phenolic-4'-hydroxyl group in drug with unsaturated fatty acids to obtain lipophilic prodrugs, soluble in lipid emulsion. The prodrug was found to be chemically stable both in buffer and in medium containing serum. The emulsion showed particle diameter of 104 nm, good physical stability and no leakage of entrapped drug. The linoleic derivative showed very much the same activity in-vitro cytotoxic activity against K562 & T-47D cancer cells as the parent drug.

Microemulsions bearing hydrophobic internal phase exhibit higher physical stability in plasma compared to vesicles. Their unique feature allows to incorporate lipophilic prodrugs into the oil phase i.e. N-(u)-3β-(oleoyloxy)androst-5-en-17β yl (pentyl)oxy)carbonyl)-N,N-bis (2-chloroethyl)amine (Lundberg, 1987) and amphiphilc prodrugs to intercalate or anchor into the surface monolayer of the microemulsion particle. The intercalation of amphiphilic drug molecules such as phenothiazines mostly depends upon the state of ionization, therefore deliberate attempts have been made to achieve such effects. Murtha & Ando (1994) established the feasibility of formulating cholesteryl ester prodrug in phospholipid microemulsion and evaluated cholesteryl ibuprofen and cholesteryl flufenamate to optimize with respect to composition and particle size. The prodrug showed slower enzymatic hydrolysis in-vitro than cholesterol palmitate or oleate ester. The microemulsions were prepared by adding 1-propanol solution of the cholesteryl ester, then lipid and phospholipid to a rapidly mixing KCl/KBr solution. The 75:25 molar ratio of DPPC : cholesteryl ester consistently gave mean particle size of 100-150 nm.

10.2.1.5 Prodrugs in solid lipid nanoparticles

Solid lipid nanoparticles (SLN) combine the advantages of both liposomes and fat emulsions (Schwarz et al, 1994). They comprise of a high melting point triglyceride (TG) as the solid core and a phospholipid (PL) coating. Their advantages over other systems are the use of natural lipids and incorporation of drug in TG core which may be applicable for prolonged release. However to achieve these goals it is desirable to incorporate the drug into innermost phase of emulsion. The incorporation of azidothymidine (AZT) in SLN was minimal (<1%) but the incorporation of AZT-palmitate ester prodrug increased with increasing phospholipid content to the maximum of 90% using high PL/TG ratio (Heitai et al, 1997).

10.2.2 Covalent binding to carriers

Alternative to incorporation of prodrugs, drugs can be directly linked to the carrier system. However, the complex must have good physical stability, cleavability and noninterference with receptor recognition.

10.2.2.1 Linking of drug to lipoproteins

The apoproteins in LDL are exposed to the external aqueous environment (Margolis & Longdon, 1966), allowing molecules to be covalently bound to the exterior of the particle (e.g. with lysine residues). The covalent linkage of anthracyclines to lysine residues of LDL resulted in a progressive decline in the affinity of the conjugate for the receptor (in-vitro) with increasing substitution (Masquelier et al, 1986). However, attachment of doxorubicin to the surface using activated spacer group, prevented crosslinking of the particles and allowed higher loading of 80 molecules per LDL particle. These LDL drug conjugate containing approximately 50 molecules of drug exhibited the same in-vivo fate as native LDL when injected intravenously into mice (Trouet et al, 1972) demonstrating that the complex is a suitable targeting system. The attachment of methotrexate to LDL using a water-soluble crosslinking agent gave a complex that also retained the in-vivo cytotoxic activity (Halbert et al, 1985).

10.2.2.2 Micelle forming polymeric prodrug

Yokoyama et al (1990) presented block copolymer composed of hydrophobic and hydrophilic segments, which can form micellar structures by their amphiphilic nature. The hydrophobic drugs can easily be bound to hydrophobic segment without precipitation which is otherwise observed in other polymers due to concentrated presence of drug molecules. As shown in Fig 10.2, hydrophobic drug binding segment forms the hydrophobic core of the micelle and the other hydrophilic segment of the copolymer surrounds this core as an outer shell. Thus, these polymeric prodrugs possess excellent water solubility, irrespective of hydrophobic drug loading because hydrophilic outer shell prevent the hydrophobic core from forming aggregates and precipitation. The system allows easy control of particle size by changing the length of the polymer chain. The stability of the polymer micelle is thought to be higher than that of liposomes since the hydrophobic segment is interwined with each other in the polymer micelle through inter- and intramolecular hydrophobic interactions, whereas the hydrophobic interaction in liposomes is limited to that between adjacent lipid. Conclusively, their distinctive character allows binding of drug, controlled drug release, preservation of drug activity during delivery to the target and desired interactions with protein cells and tissues.

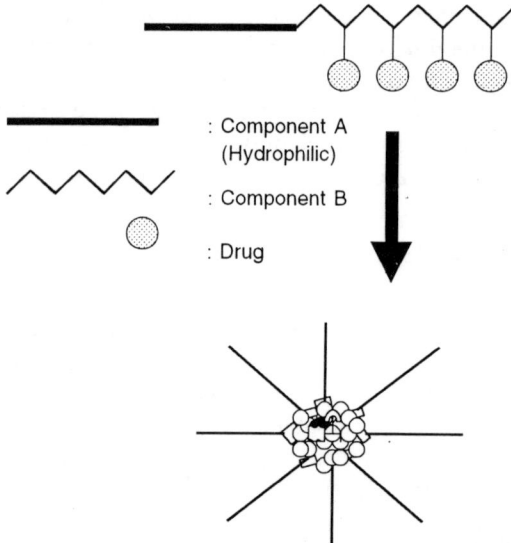

: Component A
(Hydrophilic)

: Component B

: Drug

Fig 10.2 : Concept of micelle forming polymeric prodrug (Yokoyama et al, 1990b)

The drug from polymeric prodrug may act by any of three mechanisms shown in Fig 10.3. The micelle may directly interact with cells (a); or the drug may act after releasing from the micelle (b); or there may establish equilibrium control, in which only a single polymer chain, which exists in equilibrium with micellar form, gives drug action (c). These various modes of action allow the application of the micelles forming polymeric prodrug to provide ideal pattern of drug release for desired drug.

The poly (ethylene glycol)-poly (aspartic acid) block copolymer has been widely studied. The poly (aspartic acid) segment is hydrolyzable and possesses carboxyl group for binding the drug, the other segment PEG is known to be a non-toxic and non-immunogenic water-soluble polymer and has been used in protein modification to decrease antigenicity and prolong the half-life in blood (Zalipsky, 1995). The anticancer drug, adriamycin could easily be conjugated to PEG-PASP without any precipitation in different mole ratios and 30%

of adriamycin was reproducibly bound. Its aqueous solution could be concentrated by ultrafiltration to equivalent of 20 mg ADR.HCl without any precipitate and the addition of 0.9% (w/v) NaCl did not lead to precipitation nor gelation; further it could be lyophilized without losing its water solubility in the redissolving procedure thus micelles possess good water solubility. The aqueous dispersion at different concentration showed unimodal size distribution of micelles with mean diameter of 48.5 nm. The fluorescent quenching confirmed the formation of micellar structures. The adriamycin in general binds with plasma protein, however polymeric prodrug was not at all found to bind with bovine serum albumin (Yokoyama et al, 1990b). The polymeric prodrug showed excellent in-vivo anticancer activity, judged from the increase in the ratio of the survival period of the treated mice to that of the control (T/C) from 305% for adriamycin to 490% for polymeric prodrug; Another important effect was lower toxic effects shown from body weight changes.

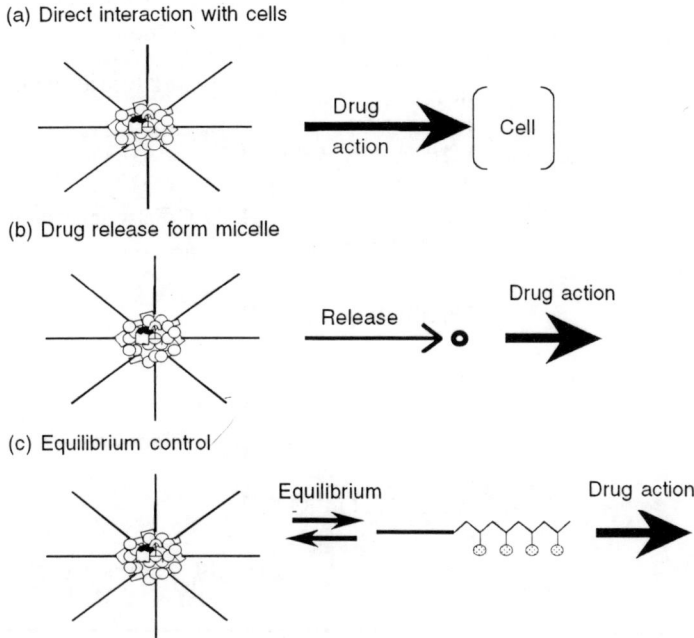

Fig 10.3: Mechanism of action of micelle forming polymeric prodrug (Yokoyama et al, 1990b).

Ohya et al (1992) coupled doxorubicin to reactive carboxyl group of poly (α-malic acid) and attached sachharide as a targeting moiety. The release of ADR from conjugate was higher in acidic conditions indicating that the amide bonds of the conjugate can be cleaved to release free ADR in lysosomal acidic conditions after uptake into tumor cell. The poly(α-malic acid)/amide/ADR/galactosamine conjugate was optimum macromolecular prodrug having high antitumor activity against hepatoma.

10.2.3 Mesomorphic prodrug as pharmacosomes

If the hydrophilic drug is conjugated with lipophilic promoiety, the prodrug becomes amphiphilic. Further, if the lipophilic part is a long chain mono- or diglyceride, the prodrug acquires mesomorphic lyotropism and assembles in the form of micellar, vesicular or hexagonal phases depending upon the lipid material and degree of hydration. The word 'mesomorphism' denotes that the system may assume several structurally different phases, while if it is due to lipid water interaction these are called lyotropic. The mechanism can be traced out to the structural similarity of prodrug with phospholipid, which have been widely studied. Any drug possessing free carboxyl group can be esterified to the hydroxyl group of the lipid; if the drug does not possess any

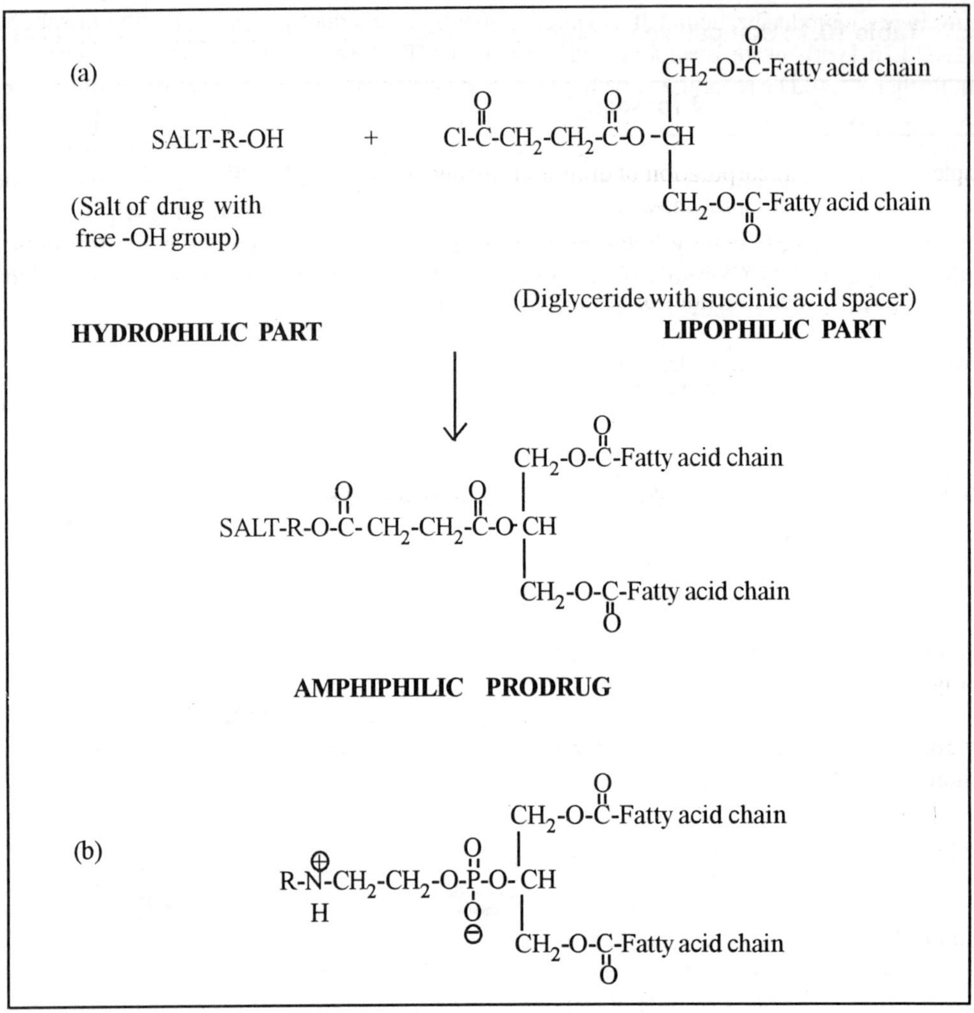

Fig: 10.4 (a) Explanatory scheme of amphiphilic diglyceride prodrug synthesis (b) Structure of phospholipids (Phosphatidylcholine,R= $(CH_3)_3$, PhosphatidyletanolamineR=H_3 etc).

free carboxyl group but another active hydrogen atom ($-OH, -NH_2$) the esterification can be accomplished by means of a spacer group. The formation of prodrug and its structural similarity with phospholipids is shown in Fig 10.4. Since the system is formed by linking of drug (pharmakon) to carrier (soma) these are called 'pharmacosomes', a word originally coined by Vaizoglu et al (1986). Pharmacosomes, therefore can be defined as the colloidal dispersion of prodrug which may exist as ultrafine vesicular, micellar or hexagonal aggregates depending on the chemical structure of the drug-lipid complex. The system was developed as alternative to liposomes, which show low entrapment efficiency (EE) and drug leakage during storage for hydrophilic drugs. The formulation of vesicular system from prodrug overcomes many constraints of liposome such as the EE is predetermined and more importantly much higher because the drug and carrier form a stoichiometrically defined unit covalently linked together. Furthermore, pharmacosomes have some practical advantages such as escaping the tedious step of removing the free from entrapped drug. Overall, a comparision of pharmacosomes to liposomes has been given in Table 10.1. This novel system is thereby discussed in detail.

Table 10.1 : Comparision of pharmacosome with liposomes (Vaizoglu et al, 1991)

	Liposomes	Pharmacosomes
Principle	Incorporation of drug in the aqueous or lipid phase of a mixture of lipid where the physicochemical properties of the carrier and release of drug will be functions of different lipids used.	-Covalent binding of a drug to a lipid where the resulting compound is the carrier and the active compound at the same time. The physicochemical properties depends on drug as well as the lipid.
Loss of drug	-Through leakage	-No leakage, since drug is covalently bound but loss of drug by hydrolysis is possible.
Manufacturing	-Cast film method -Extrusion/sonication, -Injection method -Reverse phase evaporation etc.	-Self-dispersion through moderate mixing and sonication
Separation of free drug	-Gel filtration, dialysis, Ultrafiltration, Ultracentrifugation.	-Not necessary since drug is covalently linked.
Volume of inclusion	-Decisive in incorporation of drug molecules	-Irrelevant, since the drug is covalently bound.
Surface charge	-Achieved through lipid combination	-Depends on the physicochemical structure of the drug-lipid complex.
Membrane fluidity	-Depends on lipid combination and presence of cholesterol. Fluidity influences the rate of drug release and physical stability of the system.	-Depends on the phase transition temperature of the drug lipid complex. No effect on release rate since the drug is covalently bound.
Release of drug	-Diffusion through the bilayer, desorption from the surface or release through degradation of the liposomes.	-Hydrolysis (including enzymatic)
Physical stability	-Relatively good -Aggregation through double valenced cation	-Depends on the physico-chemical properties of the drug-lipid complex.

10.2.3.1 Tensioactivity of prodrug

The judicious conjugate of drug with carrier produces a compound, which is amphiphilic in nature. The aqueous solution of these amphiphiles typically exhibits concentration dependent aggregation, which differs from that of most polar or ionic molecules. At low concentrations the amphiphile exists dispersed in the monomer state. As the more monomer are added, a critical micelle concentration (CMC) is reached, leading to dramatic changes in the concentration dependence of many physical parameters, such as osmotic pressure, surface tension and electrical conductivity. The further increment in monomers may lead to variety of structures i.e. micelles of spherical or rod like or disc shaped type or bilayered vesicles or cubic or hexagonal phases depending upon the physicochemical interactions and thermodynamic variables of amphiphile. Mantelli et al (1985) compared the effect of diglyceride prodrug on interfacial tension with the effect produced by a standard detergent dodecylamine hydrochloride, observing similar effect on surface tension lowering. Above CMC prodrug exhibits mesomorphic lyotropic behaviour and assembles in supramolecular structures.

10.2.3.2 Preparation of pharmacosomes

Because prodrugs are usually self-vesiculating, well established procedures of hand- shaking method (Mantelli et al, 1985; Vaizoglu et al, 1986) and ether injection method (Vaizoglu et al, 1986) have been utilized for preparing vesicles. In hand -shaking method, the dried film of drug lipid complex deposited in a round bottom flask upon hydration with aqueous medium readily gives vesicular suspension. In ether injection method, organic solution of drug-lipid complex was injected slowly into the hot aqueous medium, wherein the vesicles were readily formed.

10.2.3.3 Physicochemical stability of pharmacosomes

Chemical stability testing on pindolol glycerol monostearate (maleate salt) indicated no hydrolysis in any of the cases, even after two months of storage (Vaizoglu et al, 1986). Kaiser (1990) studied the effect of different electrolyte media on physicochemical stability of bupranolol hydrochloride pharmacosomes. Since polar hydrophilic head group is very sensitive towards different electrolytes, spontaneous aggregation was observed at different concentrations depending upon the valence of the electrolyte. However, aggregation in the presence of nonelectrolyte was moderate to indifferent. Best candidate for isotonization was found to be 5% glucose. For chemical stability, the half-life at 25°C in 5% glucose was found to be 111 days. Namdeo & Jain (2000) have recently formulated dry granular propharmacosomes of propranolol stearate hydrochloride by depositing the prodrug with and without egg lecithin over sorbitol. This, upon hydration and shaking readily transformed into opalescent vesicular dispersion, enabling storage for any length of time.

10.2.3.4 Applications of pharmacosomes

The approach has successfully improved the therapeutic performance of various drugs i.e. pindolol maleate, bupranolol hydrochloride, cytarabine etc. Yang et al (1982) found that CDP-diacylprodrug initially forms large vesicles which diminish in size and finally form micelles. They claim that these slow kinetics are an essential requirement for phospholipids in biomembranes in order to confer stability to the lipid bilayer and prevent the rapid exchange of lipids between separate membranes of living cells. According to Curatolo (1987), proper membrane functioning requires that the non-polar interior of the membrane be in the liquid crystalline state, which is influenced by the phase-transition temperature. The phase-transition temperature of pharmacosomes in the vesicular and/or micellar state could have significant influence on their interaction with membranes (i.e. inclusion into membrane bilayer through structural similarity and/or endocytosis). It has been shown that *Acheloplasma Laidlawii* takes up fatty acids from its environment and incorporates them directly into its membrane lipids, allowing experimental manipulation of the membrane lipid composition and fluidity (Curatolo, 1987).

The different membranes in body contain phosphatidylcholine, phosphatidyl-ethanolamine, ceramides and sphingomyeline (Curatolo, 1987). These resemble lipid prodrugs in physicochemical structure. Therefore, it can be expected that pharmacosomes can interact with biomembranes enabling a better transfer of active ingredient. This interaction can also change the phase transition temperature of biomembranes, thereby improving the membrane fluidity leading to enhanced permeation. A resume of results with different drugs linked to different carriers is presented below:

10.2.3.4.1 Pindolol: Vaizoglu & Speiser (1986) synthesized glycerol monosteatrate ester of a weak base, pindolol via spacer (succinic acid) and isolated maleate salt as two isomers. This prodrug having structural similarity with lysolecithin reduced the interfacial tension between benzene/water and opalescent vesicular dispersion could be obtained by the film method and ether injection method. The freshly prepared pharmacosomes showed a particle size of 200nm and 240 nm determined by transmission electron microscopy and photon correlation spectroscopy respectively, which upon sonication reduced to 90 nm. One weak old pharmacosomes yielded size of 213 nm.

The in-vivo fate of these vesicles was studied in beagle dogs by administering the vesicles and parent drug through oral and intravenous route and determining the plasma concentrations of unchanged pindolol. No additional exponential were significant and plasma drug profile followed the one compartment open model, indicating rapid hydrolysis in body fluids. Three to five times higher concentrations of unchanged pindolol were observed following intravenous administration of the pharmacosomes rather than free pindolol. Urine data indicated lowering of renal clearance when pindolol was administered as pharmacosomes. Oral dose yielded slightly higher plasma concentrations following administration of pindolol pharmacosomes, the difference being insignificant.

10.2.3.4.2 Bupranolol hydrochloride: Mantelli et al (1985) have synthesized the prodrug consisting of β-blocker bupranolol which is covalently linked to 1,3-dipalmitoyl-2-succinyl-glycerol. The resulting prodrug was amphipathic and dispersed readily in water above 30°C forming a smectic lamellar phase. The dispersion, similar to charged phospholipids showed continuous swelling with increasing water content and so in excess water region, the thermodynamically most stable structure was the unilamellar vesicles while oligomeric vesicles also formed. The differential scanning calorimetry indicated that dispersion undergoes order-disorder transition (phase transition temperature) at 32°C with an enthalpy change of DH = 10kcal/mol. The electron spin resonance study also indicated hyperfine splitting and order parameter also reflected the order- disorder transition.

The effect on intraocular pressure in rabbits showed enhanced biological activity compared to equimolar mother drug with the factor of 2.3 (Kaiser, 1990).

10.2.3.4.3 1-β-D- Arabinofuranosylcytosine: MacCoss et al (1982) synthesized various amphipathic liponucleotide prodrugs, 1-β-D- arabinofuranosylcytosine 5'-diacylglycerols (containing either dimyristoyl, dipalmitoyl distearoyl free fatty acid side chains) and determined the aggregational and morphological characteristics of their sonicated dispersions in relation to change in temperature. The sonication at low temperature gave turbid solutions containing large bilayer sheets. On raising the temperature, a transition temperature (t_g) was reached at which a stable three dimensional cross-linked network of small interlocking bilayer stacks was formed. Sonication at the temperature close to t_g produced small disc-shaped micellar structures. These micelles were shown to exist in another aggregational equilibrium consisting of stacking-destacking process. In contrast, the prodrug containing unsaturated fatty acid chain gave multilamellar liposomes.

Turcotte et al (Turcotte et al, 1980) reported prolonged life (93%) following intraperitoneal injection of prodrug compared to free drug (18%) against leukemia cells in mice. Herbert & Schwandender (1996) formulated stable vesicles of N4-palmitoyl-araC with matrix lipids. Evaluation on L1210 mouse lukaemia model cured 80-100% of the treated animals at a total dose of 200mmol/kg, whereas none of the mice survived that were treated with araC even at four times higher concentration.

10.2.3.4.4 Taxol Steve (1996) has synthesized and patented a drug conjugate covalently attached to a fatty acid chain of a phospholipid, glyceride, ceramide or 1,2- diacyloxypropan-3-amine. The linkage between the therapeutic agent and lipid is one which can be cleaved in-vivo. A mixture containing 1-oleoyl-2-[N-{4'-O-

(9"taxyl)-succinoyl}-11-aminoundecanoyl]-L-α-phosphatidylcholine, egg phosphatidylcholine and 1-stearoyl-L-phosphatidylcholine was dissolved in 10% methanol in benzene and then lyophilized. The resultant powder when dispersed in a buffered saline and extruded 10 times through polycarbonate filters gave particle size of 90 nm.

10.2.3.4.6 Dermatan sulfate Among the various diglycerides synthesized, poly-O-[3-(1,3-dipalmitoyloxypropane-2-oxycarbonyl propanoyl] dermatan sulfate showed tensioactivity. They formed vesicles in nanometric range. The evaluation showed some potential for improved oral bioavailability (Transmontano, 1993).

10.2.3.4.7 Azidothymidine: A monophosphate diglyceride conjugate 3'-azido-3'-dideoxythymidine-5'-phosphate diglyceride was synthesized and tested as pure prodrug vesicles or prodrug in liposomes against HIV replication in H9 cells and interaction with serum component. The compound binds very rapidly to serum components only. Following in-vivo delivery, this would be transported and biodistributed as lipoprotein complex, thereby preventing glucuronidation and filtration in the kidney resulting in significant increase in plasma lifetime (Steim, 1990).

10.2.3.4.8 Acyclovir: The lipid prodrug acyclovir diphosphate dimyristoyl glycerol forms liposomes (vesicles) and provides substantial activity against herpes simplex virus, acyclovir resistant strains of herpes simplex virus and human cytomegalo virus as compared to free acyclovir and ganciclovir (difference statistically significant $p= 0.0015$) when tested in a rabbit model of herpes simplex virus-1 retinitis. Therefore, this system, modified to improve optical clarity may allow long-acting intravitreal treatment of cytomegalovirus retinitis and other retinal diseases (Taskintuna et al, 1997)

10.3 PRODRUG BASED TARGETING

The targeted delivery achieves preferentially high local concentration of a drug at desired site to alleviate potentially dose limiting side effects and is attractive for highly toxic drugs or drugs with narrow therapeutic window. The drug targeting index (DTI) can be calculated as:

$$DTI = \frac{AUC_{R.target}/AUC_{T.target}}{AUC_{R.nontarget}/AUC_{T.nontarget}}$$

Where, $AUC_{R.target}$, $AUC_{T.target}$, $AUC_{R.nontarget}$ and $AUC_{T.nontarget}$ represent the AUCs for the response site (R) and the toxic site (T) after target delivery (target) and nontarget delivery (nontarget) respectively.

Novel prodrugs with modified properties have been designed which preferentially achieves higher concentration of biotransformed drug at the desired site such as the following.

10.3.1 Targeting to brain

Delivery of drugs to brain is limited by blood brain barrier (BBB), which allows lipophilic molecules to enter the brain but highly ionized compounds fail to cross the barrier unless actively transported. On this basis Bodor & coworkers (1981) developed dihydropyridine-pyridinium type redox system for brain specific sustained delivery of drugs. As shown in Fig 10.5 the drug containing amine group is made lipophilic by coupling to dihydropyridine promoiety, that facilitates penetration of prodrug through the BBB. In the CNS, dihydropyridine group oxidizes to polar pyridinium salt, thus becomes poorly permeable to BBB leading to retention at the site, while its cleavage provides sustained release for action. The same process in peripheral compartments readily excretes polar pyridinium salt and hydrolysed drug. This has been successfully explored for a wide variety of amine containing drugs (Pop et al, 1991). However the dihydropyridine moiety is subjected to facile oxidation,

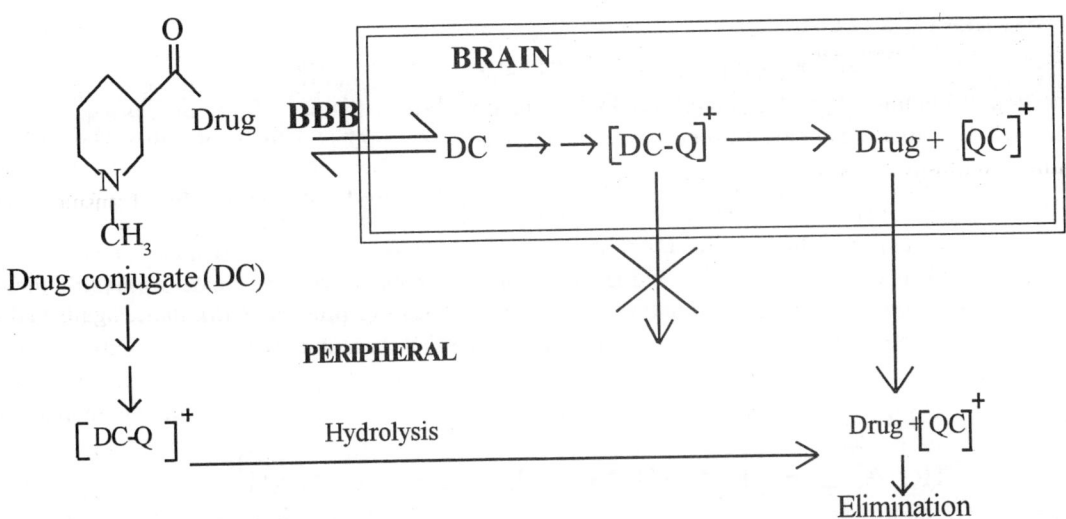

Fig 10.5 : The redox-based, prodrug mediated brain targeting system for amine containing drugs (Bodor & coworkers, 1981).

therefore, Ishikura et al (1995) developed 4-methylformylamino-3(2-propyl)dithio-3-pentenyl 2-amino 3-(3,4-dipivalyloxyphenyl) propionate prodrug involving conversion of cis-2-formylaminoethenylthio promoiety to quaternary thiazolium. The in-vivo administration of this prodrug showed 30 fold increase in AUC and 3.7 fold increase in mean residence time of DOPA in brain compared to equivalent amount of i.v. administered DOPA.

Anti-HIV drug is another important category requiring selective delivery in the CNS, where HIV virus invade early in the course of systemic infection (Yarcohan et al, 1987) and failure to stop progression leads to AIDS dementia and other neurological manifestations. Furthermore, CNS acts as a sanctuary for the HIV virus, from which periphery is continuously re-infected (Koenig et al, 1986). The drugs evolved for the treatment are primarily 2',3'-dideoxynucleoside (ddN's) encompassing five clinically approved lamivudine, zalcitabine, zidovudine, stavudine and didanosine which act by inhibiting reverse transcriptase (RT), a key enzyme in the replicative cycle of the HIV virus. Besides BBB, the endothelial cells in cerebral capillaries are tightly joined and the pinocytic vesicles are almost absent, thereby severely restricting the non-specific transport of drug into brain (Bodor, 1987). The prodrugs for improved brain delivery are primarily phosphorylated prodrugs and ester prodrugs prepared by linking promoiety to 5'-hydroxyl group in ddN's. The phosphorylated prodrugs are developed on the fact that the activity and inactivity of ddN's is crirtically dependent upon their initial conversion into 5'-O-monophosphate by nucloside kinase (after cellular uptake), therefore masked phosphate prodrugs (pronucleotides) have been designed to deliver the monophosphate species intracellularly and thus bypass the first phosphorylation step (DeClercq, 1995). The promoieties used are bis (2,2,2-trichloroethyl) (McGuigan et al, 1990) or aryloxyphosphoramide (McGuigan et al, 1993) or related groups or ether lipid (EL) conjugate (Piantadosi et al, 1991). The EL are most promising as they show selective activity, reduced toxicity and enhanced ability to cross the BBB.

The ester prodrugs have also been prepared. In the steroidal 17β-carboxyllic acid ester the steroidal acids retain some glucocorticoid features, the conjugate is expected to bind transcortin and the complex would be protected from metabolic transformation in plasma thereby prolonging the half-life of the nucleoside (Bolagopala et al, 1995). One such prodrug adamantylcarbonyl-AZT following intravenous administration showed 7-18 times higher prodrug concentration in brain than AZT (Tsuzuki et al, 1994). The retinoate, which itself inhibits HIV replication, was linked to AZT, the resulting ester prodrug was six fold more cytotoxic to H9 cells than AZT (Agrawal et al, 1990).

10.3.2 Targeting the kidney

Wilk & coworkers (1978) achieved the selective accumulation of dopamine in the kidney following the intraperitoneal administration of the double prodrug, γ-glutamyl-L-dopa to mice. The prodrug is sequentially transformed into drug by catalytic action of two enzymes that possess high activity in the kidney (Fig 10.6).

First, γ-glutamyl transpeptidase catalyzes the cleavage of the γ-glutamyl linkage; the L-dopa which is formed is then decarboxylated to dopamine by L-amino acid decarboxylase. Thus dopamine is readily available to exert its desired renal vasodilation effect in the kidney while undesired systemic blood pressure lowering effect is avoided. The levels of dopamine in kidney were found to be about five folds greater from this double prodrug then from the equimolar dose of single prodrug, L-dopa. The targeted delivery to kidney has also been achieved with the N-acyl-γ-glutamyl prodrugs of sulphmethoxazole (Wilk et al, 1980).

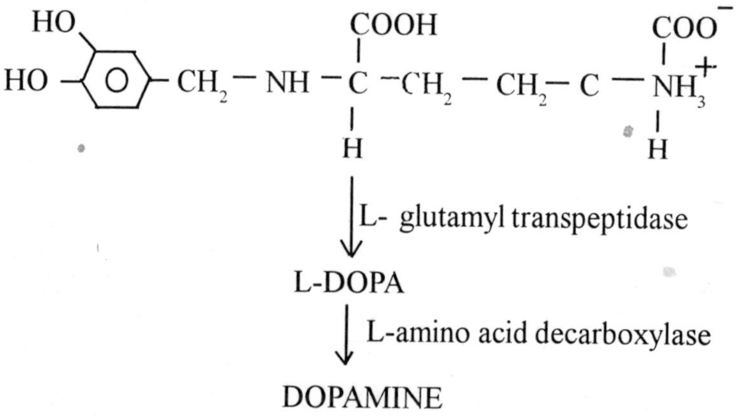

Fig 10.6 : Schematics for kidney selective delivery of dopamine (Wilk et al, 1978).

10.3.3 Liver targeting

Site selective transport pathways in the liver such as the bile acid transport system associated with the sinusoidal membrane of the hepatocytes (Anwer et al, 1976) have been exploited for the targeted delivery to liver. The bile acid prodrugs of several compounds, such as chlorambucil (Kramer et al, 1992), thyroid hormone (L-T3) (Stephan et al, 1992) have demonstrated hepatic targeting. Another transport pathway which has been frequently exploited is hepatic asiaglycoprotein receptor mediated endocytosis (Wall et al, 1980). It has been studied for targeting antiviral drugs to the parenchymal liver cells.

10.3.4 Targeting the virus

Targeting of an antiviral drug acyclovir has been achieved primarily through site selective activation by the herpes virus encoded enzyme pyrimidine deoxynucleoside (thymidine) kinase, responsible for converting acyclovir to its monoester, which is subsequently converted to triester by cellular kinases as shown in Fig 10.7.

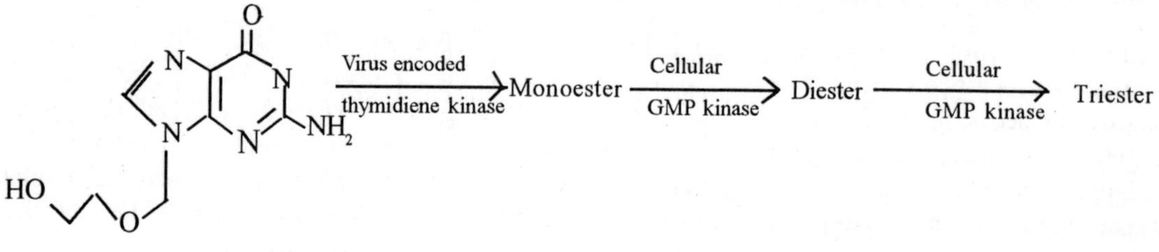

Fig 10.7: The schematics for selective delivery of acyclovir.

The triester form is pharmacologically active and the enzymatic conversion to triester occurs to a significantly greater extent in the herpes infected cells. Because of this, acyclovir displays high therapeutic activity against herpesvirus, essentially no activity against adenovirus, minimal metabolic degradation following systemic administration, and very low activity against uninfected host cells (Schaefer et al, 1978; Elion et al, 1977). An equally important advantage is that the bioconversion to the considerably more polar triester results in retention of the drug at the target site.

The structural analog of acyclovir is pencyclovir, which is phosphorylated more rapidly and produces higher triphosphate levels, and its intracellular half-life is also significantly longer than acyclovir ester (Earnshaw et al, 1992). The pencyclovir however shows poor oral bioavailability , which limits its clinical usefulness, therefore, its prodrug famcyclovir has been commercially prepared which has good oral bioavailability and shows almost complete bioconversion to pencyclovir (Hervest, 1994).

10.3.5 Targeting the colon

The targeting to colon is achieved by preparing the polar prodrug thereby decreasing the absorption in stomach and intestine while the selective cleavage by bacterial enzymes present in colon to more lipophilic drug follows fast absorption through colonic membrane (Fig 10.8). One such prodrug is sulfasalazine which is formed by coupling of diazotized 2-sulfanilamide pyridine with 5-aminosalicylic acid (ASA) (Schroder & Campbell, 1972; Peppercorn & Goldman, 1973). On oral administration, a large percentage of intact sulfasalazine reaches the colon by combination of biliary excretion and non-absorption in small intestine. The azo-reductase associated with colonic microflora now converts sulfasalazine to its constituent entities, the active species 5-ASA (Azad-Khan et al, 1977) is now available for absorption in colon, while pre-colonic absorption responsible for side effects is reduced. Another 5-ASA prodrug is azodisal (Jewel & Truelovs, 1981) which is formed by diazo-coupling of two ASA molecules. The prodrug is more polar and undergoes less pre-colonic absorption.

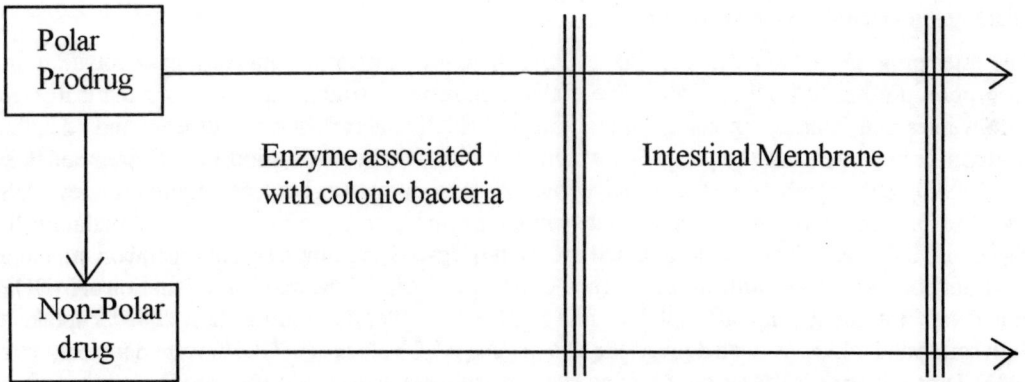

Fig 10.8 : Prodrug mediated targeted drug delivery to the colon.

The colon-specific delivery potentially improves the therapy of inflammatory bowel disease (IBD) by administration of corticosteroids (Friedman, 1989). Unless administered as enema, corticosteroids are not effective, hence targeting the colon through oral route using prodrug approach was undertaken. Glycosidic (Friend & Chang, 1984,1985) and glucuronidic (Haerberlin et al, 1993; Nolend & Friend, 1994) prodrugs of corticosteroids as dexamethasone, naloxone and menthol exploiting bacterial glycosidases and glucuronidases were utilized. Dexamethasone - β-D-glucoside was poorly absorbed in the GI tract (bioavailability < 1%) and equal efficacy was reported in lower doses of prodrug compared to drug (Friend & Tozer, 1992). Leopard & Friend (1995) studied the poly-L-aspartic acid prodrug of dexamethasone, finding greater hydrolysis in cecum and colon contents than in small intestine (p<0.01), suitable for drug targeting.

10.3.6 Prodrug based lymphatic targeting

Orally administered drugs reach the systemic circulation via portal blood or intestinal lymphatics depending upon the properties of drug and formulation. The portal blood is major absorption pathway for most of the drugs but is exposed to first-pass metabolism. The intestinal lymphatics is a specialized absorption and transport pathway for highly lipophilic compounds requiring high lipophilicity (log p>5-6) and solubility in triglyceride lipids. Such compound associate with specific lipoproteins formed by the enterocyte in response to coadministered lipid and gain access to intestinal lymphatics ultimately joining the systemic circulation at the junction of left internal jugular and left subclavian vein, thereby bypassing the first pass metabolism. Thus targeting the lymphatics is useful for (i) drugs undergoing extensive first pass liver metabolism, and (ii) for local lymphatic delivery. Other advantages are reduction in local GI toxicity and achieving sustained delivery.

The prodrug strategies involve either simple lipophilic derivatization of compounds via simple ester or ether linkages or the design of 'functionally based' promoieties such that prodrug is likely to be involved in the formation of chylomicrons by the enterocyte.

10.3.6.1 Prodrug involving ester/ether linkage

The poor bioavailability of testosterone was improved from $3.6 \pm 2.5\%$ to $6.8 \pm 3.3\%$ on administration of its undecanoate salt (Tauber et al, 1986). Only the intramuscular injection of epitiostanol (EP), an antiestrogenic compound, was approved because first pass effect precludes its oral administration (Ichihashi et al, 1991a). The ether linked prodrug mepitiostane (MP) (chemically 17-substituted methoxycyclopentane) following oral administration showed clinical profile similar to i.m. administered EP, in terms of antiestrogenic activity (Ichihashi et al, 1991b). In a thoracic duct lymph fistulated rat model study, approximately 34% of orally administered (C14) MP was recovered in lymph while 90% was associated with chylomicron and VLDL fraction of lymph (Ichihashi et al, 1991b).

10.3.6.2 Functionally based prodrug

The ester prodrugs are subjected to metabolism, therefore functional approach was evolved to mimic the absorption process of lipid products. The orally administered triglycerides are enzymatically hydrolysed within intestinal lumen to produce monoglyceride, which is absorbed by enterocyte and resynthesized as triglyceride and intercalated into lipid core of lipoproteins. On this basis, prodrugs are prepared by conjugating the drug either with 1- or 2- monoglyceride. As they mimic triglycerides, therefore they are similarly absorbed preferentially into the intestinal lymphatics and transported to systemic circulation. L-DOPA, naproxen, LK-A & LK-903, chlorambucil are such drugs undergoing first-pass metabolism and glyceride prodrug formation successfully improved their oral bioavailability. The oral administration of L-DOPA shows only 0.19% intestinal lymphatic uptake while L-DOPA diglyceride prodrug showed 8.3% uptake as parent diglyceride and 14.9% as related glyceride, the plasma AUC values of L-DOPA were doubled (Garzon et al, 1986). Different glyceride derivatives of naproxen using different spacers were prepared by Sugihara & coworkers (1988a,b) and enhanced lymphatic uptake on using spacer was reported. The glyceride prodrugs of hypolipidaemic compounds LK-A and LK-903 showed presence in lymphatic of intact prodrug (Stella & Pochopin, 1992), predicting negligible hydrolysis in lymph. This proves the efficient prodrug based lymphatic targeting.

10.3.7 Antibody based targeting

Monoclonal antibodies have been the ideal way of targeting tumor cells, therefore two approaches utilizing monoclonal antibodies have been studied as a way of selectively activating a prodrug at the tumor site. These are antibody-drug conjugates and antibody directed enzyme prodrug therapy (ADEPT).

Antibody-drug conjugates or immunoconjugates are macromolecular prodrugs, formed by covalently linking cytotoxic agent to monoclonal antibodies reactive with tumor associated antigens. As shown in Fig

10.9, the immunoconjugate binds to specific cells leading to internalization of the conjugate and drug is cleaved from the antibody intracellularly (e.g. lysosomal degradation) (Garnett et el, 1985). The approach may be limited by heterogeneity in the expression of antigen by the cancer cells, inefficient internalization of the antigen-antibody complex and/or insufficient cleavage of the linker moiety to release the free drug. This was observed for methotrexate conjugate which was found to be less potent than unconjugated drug (Kanellos et al, 1985). The approach however meets the therapeutic potential in conditions that the conjugate is highly bound and accessible to the extracellular space, the conjugate is internalized slowly and is selectively cleaved in the intracellular space, and the released drug has low egress from the intracellular space. An immunoconjugate BR6-doxorubicin has fulfilled this criteria and is currently under clinical trials (Anonymous, 1995)

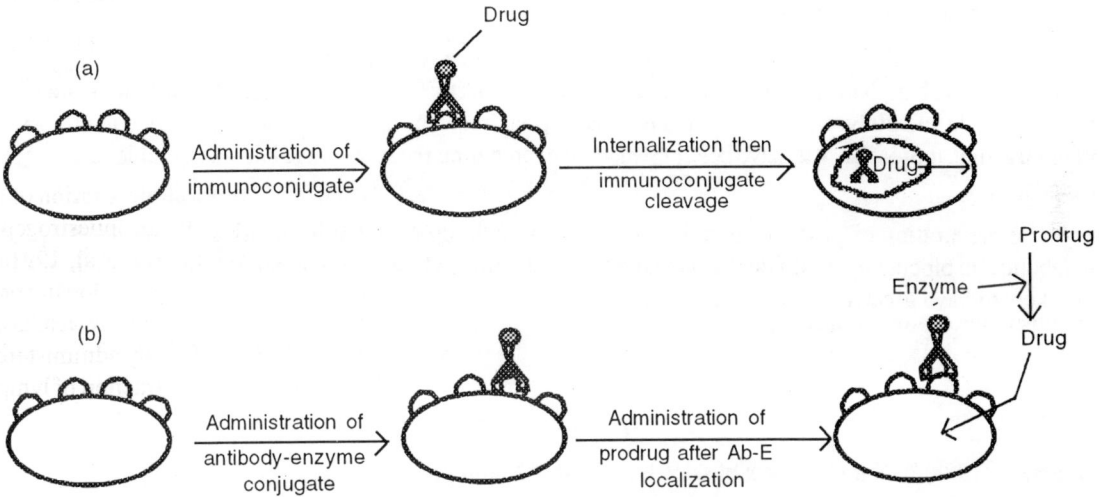

Fig 10.9 (a) Site selective delivery and activation of a monoclonal antibody-drug conjugate to a tumor cell. (b) Site selective activation of a prodrug at a tumor cell using the ADEPT approach (Kearney, 1995)

As shown in Fig 10. 6(b), the ADEPT approach involves administration of enzyme, that is covalently linked to a monoclonal antibody, which binds selectively to the respective tumor associated antigen. After the antibody-enzyme conjugate (Ab-E) has localized within the tumor and has been cleared from non-target sites, a prodrug, that is substrate for the enzyme, is administered. Upon contact with the targeted enzyme, the prodrug is converted to the drug at the tumor site (Bagshawe et al, 1994; Wallace & Senter, 1994; Springer & Niculescu-Duvaz, 1995).

An important consideration with this ADEPT approach is optimizing the time interval between administration of the Ab-E and the prodrug. To attain adequate tumor uptake, high plasma and extracellular fluid levels of the Ab-E should be maintained for several hours. Once adequate tumor levels are achieved (and prior to prodrug administration), sufficient time should be allowed for significant plasma clearance or inactivation of the non-tumor associated Ab-E to minimize prodrug activation at non-tumor sites. The approach is under clinical trials for proof of the concept (Bagshawe et al, 1991). A three-step approach is also being developed in which, Ab-E is administered first, then a galactosylated anti-Ab-E antibody is administered to remove non-tumor-associated circulating Ab-E and then the prodrug is administered (Sharma et al, 1991)

10.4 CONCLUSION

The transient modification of basic drug molecules by prodrug approach improves the physicochemical and biological properties and minimizes the number and magnitude of undesirable properties. As reviewed in this chapter, this fruitful approach has been successful in development of novel drug delivery system for drugs which were otherwise difficult to incorporate in the system. Covalent conjugation to polymeric micelles came up with manyfold advantages to solubilize the insoluble drug and also providing sustained release. Pharmacosomes bearing unique advantages over liposome and niosome vesicles have come up as potential alternative to conventional vesicles. The system yet requires greater efforts towards investigating the non-bilayer phases and exploring the mechanism of action. Furthermore, the effect of covalent linkages and addition of spacer group on rate of in-vivo hydrolysis and subsequent pharmacokinetics is to be exhaustively studied in order to exploit more advantages of this system.

The targeting through prodrug approach has been shown for some drugs yet it has to be extended to more drugs. The lymphatic targeting achieved by simple ester/ether linkage is usually not sufficient and hence monoglyceride and diglyceride derivatives have been prepared. The antibody based targeting combined with other targeting approaches will have better chances of overcoming the formidable barriers to achieving targeted drug delivery.

The preparation of prodrug should be followed by thorough screening for formulation development, metabolic and biochemical influences , hence integrated efforts which combine input from the different areas are likely to have greater chances of success.

REFERENCES

Albert, A. (1958) "Chemical aspect of selective toxicity." Nature, 182 : 421.

Agrawal, S.K.; Gogu, S.R.; Rangan, S.R.S. and Agrawal, S.C. (1990) "Synthesis and evaluation of prodrug of Zidovudine." J. Med. Chem., 33: 1505-1510.

Anonymous (1995) "Antibody based drugs for cancer (presented at ASCO meeting)" Scrip. Online, June5

Anwer, M.S.; Kroker, R and Hegner, D. (1976) "Cholic acid uptake into isolated rat hepatocytes." Hoppe-Seyler's Z. Physiol. Chem., 357 : 1477-1486.

Azad-Khan, A.K.; Piris, J. and Truelove, S.C. (1981) "An experiment to determine the active therapeutic moiety to sulphasalazine." Lancet, 2: 892-895.

Bagshawe, K.D.; Sharma., S.K.; Springer, C.J. and Rogers, G.T. (1994) "Antibody directed enzyme prodrug therapy (ADEPT)" Ann. Oncol., 5: 879-891.

Bagshawe, K.D.; Sharma., S.K.; Springer, C.J.; Antoniw, P.; Boden, J.A.; Rogers, G.T. ; Burke, P.J.; Melton, R.G. and Sherwood, R.F. (1991)" Antibody directed enzyme prodrug therapy (ADEPT): Clinical report" Dis Markers, 9: 233-238.

Bijsterbosch, M.K.; Schouten, D.; and Van Berkel, T.J.C. (1994) "Synthesis of dioleoyl derivative as iododeoxyuridine and its incorporation into reconstituted high density lipoprotein particles" Biochemistry, 33: 14073-14080.

Bodor, N.; Farag, H.H. and Brewster, M.E. (1981) "Site-specific, sustained release of drug to the brain" 214 : 1370-72.

Bodor, N. and Brewster, M. (1987) "Problems of delivery of drugs to the brain" Pharmacol. Ther., 19: 337-386.

Bolagopala, M.I.; Ollapally, A.P.; Lu, H.L. (1995) "Synthesis and anti-HIV activity of steroidal prodrugs of 3'azido-3'deoxythymidine (AZT)" Cell Mol. Biol.,41 (Suppl 1): S1-S7.

Crosasso, P.; Brusa, P.; Dosio, F.; Arpicco, S.; Pacchioni, D.; Schuber, F. and Cattel, L. (1997) "Antitumoral activity of liposomes and immunoliposomes containing 5-fluorouridine prodrugs" J. Pharm. Sci., 86(7): 832.

Curatolo, W. (1987) Pharm. Res., 4(4): 271.

DeClercq, E. (1995) "Antiviral therapy for human immunodeficiency virus infections." Clin. Microbiol. 8:200-239.

Dellamonica, P. (1994) " Cefuroxime axetil" Int. J. Antimicro. Agent., 4 : 23-36.

Earnshaw, D.L.; bacon, T.H.; Darlison, S.J.; Edmonds, K.; Perkins, R.M. and Ver Elion, G.B., Furman, P.A.; Fyfe, J.A.; De Miranda, P.; Beauchamp, L. and Schaeffer, H.J. (1977) "Selectivity of action of an antiherpetic agent, 9-(2-hydroxyehoxymethyl) guanine" Proc. Natl. Acad. Sci. USA, 74: 5716-5720.

Friedman, G. (1989) "New steroid preparations" In: Baylers, T.M. (ed) Current management of inflammatory bowel disease, D.C. Decker, Burlington, Ontario, 56-57.

Friend, D.R. and Chang, G.W. (1984) "A colon-specific drug-delivery system based on drug glycosides and the glycosidases of colonic bacteria" J. Med. Chem., 27: 261-266.

Friend, D.R. and Chang, G.W. (1985) "Drug glycosides: Potential prodrugs for colon-specific drug delivery" J. Med. Chem., 28: 51-57.

Friend, D.R. and Tozer, T.N. (1992) "Drug glycosides in colon-specific drug delivery" J. Cont. Rel., 19: 109-120.

Garnett, M.C.; Embleton, M.J.; Jacobs, E. and Baldwin, R.W. (1985) "Studies on mechanism of action of an antibody targeted drug carrier conjugate" Anti-cancer Drug Res., 1: 3-12.

Garzon-Abureh, A.; Poupaert, J.H.; Claesen, M. and Dumont, D. (1986) "A lymphotropic prodrug of L-DOPA: Synthesis, pharmacological properties and pharmacokinetic behavior of 1,3-dihexa-decanoyl-2-[(S)-2-amino-3-(3,4- dihydroxyphenyl) propanoyl] propane-1,2,3 triol" J. med. Chem., 29: 687-691.

Goundalkar,A and Mezei, M. (1984) "Chemical modification of triamcinolone acetonide to improve liposomal encapsulation" J. Pharm. Sci., 73: 834-835.

Haerberlin, B.; Rubas, W.; Nolen, H.W. and Friend, D.R. (1993) "*In-vitro* evaluation of dexamethasone-β-D-glucuronide for colon specific drug delivery." Pharm. Res., 10: 1553-1562.

Halbert, G.W.; Stuart, J.F.B. and Florence, A.T. (1984) "The incorporation of lipid-soluble antineoplastic agents into microemulsions -protein-free analogues of low density proteins." Int. J. Phar., 21: 219-232.

Halbert, G.W.; Stuart, J.F.B. and Florence, A.T. (1985) "A low density lipoprotein methotrexate covalent complex and its activity against L1210 cells in-vitro", Cancer Chemother. Pharmacol., 15: 223-227.

Heitai, H.; Tawashi, R.; Shivers, R.R. and Phillips, N.C. (1997) " Solid lipid nanoparticles as drug carriers I. Incorporation and retention of the lipophilic prodrug 3'-azo-3'-deoxythymidine palmitate" Int. J. Pharm., 146: 123-131.

Hervest, R.L. (1994) "Discovery and characterization of famciclovir (Famvirä), a novel anti-herpesvirus agent" Drugs Today, 30: 575-588.

Herbert, S. and Schwandender, R.A. (1996) "Synthesis of liposomal phospholipid - (N4 palmitoyl 1-β-D-arabinofuranosylcytosine) conjugate and evaluation of their activity against L1210 murine lukaemia." Leibig Ann, 3: 365-9.

Hodge, R.A. (1992) "Mode of antiviral action of penciclovir in MRC-5 cells infected with herpes simplex virus type 1(HSV-1), HSV-2, and varicella-zoster virus." Animicrob. Agents Chemother., 36: 2747-2757.

Ichihashi, T.; Kinoshita,H.; Shimamura, K and Yamada, H. (1991a) "Absorption and disposition of epithiosteroids in rats (1): Route of administration and plasma levels of epitiostanol." Xenobiotica, 21: 865-872.

Ichihashi, T.; Kinoshita,H. and Yamada, H. (1991b) "Absorption and disposition of epithiosteroids in rats (2): Avoidance of first-pass metabolism by lymphatic absorption" Xenobiotica, 21: 873-880.

Ishikura, T.; Senou, T.; Ishihara, H.; Kato, T. and Ito, T. (1995) Drug delivery to the brain. DOPA prodrugs based on a ring closure reaction to quaternary thiazolium compounds. Int. J. Pharm., 116 : 51-63.

Iwamoto, K.; Kato, T.; Kawahara, M.; Koyama, N.; Watanabe, S.; Miyake, Y. and Sunamoto, J. (1991) " Polysaccharide-coated oil droplets in oil-in-water emulsions as targetable carriers for lipophilic drugs." J. Pharm. Sci., 80:219-224.

Jewel, D.P. and Truelove, S.C. (1981) "Disodium azodisalicylatein ulcerative colitis" Lancet, 2: 1168-1169.

Jorge, J.C.S.; Perez-Soler, R.; Morais, J.G. and Cruz, M.F.M. (1994) "Liposomal palmitoyl-L-asparaginase: Characterization and biological activity" Cancer Chemother. Pharmacol., 34(3): 230-234.

Kaiser, R.(1990) Dissertation, ETH Zurich.

Kanellos, J.; Pietersz, G.A.; McKenzie, I.F.C. (1985) "Studies of methotrexate-monoclonal antibody conjugates for immunotherapy" J. Natl. Cancer Inst., 75: 319-332.

Kawaguchi, T.; Saito, M.; Suzuki, Y.; Nambu, N.; Nagai, T. (1985) Chem. Pharm. Bull. 33: 1652-1659.

Kearney, A.S. (1996) "Prodrugs and targeted drug delivery." Adv. Drug Del. Rev. 19:225-239.

Koenig, S.; Gendelman, H.E.; Orenstein, J.M.; Dalcanto, M.C.; Pezeshkpour, G.H.; Yangbluth, M.; Janotta, F.; Aksamit, A.; Martin, M.A. and Fauci, A.S. (1986) "Detection of AIDS virus in macrophages in brain tumor tissues from AIDS patients with encephalopathy." Science, 233: 1089-1093.

Kramer,W.; Wess, G.; Schubert,G.; Bickel, M.; Girbig, F.; Gutjahr, U.; Kowalewski, S.; Baringhaus,K.H.; Enhsen, A.; Glombik, H.; Mullner, S.; Neckermann, G.; Schulz, S. and Petzinger, E. (1992) Liver-specific drug targeting by coupling to bile acids. J. Biol. Chem., 267 : 18598-18604.

Kupchean, S.M.; Cosy, A.E. and Swintosky, J.V. (1965) "Synthesis and preliminary evaluation of testosterone derivative." J. Pharm. Sci., 54 : 515.

Leopard, C.S. and Friend, D.R. (1995) "In-vitro study for the assessment of poly (L-aspartic acid) as a drug carrier for colon specific drug delivery" J. Pharm. Sci., 126: 139-145.

Lundberg, B. (1994) "The solubilization of lipophilic derivatives of podophyllotoxins in sub-micron sized lipid emulsions and their cytotoxic activity against cancer cells in culture" int. J. Pharm., 109: 73-81.

MacCoss, M.; Edwards, J.J.; Seed, T.M. and Spragg, P. (1982) "Phospholipid nucleoside conjugates: the aggregation characteristics and morphological aspects of selected 1-β-D-arabinofuranosylcytosine-5'diphosphate-L-1,2-diacylglycerol" Biochim. Biophys. Acta., 719: 544-555.

MacCoss, M.; Edwards, J.J.; Lagocki, P. and Rahman, Y.E. (1983) "Phospholipid nucleoside conjugates.5. The interaction of selected selected 1-b-D-arabinofuranosylcytosine-5'diphosphate-L-1,2-diacylglycerol with serum lipoproteins" Biochim. Biophys. Res. Commun., 116: 368-374.

Mantelli, S.; Speiser, P. and Hauser, H. (1985) "Phase behavior of a diglyceride prodrug: Spontaneous formation of unilamellar vesicles." Chem. Phys. Lipids, 37: 329-43.

Margolis, S. and Langdon, D.G. (1966) "Studies on human serum β-lipoprotein s III enzymatic modifications" J. Biol. Chem., 241: 485-493.

Masquelier, M.; Vitols, S. and Peterson, C. (1986) "Low density lipoproteins (LDL) as a carrier of antitumour drugs: in-vivo fate of drug LDL complexes in mice" Cancer Res., 46: 3842-3847.

Matsumura, Y. and Maeda, H. (1986) "A new concept for macromolecular therapeutics in cancer chemo-therapy: mechanism of tumoritropic acuumulation of proteins and the antitumor agent." Smanc:-Cancer Res., 46: 6387-6392.

McGuigan , S.R.; Nicholl, S.R.; O'Connor, T.J. and Kinchington, D. (1990) "Synthesis of some novel dialkylphosphate derivatives of 3'-modified nucleosides as potential anti-AIDS drugs." Antiviral Chem. Chemother., 1: 355-360.

McGuigan, C.; pathirana, R.N.; Balzarini, E. and DeClercq, E. (1993) "Intracellular delivery of bioactive AZT nucleotides by aryl phosphate derivatives of AZT." J. Med. Chem., 36: 1048-1052.

Monard-Herket, G.; Teissier-Morier, F. et al (1993) "Modification of lipophilic prodrugs of ametantrone and mitoxantrone (DHAQ) inside LDL and selective uptake of prodrug LDL complex via receptor pathway" Acta. Ther., 19(4): 317-335.

Murtha, J.L. and Ando, H.Y. (1994) " Synthesis of cholesteryl ester prodrugs cholesteryl ibuprofen and cholesteryl flufenamate and their formulation into phospholipid microemulsion." J. Pharm. Sci., 83(9): 1222-1228.

Namdeo, A. and Jain, N.K. (2000) "Spontaneous vesiculation from dry granular propharmacosome containing propranolol hydrochloride." Fourth national conference of chemist and biologist, Lucknow, 23.

Nolen, H.W. and Friend, D.R. (1994) "Menthol-β-D-glucuronide: A potential prodrug for treatment of the irritable bowel syndrome" Pharm. Res., 11: 1707-1711.

Ohya, Y.; Hirai, K. and Ouchi, T. (1992) "Cell specific anticancer drug delivery using poly(α-malic acid) saccharide conjugate." Int. Sym. Cont. Rel. Bioact. Mater., 19: 68-69.

Ozaki, S.; Akiyama, T.; Ike, Y.; Mori, H. and Hoshi, A. (1989) "5-Fluorouracil derivatives XVII. Synthesis and antitumor activity of 5'-O-acyl-5-fluorouridines." Chem. Pharm. Bull., 37: 3405-3408.

Peppercorn, M.A. and Goldman, P. (1973) " Distribution studies of salicylazopyridine and its metabolites" Gastroenterology, 64: 240-245.

Piantadosi, C.J.; Marasco, C.J.; Moris-Natschke,S.L.; Meyer, R.L.; Gumus, F.; Surles, J.R.; Ishaq, K.S.; Kucera, L.S.; Iyer, C.A.; Wallen, S. and Piantadosi, S. (1991) "Synthesis and evaluation of novel ether lipid nucleoside conjugates for anti-HIV-1 activity." J. Med. Res., 34:1408-1414.

Pimm, M.V.; Perkins, A.C.; Strohalm, J.; Ulbrich, K. and Duncan, R. (1996) "Gamma scintigraphy of biodistribution of ^{123}I-labelled N-(2-hydroxypropyl) methacrylamide copolymer-doxorubicin conjugates in mice with transplanted melanoma and mammary carcinoma." J. Drug Targeting, 3:375-383.

Pop, E.; Brewster, M.E. and Bodor, N. (1991) "Site-specific delivery of the central nervous system containing amines." 16 : 919-944.

Schaeffer, H.J.; Beauchamp,L.; de Miranda, P.;Elion, G.B.; Bauer, D.J. and Collins, P. (1978) "9-(2-hydroxyehoxymethyl)guanine activity against viruses of the herpes group." Nature, 272: 583-585.

Schouten, D.; Van der Kooji, M.; Muller, J.; Pieters, M.N.; Bijsterbosch, M.K. and Van Berkel, Th. J.C. (1993) Mol Pharmacol. 44: 486-492.

Schroder, H. and Campbell, D.E.S. (1972) "Absorption, metabolism and excretion of salicylazosulfapyridine in man" Clin. Pharmacol. Ther., 13: 539-551.

Schwarz, C.; mehnert, W., lucks, J.S. and muller, R.H. (1994) "Solid lipid nanoparticles (SLN) for controlled drug delivery. I. Production, characterization and sterilization." J. Cont. Rel., 30: 83-96.

Seymour, L.W.; Ulbrich, K.; Strohalm, J.; Kopecek, J. and Duncan, R. (1990) "the pharmacokinetics of polymer-bound adriamycin." Biochem. Pharmacol., 39: 1125-1131.

Sharma, P.D. (1986) "Prodrug approach in improving drug delivery" J. Sci. & Ind. Res., 45: 534-543.

Sharma, S.K.; Bagshawe, K.D.; Springer, C.J.; Burk, P.J.; Rogers, G.T.; Boden, J.A.; Antoniw, P.; Melton. R.G. and Sherwood, R.F. (1991) " Antibody directed enzyme prodrug therapy (ADEPT): A three phase system" Dis. Markers, 9: 225-231.

Shaw, J.H.; Knight, C.G. and Dingle, J.T. (1976) "Liposomal retention of a modified anti-inflammatory steroid" Biochem. J., 158: 437-476.

Singh, M. and Revin, L.J. (1986) "parenteral emulsions as drug carrier systems." J. Parenter. Sci. Technol. 40:34-41.

Sinkula, A.A. and Yalkowski, S.H. (1975) "Rational for design of biologically reversible drug derivatives: Prodrugs" J. Pharm. Sci., 64(2): 181-209.

Springer, C.J. and Niculescu-Duvaz, I. (1995) "Antibody directed enzyme prodrug therapy (ADEPT) with mustard prodrugs." Anti-cancer Drug Design, 10: 361-372.

Steim, J.M.; Neto, C.C.; Sarin, P.S.; Sun, D.K.; Sehgal, R.K. and Turcotte, J.G. (1990) "Lipid conjugate of antiretroviral agent. I. Azidothymidine-monophosphate diglycerideanti-HIV activity, physical properties and interactions with plasma proteins." Biochim. Biopys. Res. Comm., 171(1): 451.

Stella, V.J. (1996) "Preface" Adv. Drug Del. Rev., 19 : 111-114.

Stella, V.J. and Pochopin, N.L. (1992) "Lipophilic prodrugs and the promotion of intestinal lymphatic drug transport." In: **Charman, W.N. and Stella, V.J.** (Eds) Lymphatic transport of drugs, CRC Press, Boca Raton, FL, pp 182-219.

Stephan, Z.F.; Yurachek, E.C.; Sharif, R.; Wasvary, J.M.; Steele, R.E. and Howes, C. (1992) "Reduction of cardiovascular and thyroxine-suppressing activities of L-T3 by liver targeting with cholic acid." Biochem. Pharmacol., 43 : 1969-1974.

Steve, A. (1996) "Lipophilic drug derivatives for use in liposomes." U.S. patent US S,534, 499 (Cl S14-25, A61K31/70), 9 july 1996, p11.

Sugihara, J.; Furuuchi, S.; Nakano, K. and Harigaya, S. (1988a) "Studies on the intestinal lymphatic absorption of drugs: I. Lymphatic absorption of alkyl ester derivatives and μ-monoglyceride derivatives of drugs." J. Pharmacobio-Dyn., 11: 369-376.

Sugihara, J.; Furuuchi, S.; Ando, H.; Takashima, H. and Harigaya, S. (1988b) "Studies on the intestinal lymphatic absorption of drugs: II. Glyceride prodrugs for improving the lymphatic absorption of naproxen and nicotinic acid." J. Pharmacobio-Dyn., 11: 555-562.

Taneja, D; Namdeo, A.; Mishra, P.R.; Khopade, A.J. and Jain, N.K. (2000) "High entrapment liposomes bearing 6-mercaptopurine- A prodrug approach" Drug. Dev. Ind. Pharm. (In press)

Taskintuna, I.; Banker, A.S.; Flores-Aguilar, M.; Lynn, B.G.; Alden, K.A.; Hostetler, K. Y. and Freeman, W.R. (1997) "Evaluation of a novel lipid prodrug for intraocular drug delivery: effect of acyclovir diphosphate dimyristoylglycerol in a rabbit model with herpes-simplex virus-21 retinitis" Retina, 17(1): 57-64.

Tauber, U.; Schroder, K.; Dusterberg, B. and Matthes, H. (1986) "Absolute bioavailability of testosterone after oral administration of testosterone-undecanoate and testosterone" Eur. J. Drug Metab. Pharmacokinet., 11:145-149.

Transmontano, R.J. (1993) Dissertation, ETH Zurich, 1993

Trouet, A.; Masqualier, M.; Baurain, R. and Deprez-de Campenecre, D. (1972) "A covalent linkage between desmopressin and protein that is stable in serum and reversible by lysosomal hydrolases, as required for a lysosomotropic drug-carrier conjugate: in-vitro and in-vivo studies." Proc. Natl. Acad. Sci. USA, 79: 626-629.

Tsuzuki,N.; Hama, T.; Kawada, M.; Haui, A.; Kanishi, R.; Shiwa, S.; Ochi, Y.; Futaki, S. and kitagawa, L. (1994) "Adamantane as a brain-directed drug carrier for poorly absorbed drugs. 2. AZT derivatives conjugated with the 1-adamantane moiety." J. Pharm. Sci., 83: 481-484.

Turcotte, J.G.; Srivastava, S.P.; Steim, J.M.; Calabresi, P.; Tibbetts, L.M. and Chu, M.Y. (1980) "Cytotoxic liponuclotide analog, II Antitumor activity of CDP-diacylglycerol analogs containing the cytosine arabinoside moiety." Biochim. Biophys. Acta, 619: 619-31.

Uchegbu, J.F. and Duncan, R. (1997) "Niosomes containing N-(2-hydroxypropyl) methacrylamide copolymer-doxorubicin (PK1): Effect of method of preparation and choice of surfactant on niosomes characterization and a preliminary study of body distribution" Int. J. Pharm., 155: 7-17.

Vaizoglu, O. and Speiser, P.P. (1986) "Pharmacosomes- A novel drug delivery system." Acta. Pharma Suec., 23: 163.

Van Brossum Waalkers,M. and Scerpoff,G.L. (1990) Sel. Cancer Ther. 6: 15-22.

Vasey, P.A.; Duncan, R.; Kaye, S.B. and Cassidy, J. (1996) "Clinical phase I trial of PK1 (HPMAcoplymer doxorubicin)" Eur. J. Cancer, 31A (suppl5): S 193.

Versluis, A.J.; Rensen, P.C.; Rimp, E.T.; Van Berkel, T.J.; Bijsterbosch, M.K. (1998) "Low-density lipoprotein receptor mediated delivery of a lipophilic daunorubicin derivatives to B16 tumors in mice using apoliopoprotein E enriched liposomes" Br. J. Cancer, 78(12): 1607-14.

Wall, D.A.; Wilson, G. and Hubbard, A.L. (1980) " The galactose specific recognition system of mammalian liver: the route of ligand internalization in rat hepatocyte"Cell, 21 : 79-93.

Wallace, P.M. and Senter, P.D. (1994) "Selective activation of anticancer prodrugs by monoclonal antibody enzyme conjugate" Methods Find. Exp. Clin. Makromol., 16: 505-512.

Wilk, S.; Mizoguchi, H. and Orlowski,M. (1978) "γ-glutamyl dopa: A kidney specific dopamine precursor" J. Pharmacol. Exp. Ther., 206 : 227-232.

Wilk, S.; Mizoguchi, H. and Orlowski,M. (1980) "N-acyl-γ-glutamyl derivatives of sulfamethoxazole as models of kidney selective prodrugs" J. Pharmacol. Exp. Ther, 212 : 167-172.

Yang, C.M.V.; Turcotts, G..J. and Stem, J.M. (1982) Biochim. Biophys. Acta, 689: 375.

Yarcohan, S. and Broder, S. (1987) "Development of an antiretroviral therapy for acquired immunodeficiency syndrome and ralative disorder: A progress report." N. Engl. J. Med., 316: 557-564.

Yokoyama, M.; Miyauchi, M.; Yamada, N.; Okano, T.; Sakurai, Y.; kataoka, K. and Inoue, S. (1990a) "Polymer micelles as novel drug carrier: Adriamycin-conjugated poly (ethylene glycol)-poly (aspartic acid) block copolymer" J. Cont. Rel., 11: 269-278.

Yokoyama, M.; Miyauchi, M.; Yamada, N.; Okano, T.; Sakurai, Y.; kataoka, K. and Inoue, S. (1990b) "Characterization and anticancer activity of the micelle forming polymeric anticancer drug adriamycin conjugated poly (ethylene glycol)- Poly (aspartic acid) block copolymer." Cancer Research, 50: 1693-1700.

Zalipsky, S. (1995) "Chemistry of polyethylene glycol conjugates with biologically active molecules" Adv. Drug Del. Rev., 16: 157-182.

Chapter 11

Ion-Exchange Resinates As Controlled Release Drug Delivery Systems

M. Vimala Devi, P.S.S. Krishna Babu

11.1. INTRODUCTION

Controlled release drug delivery systems are gaining momentum in the recent two decades, as the rate of delivery of drug, intensity and duration of action have been the subject of increasing multidisciplinary research. Since three decades after the appearance of spansule, a new era has started in modern therapeutics. One of the attractive methods for modified drug delivery systems preferably controlled type is ion-exchange resins as carriers for such systems. As drug release characteristics rely on the ionic environment of the resin-containing drug, they are less susceptible to environmental conditions, such as enzyme content, pH at the site of absorption. These systems can satisfactorily be achieved for zero-order release kinetics in drug delivery pattern. It is more promising for future developments in this field with ionic polymers as drug carriers in controlled delivery. Ion-exchange resins have specific properties like available capacity, acid base strength, particle size, porosity and swelling, on which, the release characteristics of drug resinates are dependent. The large pore size, the enormous surface area, the number of exchange sites and their hydrophilic nature are the favourable characteristics, that make the drug and ion-exchange complexes as superior materials for processing certain macromolecules e.g. dextran, polyacrylamide ion-exchange gels. In these favourable surroundings, macromolecules have little tendency to become destructured. Drug resinates are prepared in general, with purified resins and appropriate drugs.

11.2. ADVANTAGES AND LIMITATIONS

Ion-exchange systems are advantageous for drugs that are highly susceptible to degradation by enzymatic processes, since they offer a protective mechanism by temporarily altering the substrate. This approach to sustained release, however has the limitation that the release rate is proportional to the concentration of the ions present in the area of administration. Although the ionic concentration of the GI tract remains rather constant with limits, the release rate of drug can be affected by variability in diet, water intake and individual intestinal content (Jantzen & Robinson, 1996).

11.3. TYPES OF ION-EXCHANGE RESINS

There are two major classes of ion-exchange polymers: cation-exchangers, whose functional groups can undergo reaction with the cations of a surrounding solution; and anion-exchangers, whose functional groups can undergo reaction with the anions of a surrounding solution (Khym, 1974).

A typical cation-exchange resin is prepared by the copolymerization of styrene (I) and divinylbenzene (II) shown in Fig 11.1. During the polymerization reaction, linear chains of polystyrene are formed first and these in turn become covalently bonded to each other, at intermittent point, by divinylbenzene cross links; the result is a

Fig 11.1 : Structure of styrene (I) and divinylbenzene (II)

three-dimensional insoluble hydrocarbon network. If sulfuric acid is then allowed to react with this copolymer, sulfonic acid groups ($-SO_3^-H^+$) are introduced into most of the benzene rings of the styrene-divinylbenzene polymer, and the final substance formed is a cation-exchange resin whose structure is given in Fig 11.2.

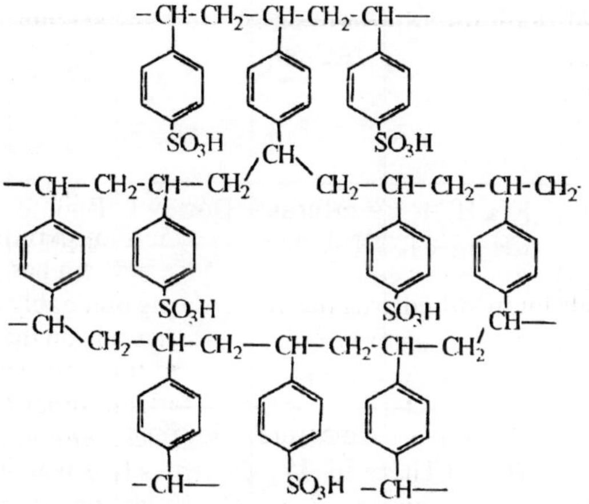

Fig 11.2 : A cation - exchange resin

A typical anion-exchange resin is prepared by first chloromethylating the benzene rings of the three-dimensional styrene-divinylbenzene copolymer to attach $-CH_2Cl$ groups and then causing these to react with a tertiary amine, such as trimethylamine. This gives the chloride salt of a strong-base exchanger, which has the structure given in Fig 11.3.

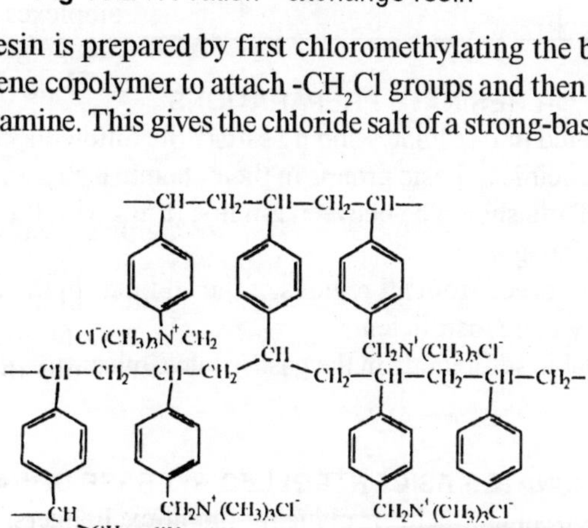

Fig 11.3 : A anion - exchange resin

Trade names and manufacturers of the most common commercially available ion-exchange resins (Khym, 1974) are given in Table 11.1.

Table 11.1: Trade names and manufacturers of the Ion-exchange resins

Resin type	Chemical constitution	Usual form as purchased	Trade names of equivalent ion-exchangers					
Strongly acidic cation-exchanger	Sulfonic acid groups attached to a styrene and divinylbenzene copolymer	ϕ-$SO_3^-H^+$	Amberlite IR-120	Dowex 50W	Duolite C-20	Lewatit S-100	Ionac C-240 (or Permutit Q)	Zeocarb 225
Weakly acidic cation-exchanger	Carboxylic acid groups attached to an acrylic and divinylbenzene copolymer	R-COO^-Na^+	Amberlite IRC-50		Duolite CC-3	Lewatit C	Ionac C-270 (or Permutit Q-210)	Zeocarb 226
Strongly basic anion-exchanger	Quaternary ammonium groups attached to a styrene and divinylbenzene copolymer	$[\phi$-CH_2N-$(CH_3)_3]^+Cl^-$	Amberlite IRA-400	Dowex 1	Duolite A-101D	Lewatit M-500	Ionac A-450 (or Permutit S-1)	Zeocarb FF (or De-Acidite FF
Weakly basic anion-exchanger	Polyalkylamine groups attached to a styrene and divinylbenzene copolymer	$[\phi$-NH-$(R)_2]^+Cl^-$	Amberlite IR-45	Dowex 3	Duolite A-7	Lewatit MP-60	Ionac A-315 (or Permutit W)	Zeocarb G

11.4. DRUGS SUITABLE FOR RESINATE PREPARATIONS
Drugs that are to be formulated into resinates should satisfy the following conditions:
1) Drugs should have acidic or basic groups in their chemical structure.
2) The biological half-life should be between 2-6 hrs; drugs with $t^{1/2} < 1$ hr or > 8 hrs are difficult to formulate into this category
3) The drug is to be absorbed from all regions of the GI tract. In the case of limited absorption zone, the bioavailability will be insufficient
4) Drugs should be stable sufficiently in the gastric juice, otherwise, their therapeutic effectiveness will drop drastically.

11.5 RATIONALE FOR RESINATES AS CONTROLLED RELEASE DOSAGE FORMS
Ion-exchange resinates of drugs can help in reducing the dose. Reduced fluctuations in blood and tissue concentrations, fewer administrations and maintenance of drug concentration below toxic level can be achieved. Resinate formulations offer an additional advantage that certain factors influencing the rate of release of drugs from ion-exchange matrixes, such as competing ions, ionic strength, pH etc. are relatively fixed by the conditions within the GI tract. By proper choice of resin characteristics such as acid or base strength, porosity, degree of cross-linkage and particle size can help to accomplish the intended purpose. However, there are quite a few negative factors associated viz., drug accumulation, if the rate of excretion and release are not balanced. In addition, long acting preparation may not be suitable when short time treatment is needed.

11.6. MECHANISM AND PRINCIPLE

Anion-exchange resins involve basic functional groups (usually a polyamine) capable of removing anions from acidic solutions. Cation-exchange resins contain acidic functional groups. Although their exact composition may vary, they usually contain polystyrene polymers with either sulfonic, carboxylic or phenolic groups.

The use of ion-exchange resins to prolong the effect of drugs is based on the principle that positively or negatively charged pharmaceuticals, combined with appropriate resins yield insoluble polysalt resinates.

$$R - SO_3^- \, H^+ + H_2N - A \Leftrightarrow R - SO_3^- \, - H_3N\text{-}A$$

$$R - N^+H_3OH^- + HOOC - B \Leftrightarrow R - N^+H_3 \, - OOC\text{-}B + H_2O$$

Where $H_2N - A$ and $HOOC - B$ represent a basic and acidic drug respectively and $R\text{-}SO_3^- \, H^+$ and $R\text{-}NH_3^+OH^-$ represent cationic- and anionic-exchange resins respectively. The slow release of drugs from ion-exchange resins was recognised by Saunders and Srivastava (1980) as a suitable approach to the design of sustained release preparations. Ion-exchange resinates administered orally are likely to spend about two hours in the stomach in contact with an acidic fluid of pH 1.2, and then move into the intestine where they will be in contact for more than six hours with a fluid of slightly alkaline pH.

In the stomach:

$$R\text{-}SO_3^- \, H_3N^+ - A + HCl \Leftrightarrow R\text{-}SO_3^- \, H^+ + A\text{-}N^+H_3Cl^-$$

$$R\text{-}N^+H_3 \, {}^-OOC\text{-}B + HCl \Leftrightarrow R\text{-}N^+H_3Cl^- + B\text{-}COOH.$$

In the intestine:

$$R\text{-}SO_3^- \, H_3N^+ - A + NaCl \Leftrightarrow R\text{-}SO_3^- \, Na^+ + A\text{-}N^+H_3Cl^-$$

$$R\text{-}N^+H_3 \, {}^-OOC\text{-}B + NaCl \Leftrightarrow R\text{-}N^+H_3Cl^- + B\text{-}COO^-Na^+$$

11.7. SOME IMPORTANT PROPERTIES OF ION-EXCHANGE RESINS

1) **Particle size and form:** The rate of ion-exchange reactions depends on the size of the resin particles. Decreasing the size of resin particle significantly decreases the time required for the reaction to reach equilibrium with the surrounding medium. (Boyd, et al., 1947; Helfferion, 1962). Most of the ion-exchange resins are sold in the form of spherical beads. When the beads are immersed in water, they imbibe a limited amount of liquid to form a homogenous gel like structure (Tompkins & Mayer, 1947; Schubert, 1956). A cross-section of a single cation-exchange bead is schematically illustrated in Fig 11.3.

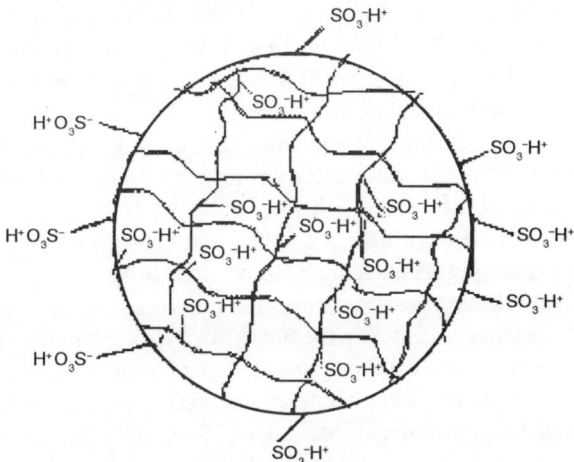

Fig. 11.3: Cation-exchange resin schematic (Reproduced from Wheaton, R.M. & Seamster, A.H., 1966).

The wavy lines represent the hydrocarbons network – the solid, insoluble, organic part of the exchanger to which the ionizable sulfonic acid groups (-H⁺) are attached. The hydrogen ions (H^+) of his group are completely dissociated in the imbibed water and are free to diffuse throughout the entire resin bead and hence can be exchanged for an equivalent amount of ions of like charge upon contact of the resin bead with a given solution.

2) **Porosity and Swelling:** Porosity is defined as the ratio of the volume of the material to its mass. The limiting size of ions, which can penetrate into a resin matrix depends strongly on the porosity. The porosity of an ion-exchanger depends not only on the amount of cross-linking substance used in polymerization but mainly on polymerization procedures (Seidl, et. al., 1967). The structural parameters considerably influence the swelling behaviour of the resin and consequently have a marked effect on the release characteristics of drug resinates. The amount of swelling is directly proportional to the number of hydrophilic functional groups attached to the polymer matrix and is inversely proportional to the degree of divinylbenzene cross-linking present in the resin.

3) **Cross-linkage:** The percentage of cross-linking affects the purely physical structure of the resin particles. Resins with a low degree of cross-linking can take up a considerable amount of water and swell into a structure that is soft and gelatinous. However, resins with a high divinylbenzene content swell very little, these particles take up only a small amount of water and consequently are somewhat hard and brittle (Dower, 1964).

4) **Available capacity:** The capacity of an ion-exchanger is a quantitative measure of its ability to take up exchangeable counter-ions and is therefore of major importance. However, in the preparation of drug resinates, the actual capacity obtained under specific experimental conditions depends on the accessibility of the functional groups for the drug of interest.

5) **Acid base strength:** The acid or base strength of an exchanger is dependent on the various ionogenic groups, incorporated into the resin (Helfferion, 1962). Resin containing sulfonic, phosphonic or carboxylic acid exchange groups have approximate pKa values of < 1, 2-3 and 4-6, respectively. Anionic-exchangers are quarternary, tertiary, or secondary ammonium groups having apparent pK_a values of >13, 7-9, or 5-9, respectively. The pK_a value of the resin will have a significant influence on the rate at which the drug will be released from resinate in the gastric fluids.

6) **Selectivity of the resins for the counter-ion:** Resin selectivity is attributed to many factors. Since ion-exchange involves electrostatic forces, selectivity at first glance should depend mainly on the relative change and the ionic radius of the (hydrated) ions competing for an exchange site (Kitchener, 1957; Kunin, 1958; Helfferion, 1962; Berg, 1963; Samuelson, 1963). Factors other than size and charge also contribute to the selection by an ion-exchange resin of one counter ion in preference to another. The extent of sorption increases with (i) the counter ion that, in addition to forming a normal ionic bond with the functional group of an exchanger, also interacts through the influence of Van der Walls forces with the resin matrix. (ii) the counter ion least affected by complex formation with its co-ion or non-exchanging ion, (iii) the counter ion that induces the greater polarization. These factors, together with the effect of the size and charge of an ion in exhibiting certain selectivity toward a resin, are at best only general rules, and as a consequence there are many exceptions to them.

7) **Stability:** The resinous ion-exchangers are remarkably inert substances. At ordinary temperature and excluding the more potent oxidising agents, vinylbenzene cross-linked resins are resistant to decomposition through chemical attack. Nevertheless, these materials are indestructible. Another limitation of these resins is their degradation and degeneration in the presence of strong gamma ray sources.

8) **Purity and Toxicity:** Since drug resin combinations contain 60% or more of the resin, it is necessary to establish toxicity of the ion-exchange resins. Commercial products cannot be used as such because they contain impurities that cause severe toxicity (Shtannikov, 1966; Makrinov, et al., 1968). Therefore careful purification of the resin prior to treatment with the drug is required.

11.8. GENERAL PREPARATION OF DRUG RESINATES

The foremost step in the preparation of drug resinates is to purify the resins carefully. Purification is generally done by cycling repeatedly between the sodium and hydrogen forms with a cation-exchanger or between the chloride and hydroxide forms in the case of anionic-exchanger. After thoroughly washing with water and subsequent air drying, the resin is sieved to get a series of fractions.

Loading of drugs: Loading of drugs is done by two ways.

a) **Column process:** A highly concentrated drug solution is eluted through a bed or column of the resin, until equilibrium is established.

b) **Batch process:** The resin particles are stirred with a large volume of concentrated drug solution.

Subsequently the resin is to be washed to remove adhering free and un-associated drug and thereafter it is air-dried. Although both prepartion modes have often been used, only few reports provide comparison between them (Chaudhry & Saunders, 1956; Strasenburgh, 1959; Kanhere, et al, 1968; Borodkin & Saunders, 1971; Thoma & Schiefer, 1975).

11.9. DRUG RESINATE DOSAGE FORMS

The interest in the use of ion-exchange resins as carriers for drug resinates commenced in early 1950s. Since then, ample work was done and patents were reported with the preparation and evaluation of resinates for a large variety of drugs. A comprehensive list is shown in the appendix to this chapter.

Keating, (1955, 1956a&b, 1961, 1964) discussed the preparation and evaluation of combinations of carboxylic, sulfonic and phosphonic acid cation-exchange resins with a variety of amine drugs, such as adrenergics, antihistaminics, antispasmodics and antitussives.

The basic principles relating to the use of ion-exchange resins in the development of sustained action dosage forms was studied by Amsel et al., (1984). In vitro properties, pharmacokinetics and bioavailability of a suspension formulation containing codeine and chlorpheniramine were described.

Preparation and in vitro release of a sustained action Belladona alkaloids dosage form based on a cation-exchange resin was reported by Chaudhry & Rai, (1984). Sustained release systems of Dapsone were prepared by Yang & Swarbrick, (1986).

Preparation of microcapsules of nylon containing ion-exchange resins using an interfacial polycondensation procedure with fluoroscein sodium as the model drug was studied by Torres, et al., (1990).

Jani, et al (1994), developed a novel delivery system for ophthalmic drugs using an antiglaucoma agent betaxolol hydrochloride as a model. The new delivery system involved both the binding and release of drug from ion-exchange resin particles. The occular comfort of betaxolol was greatly enhanced by reducing the availability of free drug molecules in the precorneal tear film.

Sustained release system of diclofenac sodium using an anion-exchange resin (Dowex- X 200) was prepared and studied by Mohamed, (1996). Oral liquid controlled release systems of salbutamol with cation-exchange resins were prepared and studied by Li, et al (1997). From this study it was found that adsorptive capacity varies with pH and drug concentration. Counter ions in drug solution had significant influence on the adsorptive capacity, which decreased with the increase of salt ion concentration.

11.10. IMPROVED RESINATE FORMULATIONS

The duration of action of drug resin combinations has ocassionally been improved by coating of the resinate particles.

Nash & Crabtree (1961) demonstrated that resinates prepared from carboxylic acid type resin and d-desoxyephedrine, release the drug very fast on oral administration in dogs. However, dosage forms consisting of desoxyephedrine hydrochloride and cellulose acetophthalate-coated carboxylic resinates gave therapeutic plasma concentration levels after less than 1 hour which were maintained for more than 12 hrs. This combination was superior to uncoated sulfonic acid type resinates. Borodkin & Sundberg (1971) using mice and rats, reported that poly (methacrylic acid) type resinates of ephedrine, pseudoephedrin, methapyrilen, and dextromethaphan, showed a slower but complete drug availability and a higher LD_{50} value when coated with cellulose ethers in comparison to the uncoated tablets.

Ion-exchange drug resinates utilising microencapsulation technique were prepared by several workers (Motycka & Nairn, 1979; Smith, 1983; Sawaya et al., 1988; Chen et al., 1992; Torres et al., 1995a&b). Most of them coated the drugs with polymeric material after resinate formation to achieve controlled drug delivery.

Motyoka, et al (1979) prepared ion-exchange resin beads in the benzoate form and coated them by microencapsulation techniques to alter and improve characteristics. The release rate of the organic anion could be controlled over a wide range, depending on the encapsulating material characteristics.

Georgia & Price, (1989) carried out evaluation of sustained release aqueous suspensions containing microcapsulated resin complexes. Chlorpheniramine-maleate, diphenydramine hydrochloride and pseudoephedrine hydrochloride resin complexes were microencapsulated and studied to determine the effects of hydration of the coating, resin type, drug type, size of the capsule, ageing, and temperature, on drug release.

Torres, et al., (1995a) prepared hydroxy propyl methyl cellulose phthalate microcapsules containing complexes of diclofenac sodium and ion-exchange resins were also prepared with various surfactants and the microcapsules were characterized in vitro. Both, the degree of cross-linking, and the presence of polymer coating significantly retarded drug release, indicating that the type of surfactant had little effect on the release rate.

11.11. EVALUATION OF DRUG RESINATES

11.11.1 In vitro tests

The *in vitro* tests demonstrate the release pattern of a drug from a resinate preparation dosage form which depends on:
i)   size of resinate,
ii)   degree of crosslinkage,
iii) ionogenic groups of the resins,
iv)   nature of the drug,
v)   the test conditions e.g., ionic strength of the dissolution medium.

A variety of methods are described for drug resinates evaluation by *in vitro* dissolution testing (Lazarus & Cooper 1959, 1961, Hersey, 1969, Sjogren, 1971; Barr et al., 1972). However, commonly employed methods to test drug resinates include the on-column and the batch exposure of the resinates to simulated gastric juice and intestinal fluids. But, both methods differ in their boundry conditions. Batch experiments are carried out with solutions of finite volume, whereas for "on-column" elution, the infinite solution volume condition is closely approached.

Typical apparatus needed for studying dissolution from ion-exchange resins was discussed by Boyd, et al., (1947), Kressman & Kitchener, (1949) and Dickel & Meyer, (1953). Boyd et al., (1947) found that the release process of ionic drug ions from resinates eluted with simulated gastric or intestinal fluids is controlled mostly by particle diffusion.

Brook & Van Noort, (1985) studied drug release from acrylic polymers via channels and cracks. Farag & Nairn, (1988) found that the capacity of the ion-exchange resin from anions, the percentage of organic anion released and the rate of release depended on the cross-linking of the anion-exchange resin, the molecular weight of the anion, and the moisture content of the resin.

Chen, et al., (1992) carried out a comparative study of doxorubicin loading, release characteristics and stability within sodium and hydrogen forms of ion-exchange resin microspheres. It was demonstrated that resins in the Na^+ form, although having lower drug loading capacity, showed similar release profiles to resins in the H^+ form, but still maintained all the drug activity. Resins in the H^+ form despite having high drug loading capacity caused drug degradation within microspheres due to their strong acidic nature. They concluded that in comparison with the H^+ form, resins in the Na^+ form can be considered as better carriers for doxorubicin in terms of sustaining the release of drug and maintaining drug activity. The parameters that help in drug release are nature of matrix materials and their influence on the drug activity and microsphere performance in vitro.

Vimala Devi & Suneeta, (1993) prepared drug resinates of glypizide with four anionic resins, i.e., IRA-416, IRA-410, IRA-400 and RDL-92-100 and studied the release parameters. In order to retard the drug release, the drug resinates were further coated with cellulose polymers. They concluded that the drug release and absorption are affected by hydrophobicity, method of preparation, nature of polymer, particle size and nature of coat. A typical example of in vitro drug release profile of uncoated and coated IRA-400 drug resinates at different percentages of coat is given in Fig. 11.4.

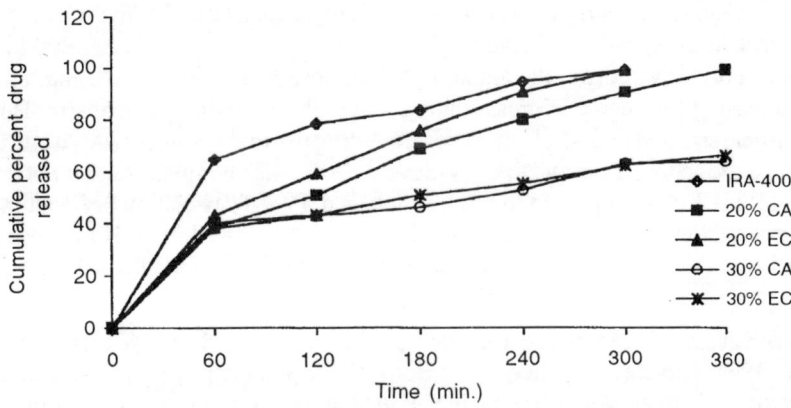

Fig 11.4 : Effect of coating on drug release rate profile

11.11.2. In vivo tests

In vivo procedures used for estimating drug activity of resinates include serum concentration level determination, urinary excretion, and toxicity studies. Blood concentration level determinations have been used frequently, but a disadvantage is that for many drugs, doses exceeding the therapeutic dose are frequently applied to facilitate chemical analysis. As an alternative measure of the physiological availability of drugs, urinary excretion has been proposed by Chapman, et al. (1957, 1959) and Campbell et al., (1957). For certain drugs a direct relationship has been shown between excretion rate and the plasma concentrations (Campbell et al., 1959).

Toxicity studies on animals have also been used for demonstrating the duration of an effect in vivo. Becker & Swift (1959) noted that the median lethal dose (LD_{50}) and the median time of death (LT_{50}) if compared with the pure drugs, were significantly increased with the resinate forms. These differences in LT_{50} and LD_{50} were attributed to slower absorption from the resinate forms. A close correlation between the delay in the time of death and the urinary excretion rate has been reported (Shenoy et al., 1959).

Torres et al., (1995b) studied the *in vivo* behaviour of enteric microcapsules containing diclofenac-resin complexes with respect to uncoated complexes and a commercial product (Dolotren Retard). The bioavailability of the diclofenac released from the microcapsules and the uncoated resins was studied in rabbits using Dolotren Retard as the reference compound. There were no statistically significant differences in maximum plasma concentration (C_{max}) and area under the plasma concentration-time curve (AUC) values among formulations.

Significant differences were found in time to achieve C_{max}. Both HPMCP microcapsules and uncoated resins exhibited a sustained-release pattern similar to the commercial dosage forms. In comparison to the uncoated product, the enteric coating led to a significantly slower apparent rate of absorption.

Conaghey et al., (1998) studied the factors affecting the release of nicotine from hydrogels containing ion-exchange resins using a Franz-types cell with artificial and human skin membranes. The overall release process across the artificial membrane was controlled by matrix diffusion through the hydrogel. The availability of ions suitable to exchange the nicotine, following their diffusion from the receptor buffer solution, substantially increased the delivery rate. The vehicles were unsuitable for passive release across human skin.

11.11.3. Correlation of in vitro-in vivo release pattern of drug resinates

This should be nearly parallel, if not totally, as *in vitro* release pattern is always an indication of release from dosage form whereas in-vivo is the pattern of drug release in biological fluids in a changing environment. However, the correlation coefficient is the only confirmation for the best performance of the developed dosage forms i.e. drug resinates.

Keating (1955, 1956a & b, 1961, 1964) demonstrated by in vitro tests that the release pattern of a drug from a resinate dosage form depends on the type of drug and on the size, degree of cross-linking and ionogenic groups of the resin. For a given drug, the amount of drug absorbed as well as the rate of release of drug decreases with increasing the degree of cross-linking and with increasing particle size. However, optimal combination of particle size and cross-linkage varies from drug to drug. Drug resinates were found to have an advantage in therapeutic action, onset and toxicity. Severe effects were nominal. Activity of the drug could be enhanced upto 8-11 hrs. Keating claimed to have established a good correlation between in vitro tests and LD_{50} studies. In general, the drug resinates releasing less than 50% of the drug in 1hr in gastric juice have an LD_{50} value at least twice that of the usual common drug salt. Others have confirmed most of the Keating's conclusions.

Many workers (Chaudhry & Saunders, 1956; Smith et al., 1959; Brudney, 1961; Nash & Crabtree, 1961; Khomyakov et al., 1964; Hirscher & Miller, 1962; Borodkin & Sundberg, 1971) have shown that polymers containing carboxylic acid groups cannot be used in making long-acting preparations of amine drugs. However, carboxylic acid ion-exchange resins have been used frequently as drug carriers e.g., in attempts to prepare tasteless dosage forms (Thoma & Schiefer 1975; Brudney, 1961; Bryan et al., 1967) which give maximal drug availability in the stomach. Phillips & Lenahan, (1961) claimed that antispasmodic compositions of a carboxylic cation-exchange resin could be useful in treating patients suffering from gastric ulcers by controlling the secretion of excess gastric acid. If the pH is below about 3, the drug is released rapidly. When the pH of the stomach content is above 3, the product is retained in the resinate. At this pH it is not desirable to administer the antispasmodic, since under these conditions sufferers from gastric ulcers and related conditions seldom have distressing symptoms. Adrenergics, antihistaminics, antitussives, barbiturates and antibacterial agents are among the drugs that were originally studied for use in ion-exchange resinates form in the 60's and 70's.

Dew et al (1983) studied the colonic release of 5-amino salicylic acid from an oral preparation coated with acrylic based resin in active ulcerative colitis, and reported that through abdominal x-rays, the preparation released its contens in the terminal ileum and proximal colon.

Jones et al (1989) studied polystyrene based ion-exchange resins as a carrier system for the sustained delivery of cytotoxic drugs. A batch ion-exchange procedure was developed for loading the drugs onto cation- and anion-exchange resins. A closed circuit in vitro drug release system was developed to measure rate at which resins released entrapped drug and reached equilibrium drug concentration. A large degree of variation in the equilibrium drug concentrations was observed between the different drug systems, but the rate at which equilibrium was attained was similar for all drugs. Doxorubicin resinate demonstrated equilibrium drug concentrations close to blood levels associated with conventional therapeutic doses. Thus doxorubicin resinate was regarded as having potential for tumor targeted drug.

11.12 SOLUBLE IONIC POLYMERS AS DRUG CARRIERS

Soluble polyelectrolytes such as polyacrylic and methacrylic acids, sulfonated and phosphorylated poly (vinyl alcohol), or polysaccharides and poly-uronic derivatives have been utilised in novel drug delivery systems to alter the release profile of the drug, also as additive in drug formulations e.g., as suspending agents or as tablet disintegrants.

According to Miller & Holland (1960) different salts of the same drug rarely differ pharmacologically. The variations are usually based on their physical properties. Although the nature of the biological responses may not differ appreciably, the intensities of the response may differ remarkably. The salt form in general and the poly salt in particular, are known to influence a number of physico-chemical properties of the parent drug, including stability, hygroscopicity, solubility and dissolution rate (Berge et al, 1977). These properties, in turn, affect the bioavailability of the drug.

The release process of a drug from a polymeric salt after oral administration can be divided in various stages: (a) penetration of the dissolving medium in the dosage form, with simultaneous liberation of a small quantity of drug; (b) swelling of the polymer with formation of a gel barrier; (c) release of the drug ion by exchange with penetrating ions and subsequent diffusion through the gel matrix and (d) eventual dissolution of the polymeric matrix with liberation of the drug by an ion-exchange process between the polymeric salt and the surrounding medium.

Ionic polymers having weak acid ionic groups are poorly soluble in gastric juice and a major release of the drug will occur in the intestine. Delivery systems of this type act as delayed action dosage forms.

11.13 EVALUATION OF POLYMER-DRUG SALT COMPLEXES

Among the first long-acting preparations, based on the formation of macromolecular salts, were combinations of antibiotics with polyacids, such as poly (acrylic acid), sulfonic or phosphorylated polysaccharides, carboxymethyl starch, and poly (uronic acids). The parenteral administration of these compounds produced low blood concentration levels of the antibiotics for long periods, while high concentration levels were attained in the lymph. In comparison, the drug sulfates gave high blood concentration levels but low concentration levels in lymph. The high uptake of the poly-salt in the lymph, attributed to the high affinity of the lymphatic system for macromolecules caused a prolonged passage of the drug through the body is because of the slow lymphatic circulation (Hoffmann, et al, 1959; Malek et al, 1958; 1959). The toxicity of macromolecular salts was substantially lower than that of the free antibisotics (Malek et al, 1958).

Streptomycin alginates have been prepared by El-shibini et al, (1971) and shown to be effective as prolonged release preparations.

Ozawa et al, (1975) claimed that streptomycin dextran sulfate injected in rabbits gradually released the antibiotic over a period exceeding 48 hours.

Malek et al, (1958, 1959) reported first about the ability of poly salts to alter the transport of drugs in the body, and hence modify the intensity and duration of the therapeutic response.

Cavallito & Jewell (1958) prepared polygalacturonates of several therapeutic amines in which the polygalacturonates served as agents for influencing the rate of release of the amines. Dialysis experiments showed that polygalacturonates can reduce the rate of release of therapeutically effective amines. This finding has applications for the preparation of oral repository drug formulations.

Poly (galacturonic acid) has also been used to prepare poorly soluble quinidine salts (Cardioquin®, Galactoquin®, Naticardina®, Sine flutter®) (Halpern, et al, 1958, 1959). They were reported to be four times less toxic orally than the sulfate. This reduction in toxicity was attributed to a slow release of quinidine from the polygalacturonate. The compound still possesses special demulcent properties and inhibits mucosal irritation, which is typical for conventional inorganic quinidine salts.

A remarkable example of a long-acting polymer-drug salt is that of pilocarpine alginate (Loucas & Haddad, 1972). When dispersed in sterile water and dried to a solid gel this preparation was found to be useful as a long-acting ophthalmic drug when tested in rabbits. While liquid preparations of alginate or hydrochloride salts had a similar miotic activity, the solid pilocarpine alginate preparations were found to increase significantly the duration of miosis. Moreover, they were more effective in constricting the pupil. In contrast to eye drops, which release pilocarpine immediately to the conjunctival fluid, the solid dose of pilocarpine diffuses slowly through the gel matrix and is available more uniformly.

An increase in duration of activity of a drug when administered as a polymeric salt is due mostly to the poor solubility of the polymer-drug complex which acts as a drug reservoir. The reduced solubility may be due to dehydration accompanying the salt formation (Ikegami & Imai, 1962) or to ionic crosslinking of the polymer by a poly functional drug.

Klaudianos, (1971) prepared long-acting preparations based on alginic acid according to a simple and economical method. Sodium alginate was mixed with calcium phosphate and a therapeutic amine and compounded into tablets. On oral administration, the GI fluids diffuse into the tablet and the soluble sodium alginate is transformed by cation-exchange into an insoluble but swellable calcium alginate. The resulting hydrogel acts as a depot from which the drug diffuses out slowly. *In vivo* experiments with caffein tablets with 8 volunteers (3 women, 5 men; ages 28 to 40) showed that the alginate tablets, in contrast to conventional tablets, were able to liberate the active substance over a period of 6 to 8 hr after their administration. In the approach of Klaudianos, it is not the drug, but a polyvalent metal ion that causes cross-linking of the polyacid. Salib, et al (1976) used an analogous procedure to obtain long-acting chloramphenicol dosage forms based on carboxymethyl cellulose to which aluminum sulfate was added as the gel-forming agent. This concept obviously can also be applied to entrap nonionogenic drugs.

Drug entrapment by polymeric flocculation, as an approach to slow release dosage forms, was further studied by Rhodes, et al (1970) and Elgindy (1976). It was shown that the polymer-drug interactions in the flocculates are complex and not caused by ionic effects only. Hydrogen bonding as well as hydrophobic drug-drug and drug-polymer interactions can be involved. This confirmed earlier reports of Kennon & Higuchi (1957), who studied the interaction of cationic drugs with the sodium salts of anionic polyelectrolytes. They concluded that the drug binding appeared to take place by (I) coacervation of oppositely charged ions, (II) additional intermolecular force phenomena, and/or (III) replacement of bound sodium by organic cations.

Effect of several salts on the adsorption of paraquat by cation-exchange resins and activated charcoal in disintegration test fluids at 37°C was studied by Honda et al (1992). In the absence of salts, cation-exchange resins showed a much greater adsorption capacity for paraquat than did activated charcoal. However, the adsorption capacity of cation-exchange resins was extremely decreased in the presence of sodium chloride, magnesium sulfate and sodium sulfate; whereas, the capacity of activated charcoal was enhanced by the salts.

11.14. DIAGNOSTIC AND THERAPEUTIC APPLICATIONS

Synthetic as well as natural polysaccharides based on ion-exchange resins have been used with good results for diagnostic determinations. e.g., of gastric acidity (Kamp, 1962). They have also found applications as adsorbents of toxins, as antacids, and as bile acid binding agents. Among other therapeutic applications they were successfully applied for the treatment of liver diseases, renal insufficiency, urolithic disease and occupational skin diseases (Leclerc, 1956; Naumann, 1958; Kamp, 1962; Schneider et al, 1979).

Chlosteramine is a quaternary ammonium anion-exchange resin with basic groups attached to a styrene-divinyl benzene copolymer by carbon-carbon bonds. Originally used to control pruritis in patients with elevated plasma bile acid concentrations, it is currently indicated as adjunctive therapy to diet for the reduction of elevated serum cholesterol in patients with primary hypercholesterolemia. Cholestipol hydrochloride is an anion-exchange resin of diethylenetriamine and 1-chloro-2, 3-epoxypropane. Cholestipol increases the fractional catabolic rate of low-density lipoproteins and decreases the (LDL) cholesterol pool as well as the content of cholesterol in the (LDL) particles. Sodium polystyrene sulfonate is a sulfonic cation-exchange resin used in the treatment of hyperkalemia. Although it is indicated for the treatment of hyperkalemia, it is best-utilized in patients whose hyperkalemia is associated with oliguria or anuria secondary to acute renal failure. The resin should be considered as an adjunct to other measures, such as restriction of diet, electrolyte intake and control of acidosis. Phentermine, a sympathomimetic amine is indicated for short-term use in the management of exogenous obesity in a regimen of weight reduction utilising caloric restriction (Kubacka, 1984).

Applications of ion-exchange resins including their use in the pharmaceutical industry for the control of cholesterol levels and potassium ion levels was reviewed by Cristal, (1985).

Table 11.2 : Summary of Exchange Resins Available in the U.S.

Drug		Dosage
Cholestyramine	Adult	: 1 packet tid to qid before meals.
	Child	: Dosage schedule has not been established by the manufacturer.
Colestipol HCl	Adult	: 15-30 g/day taken in divided doses bid to qid.
	Child	: Safety and effectiveness in children has not been established.
Sodium polystyrene	Adult	: Orally 15g, qd to qid. Rectally, 30 to 50 g, qid.
	Child	: Practical exchange rate of 1 g resin for each 1 mEq of potassium above the normal range.
Phentermine	Adult	: 15 to 30 mg daily before breakfast or 10-14 hr before retiring.
	Child	: Not recommended for children less than 12 years of age.
Hydrocodone & Phenyltoloxamine	Adult	: 1 teaspoonful (capsule or tablet) every 8-12 hrs.
	Children	: Under 1 year of age ¼ teaspoonful every 12 hrs.
	1-5 years	: ½ teaspoonful every 12 hours.
	over 5 years	: 1 teaspoonful every 12 hrs.
Dextromethorphan	Adult	: 2 teaspoonful bid.
	6-12 years	: 1 teaspoonful bid.
	Children 2-5	: ½ teaspoonful bid.

Use of ion-exchange resins in sustained action dosage forms, drug complexes and in microcapsules was reviewed by Manekar & Joshi, (1991).

A 2-phase method using guiac (guajac) and an immunochemical technique was developed by Czalbert, (1990) and it was utilised for the early detection of intestinal neoplasms.

A microdetection method for the determination of cyanide utilising the decoloration of Amberlite IRA-400 resin beads was developed by Gridinic, & Oresis, (1985). The influence of anions on the test and stability of resin grains in the presence of various agents was discussed. They also studied the conditions for the determination of various compounds utilising ion-exchange resins. Sulfur and nitrogen containing compounds were emphasized.

To elucidate conditions for the maximum separation of amino acid and peptide byproducts from medically usable protein hydrolysates, the dynamics of the ion-exchange adsorption process and desorption of nitrogenous products of blood protein hydrolysis from anion-exchange resins was studied by Chaplygina, et al, (1981).

Summary of ion-exchange resins that are available in US market was given in Table 11.2 (Kubacka, 1984).

11.15 CONCLUSIONS

Ion-exchange resinates prepared from suitable drugs and ionic polymers can help in alteration of physicochemical and biological properties of drugs. Improved therapeutic efficacy and reduced toxicity is the beneficial performance of these resinates. However, most desirable experimental designs are to obtain *in vivo - in vitro* correlation data rather than simple in vitro data. Drug-resin complexes are promising controlled delivery systems and can come to market with a manufacturing feasibility, as these can give better tolerance, more uniform delivery of the drug, and for a longer period.

11.16 ACKNOWLEDGEMENTS

Our grateful thanks are to Dr. (Mrs.) J. Vijaya Ratna, Associate Professor and Dr. P. Uma Devi, Research Associate, Dept. of Pharmaceutical Sciences, Andhra University, Visakhapatnam for their assistance.

REFERENCES

Abrahams, A. and Linnell, W.H. (1957) Lancet, 2 : 1317.

Alba, S.; Alfonse, H.; De Armas, R. and Goire, D. (1979) Rev. Cubane, Farm. 13 : 133-140.

Amsel, L.P.; Hinsvark, O.N.; Rotenberq, K. and Sheumaker, J.L. (1984) Pharm. Technol, 8 : 28-48.

Atyabi, F.; Sharma, H.L.; Mohammed, H.A. and Fell, J.T. (1996) J. Cont. Rel. 42: 25-28.

Barr, W.H.; Gerbracht, L.M.; Letcher, K.; Plant, M. and Strahl, N. (1972) J. Clin. Pharmacol. Ther. 13 : 97.

Becker, B.A. and Swift, J.G. (1959) Appl. Pharmacol. 1: 42.

Berg, E.W. (1963) In: Physical and Chemical methods of separation, McGraw-Hill Book company, Ed. 19, Inc. New York, Chaps. 10, 11.

Berg, P.R. and Strup, P. (1966) Dansk. Tidsskr. Farm. 40: 33, 55.

Berge, S.M.; Bighley, L.D. and Monkhouse, D.C. (1977) J. Pharm. Sci. 66(1) : 1.

Bharucha, E. and Hamied, Y. (1963) Indian J. Chem. 1: 233.

Borodkin, S. and Sundberg, D.P. (1971) J. Pharm. Sci. 60(10): 1523.

Boyd, G.E.; Adamson, A.W. and Myers, L.S. Jr. (1947) J. Am. Chem. Soc. 69 : 2836.

Brook, I.M. and Van Noort, R. (1985) Biomaterials, 6(4) : 281-285.

Brudney, N. (1961) U.S. Patent 2 : 987, 441.

Bryan, W.L.; Meed, B.; Nager, U.F. and Wiseloghe, F.Y. (1967) U.S. Patent 3 : 313, 686.

Burke, G.M.;Mendes, R.W. and Jambhekar, S.S. (1986) Drug Dev. Ind. Pharm. 12(5) : 713-732.

Campbell, J.A.; Chapman, D.G. and Chatten, L.G. (1957) Can. Med. Assoc. J. 77: 602.

Campbell, J.A.; Nelson, E. and Chapman, D.G. (1959) Can. Med. Assoc. J. 81 : 15.

Cass, L.J. and Frederik, W.S. (1958) Ann. Int. Med. 49 : 151.

Cavallito, C.J. and Jewell, R. (1958) J. Am. Pharm. Assoc. 47 : 165.

Chaplygina, Z.A.; Gorskaya, N.A. and Tkhorzheuskeya, Z.S. (1981) Pharm. Chem. J. (USSR) 14 : 247-250.

Chapman, D.G.; Chatten, L.G. and Campbell, J.A. (1957) Can. Med. Assoc. J. 76 : 102.

Chapman, D.G.; Shenoy, K.G. and Campbell, J.A. (1959) Can. Med. Assoc. J. 81 : 470.

Chaudhry, N.C. and Rai, D. (1984) Indian J. Hosp. Pharm. 21 : 203-207.

Chaudhry, N.C. and Saunders, L. (1956) J. Pharm. Pharmacol. 8 : 975.

Chen, Y.; Burton, M.A.; Codde, J.P.; Napoli, S.; Martins, I.J. and Gray, B.N. (1992) J. Pharm. Pharmacol. 44(3) : 211-215.

Conaghey, O.M.; Corish, J. and Corrigan, O.I. (1998) Int. J. Pharm. 170 : 215-224.

Cristal, M. (1985) Manufacturing Chemist, 56 : 50-51,53.

Czalbert, J.H. (1990) Gyogyezereszet 34 : 291-293.

Deeb, G. and Becker, B.A. (1960) Toxicol. Appl. Farmacol. 2 : 410.

Dew, M.J.; Rydes, R.E.J.; Evans, N.; Evans B.K. and Rhodes, J. (1983) British, J. Clin. Pharmacol, 16 : 185-187.

Dickel, G. and Meyer, A. (1953) Z. Electrochem. 57 : 901.

Dower, (1964) Midland, Mich, Chap.-1.

Durrani, M.J.; Whitaker, R.F.; Manji, P.A. (1997) Drug Dev. Ind. Pharm. 23(12) : 1201-1205.

El. Shibini, H.A.M.; Abdel-Nasser, M. and Motawi, M.M. (1971) Pharmazie, 26(10) : 630.

Elgindy, N.A. (1976) 934, Can. J. Pharm. Sci. 11(1) : 32.

Farag, Y. and Nairn, J.G. (1988) J. Pharm. Sci. 77(10) : 872-875.

Fiedler, W.C. and Sperandio, G.J. (1957) J. Am. Pharm. Assoc. Sci. Ed. 46(1) : 47.

Freed, S.C.; Keating, J.W. and Hays, E.E. (1956) Ann. Int. Med. 44 : 1136.

Freed, S.C. and Hays, E.E. (1959) Chem. J. Med. Sci. 238(91) : 55.

Geneidi, A.S. and Hamachar, H. (1980) Pharm. Ind. 42(2) : 198-202.

Georgia, O.L. and Price, J.C. (1989) Drug, Dev. Ind. Pharm, 15: 1275-1287.

Gridinic, V. and Oresis, L.S. (1985) Acta. Pharm. Jygosl, 35 : 261-274.

Gustus, E. (1954) U.S. Patent 2 : 697, 059.

Gyselinck, P.; Van Severen, R.; Braeckman, P. and Schacht, E. (1981) Pharmazie, 36(11) : 769.

Halpern, A.; Shaftel, N. and Monte-Bovi, A.J. (1958) Am. J. Pharm. 130 : 190.

Halpern, A.; Shaftel, N. and Schwartz, G. (1959) Antibiot. Chemother. 9 : 97.

Hays, E.E. (1962) U.S. Patent 3, 035, 979.

Helfferion, F. (1962) In: Ion Exchange, McGraw Hill, New York, Chapters 1,4,5,6.

Hersey, J. (1969) Mfg. Chem. 40 : 32.

Hirscher, D.A. and Miller, O.H. (1962) J. Am. Pharm. Assoc. NS2(2) : 105.

Hoffman, J.; Malék, P.; Herold, M.; Capková, J.; Kolc, J. and Vondrácék, M. (1959) Casopis lekaru ceskych, 98 : 965; through Chem. Abstr. (1960) 54 : 16663.

Honda, Y. Nakano, M. and Nakano, N. (1992) J. Jap. Soc. Hosp. Pharm, 18 : 100-105.

Hwa, J. and Loeffler, D. (1959) Ger. Off. 1, 070 : 381.

Ikegami, A. and Imai, N. (1962) J. Pol. Sci. 56 : 133.

Irwin, W.J.; Belaid, K.A. and Alpar, H.O. (1987) Drug Dev. Ind. Pharm. 13(9-11) : 2047-2066.

Jacks, D. (1962) Pharm. J. 188 : 581.

Jani, R.; Gan, O.; Ali, Y.; Rodstrom, R. and Hancock, S. (1994) J. Ocul. Pharmacol. 10(1) 57-67.

Jantzen M. Gwen and Robinson R. Joseph (1996) Sustained and Controlled Release Drug Delivery Systems, In: Modern Pharmaceutics- 3rd edition, Edited by Glibert S. Banker and Christopher T. Rhodes, Marcel Dekker Inc. New York, 593.

Jayaswal, S.B. and Bedi, G.S. (1980) Indian Drugs, 17(4) : 102.

Jenquin, M.R.; Liebowitz, S.M.; Sarabia, R.E. and Mc Ginity, J.W. (1990) J. Pharm. Sci. 79(9) : 811-816.

Jones, C.; Burton, M.A.; Gray, B.N. and Hodqkin, J. (1989) J. Controlled Release, 8 : 251-257.

Kamp, W. (1962) Pharm. Weekbl. 97 : 141.

Kanhere, S.S.; Shah, R.S. and Bafna, S.L. (1968) J. Pharm. Sci. 57(2) : 342.

Kanhere, S.S.; Vyas, A.H.; Bhat, C.V.; Kamath, B.R.; Shah, R.S. and Bafna, S.L. (1969) J. Pharm. Sci. 58(12) : 1550.

Keating, J.W. (1955) U.S. Patent 527 : 130.

Keating, J.W. (1956) U.S. Patent 582 : 346.

Keating, J.W. (1956) U.S. Patent 598 : 215.

Keating, J.W. (1961) U.S. Patent 2, 990 : 332.

Keating, J.W. (1964) U.S. Patent 3, 143 : 465.

Kennon, L. and Higuchi, T. (1957) J. Am. Pharm. Assoc. 46 : 21.

Khomyakov, K.P.; Virnik, A.D. and Rogovin, Z.A. (1964) Russ. Chem. Rev. 33(9) : 462.

Khym Joseph, X. (1974) In: Analytical Ion-Exchange Procedures in Chemistry and Biology; 62 : 2-4.

Kitchener, J.A. (1957) In: Ion Exchangers in Organic and Biochemistry, Interscience Publishers, Inc. New York, 195.

Klaudianos, S. (1971) Pharm. Ind. 33(5) : 296.

Kressman, T.R.E. and Kitchener, J.A. (1949) Discussions Faraday Soc. 7 : 90.

Kubacka Renee, T. (1984) U.S. Pharmacist, Jun, 36-41.

Kunin, R. (1958) In: Ion Exchange Resins, John Wiley & Sons, Inc. New York, 2nd ed. Chaps.2, 3 & 5.

Lazarus, J. and Cooper, J. (1959) J. Pharm. Pharmacol. 11 : 257.

Lazarus, J. and Cooper, J. (1961) J. Pharm. Sci. 50 : 715.

Leclerc, M. (1956) Bull. Soc. Sci. Hyg. Aliment. 44 : 251.

Li, Z.H.; Ping, Q.N.; Zhu, W.; Lin, G.J. and Zhou, J.P. (1997) J. China Pharm. Univ. 28(2): 77-81.

Loucas, S.P. and Haddad, H.M. (1972) J. Pharm. Sci. 61(6) : 985.

Makrinov, V.A.; Degtowra, K.T. and Suchukina, E.V. (1968) Tr. Voronezh. Gos. Med. Inst. 73(4) : 134; through Chem. Abstr. (1971) 74 : 84805.

Malék, P.; Kolc, J.; Herold, M. and Hoffman, J. (1958) Antibiotics Annual, 1957-1958, Medical Encyclopedia, New York, 564.

Malék, P. and Kolc, J. (1959) Casopis lekaru ceskych, 98 : 790; through Chem. Abstr. (1960) 54 : 16663.

Manekar, N.C. and Joshi, S.B. (1991) Pharma-Times, 23 : 25-27.

Miller, L.C. and Holland, A.H. (1960) Mod. Med. 28 : 312.

Mohamed, F.A. (1996) S.T.P. Pharm. Sci. 6(6): 410-416.

Moldenhauer, M.G. and Nairn, J.G. (1990) J. Pharm. Sci. 79 : 659-666.

Motycka, S.; Newth, C.J.L. and Nairn, J.G. (1985) J. Pharm. Sci. 74 : 643-646.

Motycka, S. and Nairn, J.G. (1979) J. Pharm. Sci. 68 : 211-215.

Nash, J.F. and Crabtree, R.E. (1961) J. Pharm. Sci. 50 : 134.

Naumann, G. (1958) Pharmazie, 13(4) : 139.

Nean, S.H.; Chow, M.Y. and Durrani, M.J. (1996) Int. J. Pharmaceutics, 131 : 47-55.

Ozawa, H.; Ozeki, E.; Shimizu, H. and Nishio, S. (1975) Japan Kokai, 75, 24 : 429; Chem. Abstr. (1975) 83 : 103292q.

Phillips, G.E. and Lenahan, J.G. (1961) Antispasmodic composition, U.S. Patent 3, 007 : 847.

Quinlan, J.N. (1974) Can. Pat. 946 : 742.

Raghunathan, Y.; Amsel, L.; Hinsvark, O. and Bryant, W. (1981) J. Pharm. Sci. Apr. 70(4) : 379-384.

Rety, S.P.; Linnell, W.H. and Timmington, H. (1963) U.S. Patent 3, 108, 044.

Rhodes, C.; Wai, K. and Banker, G.S. (1970) J. Pharm. Sci. 59 : 1578-1581.

Salib, N.N.; EL-Menshawy, M.E. and Ismail, A.A. (1976) Pharmazie, 31: 12.

Samsonov, G.V. and Parechnik, V.A. (1980) Russ. Chem. Rev. 38(7) : 547.

Samuelson, O. (1963) In: Ion Exchange separations in Analytical Chemistry, John Wiley & Sons, Inc. New York, Chaps. 2, 3, 4.

Saunders, L. and Srivastava, R. (1980) J. Chem. Soc. 2915.

Sawaya, A. Fickat, R. Benoit, J.P. Prisienx, F. and Benita, S. (1988) J. Microencapsul. 5(3) : 255-267.

Schacht, E.; Goethals, E.; Gyselinck, P. and Thienpont, D. (1982) J. Pharm. Belg. 37(3) : 183.

Schlichting, D.A. (1962) J. Pharm. Sci. 51 : 134.

Schneider, H.J. and Stein, G. (1979) Dtsch. Gesundheitswes. 48(34) : 2385.

Schubert, J. (1956) In: Methods of Biochemical Analysis, Interscience Publishers, Inc. New York, Vol. 3 : 247.

Schwendeman, S.P.; Amidon, G.L.; Labhasetwar, V. and Lery, R.J. (1994) J. Pharm. Sci. 83(10) : 1482-1494.

Seidl, J.; Malinsky, J.; Dusek, K. and Heitz, W. (1967) Adv. Polym. Sci. 5: 113.

Shenoy, K.G.; Grice, H.C. and Campbell, J.A. (1959) Toxicol. Appl. Pharmacol. 1 : 42.

Shtannikov, E.V. (1966) Gigiena isam (7) 59; through Chem. Abstr. (1966) 65 : 15965h.

Siegel, S.; Pettebone, R.H. and Hanus, E.J. (1961) U.S. Patent 3, 070, 503, ,

Sjogren, J. (1971) Acta. Pharm. Suec. 8(3) : 153.

Smith, H.A.; Evanson, R.V. and Sperandio, G.J. (1959) J. Am. Pharm. Assoc. 49(2) : 94.

Smith, J. (1983) Pharm. Technol. 7 (Suppl) : 26.

Strasenburgh, R.J. (1959) In: Therapeutic compositions, British Patent 824, 337.

Swift, J.G. (1960) Arch. Intern. Pharmacodynamie, 124 : 341.

Thoma, K. and Schiefer, G. (1975) Dtsch. Apoth. Ztg. 115(32) : 1165.

Tobin, L. and Weber, J. (1964) U.S. Patent 3, 121, 043.

Tompkins, E.R. and Mayer, S.W. (1947) J. Am. Chem. Soc. 69 : 2859.

Torres, D. Garcia Encina, G. Seizo, B. and VilaJato, J.L. (1995 a) Int. J. Pharm. 121 : 239-243.

Torres, D.; Garcia Encina, G.; Seijo, B. and Vila Jato, J.L. (1995 b) Eur. J. Pharm. Biopharm. 41(2) : 127-131.

Torres, D.; Garcia-Encina, G.; Seijo, B. and Vila Jato, J.L. (1993) J. Controlled Release, 23 : 201-207.

Torres, D.; Seizo, B.; Garcia Encina, G.; Alonso, M.J. and Vila Jato, J.L. (1990) Int. J. Pharm. 59 : 9-17.

Ullmann, E. (1975) Dtsch. Apoth. Ztg. 115(34) : 1240.

Veds, S. (1961) Acta Pharmacol. Toxicol. 18 : 157.

Vercammen Plaizier, J.A. (1992) Int. J. Pharm. 87 : 31-36.

Vimala Devi, M. and Suneeta, A. (1993) Ph.D. thesis "Effect of hydrophobicity in design and in vivo-in vitro release kinetics of controlled drug delivery systems", Andhra University, Visakhapatnam, India, 196-222.

Wheaton, R.M. and Seamster, A.H. (1966) In: Kirk-othmer Encyclopedia of Chemical Technology, Interscience Publishers, Inc. New York, Vol. II, 873.

Woodworth, J.R.; Liudden, T.M.; Ludden, L.K.; Shepherd, A.M. and Rotenberg, K.S. (1992) J. Pharm. Sci. 81(6) : 541-542.

Wulff, O. (1965) J. Pharm. Sci. 54 : 1058.

Yang, T.T. Swarbrick, J. (1986) J. Pharm. Sci. 75(3) : 264-270.

Chapter 12

Novel Systems for the Treatment of Cytomegalovirus Retinitis in Immuno-compromised Patients

J.K.Pandit, Romi Barat

12.1 INTRODUCTION

The eye is one of the most highly developed sensory organs, characterized by its complex structure and high resistance to foreign substances, including drugs. Due to the unique anatomical position of the eye, it is exposed to numerous offending agents and these agents can affect almost every ocular tissue. While superficial ocular diseases can be treated comparatively easily with conventional but somewhat primitive ophthalmic solution, suspension and ointment dosage forms; frequently drug entities need to be targeted to the deeper tissues within the eye. As a result, systemic administration and direct injection into the eye are two alternatives, which carry substantial risks to the patient. A virtual flood of patients undergoing immunosuppressant therapy and of AIDS patients has created a unique class of population suffering from virulent uveitis and retinopathies who need drug targeting within the globe. A very common pathogen implicated in retinopathy in such patients is the cytomegalovirus (CMV), the less common ones being herpes simplex and varicella zoster. Human cytomegalovirus (CMV) is an important pathogen in the immunocompromised patient, especially in patients with acquired immunodeficiency syndrome (AIDS). Retinitis caused by CMV in AIDS patients is a leading cause for blindness. Retinitis involves ureal infection with acute intra ocular inflammation and retinopathy. Progressive retinal necrosis results in blurring of vision and finally blindness. Evidently two modes of therapy are open for these patients. For patients on immunosuppressive drugs for organ transplantation, discontinuation of immunosuppressive medication has often been found to result in regression of CMV retinitis, if otherwise not affected by AIDS. Treatment of patients suffering from AIDS with antiviral drugs has shown limited success. It must be clearly understood that as of the present, restoration of immunity in AIDS patients is not possible. As a consequence, CMV retinitis in AIDS patients assumes a bizarre situation, in that the simultaneous threats of loss of vision and life render the affected person extremely prone to psychosis due to very poor disease prognosis. Delivery of antiviral drugs to the vitreous cavity has been attempted by various routes which suffer from some weakness or the other. Recent developments in this field have been in the form of intravitreal and transcleral implants, and iontophoretic delivery. The present chapter describes these devices and other future possibilities in the treatment of CMV retinitis.

12.2 ISSUES IN DRUG DELIVERY TO THE POSTERIOR SEGMENT OF THE EYE

In general, there are a number of ocular pathologies in the posterior part of the eye comprising the lens, sclera, vitreous humor, choroid and retina, (Fig 12.1) requiring drug treatment. Two important issues in posterior drug delivery are:

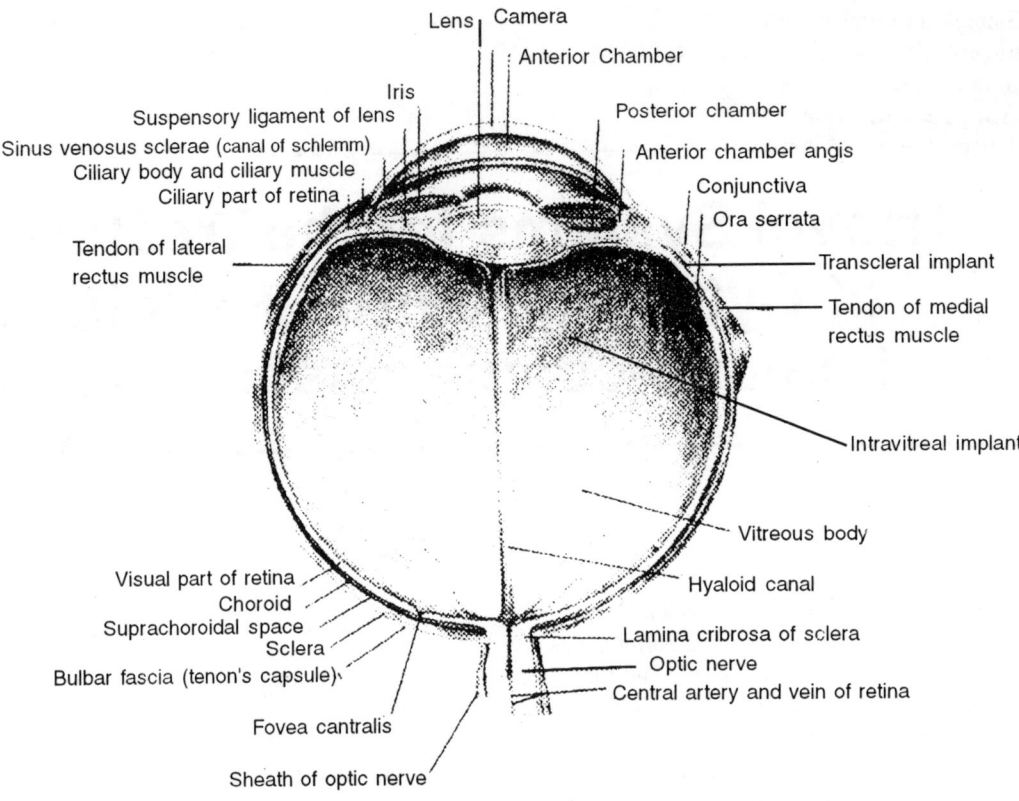

Fig 12.1 : Cross sectional view of the eye showing position of introcular implants.

(i). Drug disposition in the back of the eye has not been fully investigated and hence, is not fully under stood. Due to the low diffusional barrier of the vitreous humor to drug movement, a rapid and extensive drug loss may occur unless the availability of the drug is rate limited by release of the drug from the delivery system.

(ii). Intracameral and intravitreal devices must not interfere with the visual pathway, additionally their components must be fully compatible, both physically and chemically, with ocular tissues.

12.3 PROBLEMS ASSOCIATED WITH THERAPY OF CMV RETINITIS

Ganciclovir (GCV) and Foscarnet (FN) are effective in the treatment of CMV retinitis. GCV is a hydroxylated homolog of Acyclovir, chemically known as 9-(1,3-dihydroxy-2-propoxy-methyl) guanine ($C_9H_{12}N_5NaO_4$, mol. wt.=277.2). FN is a non-nucleoside pyrophosphate analogue chemically known as Phosphonatoformate Sodium (CNa_3O_5P, mol. wt.=192.0). These drugs are usually administered by intravenous injection, but the margin of safety of both drugs is low : long term intravenous administration is associated with neutropenia, neuropathy and bone-marrow suppression, necessitating cesation of therapy. Due to the tight junctions between retinal pigmented epithelial cells and between the endothelial cells of retinal capillaries, aqueous availability is reduced. Thus it is necessary to follow a regimen of two-week period of induction therapy and indefinite lower dose maintenance therapy. Inspite of such intensive dosage regimen, relapse is common to the extent of 9-50% of patients during the maintenance period necessitating reinduction therapy. The reasons for reactivation are twofold û since both GCV and FN are virostatic, development of viral resistance can occur and it is possible that the maintenance intravenous therapy provides drug levels inadequate for complete suppression of viral replication in the eye.

Some of the problems associated with the intravenous administration of GCV and FN can be circumvented by intravitreal injection. Intravitreal injection provides a higher intra-ocular drug concentration than systemic therapy due to low plasma protein binding and direct drug transfer from the vitreous to retina, the target tissue. Even with the intravitreal administration, the occurence of endophthalmitis, vitreous traction and retinal detachment (Saran & Maguire, 1994) and the need to deliver one or two injections per week, poor patient tolerance, militate against this mode of administration. Clearly, alternative systems of GCV and FN delivery need to be investigated.

12.4 PHARMACOKINETICS OF ANTI-CMV DRUGS

The study of intraocular pharmacokinetics of antiCMV drugs in humans needs frequent sampling of the vitreous, and is associated with the attendant risk of retinal detachment and endophthalmitis. Henry et al (1987) reported the intra-vitreal half life of GCV to be 13.3 hours and a Vd of 11.7ml, while Jabs et al (1987) calculated the half life to be 8.1 hours û both these reports are based on data of just one patient each. Clearly, the large difference is due to the smallest number of subjects. A mathematical treatment, proposed by Ashton et al (1992), (Fig 12.2) assumes that elimination of GCV from the vitreous takes place as a first order process with respect to vitreous concentration :

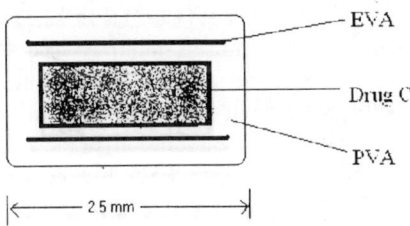

EVA

Drug C·

PVA

2·5 mm

Fig 12.2 : The device used for the drug delivery (Ashton et al 1994)

$$R_e = V_d.k.C \qquad (1)$$

where R_e is the elimination rate (µg/hr), V_d is the volume of distribution of GCV in the vitreous, C is the vitreous concentration of GCV and k is the elimination rate constant. This equation (1) may be rewritten as :

$$R_e = k_1.C \qquad (2)$$

where k_1 is a rate constant (ml/hr). Since it is much easier to use a rabbit as an experimental animal than humans, a second rate constant k_2 can be defined as :

$$k_2 = k_1 / V_a . \qquad (3)$$

where Va is the volume of vitreous. If the surface area of the retina is denoted by SR, the ratio k_2/SR gives the retinal rate constant :

$$K = k_2/SR \qquad (4)$$

where K gives an estimate of the elimination rate constant per unit area of the retina.

A perusal of the above reveals that the parameter k_1 predicts the release rate required to achieve a target concentration in the vitreous. Also, these authors (Ashton et al, 1992)·report that the retinal rate constant K being very similar, 0.017 ± 0.006 for rabbit and 0.015 ± 0.007 for diseased human, it is very likely that GCV is transported from the vitreous to the retina thus pointing towards an active trans-retinal elimination.

The mean intravitreal GCV concentrations after intravenous administration to AIDS patients is reported by Kuppermann et al (1993) to be significantly below the ID_{50}, i.e., near-steady-state subtherapeutic level of

GCV explain the difficulty of long term complete suppression of CMV retinitis. However, in a later report Morlet et al (1996) have opined that at a dose of 2mg delivered intravitreally, GCV was eliminated in about 7 days and the concentration remained at the ID_{50} for CMV (0.25 - 1.22 mg/l) for up to 7 days.

The half-life and vitreous clearance of trifluorothymidine, which demonstrates good activity against CMV, as reported by Pang et al (1992), was found to be 3.15 hours. The vitreous concentration remained above the ID_{50} for CMV for about 30 hours in non-inflamed rabbit eyes. Although these authors suggest that there would be no toxic accumulation following repeated injections, a significantly shorter half-life of intravitreal medications in the inflamed eye is reported by Kane et al (1981). The purport of this report is simple-repeated injections would still be required to keep the intravitreal concentration at inhibitory levels.

The foregoing consideration clearly points to the need to evolve newer strategies to manage CMV retinitis. AIDS patients are living longer with better disease state management, and hence the risk of CMV retinitis also has increased.

12.5 TREATMENT OF CMV RETINITIS WITH IMPLANTABLE INTRAOCULAR DRUG DELIVERY

As stated earlier, direct intravitreal injection has been observed to be better tolerated than systemic adminis-tration of GCV. However, even this mode of therapy is associated with unacceptable levels of risks of endophthalmitis and vitreous hemorrhage. Sanborn et al (1992) (Fig 12.3) reported the first human tests on GCV implant, programmed to release 2µg/hr for 4 months. It stabilized successfully CMV retinitis in 90% of the patients. The majority of these patients had received intravenous GCV but the treatment had failed due to various reasons. These authors had used the basic device designed by Smith et al (1992), who prepared a 6mg pellet of GCV coated with a small volume (350 µℓ of a 10% solution) of PVA. Two series of pellets were prepared to give 5µg/hr and 2µg/hr release rates. For the former, 3mm EVA discs coated with 10% PVA were fixed on the top and bottom of dried pellets using 2% PVA solution. The later device was prepared by coating the pellets on three sides with a film of EVA and then capped with a 3mm PVA disc coated with 10% PVA. Afterwards, both types of pellets were once again coated with 10% PVA, dried overnight and then heated to 190°C for about 5 hours.

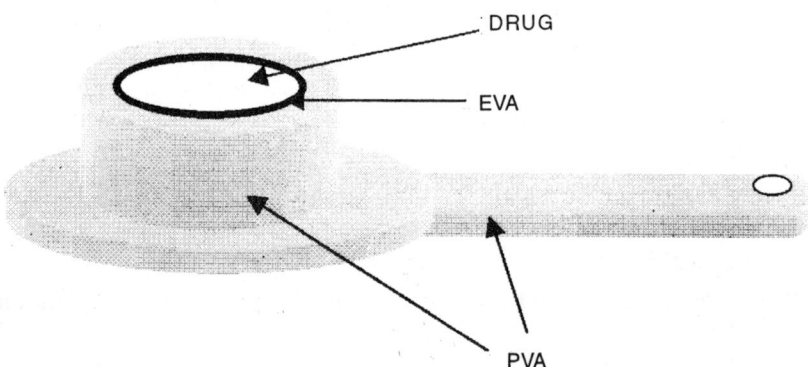

DRUG

EVA

PVA

Fig 12.3 : Intravitreal Ganciclovir device by Sanborn et al, (1992).

The in-vitro release was conducted in isotonic buffered saline at 37°C, the entire receptor fluid being changed every 20 days to maintain sink condition. New Zealand white rabbits were used for vitreous implantation of both devices (5µg/hr and 2µg/hr). Vitreous samples were obtained from the eyes at different times, and animals were sacrificed to retrieve the devices. Retinal examinations were performed before and after death. All samples were analyzed with reverse phase HPLC. To assess any potential retinal toxicity one rabbit was implanted with an uncoated 6mg pellet of GCV, retinal functions were assessed up to 48 days, and the animal was then killed. The study demonstrated that chronic low levels of GCV were maintained in the vitreous of rabbits for more than 80 days after implantation of the polymeric device and the device was well tolerated. Only a few histopathologic changes were observed, which were caused due to frequent taking of vitreous samples, and even the implantation of an uncoated 6 mg pellet of GCV did not cause irreparable damage to the retina. Both devices maintained intravitreal concentrations exceeding the ID_{50} of GCV. Using the half-life (13 hr) and distribution volume (11 ml) for GCV estimated by Henry et al (1987) in human eye, the theoritical steady state concentration in the vitreous could be calculated : the devices could be expected to maintain 8.5 mg/l and 3.4 mg/l of GCV for 50 and 125 days, respectively for the 5 µg/hr and 2 µg/hr devices. The extended duration of GCV release and the lack of inflammatory response make this non-biodegradable device a promising alternative for the treatment of CMV retinitis.

A slightly modified implantable device was evaluated in human eye by Sanborn et al (1992). A 6 mg pellet of GCV was first coated with PVA solution and then coated on all but the top surface with EVA and re-coated completely with PVA. An anchoring strut made of a strip of dried PVA was attached to the device, then heat treated and sterilized by gas. Thirteen eyes of eight patients with AIDS- related active CMV retinitis received the GCV device, surgically placed in the vitreal cavity facing the front of the eye, and the strut was firmly sutured to the sclera to make the device immobile. Follow up was done from 5 to 50 weeks or more after placement of the implant. Vitreous samples were obtained at different intervals for assay of GCV levels, which ranged from 2.7 to 18.1 m mol/l (mean 8.37m mol/l). Device release rate, ranging from 1.31 to 2.42 µg/hr, was estimated by subtracting the residual drug in the device from its initial drug content (6 mg). The mean total time of release of the device was estimated to be 137 days.

After 5 hours of administration, an intravenously administered dose of GCV produced an intraocular level of 7.16 m mol/l (Jabs et al, 1987), and is comparable to the finding of Sanborn et al (1992). However, the minimum level after 21 hours of intravenous injection was only 0.8m mol/ℓ, compared to 2.7m mol/l after 11 days of implantation. The positive aspects of the vitreous implant were its prolonged drug release in-vivo, adequate levels of GCV in the vitreous, short out-patient surgical procedure of implant fixation, absence of tissue reaction and dislocation of the device. Clinical improvement was observed in the form of regression and resolution of the retinitis in all treated eyes. The disadvantages of this device seem to be few, but as the study was conducted on a small number of patients for a short duration, it is quite likely that some more issues may become apparent in a long-term study involving larger number of eyes. Since the device was not biodegraded in-oculo it had to be removed surgically after drug evacuation, and there were a few instances of retinal detachment which needed surgical re-attachment. More studies are needed to know exactly when the drug release from the device becomes lower than the ID_{50} levels.

Martin et al (1994), using the device of Smith et al (1992), conducted clinical trial on 30 eyes of 20 patients of a 1 µg/hr GCV implant for the treatment of AIDS related CMV retinitis. *In-vivo* release rate was calculated from assay of residual drug from retrieved device, and subtracting the amount of residual drug from the original quantity (6 mg) and dividing the balance b the number of hours the device was in the eye. The in-vitro release rate did not reliably correlate with the in-vivo release rate. The investigators had anticipated that the device would last between 32.5 and 39.7 weeks, so that by re-implantation of a device at 32 weeks a constant therapeutic level of GCV would be maintained, but nine eyes developed progression of retinitis prior to 32 weeks, probably due to a wide range of in-vivo release rate. Marx et al (1996) have reported the outcome of their study on the same device conducted on 91 eyes of 70 patients. They reported that the GCV implant appears to be effective as an adjunct to systemic therapy for recurrent CMV retinitis. However in spite of the good initial response in majority of the patients, eventually about one third of the treated patients will have a relapse. Displacement of the device and retinal detachment seem to be the two limiting aspects of this device.

One important issue in the utilization of this type of device is concerned with its non-biodegradable nature and eventual retrieval of the spent device and replacement with a fresh implantable device. Morley et al (1995) have reported on the clinical implications of specifically the retrieval and re-implantation aspects and the complications associated with such procedures. The device implanted was the one reported by Smith et al was controlled in all eight patients except one, though three patients required intermittent intravenous antiCMV therapy. Most patients retained good vision after GCV implant replacement on reactivation of CMV. The GCV implants were replaced by three different methods : in the first procedure the first implant was removed and the second one was placed in exactly the same site as the first one. In the second procedure the first implant was left in place and the second device was placed contiguously (that is, the first scleral wound was lengthened and the device placed), and the third procedure involved placing the second implant at a completely different site.

In one patient wound leak developed after three implants were placed through the same incision. Sterile intraocular inflammation developed after the first device was placed due to residual ethylene oxide used in sterilization of the device. Two patients developed cataract. Late complications included retinal detachment in four eyes of three patients, and in one case one implant out of the four that were placed became dislodged into the vitreous cavity. According to these investigators, placement of the device in the original site is preferable, but the retrieval may be difficult sometimes because of enclosure of the device strut in the surrounding fibrotic tissue. A new site should be used when replacing a third or fourth implant to avoid scleral thinning and necrosis. A contiguously placed implant disrupts the circulation to the anterior segment of the eye, and the first implant is liable to be pushed or dislodged by the second implant due to strut failure. The best way to overcome these problems is to use a completely new site for the implantation of the device.

The therapeutic efficacy, toxicity and success rate of the device fabricated by Smith et al (1992) is under phase III multi-center studies in the USA. The device has been extensively tested in small groups of patients by a number of investigators (Duker et al, 1995; Charles & Steiner, 1996; Ashton et al, 1994; Anand et al, 1993).

A perusal of the available literature in the intravitreal implantable GCV device indicates that a change in design and composition of the device and a different site of placement may overcome the dangers associated with this device.

Biodegradable scleral plugs of GCV and Doxorubicin are reported to overcome a majority of the dangers and problems associated with placement of GCV- loaded non-biodegradable device in the vitreal cavity (Kunou et al, 1995; Hashizoe et al,1997; Kimura et al, 1994). The scleral plugs, 5mm length x 1-mm diameter, average weight 8-9 mg, containing the drug and various combinations of PLA and PLGA, were prepared by lyophilization and compression on a hot plate. In-vitro release study in PBS (0.1M, pH 7.4) at sink conditions showed a triphasic release profile, viz. an initial burst (first three days), a second stage of diffusional release (3 to 42 days) before erosion and swelling of the polymer, and the third stage of sudden burst due to swelling and disintegration of the polymeric matrix (42 days). The rapid release of the surface deposited drug is likely to be the cause of the initial burst release. The degradation speed of the polymer was responsible for the second, slower stage, and the final phase of release occurred at a stage of optimum swelling and near- disintegration. Rabbits were used for in-vivo release studies. The device (25% drug loading) was placed sub-sclerally, and at 1,2,4,8,12 and 20 weeks the animals were euthanized. The retrieved scleral implants and samples of ocular tissue were analyzed for GCV concentrations. Biodegradation of the device in the vitreous was estimated as weight change, represented by the relationship

$$\% \text{ Wt. Change} = \left[\frac{\text{initial wt of polymer - residual wt of polymer}}{\text{initial weight of polymer}} \right] \times 100$$

A high GCV loading (40%) resulted in almost total release of GCV in-vitro in about 20 days, whereas 10 and 25% loadings showed a triphasic release pattern.

The maximum GCV levels in the various ocular tissues were : aqueous humor, below detection limit; vitreous- 1.92 ± 2.12 µg/g at 1 week, and retina / choroid - 26.16 ± 12.70 µg/g at 2 months after implantation. The ED_{50} of GCV for human CMV is reported to be in the range $0.15 - 4.0$µg/ml by Plotkin et al (1985) in the target site, the retina / choroid. The GCV concentration was greater than or within the ED_{50} range for 5 months, while in the vitreous the GCV concentration was maintained in the ED_{50} range for 3 months. The authors explained the higher GCV concentration in the retina/choroid and the substantially lower concentration in the vitreous as due to clearance of GCV from the vitreous mainly via the retinal route. The drug release mechanism in-vivo has also been analyzed. An initial burst in the first week was followed by a diffusional phase for 2 months, the GCV release being complete in three months. The weight loss profiles in-vivo occurred in two phases. In the first phase, the lag phase, the weight did not change for a few days, but the drug diffused through the water channels in the polymer matrix. The second phase of remarkable weight change is indicative of erosion and production of soluble oligomers. The retrieved devices showed only slight deformation during 2 months after implantation, but in 10 weeks the implants showed fragmentation and were displaced into the vitreous. At 3 months the swollen implants began to disintegrate in the vitreous and eventually completely disappeared at 5 months after implantation. The implants did not produce any inflammatory response in the ocular tissues, neither any retinal detachment was noted. This pioneering work on biodegradable scleral implant was followed by the investigations of Hashizoe et al (1997), who have reported almost similar findings.

Obviously, the scleral implant apparently provides a number of advantages over the vitreous implant. besides providing the advantages of a biodegradable system, like there is no need to remove the spent device, the surgical procedure of implantation itself is much less traumatic to the patient and is less invasive. Although the scleral implant has only been studied in rabbits, experiments on the vitreal implants in rabbit showed incidences of retinal detachment, while in humans it has given rise to strut failure, leakage and problems have arisen when re-implantation is needed. Moreover, the displacement of the vitreous implant into the suprachoroidal area is likely to cause visual obstruction. These inadequacies of the vitreal implant are probably not balanced by the zero-order GCV release. The only drawback in the scleral implant that can be visualized as of the present is its shorter duration of residence in the eye, and its triphasic drug release pattern. These are not serious drawbacks and can be overcome with the use of other polymers in device fabrication.

One such polymer worthy of attention is gellan, a microbial exopolysaccharide. Gellan forms strong, brittle gels with various cations, that is, a phase-transition system. Its ocular tolerance and use in eye drops have been investigated and reported by a number of investigators (Sutherland, 1998; Nelson et al, 1996; Greaves et al, 1990; Mesegner et al, 1996; Chasting et al, 1995; Grove et al, 1992). a superior residence time (up to 100 minutes) for gellan in man has been shown compared to traditional viscous vehicles (HEC, HPMC, PVA).

Based on these results we hypothesized that a scleral implant of GCV made using gellan gum would provide a number of advantages over PLA /PLGA based devices reported by Kunou et al, 1995. Briefly, the gellan based device forms a gelled mass in presence of cation which erodes slowly but does not form fragments. The in-vitro drug release profile is expected to be biphasic. Since the device will not fragment, displacement into the vitreous will not occur.

12.6 OTHER MEANS OF INTRAVITREAL DELIVERY GCV.

12.6.1 Liposomally encapsulated GCV

With an aim to confine GCV in the vitreous and thereby increase the amount of drug delivered to the choroid / retina, Peyman et al, (1987) were the first investigators to report the utility of liposomally encapsulated GCV in the treatment of GCV retinitis. They showed that liposomal GCV, delivered intravitreally, decreased intraocular side effects through a controlled release depot effect, and this specialized formulation was superior to intravitreal injection of GCV solution in many ways. The liposomal GCV was retained upto 24 days after injection of 0.25 ml (1 mg GCV) in a concentration higher than ID_{50} of CMV (Akula et al, 1994). In humans, though a vitreal haze was observed due to dispersal of the liposomal particles in the vitreous but no progression or occurrence of retinitis was observed. Diaz-Llopis (1992) reported complete remission of the CMV retinitis at the third injection of 0.5 mg GCV administered once per week. No relapse was reported upto 4 months of follow up. Though the duration of action of the liposomal GCV is substantially shorter compared to vitreous or scleral implants, the absence of a surgical procedure makes this formulation an interesting alternative to the implants. The vitreal haze, poor entrapment of the hydrophilic GCV and poor physiochemical stability of liposomal GCV need to be addressed in more concerted studies, since these are intrinsically releated to all liposomal systems.

12.6.2 Transcleral iontophoresis for the intravitreal delivery of GCV

Lam et al (1994), based on their study, have reported that a therapeutic dose of GCV could be delivered to intraocular tissues through transcleral iontophoresis. Transcleral iontophoresis was performed in albino New Zealand rabbits at 1.0mA for 15 minutes with a 20% aqueous solution of GCV. After iontophoresis the vitro-retinal level of GCV was $74 \pm 17 \mu g/ml$ at 2 hour and $4.2 - 0.6 \mu g/ml$ after 24 hour, which was above the ID_{50} of GCV. It is possible to deliver higher amounts of GCV for a longer period by manipulating the different parameters of iontophoresis. Though minimal retinal lesions were noted, the effects of repeated iontophoretic application have not been studied.

12.7 FUTURE PROSPECTS

Although no future trends can be accurately surmized, two clear areas in the development of intraocular delivery of anti-CMV drugs are seen. One is that of drugs with higher activity and/ or prolonged drug release half-life. Neutral salt of the cyclic phosphate derivative of GCV, 2'- nor- cyclic GMP, was reported by Shakiba et al (1993) to be extremely water soluble, and it can be encapsulated into a MLV liposome system due to the charged phosphate group at neutral pH. They reported an in-vitro drug release half- life of 1,000 hr, and intravitreally injected at 10 μg dose, which is greater than 20 times the ID_{50} to inhibit CMV, is not toxic to the rabbit retina.

The second aspect is concerned with the development of an animal model of acute viral retinitis. Since all preliminary evaluations are done in healthy rabbitsÆ eyes, it is difficult as well as highly speculative to upgrade the data to CMV- retinitis affected eye in humans. Freeman et al (1993) have reported the development of a rabbit model which mimicks many similarities to viral retinitis (herpes simplex, zoster and CMV) in humans. Further development of the animal model is needed.

ACKNOWLEDGEMENT

Assistance rendered in the preparation of this manuscript by Mr. J.Balasubramaniam is gratefully acknowledged.

REFERENCES

Akula, S.K.; Ma, P.E.; Peyman, G.A.; Rahimy, M.H.; Hyslop Jr., N.E.; Janney, A. and Ashton, P.(1994) "Treatment of Cytomegalovirus retinitis with intravitreal injection of liposome encapsulated Ganciclovir in a patient with AIDS." Brit. J. Ophthalmol. 78: 677-680.

Anand, R.; Font, R.L.; Fish, R.H.and Nightingale, S.D. (1993)"Pathology of cytomegalovirus retinitis treated with sustained release intravitreal Ganciclovir." Ophthalmology, 100 : 1032 - 1039.

Ashton, P.; Blandford, D.L.; Pearson, P.A.; Jaffe, G.J.; Martin, D.F. and Nussenblatt, R.B. (1994) "Review: Implants." J.Ocul. Pharmacol., 10: 691- 701.

Ashton, P.; Brown, J.D.; Pearson, P.A.; Blandford, D.L.; Smith T.J.; Anand, R.; Nightingale, S.D. and Sanborn G.E.(1992) "Intravitreal Ganciclovir Pharmacokinetics in Rabbits and Man." J.Ocul. Pharmacol., 8 : 343-347.

Barza, M.; Kane, A. and Baum, J. (1982) "Effects of infection and probenecid on the transport of carbenicillin from the rabbit vitreous humour." Invest. Ophthalmol. Vis.Sci : 22:720-726.

Charles, N.C. and Steiner, G.C (1996) "Ganciclovir intraocular implant. A clinicopathologic study." Ophthalmology, 103: 416-421.

Chastaing, G.; Rozier, A.; Plazonnet,B. and Grove, J. (1995) "Gelrite enhances the ocular

penetration of pilocarpine in the pigment rabbit." Invest. Ophthalmol., 36 : S159-162.

Capparellli, E.V.; Sherwood, C.H. and Freeman, W.R. (1993) "Intravitreal Ganciclovir concentration after intravenous administration in AIDS patient with cytomegalovirus retinitis. Implications for therapy." J. Infect. Dis., 168: 1506-9.

Diaz-Llopis, M.; Martos, M.J.; Espana, E.; Cervera, M.; Vila, A.O.; Navea, A.; Molina, F.J. and Romero, F.J. "Liposomally entrapped Ganciclovir for the treatment of cytomegalovirus retinitis in AIDS patient. Experimental toxicity and pharmacokinetics and clinical trial." Doc Ophthalmol., 82 : 297-305.

Duker, J.S.; Robinson, M.; Anand, R. and Ashton, P. (1995) "Initial experience with an eight month sustained release intravitreal ganciclovir implant for the treatment of CMV retinitis associated with AIDS." Ophthalmic-Surg-Laser, 26: 442-448.

Freeman, W.R.; Schneiderman, T.E.; Wiley, C.A.; Listhaus, A.D.; Svendsen, P.; Mungia, D. and Bergeron-Lynn, G. (1993), "An animal model of focal, subacute, viral retinitis", Retina : 13, 214-221.

Greaves, J.L.; Wilson, C.G.; Rozier, A.; Groves, J. and Plazonnet, B (1990) "Scintigraphic assessment of an ophthalmic gelling vehicle in man and rabbit" Curr. Eye Res., 9: 415-420.

Grove, J.G.; Chastiang, G.; Rozier, A. and Plazzonet, B. (1992) "Ophthalmic Gelrire increases ocular bioavailability of indomethacin." Exper. Eye Res., 55: S54-57.

Hashizoe, M.; Ogura, Y.; Takanashi, T.; Kunou, N.; Honda, Y. and Ikado, Y (1997) "Biodegradable polymeric device for sustained intravitreal release by Ganciclovir in rabbits." Curr. Eye Res., 16, 663-669.

Henry, K.; Cantrill, H.; Fletcher, C.; Chinnock, B.J. and balfour, H.H. (1987) "Use of ganciclovir (dihydroxy propoxy methyl guanine) for cytomegalovirus retinitis in a patient with AIDS." Am. J. Ophthalmol. 103: 17-23.

Jabs, D.A.; Newman, C.; Buston, D.S. and Polk, B.F. (1987) " Treatment of cytomegalovirus retinitis with ganciclovir." Ophthalmology, 94, 824-880.

Kane, A.; barza, M. and Brown, J. (1981) " Intravitreal injection of gentamicin in rabbits: effect of inflammation and pigmentation on half-life and ocular distribution." Invest. Ophthalmol. Vis. Sci., 20: 593-597.

Kimura, H.; Ogura, Y.; Hashizoe, M.; Nishiwaki, H.; Honda, Y. and Ikada, Y. (1994) "A new vitreal drug delivery system using an implantable biodegradable polymeric device." Invest. Ophthalmol. Vis. Sci., 35: 2815-2819.

Kunou, N.; Ogura, Y.; Hashizoe, M.; Honda, Y.; Hyon, S. and Ikada, Y. (1995) "Intravitral ganciclovir concentration after intravenous administration in AIDS patients with cytomegalovirus retinitis: Implications for therapy." J. Cont. Rel., 37: 143-150.

Kuppermann, B.D.; Quecino, J.I.; Flores-Aguilar, M.; Connor, J.D.; Capparelli, E.V.; Sherwood, C.H. and Freeman, W.R. (1993) "Intravitreal ganciclovir concentration after intravenous administration in AIDS patient with cytomegalovirus retinitie. Implications for therapy." J. Infect. Dis., 168: 1506-1509.

Lam, T.T.; Fu, J.; Chu, R.; Stojack, K.; Siew, E. and Tso, M.O.M. (1994) " Intravitreal delivery of ganciclovir in rabbits by transdermal iontophoresis." J. Ocul. Pharmacol., 10: 571-575.

Martin, D.F.; Parks, D.J.; Mellows, S.D.; Ferris, F.L.; Walton, R.C.; Remaley, N.A.; Chew, E.Y.; Ashton, P.; Davis, M.D. and Nussenblatt, R.B. (1994) "Treatment of cytomegalovirus retinitis with an intraocular sustained release ganciclovir implant - A randomised controlled clinical trials" Arch Ophthalmol., 112: 1531-1539.

Marx, J.L.; Kapusta, M.A.; Patel, S.S.; LaBree, L.D.; Walonker, F.; Rao, N.A. and Chang, L.P.

(1996) "Use of ganciclovir implant in the treatment of recurrent cytomegalovirus retinitis." Arch. Ophthalmol, 114: 815-820.

Meseguer, G.; Buri, P.; Plazonnet, B.; Rozier, A. and Gurny, R. (1996) "Gamma scintigraphic comparisions of eyedrops containing pilocarpine in healthy volunteers." J. Ocular. Pharmacol. Ther., 12: 481-488.

Morlet, N.; Young, S.; Naidoo, D.; Graham, G. and Coroneo, M.T. (1996) "High dose intravitreal ganciclovir injection provides a prolonged therapeutic intraocular concentration." Brit. J. Ophthalmol, 80: 214-216.

Morley, M.G.; Duker, J.S.; Ashton, P. and Robinson, M.R. (1995) "Replacing ganciclovir implants." 102: 388-392.

Pang, M.P.; Branchflower, R.V.; Chang, A.T.; Peyman, G.A.; Blatt, H. and Minatoya, H.K. (1992) "Half life and vitreous clearing of trifluorothymidine after intravitreal injection in rabbit eye." Can. J. Ophthalmol., 27: 6-9.

Peyman, G.A.; Khoobehi, B.; Tawkol, M.; Schulman, J.A.; Mortada, H.A.; Alkan, H. and Fiscella, A. (1987) "Intravitreous injection of liposome encapsulate ganciclovir in rabbit model." Retina, 7: 227-229.

Plotkin, S.A.; Drew, W.L.; Felsenstein, D. and Hirsch, M.S. (1985) "Sensitivity of clinical isolates of human cytomegalovirus to 9-(1,3-dihydroxy-2-propoxymethyl)guanine." J. infect. Dis., 152: 832-834.

Sanborn, G.E.; Anand, R.; Torti, R.E.; Nightingale, S.D.; Cal, S.X.; Bradley, Y.; Ashton, P. and Smith, P. (1992)" Sustained release of ganciclovir therapy for treatment of cytomegalovirus retinitis-use of an intravitreal device." Arch. Ophthalmol., 110: 188-195.

Saran, B.R. and Maguire, A.M. (1994) retinal toxicity of high dose intravitreal ganciclovir, 14: 248-252.

Shakiba, S., assil, K.K., Listhaus, A.D., Mungwa, D., Flores-Aguilar, M., Vuong, C., Wiley, C.A.; Tolman, R.L.; karkas, J.D.; Bergeron-Lynn, G. and Freeman, W.R. (1993) "Evaluation of retinal toxicity and liposome encapsulation of the Anti-CMV drug 2'-norcyclic GMO." Invest. Ophthalmol. Vis. Sci., 34: 2903-2910.

Smith, T.J.; Pearson, P.A.; Blandford, D.L.; Brown, J.D.; Goins, K.A.; Hollins, J.L.; Schmeisser, E.T.; Glavinos, P.; Baldwin, L.B. and Ashton, P. (1992) "Intravitreous sustained release ganciclovir." Arch. Ophthalmol., 110: 155-258.

Sutherland, I.W. (1998) "Novel and established applications of microbial polysaccharide." Tibtech, 16: 41-46.

Chapter 13

Aquasomes as Drug Carrier

Sanjay K. Jain, N.K. Jain

In recent years, much revolutionary explorations were come across the formulation and development of dosage forms of small size to improve the performance of the drug (Bhave et al., 1989). Colloidal drug delivery systems include microcapsules (Bakan & Anderson, 1976), macromolecular complexes (Batz et al.,1974), microspheres (Gupta & Hung, 1989), liposomes (Ramachan & Jayesh, 1995), nanocapsules and nanoparticles (Oppenhein, et al 1982). Nanoparticulate carriear systems constitute one of the self-assembling approach for the delivery of bio-active agents. Nanoparticles can be fabricated from either polymers or ceramics. The pharmacologically active molecule can be incorporated into them either by co-polymerization within self-assembling nanoparticulate matrix or diffusion into pre-assembled nanoparticulate matrix or adsorption to the surface of pre formed nanoparticles.(Kossovsky et al.,1993). Polymeric nanoparticles can be made from quasi-biologicals like albumin or gelatin or from organics like acrylates. British Biotech developed polymeric self-assembling virus-like particles by engineering yeast retrotransposons to produce HIV core proteins, likewise crystalline carbon and calcium phosphate based nanoparticles are proved to be effective self-assembling vehicles. Drugs are allowed to adsorb on the surface of nanoparticles in the presence of carbohydrates film that prevents soft drugs from changing shape and being damaged when surface bound. These carbohydrate stabilized nanoparticles of ceramics/calcium phosphate are known as "Aquasomes", which was first developed by Nir kossovsky (Kossovsky et al., 1993). It represents a marriage of principles from microbiology, food chemistry, biophysics and many Nobel prize winning discoveries including solid phase synthesis, supramolecular chemistry, molecular shape change and self-assembly (Kossovsky, 1996). Nature is the sole example for most of these discoveries. The Baker's yeast cells provide inspiration for aquasomes discovery for stabilizing drug activity during delivery.

Aquasomes are like "bodies of water" and their water like properties help to protect and preserve the fragile biological molecules. It is comprised of a solid phase nanocrystalline core coated with oligomeric film to which the drug moieties or biochemically active molecules are adsorbed with or without modification. These three layered structures are self-assembled by non-covalent and ionic bonds (Fig 13.1).

13.1 SELF-ASSEMBLY AND SELF-ASSEMBLED NANOSTRUCTURES

Nature again exemplify the self-assembly i.e., first thermodynamic self-assembly shown by the rain drops. The liquid assumes the smooth curved surface between liquid and air and thereby maximizes its energetic stability. The second is the embryo which exemplifies the coded self-assembly (Whitesides, 1995). Liposomes are examples of self-assembling natural vehicle. They mimic cell membrane and micelles. During its preparation,

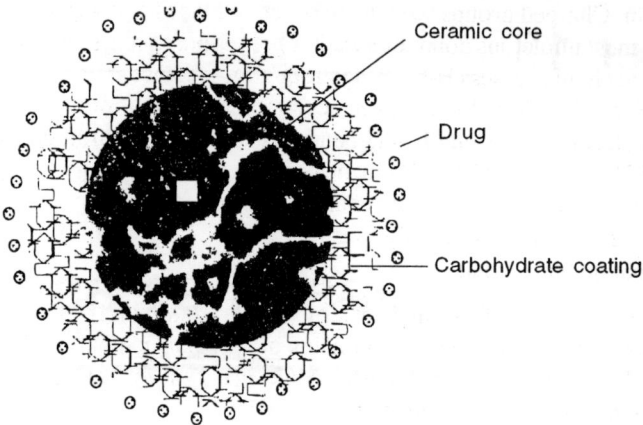

Fig 13.1 : Schematic view of aquasome

the addition of hydrophilic solution to thin layer of hydrophobic lipid film and resulting amphipathic membrane self- assembles into multilayered liposomes.

Molecules are also capable of self-assembly. Molecular self-assembly is the spontaneous association of molecules under equilibrium condition into stable, structurally well-defined aggregates joined by non-covalent bonds. Approaches based on chemical synthesis are less highly developed than approaches through micro-fabrication. Chemical synthesis , however, offer a level of control over the selection and placement of individual atoms to a high extent than other methods of fabrication (Whitesides et al., 1991). Molecular self-assembly has the additional attraction that it generates structures which occupy thermodynamic minima. These structures are robust and intrinsically very resistant to the incorporation of impurities.

13.1.1. Principle of self-assembly

Synthetic products are self-assembling if the constituent parts assume spontaneously prescribed structural orientation in two or three dimensional space. In aqueous biological environments, the assembly of macromolecule is governed basically by three physico-chemical processes: the interaction of charged groups, hydrogen bonding and dehydration effect, and structural stability (Kossovsky et al., 1994a).

13.1.1.1. Interaction between charged groups

Most biological and synthetic surfaces are charged due to intrinsic chemical groups or adsorbed ions from the biological milieu. The interaction of charged groups, such as amino, carboxyl, sulphate, phosphate groups facilitate the long range approach of self-assembling sub-units. The long range interaction of constituent sub-units and their gradual attraction is the necessary first phase of self-assembly.

Natural self-assemblies that are driven strongly by interactions of charged groups include crystal lattice formation and bone mineralization. Charged groups also play a role in stabilizing tertiary structures of folded proteins. Examples of ion pairs include drug carboxylated or phosphate groups bound to ionized arginine or lysine side chains of the protein, ionized drug nitrogen atoms binding to protein carboxylates, and metal ions co-ordinated to protein side chains or bridging between protein and ligand.

13.1.1.2. Hydrogen bonding and dehydration effects

Hydrogen bonds are formed between hydrogen atom attached to an electronegative donor atom (e.g. O, N) and an electronegative or basic acceptor (e.g. carbonyl oxygen). Either donor or acceptor can be ionised. Both donor and acceptor can be involved in more than one H-bond at a time, though unshared hydrogen bonds are most common. Charged groups seem to be better at donating or accepting multiple H-bonds. With regard to proteins, the most numerous donor or acceptor groups are of course N-H and O=C, respectively, but several of the amino acid chains possess H-bonding groups, for instance $-NH^{+3}$ (from Lys), $-CO_2-$ (from Asp., Glu) and -OH- (from Ser., Thr., Tyr). Water molecules attached to such groups are often available for further H-bonding with small molecules. The length of H-bonds also show some variation with O(H).... and O(H)....N at about 2.7Å and N(H).....O and N(H)....N at nearer 3Å. The more electronegative the acceptor and the more electropositive the hydrogen the shorter and stronger bond in every case. It is very uncommon for a H-bond to be less than 2.5Å while it is usually considered that 3.5Å is the limit, beyond which the energy of interaction is so small that no bond exists.

The lion's share in self-assembly of structures is contributed by hydrogen bonds. It is the most important molecular interaction. Hydrogen bond helps in base pair matching and stabilization of secondary protein structure such as α helices and β sheets. Molecules that form hydrogen bonds are hydrophilic and these molecules confer a significant degree of organisation to the surrounding water molecules. On the other hand, hydrophobic molecules are incapable of forming hydrogen bonds. However, their tendency to repel water helps to organize the moiety to the surrounding environment. The organized water decreases the overall level of disorder/entropy of the surrounding medium. Since, organized water is thermodynamically unfavourable, the molecules loose water/dehydrate and get self-assembled. This is the core of self-assembly.

13.1.1.3 Structural stability

Molecules that carry less charge than formally charged groups exhibit a dipole moment. The forces associated with dipoles are known as van der Waals forces. The structural stability of proteins in the biological environment is determined by the interaction between charged groups and hydrogen bonds largely external to the molecule and van der Waals forces largely internal to the molecule. The van der Waals forces, most often experienced by the relatively hydrophobic molecular regions that are shielded from water play a subtle but critical role in maintaining molecular shape or conformation during self-assembly.

The van der Waals forces are largely responsible for the "hardness" or "softness" of molecules. The van der Waals interaction among hydrophobic side chains promotes stability of compact helical structures which are thermodynamically unfavourable for expanded random coils. It is the maintenance of internal secondary structures, such as helices which provide sufficient softness, that enable molecules to maintain conformation during self-assembly, small changes are necessary for successful antigen-antibody interactions.

In biotechnological self-assembly, this can lead to altered molecular function and biological activity. Thus, the van der Waals forces are to be buffered for maintaining the optimal biological activity. In case of aquasomes, the sugar helps in the molecular plasticization.

Permanent dipoles can interact with other permanent dipoles or with point charges. The most common dipole in proteins are those formed by the amide linkage in the main chain where the configuration is helical, these line up to reinforce each other, so generating a large overall dipole moment.

Van der Waals forces arise from the interplay of dipoles induced in the electron clouds of non-bonding atoms when in close proximity. These are the weakest but most ubiquitous of interactions between molecules. At long distances, they are attractive with maximum binding when the atoms are separated by the sum of their so-called van der Waals radii. On closer approach a repulsive element due to the overlap of non- or anti-bonding electron clouds rapidly takes over so that forcing, two hydrogen only 0.5 Å closer than optimum requires several K Cal Mol^{-1} of energy.

13.2 STRATEGIES USED IN CHEMICAL SYNTHESIS OF NANOSTRUCTURES

Aquasomes are self-assembled three layered nanostructures. Therefore the strategies involved in chemical synthesis of nanostructures need elaboration. The strategies normally used in the chemical synthesis of nanostructures are discussed below.

13.2.1 Sequential covalent synthesis

This can be used to generate arrays of co-valently linked atoms with well-defined composition, connectivity and shape i.e., vitamin B12 (Woodward 1973; Eschenmoser & Wintner, 1977). It can generate structures that are far from the thermodynamic minimum for that collection of atoms. It nonetheless illustrates the basic strategy of nanostructures synthesis : the use of reversible interactions (hydrogen bonds) to bind the participating molecules in the aggregate; preorganization of the interacting group through network of covalent bond to control the entropy of association and to determine the shape of the aggregate; choice of the components so that they recognize each other with high selectivity and design of the system to show positive cooporativity.

13.2.2 Covalent polymerization

This is the most important strategy for the preparing molecules with high molecular weight (Bovey & Winslow, 1978; Seymour & Carraher, 1988). Here a relatively simple, reactive low molecular weight substances (a monomer) is caused to react with itself in a process that produces a molecule (a polymer) comprising many covalently connected monomers, e.g. formation of polyethylene from ethylene. The molecular weight of polyethylene can be high (> 106 daltons), and it is easily prepared, but the molecular structure is simple and repetitive and the process by which it is formed offers only limited opportunity for controlled variation in this structure or for control of its three dimensional shape. Polymerization indirectly provides synthetic routes to stable nanostructures e.g. phase separated polymers (Shull et al., 1991; Frankel et al., 1989).

13.2.3 Self-organizing synthesis

The third synthetic strategy widely used abandons the covalent bond as a required connection between atoms and relies instead on weaker and less directional bonds such as ionic bonds, hydrogen bonds and van der Waals interaction to organize atoms, ions or molecules into structures. The different types of structures prepared by this strategy include molecular crystals, ligand crystals, colloids, micelles, emulsions, phase-separated polymers, Languir-Blodget films and self-assembled monolayers. Self-organization is the peculiar feature of these methods. The molecules or ions adjust their own position to reach a thermodynamic minimum. By self-organization, true nanostructures can be prepared.

13.2.4. Molecular self-assembly

It is the spontaneous assembly of molecules into structured, stable, non-covalently joined aggregates. Molecular self-assembly combines the features of each of the preceding strategies to make large structurally well-defined assemblies of atoms : (1) formation of well defined molecules of intermediate structural complexity through sequential covalent synthesis; (2) formation of large, stable structurally defined aggregates of these molecules through hydrogen bonds, van der Waals interactions or other non-covalent links; and (3) use of multiple copies of one or several of the constituent molecules, or of a polymer, to simplify the synthetic task. The key to this type of synthesis is to understand and overcome the intrinsically unfavourable entropy together in a single aggregate.

For the final assembly to be stable and to have well-defined shape, the non-covalent connection between the molecules must be collectively stable. The strength of the individual van der Waals interactions and hydrogen bonds are weak (0.1 to 5 kcal/ mol) relative to typical covalent bonds (40 to 100 kcal/mol) and comparable to thermal energies (RT$\cong$0.6 kcal/ mol at 300 K). Thus, to achieve acceptable stability, molecules in self-assembled aggregates must be joined by many of these weak non-covalent interaction or by multiple hydrogen bonds or both.

13.3 RATIONAL BEHIND DEVELOPMENT OF AQUASOMES

Over the last three-decades much competing developments have been reported in the pharmaceutical field specially in the case of drug delivery with the intention of reducing the drug toxicity and dosage requirement, enhance cellular targeting and improve shelf-life. Hnatyszyn et al. (1994) have explained the three competing systems like prodrug or zymogen-like systems, simple soluble macromolecular systems and complex particulate multicomponent systems.

The carriers like prodrugs, macromolecules and liposomes have served to attain the intended purpose. However, all these are prone to have biophysical constraints. The destructive interactions between the drug carrier and the drug are often inevitable and these always bring limitation to the drug delivery system. In such a circumstance, the aquasomes are worth promising carrier, which are comprised of solid carriers whose surface has been treated with a film of carbohydrate to prevent destructive denaturing drug interactions.

Molecular conformation is an important attribute as molecular composition in most biochemical processes (Stryer, 1988). Normally, the pharmacological molecules exhibit three activity related spatial qualities: a unique three-dimensional conformation, a freedom of internal molecular rearrangement induced by molecular interactions, and a freedom of bulk movement. This is to be maintained for optimum pharmacological activity. Dehydration, degradation and decomposition can change these spatial qualities. Many of the biological molecules like proteins undergo irreversible denaturation and become non-functional when desiccated (Carpenter et al., 1986; Hellman et al., 1983), at the same time, they are not resistant to denaturation for a long time in aqueous state. In the aqueous state pH, temperature, solvents, salts, etc., can cause denaturation. So the challenge is to maintain a water like circumstance otherwise it may lead to dehydration and conformational changes, which in turn leads to degradation and alteration of chemical composition. This can not be appreciated when one is aware that the pharmacologically active molecules derive their structural and functional properties from their chemical composition.

The intrinsic biophysical constraints, dehydration and conformational changes caused by the drug delivery system can lead to adverse or allergic reaction with suboptimal pharmacological activity (Hnatyszyn et al., 1994; Haberland et al., 1992). By incorporating such biological molecules on aquasomes with natural stabilizers, one can preserve the molecular conformation since these natural sugars act as dehydroprotectants.

Many reports are there to support the dehydroprotectant activity of natural sugars (Back et al., 1979; Lee & Timasheff, 1981). Fungal spores producing ergot were stabilized by sucrose rich solution (Loo & Lewis, 1955; Lewis, 1948; Arakawa & Timasheff, 1982). Desiccation induced molecular denaturation is reported to be prevented by certain disaccharides like trehalose (Crowe, 1971; Crowe et al., 1988). Back et al. (1979) reported that sugars and polyols stabilize protein against heat denaturation and it is argued that this stabilization is due to the effects of sugars and polyols on hydrophobic interactions. The extent of stabilization by different sugars and polyols is explained by their different influences on the structure of water. The hydroxyl groups on the carbohydrate interact with polar and charged groups of the biological molecules in a manner similar to water molecules alone and preserve the aqueous structure of biological molecules like proteins on dehydration (Prestelski et al., 1993). Since these disaccharides are rich in hydroxyl groups and help to replace the water around the polar residues in proteins, thus maintaining their integrity in the absence of water. The free bond mobility associated with a rich hydroxyl component creates a unique hydrogen binding substrate that produces a glassy aqueous state (Quiocho, 1988; Johnson et al., 1988; Green & Angell, 1989; Levine & Slade, 1992; Kossovsky et al., 1994a; 1994b; 1994c; Franks, 1994; Peleg, 1994). Presence of the sugar, trehalose, both inside and outside liposome bilayers reveals that almost 100% of trapped solute retained in rehydrated vesicles having been freeze dried with 1.8 g of trehalose per gram of drug phospholipid (Debolt et al., 1976). Other sugars, which exhibit similar dehydroprotectant activity, include cellobiose, sucrose, glucose, maltose, lactitol and raffinose (Crowe et al., 1984).

There are many systemic biophysical and intrinsic biophysical constraints, which tend to destabilize the drug. The intrinsic biophysical constraints caused by the delivery systems can be removed by using natural molecular stabilizers like sugar.

13.3.1 Systemic biophysical constraints

There are physical and chemical degradative agents, which cause compositional changes and loss of spatial activity by breaking chemical bonds in the drug candidate. Such agents include UV radiation, heat, ozone, peroxide and other free radicals. Likewise, mammalian body also contains certain agents viz.. inflammatory peroxides, free radicals and degradative enzymes related to serine proteases (Franks,1994). Other than these physical and chemical degradative agents, those agents that promote dehydration also cause molecular inactivation. Since water is a critical structural component of most biochemically reactive molecules, its loss leads to change in energies and results in altered molecular conformation and impaired spatial qualities (Dunitz, 1994; Ragone & Colonna, 1994; Bryan, 1994). Exposure and surface immobilization often promotes dehydration. Degradative agents present in mammals can destroy rapidly complex and expensive polypeptide biopharmaceuticals, while denaturation during dehydration can impair polypeptides on long term storage (Norde & Lyklema, 1992).

13.3.2 Intrinsic biophysical constraints

The intrinsic biophysical constraints are normally imposed by drug delivery system. When drug candidates are immobilized to nanoparticulate substrate, it can cause surface induced dehydration and, in turn, molecular conformation. The altered molecular conformation can produce adverse or allergic reaction with suboptimal pharmacological activity. (Hnatyszyn et al., 1994; Hubbard et al., 1993; Hoff et al., 1992).

In short, biochemically active molecules loose their functional properties in either case, means in a "dry" and "wet" state. At the same time, a water environment is vital for molecular activity. Therefore, the challenge is to store and transport promising and useful biomolecules in the dry state without causing them to loose too much of their potential activity.

In such a situation, the aquasomes with natural stabilizers are promising. The different polyhydroxy oligomers/sugars act as a dehydroprotectant and thereby help to preserve the molecular conformation of bioactive molecules in dry solid state. The stabilization efficiency of sugars are reported in literature. Fungal spores producing ergot alkaloids were stabilized by sucrose-rich solution (Lewis, 1948; Loo & Lewis, 1955). Desiccation-induced molecular denaturation is reported to be prevented by certain disaccharides (Crowe et al., 1988).

13.3.3 Role of disaccharides in preserving molecular structure

The hydroxyl groups on the carbohydrate interact with polar and charged groups on the proteins, in a similar manner to water molecules alone and preserve the aqueous structure of proteins on dehydration (Prestelski, 1993). Disaccharides such as trehalose are reported to have stress tolerance in fungi, bacteria, insects, yeast and some plants. Trehalose works by protecting proteins and membranes within plant cells during the desiccation process (Crowe, 1971; Crowe et al., 1988) and thereby preserves cell structures, inherent flavours, colours and textures. These disaccharides are rich in hydroxyl group and help to replace the water around polar residues in proteins, thereby maintaining their integrity in the absence of water. The free bond mobility associated with a rich hydroxyl component creates a unique hydrogen binding substrate that produces a glassy aqueous state (Kossovsky et al., 1994a, 1994b, 1995b; Franks.1994; Levine & Slade, 1992; Green & Angell, 1989).

The first studies, indicating that the structure and function of cellular components could be protected by sugar during lyophilization, were conducted with Ca-transporting microsomes isolated from rabbit muscles (Sreter et al., 1970) and lobster muscles (Crowe et al., 1983). When Ca-transporting microsomes are lyophilized without stabilizing sugar, the rehydrated vesicles show greatly reduced Ca-uptake and uncoupling of ATPase activity. Vesicles lyophilized in presence of as little as 0.3 g trehalose per g membrane upon rehydration are morphologically distinguishable from freshly prepared vesicles (Crowe et al. 1983, 1984). Green & Angell

(1989) reported that the trehalose/water system passes into the glassy state and thereby arrests all long range molecular motion. Denaturation is thus impeded. Presence of trehalose both inside and outside liposome bilayers reveals that almost 100% of trapped solute retained in rehydrated vesicles having been freeze dried with 1.8g of trehalose per g of dry phospholipid (Debolt et al., 1976). Rozhkov (1991) described a similar stabilizing protein activity by saccharose. The glass transition temperature of the most common natural dehydroprotectants, trehalose and sucrose, are 79° and 70°C, respectively; and that of cellobiose is 77°C. Other sugars, which exhibit similar dehydroprotectant activity, include cellobiose, sucrose, glucose, maltose, lactitol and raffinose (Crowe et al., 1984).

Timasheff and his colleagues have determined the mechanism by which sugars exert their protective influence. It is well established that sugars stabilize protein solution against such perturbations like thermally induced unfolding and pH-induced dissociation (Back et al., 1979; Lee & Timasheff, 1981; Arakawa & Timasheff, 1982).

Many organic compounds are known to stabilize proteins in solutions. Sugars, polyols and amino acid have also been used as effective cytoprotectants for soluble proteins (Carpenter et al., 1986; Shikama & Yamazaky, 1961; Chilson et al., 1965; Brandts et al. 1970).

13.4. METHOD OF PREPARATION OF AQUASOME

By using the principle of self-assembly, the aquasomes are prepared in three steps i.e., preparation of core, coating of core, and immobilization of drug molecule. It is well known that the aquasome is an aqueous colloid comprised of small solids formed from relatively few atoms clustered in solid crystals to which glassy carbohydrates are then applied as surface coating. The carbohydrate coated core serves as non-denaturing solid phase for the subsequent attachment of the active drug candidate which then individually confer the final properties of colloids. The three layered solid phase of the colloid (aquasomes), is fully self-assembling and is maintained through both ionic and non-covalent bonds, van der Waals forces and entropic forces (Fig 13.2).

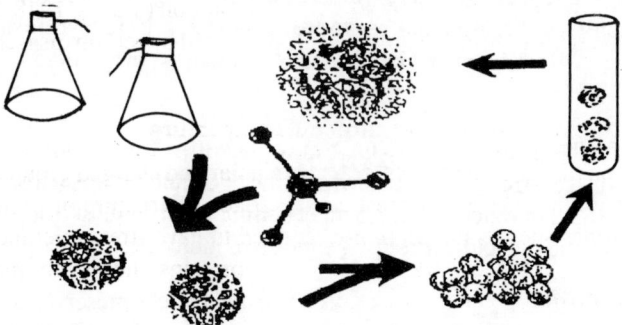

Fig 13.2 : Diagramatic representation of aquasome preparation

13.4.1 Preparation of the core

The first step of aquasome preparation is the fabrication of the ceramic core. The process of ceramic core preparation depends on the selection of the materials for core. These ceramic cores can be fabricated by colloidal precipitation and sonication, inverted magnetron sputtering, plasma condensation and other processes (Kossovsky et al., 1994a).

For the core, ceramic materials were widely used because ceramics are structurally the most regular materials known. Being crystalline, the high degree of order in ceramics ensures that any surface modification will have only a limited effect on the nature of the atoms below the surface layer and thus the bulk properties of the ceramic will be preserved. The high degree of order also ensures that the surfaces will exhibit high level of surface energy that will favour the binding of polyhydroxy oligomeric surface film. Two ceramic cores that are most often used are diamond and calcium phosphate. The freshly prepared particles have good properties to adsorb environmental molecules within fraction of a second (Ca 10^{-6}S). Colloid chemistry is able to precipitate small uniform crystals of inorganic solids with astonishing regularity in size and properties.

13.4.1.1 Synthesis of nanocrystalline tin oxide core ceramic

It can be synthesized by direct current reactive magnetron sputtering. Here, a 3 inches diameter target of high purity tin is sputtered in a high pressure gas mixture of organ and oxygen. The ultrafine particles formed in the gas phase are then collected on copper tubes cooled to 77°K with flowing nitrogen.

13.4.1.2 Self-assembled nanocrystalline brushite (Calcium phosphate dihydrate)

These can be prepared by colloidal precipitation and sonication by reacting solutions of disodium hydrogen phosphate and calcium chloride.

1.4.1.3 Nanocrystalline carbon ceramic, diamond particles

These can also be used for the core synthesis after ultra cleansing and sonication.

The common feature of the various cores is that they are crystalline and that when they are introduced into the synthetic processes, they measure between 50-150nm and exhibit extremely clean and therefore reactive surfaces (Norde & Lyklema, 1992; Israelachvili, 1985; Horbett & Brash, 1987).

13.4.2 Carbohydrate coatings

The second step involves coating by carbohydrate on the surface of ceramic cores. There are number of processes to enable the carbohydrate (polyhydroxy oligomers) coating to adsorb epitaxially on to the surface of the nanocrystalline ceramic cores (Kossovsky et al., 1990; 1991; 1993; Kossovsky & Millett, 1991) The processes generally entail the addition of polyhydroxy oligomer to a dispersion of meticulously cleaned ceramics in ultrapure water, sonication and then lyophilization to promote the largely irreversible adsorption of carbohydrate on to the ceramic surfaces. Excess and readily desorbing carbohydrate is removed by stir cell ultrafiltration. The commonly used coating materials are cellobiose, citrate, pyridoxal-5-phosphate, sucrose and trehalose (Blifield et al., 1991; Bauman & Gauldie, 1994; Kossovsky et al., 1995a). (Fig 13. 3).

13.4.2.1 Cellobiose

It is 4-0-ß-D-glucopyranosil-D-glucose [$C_{12}H_{22}O_{11}$, m.w. 342.30]. It does not occur free in nature or as glycoside. It is prepared from cell-free enzymatic hydrolyzate of cellulose. It is with an indifferent taste. One gram cellobiose dissolves in 8 ml of water and in 1.5 ml of boiling water, almost insoluble in alcohol and ether. It reduces Fehling's solution and on acid hydrolysis, yields two molecules of ß-D-glucose.

13.4.2.2 Pyridoxal-5-phosphate

It is 3-hydroxy 2 methyl-5-[(phosphonoxy)methyl]-4-ester or 3 hydroxy 5-(hydroxy methyl)-2-methyl isonicotinaldehyde 5-phosphate. [$C_8H_{10}NO_6$, m.w. 247.14]. It is prepared by the action of phosphorous oxychloride on pyridoxal in aqueous solution and by phosphorylation of pyridoxamine with 100% H_3PO_4 followed by oxidation. It is colourless in acid solution and bright yellow in alkaline solution. Alkaline solution gives a U.V. maxima at 390 nm (Emax 3.7) and in acid solution it is 295 nm (Emax 5.1). It gives a negative 2,6-dichloroquinone chlorimide test. On oxidation with hydrogen peroxide in alkaline solution, it yields [(2-methyl 3,4-dihydroxy-5-pyridyl)methyl] phosphoric acid.

13.4.2.3 Trehalose

It is α-D glucopyranosil α-D glucopyranoside [$C_{12}H_{22}O_4$, m.w. 342.30]. It is found in the parasite beetle,

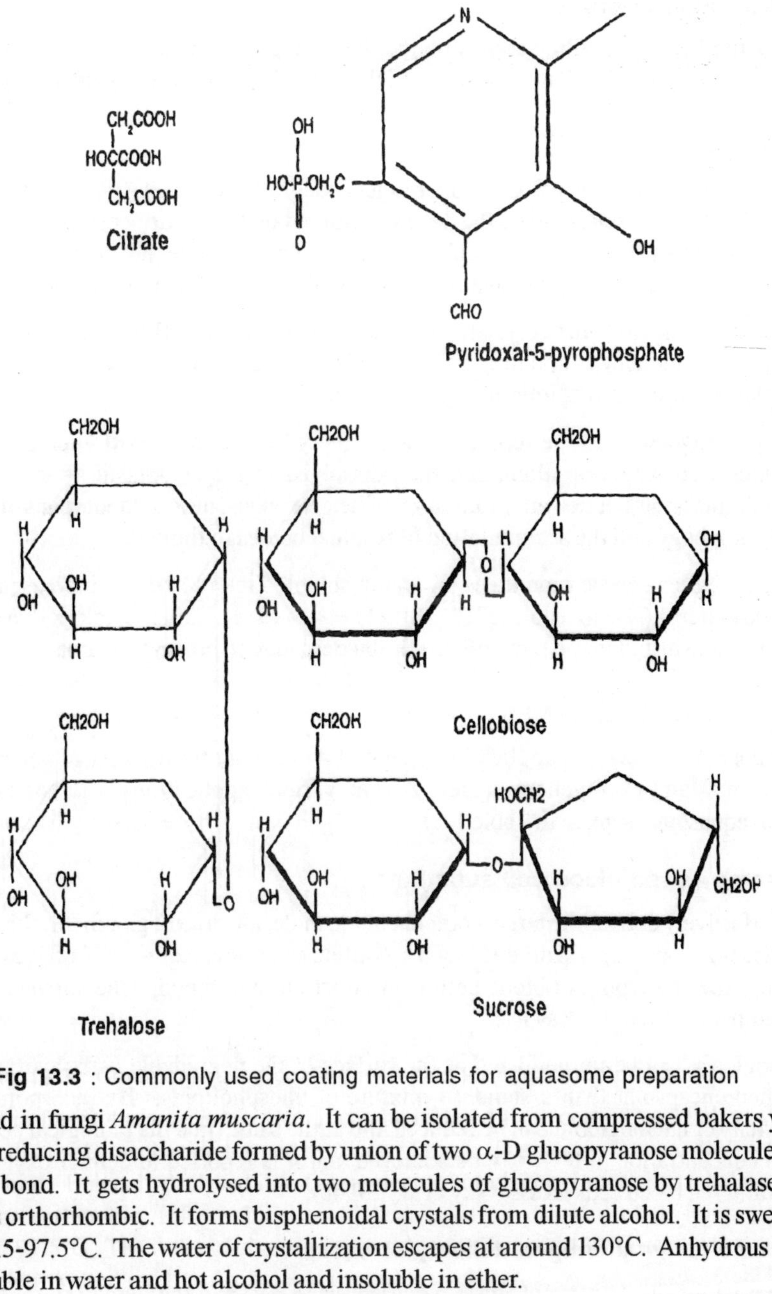

Citrate

Pyridoxal-5-pyrophosphate

Cellobiose

Trehalose

Sucrose

Fig 13.3 : Commonly used coating materials for aquasome preparation

Larinus species and in fungi *Amanita muscaria*. It can be isolated from compressed bakers yeast. This is a symmetrical, non-reducing disaccharide formed by union of two α-D glucopyranose molecules connected by an α-α glucosidic bond. It gets hydrolysed into two molecules of glucopyranose by trehalase or by mineral acids. Dihydrate is orthorhombic. It forms bisphenoidal crystals from dilute alcohol. It is sweet in taste. The melting point is 96.5-97.5°C. The water of crystallization escapes at around 130°C. Anhydrous trehalose melts at 203°C. It is soluble in water and hot alcohol and insoluble in ether.

13.4. 2.4 Sucrose

Sucrose or cane sugar is a disaccharide composed of one molecule of α-D-glucopyranose and one molecule of ß-D-fructofuranose. There is no free aldehyde or ketone group in sucrose molecule. Thus, it is a non-reducing sugar and does not undergo mutarotation. It can be hydrolysed by dilute mineral acids on heating. Sucrose is also hydrolysed by invertase and the equimolar mixture of glucose and fructose due to its change in optical rotation.

13.4.3 Immobilization of drugs

The surface modified nanocrystalline cores provide the solid phase for the subsequent non-denaturing self-assembly for broad range of biochemically active molecules. The drug can be loaded by partial adsorption.

13.5 FATE OF AQUASOME

The drug delivery vehicle aquasome is colloidal range biodegradable nanoparticles, so that they will be more concentrated in liver and muscles. Since the drug is adsorbed on to the surface of the system without further surface modification as in case of insulin and antigen delivery, they may not find any difficulty in receptor recognition on the active site so that the pharmacological or biological activity can be achieved immediately.

In normal system, the calcium phosphate is a biodegradable ceramic. Biodegradation of ceramic in vivo is achieved essentially by monocytes and multicellular cells called osteoclasts because they intervene first at the biomaterial implantation site during inflammatory reaction.

Two types of phagocytosis were reported when cells come in contact with biomaterial, either calcium phosphate crystals were taken up alone and then dissolved in the cytoplasm after disappearance of the phagosome membrane or dissolution after formation of heterophagosomes. Phagocytosis of calcium phosphate coincided with autophagy and the accumulation of residual bodies in the cell.

Monocytic activities can be modulated by many soluble factors and are increased by IFN-g or 1,25 dihydroxy cholecalciferol (Kreutz et al., 1993; Blifield et al., 1991). Other cytokines can also contribute to inflammatory mechanism and may be involved in the biodegradation process (Bauman & Gauldie, 1994).

13.6. APPLICATIONS OF AQUASOMES

Aquasome has got a quite versatile application potential as a carrier for delivery of vaccines, haemoglobin, drugs, dyes, enzymes and even genetic material. The various applications with the rationale behind its incorporation on aquasome is given in Table 13.1.

13.6.1. Aquasome as red blood cell substitute

Aquasome can effectively deliver the large, complex labile molecule, haemoglobin. In this form, many of the biological hurdles for producing a synthetic blood substitute can be overcome. This solves the major problem of incompatibility thereby typing of blood before administration of blood. The surrogate produced can be easily stored and freeze dried for easy use.

The haemoglobin can be immobilized at the surface of the degradable carbohydrate coated diamond particles and then encapsulated in a standard mixture of phospholipids. By incorporating in aquasome carriers, the toxicity of haemoglobin can be reduced and at the same time the biological activity is preserved. A haemoglobin concentration of 80% can be achieved and it is reported to deliver oxygen in a non-linear manner like natural red blood cells (Kossovsky et al., 1994c).

13.6.2. Aquasome for viral antigen delivery or vaccine:

Aquasomes are used for the delivery of Epstein-Barr virus (EBV) and the human immune deficiency virus (HIV). For the B-cell stimulation, the protein antigens should be in their native conformational state. Using surface modified carbon and calcium phosphate ceramic particulates, the nonnuclear material extracted from HIV-1 is immobilized. Here, the cleaned ceramic was coated with the disaccharide cellobiose and mixed with the emulsified viral protein and then dialyzed into the final delivery vehicle. The HIV decoys could elicit both humoral and cellular immune responses similar to that evoked by whole (live) HIV virus (Kossovsky et al., 1995b).

In case of EBV, the solid phase core is tin oxide with cellobiose coating and the biological agent is the major glycoprotein, gp 350, (glycoprotein of molecular weight 350,000) of the envelope of the EBV. The whole virus is solubilized, genetic material removed and the remaining proteins cleaned and isolated and then immobilized on the surface modified cores. The self-assembled viral decoys exhibited both physiological and immunological similarities with native EBV. They could evoke 4 and 3.5 fold greater responses than that evoked by infections of pure viral envelope, gp 350, and Freund's complete adjuvant plus gp 350, respectively.

Mussel adhesive protein (MAP) was also immobilized in a similar way on cellobiose coated diamond particles (Kossovsky et al., 1995a). Antibodies raised against the aqueous conformation of MAP bind avidly to MAP immobilized on a hydrophilic surface (treated polystyrene) and substantially less avidly to MAP immobilized on a hydrophobic surface (siliconized).

In the case of antigen delivery, recognition of antigens by immunocompetent cells involves interactions that are specific to the chemical sequence and conformation of the epitope. These aquasome delivery vehicles provide conformational stabilization as well as a high degree of surface exposure to protein antigens (Kossovsky et al., 1995b).

13.6.3. Aquasomes for Insulin delivery

The colloidal precipitation and sonication of a solution of disodium hydrogen phosphate and calcium chloride prepare the calcium phosphate dihydrate core. This core is then further coated with coating materials like cellobiose, citrate, pyridoxal-5-phosphate and trehalose under sonication and the drug is loaded to these coated nanoparticles or aquasomes by partial adsorption mechansim at low temperature or lyophilization. By microporating insulin via this delivery vehicle, the three dimensional structure and chemical integrity could be preserved and the pharmacological activity could be increased to 60% with the same dose of insulin on intravenous administration (Cherian and Jain, 2000; Kossovsky, 1996).

Further, aquasomes can be used for the efficient delivery of enzymes like DNAse, genetic material and pigments/dyes/cosmetics.

Table 13.1: Applications of Aquasome

Use	Protein/surface	Rationale macromolecules
Vaccines	Antigenic envelope	To be effective protein protective antibodies must be raised against conformationally specific target molecules .
Blood substitutes	Haemoglobin	Physiological binding and release of O_2 by haemoglobin is conformationally sensitive
Pharmaceuticals	Active drug	Drug activity is conformationally specific
Pigents/dyes	Dye agent	Wavelength absorption and reflection / cosmetics properties of natural pigments are sensitive to molecular conformation
Enzymes	Polypeptide	Activity fluctuates with molecular conformation. Gene therapy Genetic Targeted intracellular material delivery

13.6 CONCLUSION

Aquasomes represent one of the simplest yet a novel drug carrier based on the fundamental principle of self-assembly. The drug candidates delivered through the aquasomes show better biological activity even in case of conformationally sensitive ones. This is probably due to the presence of the unique carbohydrate coating the ceramic. This molecular plasticizer, carbohydrate prevents the destructive drug-carrier interaction and helps to preserve the spatial qualities. Moreover, the crystalline nature of the core gives structural stability and overall integrity. In conclusion, aquasomes appear to be promising carriers for the delivery of a broad range of molecules including viral antigens, haemoglobin and insulin. This strategy may be beneficially extended to the novel delivery of other bioactive molecules. However, the roles of molecular plasticizers and core crystallinity need further extensive investigations.

REFERENCES

Arakawa, T. and Timasheff, S.N. (1982) "Stabilization of protein structures by sugars." Biochemistry 21: 6536-6544.

Back, J.F.; Oakenfull, D. and Smith, M.B. (1979) "Increased thermal stability of proteins in the presence of sugars and polyols." Biochemistry, 18: 5191-5196.

Bakan, J. A. and Anderson, J. L. (1976) In "Theory and practice of industrial pharmacy", Lachman L., Lieberman, H.A. and Kannig, J.C., Eds. , 2nd edition, Lea and Febigen, Philadelphia, pp 420.

Batz, H.G.; Ringsdrof, H. and Ritter, H. (1974) "Pharmacologically Active Polymers", Macromol. Chem, 175 (8) : 2229-2239.

Bauman, H. and Gauldie, J. (1994) " The acute phase response." Immunol. Today. 15: 74-88.

Bhave, S.; Sewak, P. and Saxena, J. (1989) "Nanoparticles. A new colloidal drug delivery system." The Eastern Pharmacist, Oct. 17-21

Blifield, D.C.; Prehn, J.L. and Jordan, S. (1991) "Stimulus- specific $1,25 (OH)_2D_3$ Modulation of TNF and Il-1 beta gene expression in human peripheral blood mononuclear cells and monocytoid cell lines." Transplantation, 51: 498-503.

Bovey, F.A. and Winslow, F.H. (1978) " Macromolecules", Academic Press., New York.

Brandts, J.F.; Fu, J. and Nordin, J.H. (1970) In " The Frozen Cell", Wetnhme,G.E.W. and O'Conner, M., eds., Churchill, London, pp. 189-212.

Bryan, W.P. (1994) Science, 266: 1726.

Carpenter, J.F.; Hand, S.C.; Crowe, L.M. and Crowe, J.H. (1986) "Cryoprotection of phosphofructokinase with organic solute : characterization of enhanced protection in the presence of divalent cations." Arch. Biochem. Biophys., 250: 505-512.

Cherian, A. and Jain S. K. (2000) "Self assembled carbohydrate stabilized ceramic nanoparticles for the parenteral delivery of insulin." Drug Dev. Ind. Pharm., 26: 459-463.

Chilson, O.P.; Costello, L.A.; Kaplan, N.O. (1965) Fed. Proc., 24: 825.

Crowe, J.H. (1971) "Anhydrobiosis: An unresolved problem." Am. Nat. 105: 563-574.

Crowe, J.H.; Crowe, L.M. and Jackson S.A. (1983) "Preservation of structural and functional activity in lyophilised sarcoplasmin reticulum." 220 (2) : 477-484.

Crowe, J.H.; Crowe, L.M. and Chapman, D. (1984) "Infrared spectroscopic studies on interactions of water and carbohydrate with a biological membrane." Arch. Biochem. Biophys. 232: 400.

Crowe, J.H.; Crowe, L.M.; Carpenter, J.F.; Rudolph, A.S.; Wistrom, C.A.; Spargo, B.J. and Acnhordoguy, T.J. (1988) "Interaction of sugars with membrane." Biochim. Biophys. Acta, 947: 367-384.

Debolt, M.A.; Easteal, A.J.; Macedo, P.B. and Moynihan, C.T. (1976). "Analysis of structural relaxation in glass using rate heating data." J. Am. Ceramic Soc., 59: 16-21.

Dunitz, J. D. (1994) "The entropic cost of bound water in crystals and biomolecules." Science, 264, 670.

Eschenmoser, A.E. and Wintner, C.E. (1977) "Natural product synthesis and Vit B12." Science, 196:1410.

Frankel, D.A.; Lamparski, H.: Liman, U.; O'Brien, D. F. (1989) "Photoinduced destabilization of bilayer vesicles." J. Am. Chem. Soc., 111: 9262.

Franks, F. (1994) "Long term stabilization of biologicals." Bio/Technology, 12: 253.

Green, J.L. and Angell, C.A. (1989) "Phase relations and vitrification in sacharide water solutions and trehalose anomaly." J. Phys. Chem. 93: 2880-2882.

Gupta P.R. and Hung, C.P. (1989) "Albumin microspheres I : Physicochemical characteristics." J. Microencap. 6: 427.

Haberland, M.E.; Fless, G.M.; Scanu, A.M. and Fogelman, A.M. (1992) "Malondialdehyde modification of lipoprotein (a) produces avid uptake by human monocyte-macrophages." J. Biol. Chem., 267: 4143-4151.

Hellman, K.; Miller, D.S. and Cammack, K.A. (1983) "The effect of freeze drying on the quaternary structure of L-asparaginase from Erwinia carotovora." Biochim. Biophys. Acta. 749: 133-142.

Hnatyszyn, H.J.; Kossovsky, N.; Gelman, A. and Sponsler, E. (1994) "Drug delivery systems for the future." PDA J. Pharm. Sci. Technol., 48(5) : 247-254.

Hoff, H.F.; Whitaker T.E. and O'Neil J. (1992) "Oxidation of low density lipoproteins leads to particle aggregation and altered macrophase recognition." 267 (1) : 602-609.

Horbett, T.A.; Brash, J.L. (1987) "Proteins at interfaces : Current issues and future prospects." In: Brash, J.L. and Horbett, T.A. (eds.), "Proteins at interfaces : Physicochemical and Biochemical Studies." ACS symposium Series, 343: Washington : ACS, pp 1-33

Hubbard, A.K.; Lorh, C.L.; Hastings, K. (1993) Immunipharm. Immunitoxicol., 15: 621-637.

Israelachvili, J. N. (1985) "Intermolecular and surface forces." New York Academic Press.

Johnson, L.N.; Cheetham, J.; McLaunghlin, P. J.; Acharya, K. R.; Barford, D. and Philips, D. C. (1988) "Protein-oligosaccharide interactions : lysozyme, phophorylase, amylases." Curr. Top. Microbiol. Immunol. 139: 81-134.

Kossovsky, N. (1996) "Perfecting delivery." Chemistry in Britain, 43-45.

Kossovsky, N. ; Millett, D.; Gelman, L.A.; Sponsler, E.D. and Hnatyszyn, H.J. (1993) "Self-assembling nanostructures." Biotechnology, 11: 1534.

Kossovsky, N. and Millett, D. (1991) "Materials biotechnology and blood substitutes." Matr. Res. Soc. Bull., Sept.: 78-81.

Kossovsky, N.; Bunshah, R. F.; Gelman, A.; Sponsler, E.D.; Umarjee, D.M.; Sulr, T.G.; Prakash, S.; Doer, H. J. and Deshpandey, C.V. (1990) "A non-denaturing solid phase pharmaceutical carrier comprised of surface-modified nanocrystalline materials." J. Appl. Biomater., 1: 289-294.

Kossovsky, N.; Gelman, A. and Sponsler, E.E. (1994c) "Cross linking encapsulated haemoglobin with solid phase supports : lipid enveloped haemoglobin adsorbed to surface modified ceramic particles exhibit physiological oxygen lability. Artif. Cells Blood Sub." Immobil. Biotech. 223: 479-485.

Kossovsky, N.; Gelman, A.; Hnatyszyn, H.J.; Rajguru, S.; Garrel, R.L.; Torbati, S.; Freitas, S.S. and Chow, G.M. (1995b) "Surface modified diamond nanoparticles as antigen delivery vehicles." Bioconjug. Chem. 6, 5: 507-511.

Kossovsky, N.; Gelman, A.; Sponsler, E.; Rajguru, S.; Torres, M.; Mena, E.; Ly, K. and Festekjian, A. (1995a) "Preservation of surface-dependent properties of viral antigens following immobilization on particulate ceramic delivery vehicles." J. Biomed. Mater. REs., 29,5:561-573.

Kossovsky, N.; Gelman, A.; Sponsler, E.D.; Millett, D. (1991) "Nano-crystalline Epstein-Bar Virus decoys." J. Appl. Biomater., 2: 251-259.

Kossovsky, N.; Gelman, A.; Sponsler, E.E.; Hnatyszyn, A.J.; Rajguru, S.; Torres, M.; Pham, M.; Crowder, J.; Zemanovich, J.; Chung, A. and Shah, R. (1994a) "Surface modified nanocrystalline ceramic for drug delivery applications." Biomaterials, 15: 1201-1207.

Kossovsky, N.; Nguyen, A.; Sukiassians, K.; Festekjian, A.; Gelman, A. and Sponsler, E. (1994b) "Secondary structure of albumin acquired rapidly by modified conventional ATR-FTIR is comparable CD spectral data." J. Colloid. Interface Sci., 166: 350-355.

Kreutz, M.; Andreesen, R.; Krause, S.; Szabo, A.; Ritz E. and Reichel, H. (1993) "Dihydroxy vitamin D3 production and Vitamin D-3 receptor expression are developmentally regulated during differentiation of human monocytes into macrophages." Blood, 82: 1300-1307.

Lee, J.C. and Timasheff, S.N. (1981) "The stabilization of proteins by sucrose." J. Biol. Chem. 256: 7193-7201

Levine, H. and Slade, L. (1992) "Another view of trehalose for drying and stabilizing biological materials." Biopharm. May: 36-40.

Lewis, R.W. (1948) "Artificial inoculation of rye with Erogt. A susceptible rye and the control of Ergot beetles." J. Am. Pharm. Assoc. 37: 511-512.

Loo, Y.H. and Lewis, R.W. (1955) "Alkaloid formation in Ergot sclerotia." Science, 121: 367-369.

Norde, W. and Lyklema, J. (1992) "Why proteins prefer interfaces." In: Bamford G.H.; Cooper, S.L.; Tsuruta, T. eds. "The Vroman Effect." Utrecht: VSP

Oppenheim, R. C.; Stenwart, N. F.; Gordon, L. and Patel, H.M. (1982) "Drug Dev. Ind. Pharm." 8: 513.

Peleg, M. (1994) "A Model of Mechanical Changes in Biomaterials at and around their glass transition." Biotechnol. Prog. 10: 385-388.

Prestelski, S.J.; Tedeschi, N.; Arakawa, T. and Carpenter, J.F. (1993) "Dehydration induced conformational transitions in proteins and their inhibition by stabilizers." Biophys. J., 65: 661-671.

Quiocho, F.A. (1988) "Molecular features and basic understanding of protein-carbohydrate interactions : the arabinose-binding protein-sugar complex." Curr. Top. Microbiol. Immunol. 13 : 81-134.

Ragone, R. and Colonna, G. (a1994) "The role of conditional hydration on the thermodynamics of protein folding." J. Am. Chem. Soc., 116: 2677.

Ramchan, M.W. and Jayesh, R.B. (1995) "Manufacture of liposomes : A review." Current Science, 68:715.

Rozhkov, S.P. (1991), Biofizika, 36: 571.

Seymour, R.B. and Carraher, C.E. Jr. (1988) "Polymer Chemistry ", Dekker, New York.

Shikama K. and Yamazaki I (1961) "Denaturation of catalase by freezing and thawing". Nature 190 (1) : 83-84.

Shull, K.R.; Winey K.I.; Thomas E.L. and Kramer E.J. (1991) "Segregation of block co-polymer micelles to surfaces and interfaces". Macromolecules, 24 (10) : 2748-2751.

Sreter, F.; Ikemoto, N. and Gergeley J. (1970) "The efffect of lyophilization and dithiothreitol on vesicels of skeletal and cardiac muscel sarcoplasmic reticulum." Biochem. Biophys. Acta. 203 : 354-357.

Stryer, L., Ed., (1988) Biochemistry, III Edition, W. H. Freeman & Co. New York, 15-41.

Whitesides, G.M. (1995) "Self-assembling materials." Scientific American, 114-117

Whitesides, G.M.; Mathias, J.P. and Seto C.T. (1991) "Molecular self-assembly and nanochemistry : A chemical strategy for the synthesis of nanostructures." Science, 254: Nov. 1312-1319.

Woodward, R.P. (1973) "The total synthesis of vitamin B_{12}", Pure Appl. Chem., 3 (1) : 145-177.

Chapter 14

Engineered Nanoerythrosomes as a Novel Drug Carrier

Sanjay Jain, N. K. Jain

14.1. INTRODUCTION

The inadequacy of therapeutic armentorium of drugs used conventionally and their inability to perform upto a desirable level, have drawn the attention of pharmaceutical community. Profound undesirable side effects, lack in efficacy, inconvenience due to multiple dosing are some of the glaring situations that need immediate redressal. Improper drug distribution inside the biological system not only causes the distresses to the other body tissues but also demands more number of therapeutic molecules to evoke the needed effect consequently exaggerating the conditions. Frequent and repeated dosing is required to maintain a therapeutic drug level due to drug's instability in biological milieu. Drugs have often been observed to be ineffective due to their lack of interaction with the receptors and the development of resistance by the microorganisms. In these perspectives, treatment of various diseases reflects a compromise between the beneficial and hazardous effects and after a level, drugs are required to be withdrawn from the therapy. Thus an improvement and development of the drugs are of utmost importance for their better utilization. So, current research in drug delivery is aimed at maximizing the therapeutic efficacy of drugs and minimizing the side effects. Targeted drug delivery is a means of achieving this objective. In the past years, there has been a growing interest in the design and evaluation of novel and controlled release systems for target oriented delivery of drugs.

Selective drug delivery and targeting seek to improve the risk/benefit ratio associated with drugs. Ideally a drug intended for clinical use should have a high therapeutic index. Many drugs particularly chemotherapeutic agents have narrow therapeutic window and their clinical use is limited and compromised by dose limiting toxic effects. Approaches are being adapted either to control the distribution of drug by incorporating it in a carrier system or by altering the structure of the drug at the molecular level, or to control the input of the drug into the bioenvironment to ensure an appropriate profile of biodistribution.

Biotechnological developments led to the concept of conferring selectivity to drugs through targeted delivery. Currently drug delivery technology has infused new interest in seemingly ineffective or inefficient drugs by targeting them specifically to the desired site of action. Also in new millennium, target oriented drug administration systems with improvement in therapeutic efficacy, reduction in side effects and compliance in dosing regimen, shall be the leading trends in the area of therapeutics.

The concept of designing specified delivery system to achieve drug targeting has originated from the perception of Paul Ehrlich, who imagined drug delivery as a "magic bullet", describing targeted drug delivery system as an event where a drug carrier complex delivers drug(s) exclusively to the preselected target cells in specific manner. Bangham's (1965) observation on phospholipid hexagonal crystals, that they are preselective to the ions in a manner similar to biomembrane, led to the discovery of artificial somatic system based on

phospholipid amphiphiles. Gregoriadis (1972) described targeting with the help of novel drug delivery systems as 'old drugs in new clothes'.

Among the various carriers used for targeting of drugs to various body tissues, the cellular carriers meet several criteria desirable in clinical applications, among the most important being biocompatibility of carrier and its degradation products. Leukocytes, platelets, erythrocytes and nanoerythrosomes etc. have been proposed as cellular carrier systems. Among these, the erythrocytes have been the most investigated and have been found to posses great potential in drug delivery. In its infancy, erythrocyte encapsulation attracted many scientists who were enamored with the idea of RBC encapsulation. In the past two decades many claims and disclaims have been made about RBC as useful carriers for enzyme and other exogenous agents. Here a new derivative of erythrocytes, nanoerythrosomes, have been proposed as a new carrier which seemingly has a lot of potential in it.

14.2. HISTORICAL ASPECTS

Red blood cells remained to be an enigma for a long period after their discovery in 1658 because there were no established methods for blood analysis. It took over nearly 60 years before the importance of RBC was realized. It was not until 200 years later that erythrocytes were shown to stem from colorless nucleated cells in the bone marrow. Thus, the developing RBC has the capacity to synthesize hemoglobin, the adult erythrocytes however lose this capacity and serve only to carry hemoglobin. The membrane mainly encloses cytoplasm and a red pigment called hemoglobin. Some of the hemoglobin is lost and other cellular constituents are retained, the cells on resealing lose some of the properties of normal erythrocytes and referred to as "resealed erythrocytes" or "engineered erythrocytes". The attempts towards encapsulation of substances in erythrocytes and other carrier systems began in early 1970's. Ihler et.al., (1973) and Zimmerman et. al., (1973, 1975) independently suggested that resealed erythrocytes could be useful as drug carriers. The term carrier RBC was first introduced in 1979 (DeLoach, 1979). Such erythrocytes which contain no or little hemoglobin are called "ghosts". Pink ghosts are superior to white ghosts as slow release carrier (DeLoach, 1986). Jain & Jain (1997h, 1998a) have extensively reviewed the topic of engineered erythrocytes. Recently, a derivative of erythrocytes ghosts, nanoerythrosomes (nEs) have been proposed and patented as a new carrier which could be useful as drug carrier.

14.3. ADVANTAGES

Nanoerythrosomes have many advantages of a biological carrier:

(a) They are the natural products of the body, which are biodegradable in nature.

(b) Isolation of nanoerythrosomes is easy and larger amount of drug can be loaded in a small volume of cells.

(c) The loading of drugs does not require the chemical modification of the substance to be loaded. This is in contrast with other systems, which involve covalent coupling of the drug and carrier, which may affect the inherent biological activity of the parent drug.

(d) They are non-immunogenic in action and can be targeted to diseased tissue/organ.

(e) They prolong the systemic activity of drug while residing for a longer time in the body.

(f) They protect the premature degradation, inactivation and excretion of proteins and enzymes and act as a carrier for number of drugs.

(g) They can target the drugs within reticuloendothelial system (RES) as well as non-RES organs/sites.

(h) The techniques for collecting and storing cellular carriers are very well known.

(i) Nanoerythrosomes are biocompatible provided that compatible cells are used in patients, there is no possibility of triggered immunological response.

(j) In nanoerythrosomes, the drug is chemically bonded with the protein of the erythrocyte membrane.

(k) These are less prone to aggregation and fusion and flexibility of membrane allows them to escape RES for longer periods (Widder et al, 1978; 1980).

14.4. THE ERYTHROCYTE AND ERYTHROCYTE MEMBRANE

The erythrocyte membrane's relative simplicity, availability and ease of isolation have made it the most extensively studied and best understood biological membrane. It is therefore a model for the more complex membranes of other cell types. A mature mammalian erythrocyte is devoid of organelles and carries out few metabolic processes; it is essentially a membranous bag of hemoglobin. Erythrocyte membranes can therefore be obtained by osmotic lysis, which causes the cell contents to leak out. The resultant membranous particles are known as erythrocyte ghosts because, upon return to physiological conditions, they reseal to form particle that retain their original shape. Indeed, by transferring sealed ghosts to another medium their contents can be made to differ from the external solution. Erythrocyte membranes contain a variety of proteins.

The erythrocytes membrane has a more or less typical plasma membrane composition of about one-half protein (Fig 14. 1), somewhat less lipid (Fig 14. 2), and the remainder carbohydrates. Its proteins may be separated by sodium dodecyl sulfate (SDS) polyacrylamide gel electrophoresis after first solubilizing the membrane in a 1% SDS solution. The resulting electrophoretogram for a human erythrocyte membrane has seven major and many minor bands when stained with Coomassie brilliant blue. If the electrophoretogram is instead treated with periodic acid Schiff's reagent (PAS), which stains carbohydrate, four so called PAS bands become evident. The polypeptide corresponding to bands 1, 2, 4.1, 4.2, 5 and 6 are readily extracted from the membrane by changing the ionic strength or pH and hence are peripheral proteins. These proteins are located on the inner side of the membrane as is indicated by the observation that they are not altered by the incubation of intact erythrocytes or resealed ghosts with proteolytic enzymes or membrane impermeable protein labeling reagent. These proteins are altered, however, if 'leaky' ghosts are so treated.

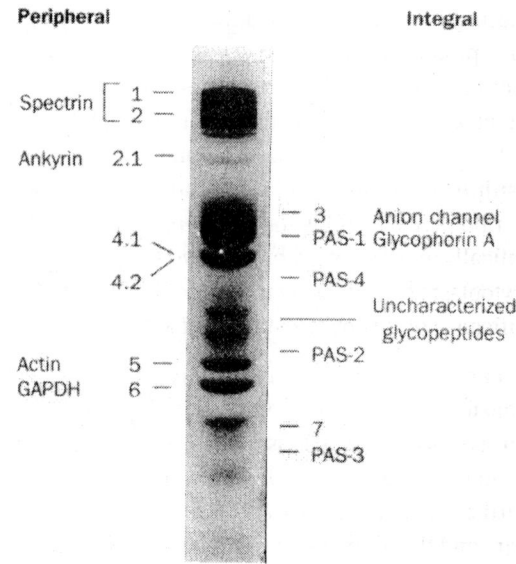

Fig 14.1. A SDS polyacrylamide gel electrophoretogram of human erythrocyte membrane proteins

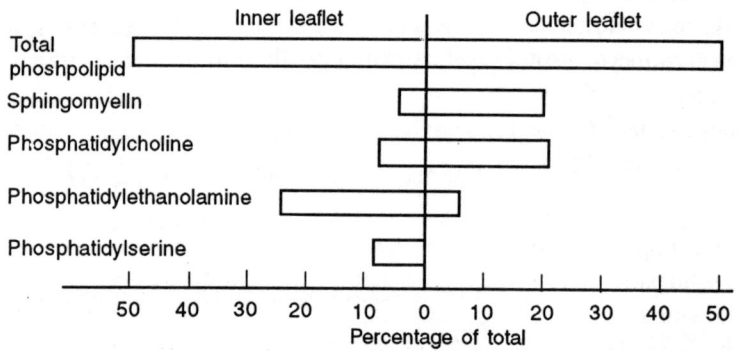

Fig 14. 2. The asymmetric distribution of phospholipids in human erythrocyte membranes

In contrast, bands 3, 7 and all four PAS bands correspond to integral proteins; they can be released from the membrane only by extraction with detergents or organic solvents. Of these, band 3 and PAS bands 1 and 2 correspond to transmembrane proteins as indicted by their different labeling patterns when intact cell are treated with membrane impermeable protein-labeling reagents and when these reagents are introduced inside sealed ghosts.

The transport of CO_2 in blood requires that the erythrocyte membrane be permeable to HCO_3^- and Cl^- (the maintenance of electroneutrality requires that for every HCO_3^- to enter a cell, a Cl^- or some other anion must leave the cell). The rapid transport of these and other anions across the erythrocyte membrane is mediated by specific anion channel of which their are ~1 million/cell (comprising > 30% of membrane protein). Band 3 protein (929 residues and 5-8% carbohydrate) specifically reacts with anionic protein labeling reagents that block the anion channel thereby indicating that the anion channel is composed of band 3 protein. Furthermore, crosslinking studies with bifunctional reagents demonstrate that the anion channel is at least a dimer hemoglobin and the glycolytic enzymes (glucose-metabolizing) aldolase phosphofructokinse and that band 6 protein glyceraldehyde 3 phosphate dehydrogenase, all specifically and reversibly bind to band 3 protein on the cytoplasm side of the membrane. The functional significance of this observation is unknown.

The erythrocyte's membrane skeleton is responsible for its shape. A normal erythrocyte's biconcave disclike shape assures the rapid diffusion of O_2 to its hemoglobin molecules by placing them no further than 1 μm from the cell surface. However the rim and the dimple regions of an erythrocyte do not occupy fixed positions on the cell membrane. This had been demonstrated by anchoring erythrocytes to a microscope slide by a small portion

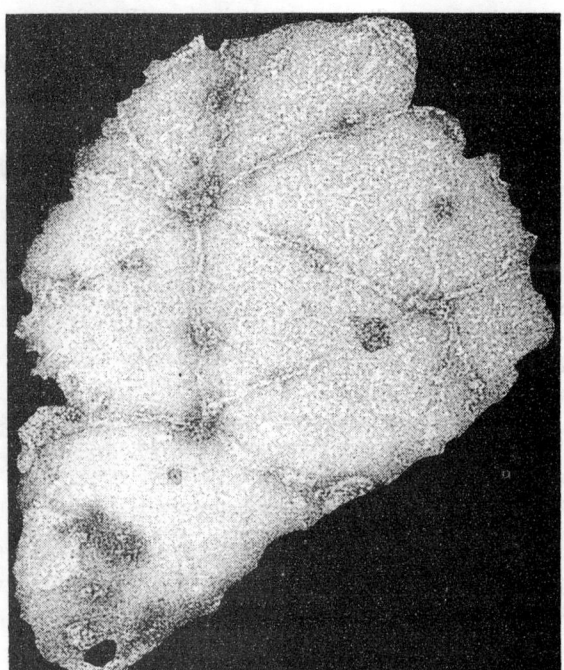

Fig 14. 3: Electron micrograph of an erythrocyte membrane skeleton

of its surface and inducing the cell to move laterally with a gentle flow of isotonic buffer. Evidently, the membrane is rolled across the cell while maintaining its shape much like the thread of a tractor. This remarkable mechanical property of the erythrocyte membrane results from the presence of submembranous network of proteins that function as a membrane skeleton. Indeed this property is partially duplicated by a mechanical model consisting of a geodesic sphere (a spheriodal cage) that is freely jointed at the intersections of its struts but constrained from collapsing much beyond a flat surface. When placed inside an evacuated pulsatile bag this cage also assumes a biconcave disclike shape.

The fluidity and flexibility imparted to an erythrocyte by its membrane skeleton has important physiological consequences. A slurry of solid particles of a size and concentration equal to that of red cells in blood has the flow characteristics approximating that of sand. Consequently, in order for blood to flow at all, much less for its erythrocytes to squeeze through capillary blood vessel smaller in diameter than they are, erythrocyte membranes, with their membrane skeletons, must be fluid-like and easily deformable (Fig 14. 3, 4 and 5).

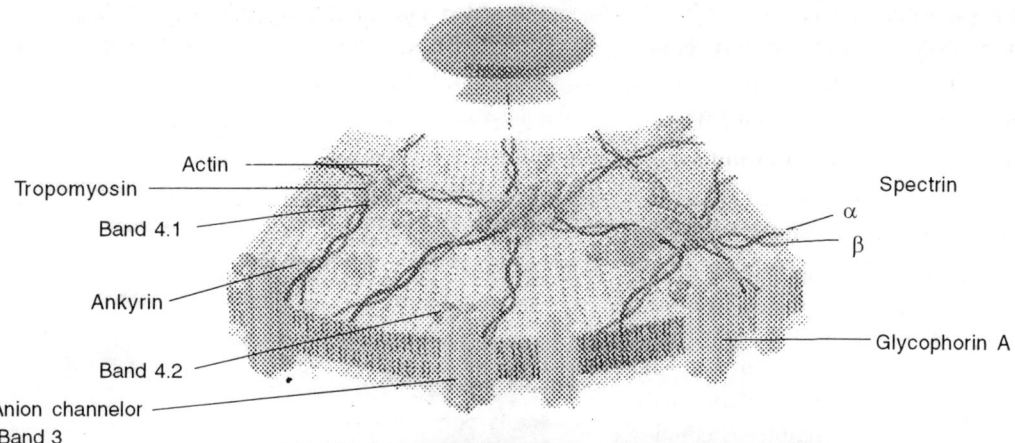

Actin

Tropomyosin

Band 4.1

Ankyrin

Band 4.2

Anion channelor
Band 3

Spectrin

α

β

Glycophorin A

Fig 14. 4: A model of the erythrocyte membrane skeleton

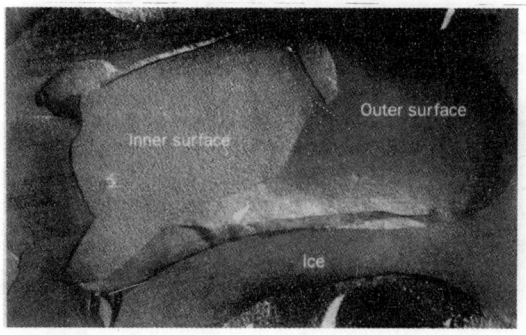

Fig 14. 5: A freeze-etch electron micrograph of a human erythrocyte plasma membrane

The protein spectrin, so called because it was discovered in erythrocyte ghosts, accounts for ~75% of the erythrocyte membrane skeleton. It is composed of two similar polypeptide chains, band 1 (α subunit, 220 kD) and band 2 (ß subunit; 240 kD), which sequence analysis indicates each consist of repeating 106 residue segments that are predicted to fold into triple stranded α helical coiled coils. Electron microscopy indicated that these large polypeptides are loosely intertwined to form a flexible worklike aB dimer that is 1000 Å long. Two such heterodimers further associate in a head to head manner to from an $(\alpha\beta)_2$ tetramer. These tetramers, of which their are 100,000/cell are crosslinked at both ends by attachments to bands 4.1 and 5 to form an irregular protein meshwork that underlies the erythrocyte plasma membrane. Band 5, a globular protein that forms filamentous oligomers, had been identified as actin, a common cytoskeletal elemental in other cells and a major component of muscles. Spectrin also associates with band 2.1, a 215-kD monomer known as ankyrin, which in turn binds to band 3, the anion channel protein.

This attachment anchors the membrane skeleton to the membrane. Indeed, upon solubilization of spectrin and actin by low ionic strength solutions erythrocyte ghosts lose their biconcave shape; their integral proteins that normally occupy fixed position in the membrane plane become laterally mobile. Immunochemical studies have recently revealed spectrin like, ankyrin like, and band 4.1 like proteins in a variety of tissues (Voet & Voet, 1990).

The erythrocyte membrane contains about equal weight of protein and lipid. Some membrane components contain carbohydrates, which are responsible for some of the surface antigenic properties. The outer surface of the membrane bears a net negative charge due largely to carboxyl groups of sailic acid. The isoelectric point is about pH 2, which is raised to pH 4-5 after quantitative removal of the sialic acid with neuraminidase. There are about 2.4×10^7 N-acetyl-neuraminic acid residues per human erythrocyte (Eylar et. al., 1962). The negative surface charge maintains a sufficient distance between erythrocytes so that they are prevented from coming into direct contact and hence they cannot be readily agglutinated with IgG. Consequently it is possible to treat erythrocyte with IgG for the purpose of activating erythrocytes for uptake by phagocytic cells without agglutination. IgM antibodies, on the other hand, can span the gap between erythrocytes.

The phosphoglyceride content of the membrane is about 50% of the total lipid content, phosphatidylcholine, phosphatidylethanolamine and phosphatidylserine being predominant species. The other major lipid constituents of the membrane are sphingomylin and cholesterol. Glycolipids are minor constituents, the principle one being globoside (GL-4), or N-acetylgalactosaminyl-galactosyl-glucosyl ceramide.

The erythrocytes do not have the ability to synthesize lipid *de novo*, but have the capacity for lipid turnover and replacement using plasma lipids. Cholesterol as well as other lipids can be acquired from or lost to plasma (Ihler, 1983).

14.5. REQUIREMENT FOR ENCAPSULATION

Nanoerythrosomes are patented nano-vesicles (Dignocure Inc., Canada) derived from red blood cell membranes through a process of hemodialysis through filters of defined pore size. These vesicles have the ability to be loaded with a diverse array of biologically active agents including proteins. The nanoerythrosome's membrane is a most versatile natural membrane structure, which is composed of proteins, phospholipids and cholesterol.

The presence of membrane is particularly advantageous since it permits the conjugation, using simple and well-known chemistry of polyethylene glycols and proteins, for example, monoclonal antibodies. Additionally, natural membrane stability allows the insertion of recombinant ligands providing another method for incorporating targeting moieties into the nanoerythrosomes.

A wide variety of biologically active substances can be loaded with nanoerythrosomes. Generally, the molecules should be polar or hydrophilic but non-polar molecules have also been successfully entrapped. The erythrocyte membrane contains approximately 60% protein and 40% lipid by dry weight. A wide variety of drugs having hydroxyl group, amino group and or carboxyl group are good candidate for drug conjugation.

14.6. ISOLATION OF ERYTHROCYTES

14.6.1 Collection and Storage of Blood

Blood samples can be collected from animal by cardiac puncture (rats, mice etc.) / vein puncture (rabbit, human etc.) into a syringe containing heparin sodium (100 I.U./ml in 0.9% saline). The freshly collected blood is stored in a refrigerator at $4\pm1°C$.

14.6.2 Separation and Washing of Erythrocytes from Blood

The freshly collected blood is centrifuged in a refrigerated centrifuge at 1000 rpm for 10 minutes at $4\pm1°C$. The plasma and buffy coats are discarded and sedimented erythrocytes are washed with washing buffer (pH 7.4). These washed cells are stored under refrigeration at $4\pm1°C$ (Fig 14. 6).

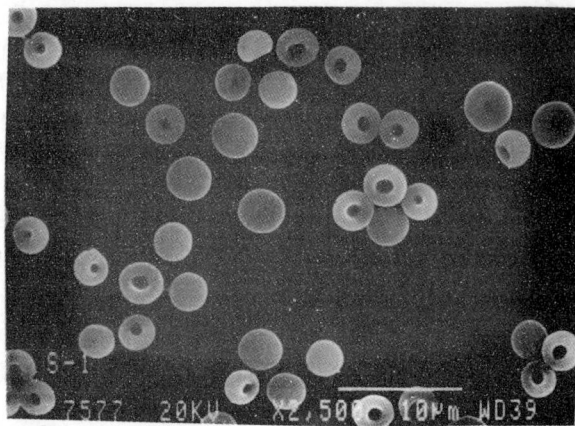

Fig 14. 6: Photomicrograph of normal erythrocytes (x 1500)

14.6.3 Preparation of Erythrocyte Ghosts

Hypotonic osmotic lysis method described by DeLoach et. al., (1994) is used for the preparation of ghost suspension. The cells are lysed and washed several times with hypotonic saline solution. After each wash, the solution is centrifuged at 1000 rpm for 10 minutes at 4±1°C in a refrigerated centrifuge and the supernatants are aspirated and discarded. The ghost suspension is finally obtained when supernatant becomes colorless. Packed ghost cells suspension is diluted with 0.9% saline to obtain 50% hematocrit and stored at 4±1°C until used (Jain & Jain, 1998d).

Erythrocyte ghosts can also be prepared as reported by Sprandel et. al., (1987). Briefly, a volume of red blood cells is washed with an isotonic phosphate buffer solution. The suspension of erythrocytes is centrifuged at 1000 rpm for 20 min. The supernatant is aspirated and discarded. The sedimented erythrocytes are treated with a hypotonic buffer solution. The mixture is then centrifuged for 20 min at 23,500 x g. The supernatant is aspirated and discarded. The addition of the hypotonic buffer solution is repeated several times until the supernatant becomes colorless. The erythrocyte ghosts are stored in the refrigerator for further use .

14.6.4 Preparation and loading of nanoerythrosomes

The nanoerythromes can be prepared using extrusion, sonication and electrical breakdown methods.

In extrusion method erythrocytes ghosts are passed through polycarbonate membrane filter which causes them into smaller vesicles, nanoerythrosomes (nEs); in sonication method erythrocyte ghosts are converted into small vesicles using dismembrator; the electrical breakdown method is used to convert ghosts into small vesicles under the influence of electrical potential. Out of the three methods nEs prepared by extrusion method yield vesicles of more uniform size. It is a quicker and cheaper method in comparison to sonication and electrical breakdown methods. Furthermore, in case of sonication and electrical breakdown methods, heat generated during preparation if not controlled, may also modify membrane.

Drug is conjugated to nEs with the help of a crosslinker. Nanoerythrosome concentration is determined by quantitation of protein by a reported method (Lowery et. al., 1951).

Methotrexate (MTX) was loaded on nanoerythrosomes by three methods, namely - extrusion [E], sonication [S] and electrical breakdown [EB]. Jain & Jain, (1999a,b) have reported electrical breakdown method. Various process variables that could affect the preparation and properties of the nEs were established, identified and optimized. The preparation procedure was accordingly optimized and validated. In vitro characterization was done on MTX loaded nanoerythrosomes for various pharmaceutical and physiochemical attributes. A brief review of this work is presented below (Jain, 1999; Jain & Jain, 1996a,b; 1997a,b,c; 1999a,b; 2000).

14.6.4.1 Extrusion Method

Extrusion method reported by Lejeune et. al., (1994) and Jain & Jain (1996 b) was used with little modification for conjugation of drug with nEs. The erythroycte ghosts suspension (50% Hct) was extruded through a polycarbonate membrane filter (0.4 μm) attached to an adapter. nEs were obtained by 8 consecutive extrusions and the final preparation was stored at 4±1°C in the refrigerator. Extrusion was done under nitrogen pressure. The yield was more than 80% as determined by protein recovery.

Drug Nanoerythrosome Conjugation: MTX was conjugated to nEs membrane using gluteraldehyde (G) as a crosslinker. Two thousand five hundred micrograms of drug was added to 2ml of nEs preparation (50% Hct) in presence of 0.03% gluteraldehyde (in 0.9% saline) in a final volume of 3ml. The mixture was incubated for 45 min. at 4±1°C and then reaction was discontinued by addition of 1ml of 15% glycine solution in isotonic saline. The suspension was centrifuged at 20,000 x g for 20 min. at 4±1 °C. The nEs-G-MTX were washed four times with 5ml of PBS until no free MTX was detected in the supernatant. The MTX-G-nEs complex was separated from free MTX by centrifugation. Finally the preparation was stored at 4±1°C in the refrigerator until used. All manipulations were done under sterile conditions.

Control Experiment: To check the membrane binding of MTX on nEs, samples were treated identically except that crosslinker was not used.

Optimization of Formulation

The effect of following variables were investigated under extrusion method:

Drug concentration: In order to investigate the effect of drug concentration on conjugation the various concentrations representing 1.0, 2.0, 2.5 and 3.0 mg/ml of MTX were used. Other experimental conditions were pore diameter of membrane: (0.4μm); type and concentration of crosslinker, gluteraldehyde concentration (0.030%), incubation period (45 min.) and temperature (37°C). The effect of variable drug concentrations was optimized for effective conjugation of drug on nEs. Nearly 1.0-2.5% of MTX was found to be associated with the cells when estimated in the control experiment, which could be ascribed to the adsorption of the drug on nEs.

Pore size of membrane: Membranes with pore diameter ranging from 2.0μm to 0.1μm were employed for the preparation of nEs. It was observed that membranes with pores of 2μm do not break down the erythrosomes. This is not surprising since in physiological conditions the erythrocytes undergo repeated passage through narrow capillaries and through membranes having sinusoids. However, when passed through membranes having pores of 1μm in diameter, the erythrosomes were fragmented into small vesicles. Nanoerythrosomes (nEs) are spheroid closed vesicles having a mean diameter of 0.1-0.2μm. The extrusion of erythrosomes through filters having pores of 0.4μm in diameter did not lead to small particles. It is likely that extrusion of erythrosomes through pores having a diameter equal or smaller than 1μm break the erythrosomes membrane spontaneously to form small vesicles.

Polycarbonate membrane filters with pore size 1.0μm and 0.4μm gave the same results while 2.0μm filters were not considered suitable for the preparation of nanoerythrosomes. Polycarbonate membrane filters with pore size 0.4μm were used in all the studies.

Type and concentration of crosslinker: The effect of type and concentration of crosslinkers was optimized for effective conjugation of drug on nEs. The effect of crosslinker (gluteraldehyde, cis-aconitic and itaconic anhydride) on the degree of conjugation indicated that maximum drug conjugation was observed in case of gluteraldehyde. The 0.030% concentration of gluteraldehyde was found to be optimum. Moreover, the crosslinker cis-aconitic and itaconic anhydride have been reported to be pH sensitive (Lejune et. al., 1994). The percent conjugation increases as concentration of crosslinker increases from 0.010 to 0.030%. Nearly same % drug conjugation was obtained on further increase in concentration of crosslinker indicating saturation of conjugation sites. The % drug conjugation using 0.030% of gluteraldehyde was 210ng/μg protein.

Preparation of cis-aconityl-MTX (C-MTX) and itaconyl-MTX (I-MTX): These were prepared according to the method reported by Moorjani et. al., (1996). One mg of MTX was dissolved in 1ml of 7% NaHCO$_3$ solution. The solution was kept on ice and 2.0 mg cis-acotinic anhydride or itaconic anhydride was added over a period of 60 minutes to the stirred solution. The untreated MTX was extracted with 5.0ml of dichloromethane. Afterwards, five ml of ethyl acetate was added to the aqueous solution, and solution of chlorhydric acid (1.0 N) was added dropwise until the free carboxylic derivatives were extractable by the organic phase. The aqueous phase was re-extracted twice with 5ml of ethyl acetate. The organic phase was pooled and evaporated under a stream of dry nitrogen. The C-MTX and I-MTX derivatives were dissolved in anhydrous dimethyl sulfoxide (DMSO) and kept frozen at -20°C. These derivatives were later conjugated to nEs membrane by the addition of 200μg of the MTX derivative and 7.25mg of 1(3-dimethyl-aminopropyl)-3-ethylcarbodiimide HCl (EDCI) (EDCI: MTX derivative ; 100 :1) to 500μg of nEs equivalent protein. The mixture was incubated for 2hr at 37°C. The nEs-C-MTX or nEs-I-MTX conjugates were then separated by centrifugation.

Incubation period: The effect of incubation period was seen for maximum conjugation of drug on nEs. The data also show a higher uptake of MTX at 37°C for 45 minutes .

Temperature: The effect of variable temperature was optimized for maximum conjugation of drug on nEs. The data also show a higher uptake of MTX at 37°C for 45 minutes than at room temperature and 4°C upon incubation. It indicates higher activity at 37°C.

Preparation of Nanoerythrosomes (Jain & Jain, 1996)

Normal erythrocytes

↓ depletion of hemoglobin

Preparation of erythrocytes ghost

↓ extrusion/sonication/ electrical breakdown

Nano vesicles

↓ staining with 0.1% Uranyl actate

and microscopical examination

Nanoerythrosomes

The formulation was prepared using optimum parameters. The maximum drug conjugation using optimized variables was found to be 210ng/μg protein.

14.6.4.2 Sonication method

Sonication procedure reported by Achi & Green wood (1993a & b) and Jain & Jain (1996a) be used for the preparation of nEs.

The erythrocyte ghost suspension (50% Hct, in 0.9% saline) was sonicated at an energy level of 50 W for 5 minutes using dismembrator. During the experiment, the temperature was maintained at 4±1°C and finally nEs were stored at 4±1°C in the refrigerator. Drug-nanoerythrosome conjugation is done as described under extrusion method.

Optimization of formulation

The various formulations prepared by sonication method were optimized for following parameters:

Drug concentration: The effect of variable drug concentrations was optimized for effective conjugation of drug on nEs. The drug concentration 2.5mg/ml was adjudged to be optimum for drug conjugation.

Sonication time: The sonication time for formulation was varied from 1-5 min and its effect on particle size was noted as a function of turbidity. Turbidity measurement is based on the fact that change in particle size can be assessed as a function of turbidity. For turbidity measurement, the absorbance (abs) of an appropriate diluted sample was measured at 450nm in a spectrophotometer. Absorbance was then converted to turbidity by using following formula (Wheeler et. al., 1995).

$$\text{Turbidity} = 10^{abs}$$

Sonication of erythrocyte ghosts at 50W for 3 minutes was considered suitable for the preparation of nanoerythrosomes. As sonication increases turbidity also decreases. Nearly 1.0-2.3% of MTX was found to be associated with the cells when estimated in the control experiment, which could be ascribed to the adsorption of the drug on nEs.

Type and concentration of crosslinker: The effect and concentration of crosslinker was optimized for effective conjugation of nEs. The effect of crosslinker (gluteraldehyde, cis-aconitic and itaconic anhydride) on the degree of conjugation indicated that maximum drug conjugation was observed in case of gluteraldehyde. The 0.030% concentration of gluteraldehyde (G) was found to be optimum.

Incubation period: The effect of incubation period was also seen for maximum conjugation of drug. The data also show a higher uptake of MTX at 37°C for 45 min incubation.

Temperature: The effect of variable temperature was optimized for minimum conjugation of drug on nEs. The data also show a higher uptake of MTX at 37°C for 45 min than at room temperature and 4°C after incubation.

The maximum drug conjugation using optimized variables was found to be 175ng/µg protein using sonication method.

14.6.4.3 Electrical Breakdown Method

The erythrocyte ghost suspension (50% Hct in 0.9% saline) was subjected to variable electrical voltage for 100µs. During the experiment the temperature was maintained at 37°C and finally nEs were stored at 4±1°C in the refrigerator. MTX-G-nEs were separated by centrifugation. Drug was conjugated to nanoerythrosome as described under extrusion method.

The various parameters optimized under electrical breakdown method were:

Drug concentration: The effect of variable drug concentration was optimized for effective conjugation of drug on nEs. The drug concentration 2.0mg/ml was adjudged to be optimum for the drug conjugation.

Effect of voltage: The effect of variable voltage was optimized for effective conjugation of nEs. A voltage of 2KV/cm for 200 µs was found to be the optimum

Effect of type & concentration of crosslinker: The effect of type and concentration of crosslinker was optimized for effective conjugation of drug on nEs. The effect of crosslinker (gluteraldehyde, cis-aconitic and itaconic anhydride) on the degree of conjugation indicated that maximum drug conjugation was observed in case of gluteraldehyde. The 0.030% conc. of gluteraldehyde (G) was found to be optimum.

Effect of incubation time: The effect of incubation period was also seen for maximum conjugation of drug. The data show a higher uptake of MTX at 37°C for 45 min.

Effect of temperature: The effect of variable temperature was optimized for maximum conjugation of drug on nEs. The data show a higher uptake of MTX with incubation at 37°C for 45min. The maximum drug conjugation using optimized variables was found to be 160ng/µg protein.

14.6.5 Inside-Out Red cell membranous vesicles (Steck et al, 1970):

Preparation and purification: The plasma membrane deals with two distinctly different compartments. Investigation of the biochemical specialization across this membrane has been limited by the inaccessibility of its inner surface to direct examination. This problem was approached by promoting the budding of red cell plasma membrane ghosts into their cytoplasmic vesicles whose outer faces are the cytoplasmic space thereby generating inside-out vesicles whose outer faces are the cytoplasmic aspects of the parent membranes. Conversely, normally oriented vesicles are formed when a surface membrane buds into the extracellular space. They have presented methods for the preparation and purification of inside out and right side out red cell membrane vesicles suitable for the direct comparative analysis of the membrane's two faces (Fig 14. 7). Fig 14. 8 shows electron micrograph of carbon-platinum replicas of freeze-cleaved red cell ghosts and vesicles. (Left). Two distinct surfaces are visualized for ghost membranes. Fracture face A is covered with many 100-An particles (double arrows) and is oriented toward the extracellular space (ECS). Face B has fewer particles and is oriented toward the cytoplasmic region (CR). The encircled arrow indicates the direction of carbon-platinum shadowing (x 60,000)(upper right). Vesicles in the bottom band formed by exocytosis. Face A is convex (An) and faces outward while face B is concave (Bu) and faces the vesicle's interior (x 50,000). (Lower right) Vesicles from the top band formed by endocytosis. The usual morphologic relationships are now reversed. Face A is concave (Au) and face B convex (Bn), indicating membrane inversion (x 60,000).

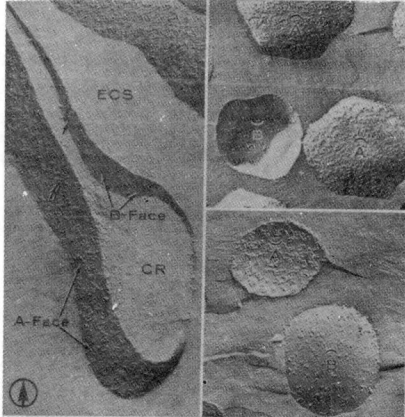

Fig 14. 7: Electron photomicrograph of carbon-platinum replicas of freeze-cleaved red cell ghosts and vesicles

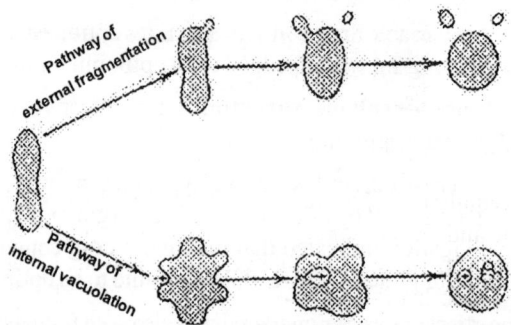

Fig 14. 8: Representation of two mechanisms leading from a normal biconcave disc to a sphere with reduced surface area.

Ethylenediaminetetraactate [EDTA] was added in a concentration of 0.0010M to freshly drawn human blood. The red cells were washed three times with cold 0.14 NaCl in 0.005M sodium phosphate buffer, (pH 8.0). Each milliliter of packed red cell was lysed by resuspension in 40ml of cold 0.005M phosphate buffer (pH 8.0). The plasma membranes were centrifuged at 20,000g for 10 minutes to form pellets, which were further washed twice with the same buffer. The resulting pellets were white and were comprised of intact membrane ghosts.

Each pellet was resuspended in 20 ml of cold 5×10^{-4} M sodium phosphate buffer, pH 8.0 for 1 hr or more, and then sedimented at 10500 g for 30 minutes. As judged by phase contrast light microscopy and thin section electron microscopy the membrane appeared to be budding spontaneously into the ghost interior leading to an accumulation of many small vesicles within each parent ghost. Gentle homogenization by pestle or by passage through a 27-gauge hypodermic needle reduced the residual ghost membrane to small vesicles and liberated the entrapped vesicles. The prior addition of divalent cation such as 1×10^{-4} M to 5×10^{-4} M phosphate buffer stabilized the ghosts against spontaneous vesiculation. Homogenization of these stabilized ghosts caused them to vesiculate, primarily by budding into the extracellular space.

Right - side - out vesicles were separated on linear gradients of Dextran-110 density (1.01 to 1.07 g/cm^3) containing 5×10^{-4} phosphate buffer, pH 8.0 and 1×10^{-4} M MgSO$_4$ (added to solubilize the vesicle). Homogenates were layered on the gradients and centrifuged to equilibrium at 10500 g for 16 hrs. Roughly 90 percent of the membrane protein was recovered in three zones (i) a bottom band at the density of intact ghosts 1.050 to 1.065, (ii) a top band at a density of approximately 1.01, and (iii) a scant zone spreading diffusely between 1.020 and 1.035. The middle zone becomes enriched at the expense of top band material when NH$_4$HCO$_3$ or tris aminomethanhydrochloride (tris HCl) is substituted for phosphate buffer throughout the procedure. About 80 percent of the vesicles formed by homogenization in the presence of MgSO$_4$ were recovered in the bottom band while 60 percent of the vesicles formed in the absence of MgSO$_4$ were found in the upper two zones (1.01 to 1.033) (Fig 14.9).

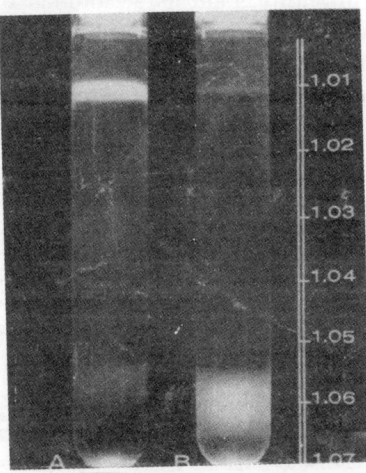

Fig 14. 9 : Equilibrium dextran density gradient centrifugation of red cell membrane

Almost all of the vesicles equilibrating between the densities of 1.01 and 1.035 were inside-out according to the following biochemical and morphologic criteria. It had been reported that the sialic acid of red cells is localized on the outer aspect of plasma membrane. They reasoned that right-side-out vesicles would present no barrier to the enzymatic hydrolysis of this surface marker but a sealed in-side-out vesicle would shield the internalized sialic acid from enzyme attack. They therefore characterized the vesicle fractions by the accessibility of their sialic acid to release by sialidase and their sialoprotein to trypsin hydrolysis. The vesicles in the upper zone had nearly the same specific sialic acid content as the input homogenate and the bottom band but only 15 percent of this marker was released by sialidase and 12 percent by trypsin. In contrast the material in the bottom band was quite sensitive to hydrolysis by both enzymes.

Morphologic evaluation of the orientation of vesicle membranes was carried out by freeze cleave electron microscopy because it was demonstrated by this technique that the red cells membrane has two readily distinguished surfaces. The fracture face normally oriented toward the extracellular space is covered by many 100-α particles while the surface oriented toward the cell interior bears only 20 to 25 percent as many particles. Although the precise location and function of the membrane associated particles is unknown their distribution nevertheless serves as a distinctive indicator of membrane orientation thus right-side-out vesicles are those which retain the orientation of the parent membrane while the inside-out species show an inversion of these morphologic markers.

By these criteria 98 percent of the top-zone vesicles were inside-out. Evaluation of the bottom band was complicated by the strong tendency of these vesicles to continue inverting during preparation for electron microscopy. Thus vesicles in bottom band generated in the presence $MgSO_4$ of appeared 60 to 80 percent right- side- out while most vesicles in the bottom band formed without $MgSO_4$ were inside-out.

The morphologic data suggest greater purity of the top (inside-out) fraction than do the biochemical results. Other than reflecting cross-contamination, the sialic acid released from the vesicles in the top zone might represent (i) the presence of small amounts of this marker on the inner aspect of the red cell membrane or (ii) partial permeability of the vesicles to the enzymes. The slight inaccessibility of the sialic acid in the bottom band to enzymatic release seems related to the observed tendency of the vesicles in the lower band to continue inverting after removal from the dextran gradient. In any case by both biochemical and morphologic criteria, more than 85 percent of the vesicles in the upper zone are inside-out.

The conditions for vesicle separation were predicted by a theoretical analysis of the factors determining the buoyant equilibrium of vesicles in density gradients. According to the proposed model the prevalence of fixed charges on the inner membrane surface is major determinant of the vesicle density in discerning gradient systems. The outer surface of the red cell membrane is enriched in sialic acid anions. It was reasoned that internalizing this excess of negative charge would produce vesicles of lower density than the parent ghost would. The model further indicates that resolution is optimal in gradients of low osmotic activity, such as dextran. Consistent with the prediction, neither sucrose nor glycerol gradients has afforded satisfactory separation of right-side-out and inside-out vesicles.

Another useful theoretical prediction was that the size of the vesicle membrane should not influence the equilibrium density of the vesicle, within its elastic limits. This was borne out by observation that intact ghosts and vesicles sharing their membrane orientation achieved buoyant equilibrium at the same density. Various treatments have been reported to promote inversion of the red cell membrane and the inner mitochondrial membrane. An electrostatic mechanism appears to be involved in their endocytosis procedure. They have looked for alteration other than topological in the inverted vesicles but have detected no significant perturbation in their fine structure, their sialic acid content and the specific activity of certain enzymes. The protein electrophoretic patterns of the inside-out and right- side-out vesicles were the same, but both species were greatly depleted of major, high molecular weight protein (spectrin) found in intact ghosts. The release of spectrin to the medium occurred only under conditions of pH, ionic strength, and divalent cation concentration, temperature and incubation time that fostered endocytosis (Steck et. al., 1970).

14.7. IN VITRO CHARACTERIZATION (Jain & Jain , 1995, 96, 97, 98, 99)

The final formulations (optimized) were prepared using the optimized parameters. These optimized formulations were subjected to in vitro characterization for evaluation of their suitability as drug carriers.

14.7.1 Percent recovery/protein content

Nanoerythrosomes concentration is determined by quantitation of the protein content by a method reported by Lowery et. al., (1951).

The mean particle size was found to be 130±26, 170±30 and 190±25 nm, respectively for MTX-G-nEs (E), MTX-G-nE(S) & MTX-G-nEs (EB). These vesicles were closed spheroidal in shape. The percent recoveries of nEs were found to be nearly 80.8%, 76.6% and 76.42% in case of extrusion, sonication and electrical breakdown methods, respectively.

14.7.2 Morphological examination

The shape and size of MTX-G-nEs are determined using SEM and TEM after proper dilution. Mean values and standard deviation for overall particles are determined after staining with uranyl acetate. Fig 14.10 show morphology of ghost cells and nEs respectively. The electron microscopical examination of nEs and MTX-G-nEs (Fig 14. 11) revealed that these are spheroid closed vesicles. The same observations were made invariably at all drug concentration, the control nEs also exhibited the similar characteristics. TEM microphotographs (Fig 14.12, 13) represent samples of MTX-G-nEs[S] and MTX-G-nEs[EB] respectively. MTX-G-nEs[E] are more uniform in size in comparison to MTX-G-nEs[S] and MTX-G-nEs[EB].

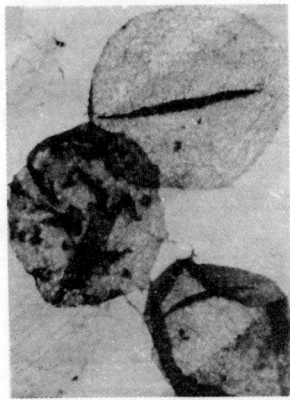

Fig 14. 10 : Electron microphotograph of ghost cells (x10,000)

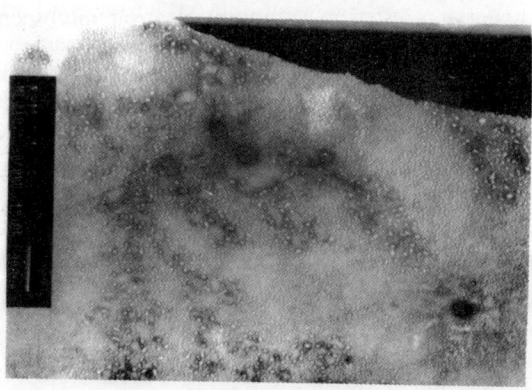

Fig 14. 11 : TEM of MTX loaded nanoerythrosomes (Extrusion method) (x10,000)

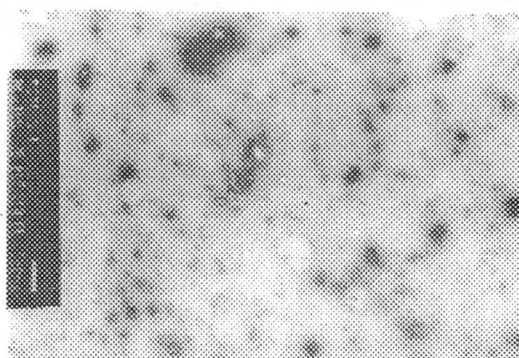

Fig 14. 12: TEM of MTX loaded nanoerythrosomes (Sonication method) (x10,000)

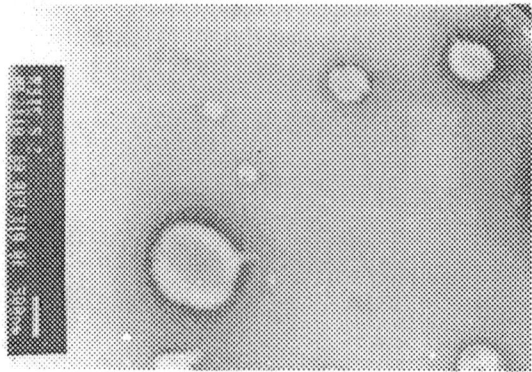

Fig 14. 13: TEM of MTX loaded nanoerythrosomes (Electrical breakdown method) (x10,000)

14.7.2.1 Scanning Electron Microscopy of nEs

Ghosts/erythrocyte-vesicles are diluted with saline water by mixing two parts of ghosts or erythrocyte-vesicles suspension with 25 parts of saline buffer. The formulation is dehydrated and dried to critical point by using elevated concentrations of alcohol. One drop of the diluted mixture is placed on a silver coated copper grid, then coated with gold. The material is tested on a scanning electron microscope.

14.7.2.2 Transmission Electron Microscopy of nEs

Ghosts/erythrocyte-vesicles are diluted with distilled water by mixing two parts of ghost or erythrocyte-vesicular suspension with 25 parts of saline buffer. One drop of the diluted mixture is placed on a coated copper grid and negatively stained with 1% uranyl acetate (pH 7.0). The material is tested on a transmission electron microscope.

14.7.3 Percent drug conjugation/ Degree of conjugation/Entrapment efficiency

MTX-G-nEs (0.2 ml) are deproteinized using acetonitrile after centrifugation at 20,000xg for 15 min. The clear supernatant is withdrawn and percent drug conjugation is estimated using following equation:

$$\text{Percent drug conjugation} = \frac{\text{Amount of drug loaded}}{\text{Amount of drug added}} \times 100$$

14.7.4 Centrifugal stress

For centrifugal stress study, MTX-G-nEs (10% Hct) are centrifuged at variable rpm in a refrigerated centrifuge at 4±1° C for 15 min. Drug leakage in supernatant solution is estimated.

The formulations are stable against centrifugal stress, as only 2.62 % , 2.92 % and 3.20% of drug could be released after centrifugation at 7500 rpm for 15 minutes from MTX-G-nEs(E), MTX-G-nEs(S) and MTX-G-nEs(EB), respectively. Centrifugal stress is the reliable parameter for the in vitro evaluation of nEs with respect to shelf-life , in vivo survival and the effect of the encapsulated substances.

14.7.5 Turbulence shock

The formulations are passed through a 25 gauge hypodermic needle at the rate of 8-10 ml/minute and drug leakage in supernatant is estimated after fixed no. of passes.

MTX-G-nEs(E), MTX-G--nEs(S) and MTX-G-nEs (EB) were found to withstand turbulence shock as only 0.882 %, 0.991 % and 1.66% of drug could be released after 15 passes through 26 gauge needle. It is a measure of simulating destruction of loaded nEs during injection.

14.7.6 Viscosity

A rotatory viscometer (Brookfield Synchro-Lectic LVT, USA) was used to determine the viscosity of the formulation. The viscosity of MTX-G-nEs(E), MTX-G-nEs(S) and MTX-G-nEs(EB) was found to be slightly higher than viscosity of nEs.

14.7.7 Relative density

The relative density of the formulation was determined using relative density bottle. The relative density of MTX-G-nEs(E), MTX-G-nEs(S) and MTX-G-nEs(EB) was found to be slightly higher than relative density of nEs.

14.7.8 Sedimentation volume

Sedimentation volume of the formulations is measured in a graduated measuring cylinder from the height of sediment using following formula:

$$F = \frac{V_u}{V_o}$$

where F - Sedimentation volume; V_u - Ultimate volume of sediment ; V_o - Original volume of the formulation

Sedimentation volume of unity in each case revealed very good stability of the formulation. It has been reported that polystyrene latex particles of size less than 500nm do not settle even upon one month storage (Vanderhoff & El Assar, 1988).

14.7.9. In vitro release

In vitro release studies were conducted using dialysis tubing (Sigma, USA). The tubing was washed with running water for 3 to 4 hr. to remove free glycerin followed by treatment with 0.3% w/v solution of sodium sulfite at 80°C for 1 minute to remove sulfur. The tube was washed with hot water at 60°C for 2 min, followed by acidification with 0.2% v/v solution of sulfuric acid. Finally, the tube was washed with hot distilled water and was kept immersed in PBS until used.

Free drug from the formulation was removed by ultra-dialysis against normal saline at 4°C by centrifugation at 20,000xg for 20 min. at 4±1°C. After removal of free drug, 1 ml of formulation was introduced into prewashed dialysis tubing and it was placed in a beaker containing 100 ml of PBS buffer.

The suitable condition was maintained by constantly stirring the buffer with the help of magnetic stirrer. Sample aliquots (0.2 ml) were withdrawn periodically from the beaker and analyzed.

The in vitro drug release of methotrexate-glutaradehyde-nanoerythrosomes [extrusion method] MTX-G-nEs[E], methotrexate-glutaradehyde-nanoerythrosomes [sonication method] MTX-G-nEs[S] and methotrexate-glutaradehyde-nanoerythrosomes [electrical breakdown method] MTX-G-nEs[EB] found to be 16.1, 22.2 & 25.1%, respectively after 8 hr. Drug release pattern followed first order release.

14.7.10. Antineoplastic activity

The cytotoxic activity of both free and conjugated MTX was determined on Leukemia cell line (L-1210) obtained from National Centre for Cell Sciences (NCCS) (Pune, India) maintained in Dulbecco's modified eagle's medium (DMEM) supplemented with 10% v/v fetal calf serum, penicillin 100 IU/ml and streptomycin 100μg/ml. Cells are obtained as monolayer culture in plastic Roux bottles (Udupa, 1995).

Culture: Cells were harvested using Trypsin Versine Glucose (TVG) in the experimental growth phase from the normal medium preincubated at 37°C for 24hr. The cells were centrifuged to adjust initial cell concentration at 2×10^5 cells /ml. One ml of concentrated cell suspension was seeded into multiwell tissue culture plate (Corning plastics) (2x105 cells/well). DMEM (0.5ml) was added to each well incubated with nEs containing varying concentration of MTX viz 10, 50 and 100 μg/ml. It was compared with cells containing MTX solution with similar supplements. The plate was incubated at 37±1°C in incubator at 95% RH and 5% CO_2 atmosphere for variable time intervals. Cell counts were made in haemocytometer (Neubaur chamber, Japan) before the start of experiment and at 4th, 12th and 48th hr.

Cytotoxicity assay : Cytotoxicity studies were performed according to the method reported by Fretiney (1994). Cell viability was measured by tryphen blue extrusion test, which is based on the ability of tryphen blue to stain dead cell. A drop of culture was added on haemocytometer and no. of stained, non-stained and total no. of cells were counted.

$$\text{Percent Inhibition} = \frac{\text{No. of viable cells - No. of visible cells after treatment}}{\text{No. of viable cells without treatment}}$$

MTX-G-nEs have higher cytotoxic and neoplastic activity than free drug as seen in in vitro studies on Leukemia cells (L-1210). In vitro Leukemia cell (L-1210) toxicity studies demonstrated that toxicity of nanoerythrosomes increased in proportion to the concentration of the drug.

14.7.11. Mechanism of action

An attempt was made to evaluate drug-cell line interaction. Cell line (Leukemia, L-1210) and formulation were incubated and studied by microscopy. Using microscopical studies it was observed that the MTX-G-nEs neither diffused through the cell membrane nor entered the cell by endogenesis. The MTX-G-nEs are rapidly absorbed on the cell membrane. Free MTX was then slowly released by hydrolysis of the gluteraldehyde linking arms, producing a high concentration of free drug in the cell vicinity over a prolonged period of time. The cytotoxicity of MTX conjugated to nEs-MTX is mediated by attachment of nEs complex to the cell membrane, slow hydrolysis of the linking arm, protection of a high concentration of drug around the cell periphery that will penetrate into the cells over a long period of time.

Lejune et. al., (1994) had studied localization of daunorubicin (DNR) in P388D$_1$ cells exposed to 5 ug/ml of free and nEs conjugated drug after exposure of 30 min, 1hr and 4hr. The results indicate that cytotoxic activity of nEs-DNR complex is much more as compared to free drug (Fig 14. 14 & 14. 15).

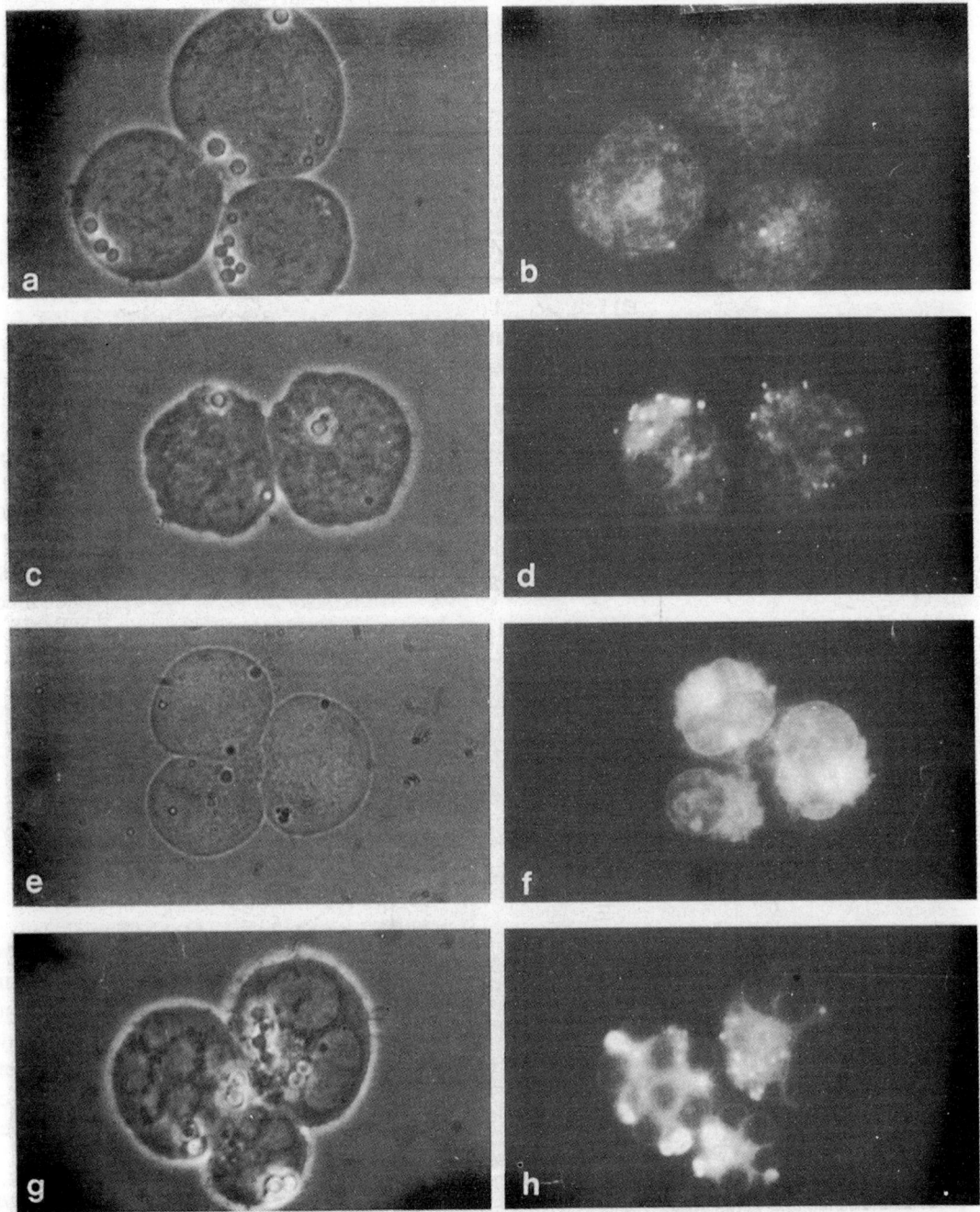

Fig 14. 14 : Localization of DNR in P388D$_1$ cells exposed to 5μg/ml of free DNR. a,b- after 15 minutes
exposure; c,d - 30minutes; e,f- 1hour; g,h- 4hours. Right column: observation with
fluorescence microscope; left column: view of the corresponding cells with light microscopy.

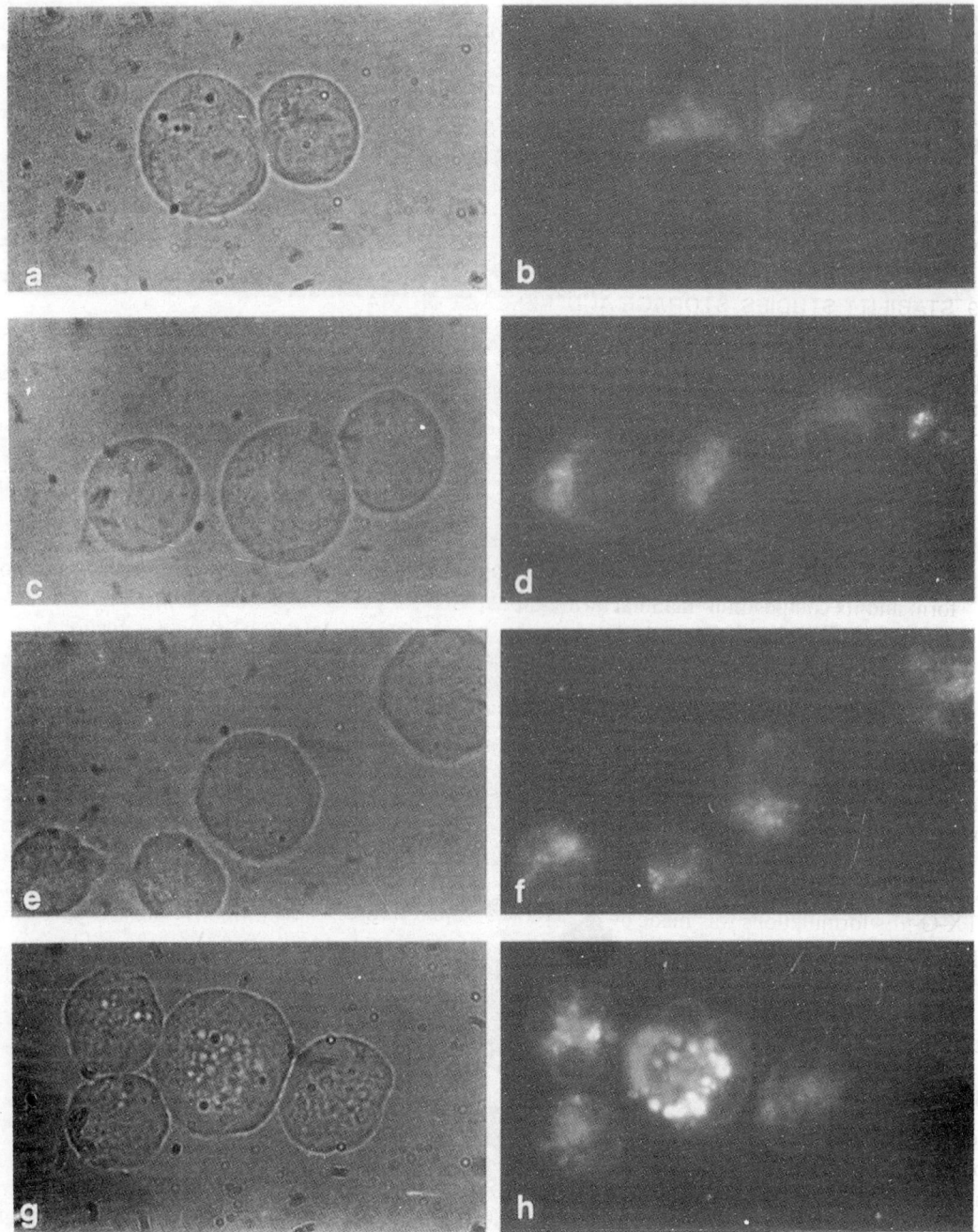

Fig 14. 15 : Localization of DNR in P388D$_1$ cells exposed to 5µg/ml of DNR conjugated to nEs. a,b- after
15 minutes exposure; c,d,- 30minutes; e,f- 1hour; g,h- 4hours. Right column: observation with
fluorescence microscope; left column: view of the corresponding cells with light microscopy.

14.7.12.Others

The spectroscopic based characterization of nEs has been reported by some workers at Canada [ulavel.ca/urr/rech/proj 62237.html].

14.8 ROUTES OF ADMINISTRATION

The in vivo evaluation of drug-carrier nanoerythrosmes preparation is normally conducted in laboratory animals, which include mice, rats and rabbits. The carrier cells are normally injected intravenously or intraarterially however, the intraperitional and subcutaneous routes can also be utilized.

14.9 STABILITY STUDIES, STORAGE AND RELEASE CHARACTERISTICS

The ability of a drug to retain properties within specified limits throughout its shelf-life is referred as stability. Improper storage of pharmaceutical products can lead to their physical deterioration and chemical degradation resulting in reduced activity and occasionally in the formation of toxic degradation products. Degradation is particularly likely to occur under tropical conditions of high ambient temperature and humidity. The most important factors which influence the rate and degree of degradation are (Garret, 1965):

(a) Environmental factors such as heat, moisture, light and any other form of physical stress like freezing, thawing and vibrations etc.

(b) Product related factors such as physiochemical properties of drug substance and the excipients, dosage form and its composition, manufacturing process and packaging and storage condition. A stable drug delivery system should maintain its integrity and morphology, and at the same time should preserve various characteristics such as nature of the entrapped drug, drug content, drug release profile etc.

Stability of a formulated product on shelf becomes an important factor in successful development of a dosage form. Very few reports are available on shelf-storage of carrier erythrocytes. Most of the workers have encapsulated their preparations and administered in circulation immediately. Lewis & Alpar (1984) have reported that encapsulated preparations (non-chemical treated cells) can be stored without loss of physical integrity when suspended in HBSS at 4°C for 2 weeks. Similar results were obtained upon storage of cells impregnated in soft bloom gelatin. Jain & Talwar (1992) and Jain & Jain (1998a) have reported drug loaded lyophilized erythrocytes bearing primaquine phosphate and meglumine antimonate respectively. A rapid assessment of MTX-G-nEs formulations was made by measuring changes in suspension turbidity. Relative turbidity was expressed as the ratio of the turbidity at time 't' to the initial turbidity. Changes in turbidity can occur when particles fuse, resulting in a transient increase in turbidity, due to large particle size. This, in turn, is followed by a decrease in turbidity as the larger particles float to the surface of suspension. Time dependent changes either increase or decrease, and can therefore be used as a measure of formulation stability.

14.9.1 Effect of aging

Storage stability was assessed at different temperatures viz. 4±1°C, room temperature and 37±1°C. Formulations [MTX-G-nEs(S), MTX-G-nEs(E) and MTX-G-nEs(EB)] were kept at variable temperature and change in particle size, sedimentation volume and relative turbidity were noted periodically. Stability of these formulations were also assessed at 4±1°C, R.T. and 37±1°C over time. Formulations exhibited little change in relative turbidity at 4±1°C but more at r.t. and 37±1°C. The effect of temperature on sedimentation volume with aging was negligible.

14.9.2 Effect of mice serum

Mice serum (0.1 ml) was added to 1.0 ml of the formulation and incubated at 37±1°C for 24 hr. The change in formulation before and 24 hr. after addition of mice serum were measured and compared. In addition to particle stability of these formulations over time at different temperatures, these were also assessed after incubation at

37±1°C in the presence and absence of serum to have an idea about in vivo stability. These formulations exhibited better stability in the presence of serum as revealed from turbidity measurement.

14.9.3 Effect of centrifugation

Each formulation was taken in centrifuge tubes and centrifuged at different rpm for 20 minutes and sedimentation volume was noted. After centrifugation at 2500 to 10000 rpm for 15 minutes, sedimentation volume of these formulations remained unity. This indicated stability of formulation upon centrifugal stress.

14.9.4 Separation of formulations in powder form

The MTX-G-nEs were collected by centrifugation and dried in vacuum (at 200 mm of Hg) for 10 hrs. The MTX-G-nEs suspension was filled in vials and lyophilized at -40°C to 0.01 torr using a laboratory lyophilizer (SICO, India). The dried powder thus obtained was filled in amber colored glass vials, sealed and stored at 4°C in a refrigerator. The MTX loaded nEs were easily transformed into dry powder form by vacuum drying and lyophilization. The morphological examination of the dry vesicles under electron microscopy (Fig 14.16) exhibited no alteration in the vesicle morphology as compared to the vesicles not subjected to drying.

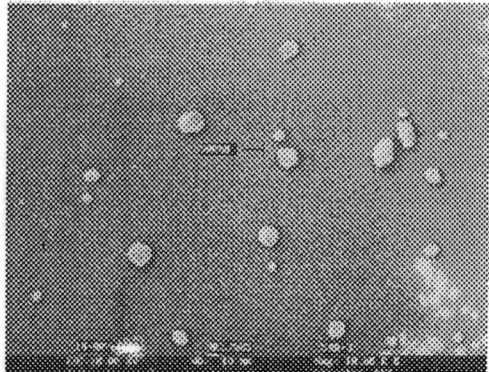

Fig 14. 16: SEM of MTX loaded lyophilized nEs.

14.9.5 Determination of drug content

The drug content of lyophilized erythrocytes powder was monitored for drug content every month, for 4 months by the following procedures :

14.9.5 Quantitation of MTX

The MTX-G-nEs were suspended in PBS (10% Hct). To 1 ml of MTX-G-nEs suspension (10% Hct), 1 ml of acetonitrile was added. From the resulting suspension, MTX was estimated to check the drug recovery. The experiment was performed using normal MTX-G-nEs and spiked with known amounts of drug . The drug recoveries of 98.23 to 99.32% were recorded. The drug content of stored cells estimated periodically for 6 months remained constant.

14.9.6 Morphological examination of powder vesicles

Morphological examination was carried out on an electron microscope.

14.9.7 In vitro release of MTX from powder cells

Following 1, 2 and 4 months of storage of the lyophilized powder, the cells were suspended in PBS (5% hct). Periodically, clear supernatant were withdrawn with the help of centrifugation and estimated for MTX release.

In vitro release profiles of MTX after 1, 2 and 4 months of storage were recorded The dried formulation (loaded) exhibited release of 12.10 to16.42% of drug upon storage for 4 months. Thus no significant variations could be detected in release of conjugated MTX from freshly prepared formulations which exhibited the release of 12.10 to 16.36% of MTX.

Thus a major problem encountered with the nEs carrier i.e. shelf-stability could be resolved by storing them in a powder form. Further the shelf-life of the carrier may be enhanced to months as compared to normal nEs. Furthermore, MTX-G-nEs as powder could be considered and may be highly promising stable carrier for MTX to be used for sustained delivery and localization especially in different organs on the basis of their particle size. However, extensive studies are required in order to investigate the biochemical changes of drug loaded nEs upon storage for prolonged periods of time, the effect of storage on in vivo disposition of nEs etc.

14.9.8 In vivo studies and toxicity

The in vivo studies of a designed formulation are very important criteria in successful development of a drug carrier system. In the case of target oriented systems, in vivo studies are conducted to ascertain the delivery of drug at the target site in the desired concentrations with minimum exposure of the drug to the non-target tissues. There are at least eight approaches for in vivo study of any sustained release dosage form namely pharmacological response, clinical level data, blood level data, nutritional studies, urinary excretion data, toxicity studies, roentgen technique and radioactive tracer technique (Robinson & Swintosky, 1959).

The in vivo evaluation study on erythrocyte carriers depends upon the properties expected from the developed system. In the system designed for prolonged dissemination of drug in the circulation, the blood levels of the encapsulated agent are measured over prolonged periods of time. DeLoach et. al., (1989) have estimated the imidiocarb blood levels following administration of imidiocarb dipropionate loaded erythrocytes in animals and compared with free drug administration. If the system is designed for targeting of the encapsulated agent to the RES system or other body site(s) the drug levels in the target tissues are measured over prolonged periods of time. Zocchi et. al., (1988) have studied tissue distribution of adriamycin encapsulated in erythrocytes and have compared it with conventional I.V. administration. In the case of enzyme-loaded erythrocytes designed to function as circulatory bioreactors the circulation level of substrate (which is to be metabolized) are monitored. Magnani et. al., (1989) measured blood levels of acetaldehyde in mice after injecting acetaldehyde-dehydrogenase loaded erythrocytes.The selected formulations (on the basis of in vitro studies) were further evaluated for in vivo performance. The drug encapsulated erythrocyte products were evaluated for their tissue distribution following I.V. administration, and were compared with the tissue distribution of plain drug solution. Jain et al., (1995a, 1997c) have successfully reported magnetically guided resealed erythrocytes bearing isoniazid.

To evaluate selectivity and specificity of the loaded cells for the target tissue, 'drug localization index' or 'drug targeting index' was determined at various time(s) using the simple equation described by Gupta & Hung (1989). The equation is:

$$\text{Drug localization index} = \text{or drug targeting index} = \frac{\text{\% drug concentration in target tissue at time t' after administration of crosslinked erythrocytes}}{\text{\% drug concentration in target tissue at time 't' after administration of drug as solution.}}$$

The value of index, if greater that 1, indicates high specificity and selectivity of the carrier for the target tissue.

The formulated products with promising (MTX-G-nEs[E]) in vitro performance were further evaluated for their in vivo performance on albino mice (Jain, 1999).

14.9.9 Pharmacokinetic profile

The albino mice of either sex (average weight 20-25 g; same size and weight) were divided into five groups each comprising of four mice. First group was administered drug solution equivalent to 200 µg of MTX (calculated at dose level of 8 mg/kg). The second to fourth groups were administered with formulation. The third group was kept as control. The blood samples were collected at different time intervals from retro-orbital plexus using heparinized syringe, the samples were centrifuged and plasma was collected. To the plasma, 2.0 ml of acetonitrile : water mixture (9:1) was added. The drug was extracted using acetic acid : ethyl acetate mixture (1:2). The samples were centrifuged and supernatants were analyzed.

14.9.10 Tissue distribution studies

Albino mice of either sex weighing about 20-25 g were used to study the organ distribution of MTX. The mice were divided into five groups each containing four mice. The animals of first group were given drug solution (equivalent to 200 µg of MTX) through caudal vein. The animals of second, third and fourth group were given MTX-G-nEs(E), MTX-G-nEs(S) and MTX-G-nEs(EB) formulations (equivalent to 200 µg MTX respectively) through caudal vein. The fifth group was kept as control. After 1 and 24 hr mice of each group were scarified. The body organs (liver, spleen, kidney, bone marrow, plasma and kidney) were removed. The body organs were washed to remove adhering debris and dried with tissue paper. The organs were homogenized and drug was extracted using acetic acid : ethyl acetate mixture (1:2). The samples were centrifuged and supernatants were analyzed.

14.9.11 Biochemical tests of liver function

The method reported by Reitman (1974) was used for the estimation of serum glutamate pyruvate transaminase (SGPT) and method reported by King & King (1954) was used for the estimation of serum alkaline phosphatase (SALP). All the estimations were done on an autoanalyser [RA-50, Technion, USA].

The blood MTX levels following the administration of MTX in free and MTX-G-nEs form were recorded. At 1 hr post administration, the free methotrexate level in blood was reduced to 50% and only 1.5% of the administered dose was present at 24 hr post dosing. Blood levels of MTX-G-nEs administration were clearly sustained as compared to free drug. This establishes the efficacy of nEs in prolonging the release of entrapped drug, as also the structural integrity of the nEs. If the nEs would not have maintained their integrity in vivo, they would have been excreted rapidly. The observation of the organ distribution and blood level study lead to the conclusion that upon in vivo administration, the nEs were localized preferentially in the liver, spleen and bone marrow by virtue of phagocytic uptake by the RES. They maintained their structural integrity and continued to release the entrapped drug over a prolonged period of time.

In order to evaluate the systemic availability, organ specificity and in vivo performance of developed erythrocyte systems, tissue distribution of drug following I.V. administration as drug solution of MTX-G-nEs were estimated in various organs.

The tissue distribution of unmetabolised MTX (represented as percent of dose injected) was recorded. After 1hr of administration of drug solution 1.47, 3.24 and 1.10 µg/g of drug was found in liver; kidney and spleen respectively, which declined by 24 hr. From bone marrow 0.22% of the MTX was recovered after 1hr. The drug level in bone marrow also declined after 24 hr when less than 1 µg/g of the drug was recovered in all the organs except spleen. Following administration of MTX-G-nEs higher hepatic, splenic, kidney and bone marrow localization of MTX was noted.

MTX-G-nEs are reported to be cleared from circulation by RES recognition [Jain & Jain, 1998], by phagocytosis in the liver, by the kupffer cells resulting in sustained drug release from these cells. The drug is made available to the parenchymatous cells and hepatocytes and metabolized following its slow release from the kupffer cells. The nEs administration thus provides an intra-hepatic slow release system of MTX with possible modification of metabolism kinetics.

The administration of developed system resulted in an elevation in the level of unmetabolised MTX, suggesting the improvement in prophylactic and therapeutic efficacy of the drug. The efficacy may be related to the more amounts of unmetabolised drug available for activity against the cancer. In order to assess the selectivity of the erythrocytes for the RES, the drug localization index was determined at various times using the equation described by Gupta & Hung (1989). The values were found to be greater than 1, indicating high specificity and selectivity of the erythrocyte carrier for the liver tissue. The value of index increases with time, which could be due to the slow release of drug in liver.

The tissue drug concentration data indicate the rapid clearance of MTX solution by spleenocytes after 1hr followed by decrease after 24hr, while the spleenic clearance of MTX-G-nEs after 24hr was found to be increased indicating higher circulation life of MTX-G-nEs.

On the basis of in vivo studies it is clear that the nEs carrier resulted in higher concentration of the MTX in the RES (liver, spleen and bone marrow), with slower elimination of drug as compared to the free drug administration. The higher concentration achieved in the RES and for prolonged time(s) may result in improvement in therapeutic efficacy of MTX against the liver tumors as higher amount of drug would be available for longer time for activity, thus aiding in cure of the disease by completely destroying the cancer cells. MTX-G-nEs can be utilized for prophylaxis of all forms of tumors of RES as well as for cure. The organ localization of the drugs may result in lowering of toxic manifestations, which confront their therapy.

Biochemical test of liver function indicated no significant change in values as compared to normal cells indicating no detrimental effect of treated cells on liver.

14.9.12 Acute toxicity studies

The method reported by Udupa (1995) was used for these studies. Acute toxicity in terms of body weight was determined in albino mice.

14.9.13 Hematological toxicity studies

Hematological toxicity of free and formulated MTX was determined by injecting (I.V.) 8.0 mg/kg of free and formulated MTX to albino mice. The peripheral and bone marrow counts of WBC were carried out at definite time intervals post injection.

The study of acute toxicity revealed improving weight loss of animals 5 days after receiving MTX-G-nEs (E) in comparison to MTX solution. The WBC suppressive characteristics of MTX-solution and MTX-G-nEs were recorded. The peripheral and bone marrow WBCs responded similarly to MTX solution and MTX-G-nEs at a dose of 8.0mg/Kg. The drug induced decrease in WBC population was observed first in the bone marrow, followed by a decrease in the peripheral count. The least peripheral WBC count was seen on day 3 for both MTX-solution and MTX-G-nEs values occurred on the second day. Both peripheral and bone marrow WBC count reached almost normal values on day 9.

Thus, it is concluded that drug loaded nanoerythrosomes can be successfully used as drug carrier for controlled and targeted delivery of methotrexate.

14.10. IMMUNOLOGICAL CONSIDERATIONS

The immunological characteristics of a drug carrier are of two types: the immunogenicity of the carrier itself and the ability of the carrier to protect an entrapped drug from immunological detection.

The autologous erythrocytes are not immunogenic. However, there is concern that the lysis procedure utilized for drug entrapment might elicit some cryptic antigens. Fiddler et. al., (1977) and Desnick et. al., (1978) examined this phenomenon and found no immunological response against resealed erythrocytes. Further they examined the immunological response in mice to bovine ß-glucuroxidase bearing autologous erythrocytes.

The repeated I.V. administration of cells entrapping ß- glucuroxidase did not elicit any detectable antibody against ß-glucuroxidase in control mice and those previously sensitized to ß-glucuroxidase. There was no difference in tissue distribution or survival of administered ß-glucuroxidase between the control and sensitized animals. Similar results can be expected in case of drug loaded nEs, as these are derivative of erythrocyte ghost.

14.11. TARGETING POTENTIAL

Conner et. al., (1987), DeLoach et. al., (1977), Talwar & Jain (1992), Jain & Jain (1996a) and Tonetti et. al., (1994) selectively targeted drug loaded erythrocytes after gluteraldehyde treatment to the liver or spleen. They found that gluteraldehyde fixation of erythrocytes renders them resistant to both osmotic shock and turbulence induced lysis.

Another novel approach is to magnetize the carrier so that the carrier cells can be retained at or guided to the target site by the application of an external magnetic field of an appropriate strength (Widder et. al., 1978, 1979; Sprandel et. al., 1987). Retention of magnetic carrier at target site will delay recticuloendothelial clearance and prolong the action of drug. This method was first suggested by Zimmerman & Pilwat [1976] and Frei [1970] who proposed that erythrocytes or lymphocytes containing fine ferromagnetic particles are targetable to a desired target site with the help of an external magnetic field.

Static magnetic fields of high strength and gradient do not seem to produce any severe side effects. On the other hand the time of application of the magnetic field may tend to induce electrical potentials and currents in the body which in turn may cause undesirable side effects.

Since magnetite is known to cause varying extent of hemolytic and cytotoxic effect on cell wall of erythrocytes, it necessitates the modification of magnetite before its entrapment in erythrocyte. Zimmermann (1982) suggested a method for prevention of hemolysis by silicone oil taking on cobalt ferrite particles (0.1-1.0 μm dia.). The coating of silicone oil prevents aggregation of the particles in electrolyte solutions. These particles can be entrapped in erythrocytes with the help of electrical breakdown method. The magnetic erythrocytes were actively accumulated specifically in the foreleg of a mouse with the aid of external magnetic field. However because of their small average size and narrow size distribution, the use of Fe_3O_4 particles (10-20 nm dia) is preferable over cobalt ferrite. Investigations with the electron microscope have revealed that magnetic particles can be entrapped in ghost cells. The membrane lysis was carried out in isotonic solutions of sucrose, mannitol or glucose using a field intensity of 1.5 KV/cm and a pulse length of 50μ sec. Some of the magnetic particles were observed to be adsorbed over the outer membrane surface. Jain & Jain (1996c, 1997c) have also reported mannan coated erythoctyes for lung targeting and lectinised erythrocytes for tumor targeting.

In in vitro experiment, with the aid of a permanent external magnet (8000 oestered), the 'magnetic' erythrocytes can be accumulated when they are allowed to flow at a rate identical to that of the blood stream (Jain & Vyas, 1994 a,b). Colloidal magnetite suspensions were sonicated prior to encapsulation, which was found to be 10-15% followed by susceptibility measurements. In vitro experiments showed that red blood cells loaded with magnetic particles might be directed to exact points by the use of magnetic fields. Khopade et. al., (1997) have reported magnetic cellular nanovesicles for delivery of a bioactive agent. The same approach may find application in case of nEs.

14.12 APPLICATIONS OF NANOERYTHROSOMES

nEs have been proposed for a variety of applications in human and veterinary medicine. Various applications can be summarized as under:

Most of technologies developed by Diagnocure Inc., Canada involve an antibody as vehicle for delivery of nanoerythrosomes, which are tiny spheres loaded with general application drugs or toxic agents used specifically to destroy selected carrier cells (Diagnocure.com).

Lejune et. al., (1994) reported that doxorubicin - nanoerythrosome conjugates have higher antineoplastic activity than the free drug on CDF$_1$, leukemia tumors. They have reported covalent binding of daunorubicin to proteins using various crosslinkers (Fig 14.17 & 14.18).

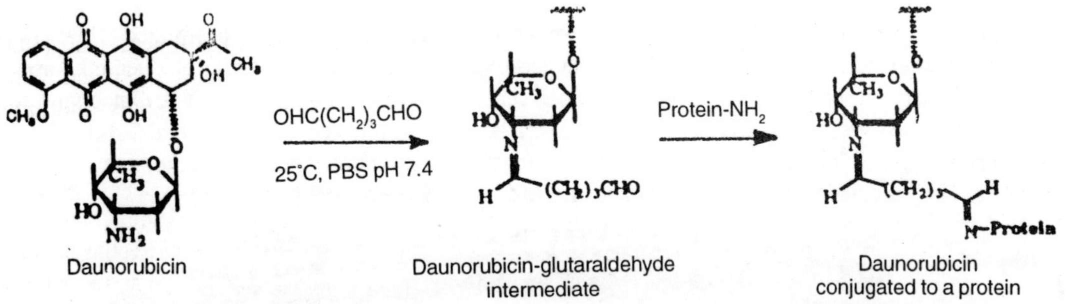

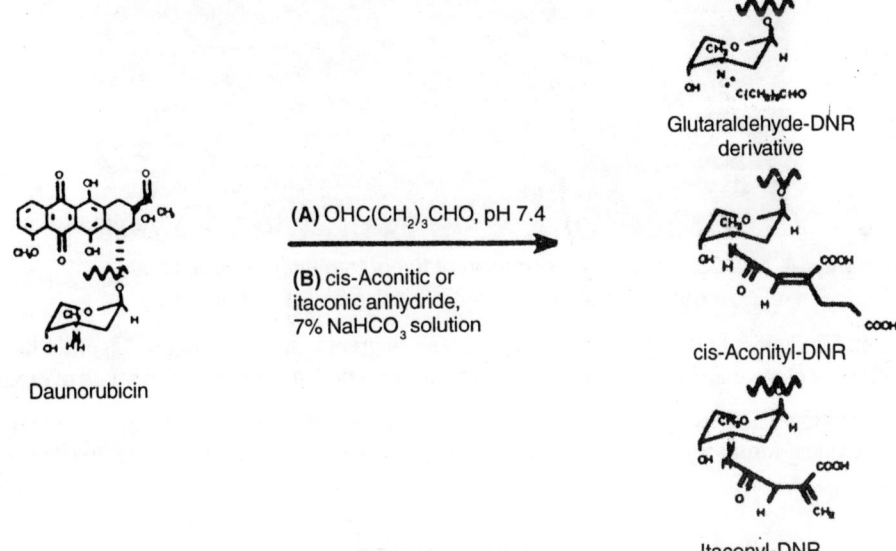

Fig 14.17: Covalent binding of daunorubicin to protein using glutaraldehyde as crosslinking agent.

Daunorubicin   Daunorubicin-glutaraldehyde intermediate   Daunorubicin conjugated to a protein

(A) OHC(CH$_2$)$_3$CHO, pH 7.4

(B) cis-Aconitic or itaconic anhydride, 7% NaHCO$_3$ solution

Daunorubicin

Glutaraldehyde-DNR derivative

cis-Aconityl-DNR

Itaconyl-DNR

Fig 14. 18 : Chemical synthesis of nEs-daunorubicin derivatives using either glutaradehyde, itaconic or aconitic acid as linking arms.

Moorjani et al (1997) reported the mechanism of action of drug loaded nanoerythrosomes.

Al-Achi et al (1990, 1993a,b) have successfully reported erythrocyte membrane vesicular delivery of insulin and doxorubicin.

Jain & Jain (1996, 1997) have reported nanoerythrosomes based delivery of mitomycin-C, hydroxyurea and 6-mercaptopurine.

Jain & Jain. (1997b) have reported inside-out and rightside-out vesicles.

Mishra & Jain (2000) have reported reverse biomembrane vesicles bearing doxorubicin.

The nEs based drug delivery systems have excellent potential for clinical applications.

14.13. ADVANCES, CONCLUSION AND FUTURE PROSPECTS

Until other carrier systems come of age, nanoerythrosomes technology will remain an active arena for the further research. A company that is developing products for human use (< biblio >) is currently testing the commercial medical applications of nEs in Canada. The coming years represent a critical time in this field as commercial applications are explored. In near future, nEs based delivery system with their ability to provide controlled and site specific drug delivery may revolutionize disease management.

Diagnocure Inc. has recently been granted a patent from US patent office for a prolonged release system that it developed to reduce the destructive adverse effects experienced by cancer patients on chemotherapy. The system uses nanoerythrosomes developed using red blood cells. According to the company, these nanoerythrosomes allow the delivery to affected part, instead of affecting both healthy and affected cells. In animal testing, they have proven to be valuable in detecting pathology. The nanoerythrosomes coupled with antibodies can increase test sensitivities. The system is projected to be available in 3 to 5 years (Woolley, 1997) (Fig 14. 19).

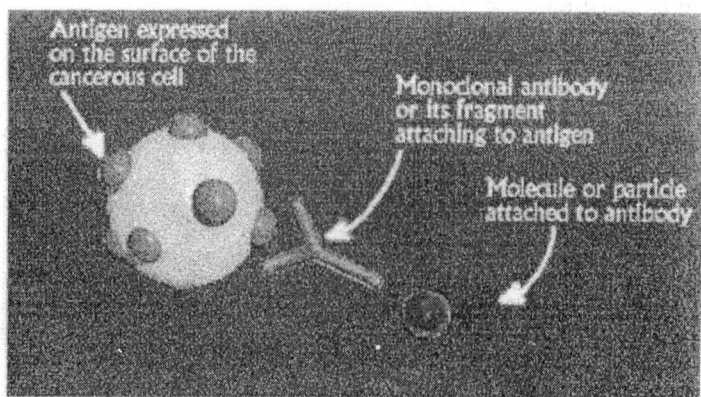

Fig 14. 19 : Schematic representation of tumor targeting using antibody coated nanoerythrosomes bearing an anticancer drug.

To this end Diagnocure Inc., Canada has an exclusive agreement with Seragen/Ligand Pharmaceuticals for the exploitation of recombinant proteins derived in part from the transmembrane domain of diphtheria toxin.

The International Society For the Use of Resealed Erythrocytes [ISURE] through its biannual meetings provides an excellent forum for exchange of information to the scientists in this exiting and rewarding field of research.

REFERENCES

Alpar, O. H. and Lewis, D.A. (1984) Int. J. Pharm., 22:137.

Al-Achi, A. and Boroujerdi, M. (1990) Drug Dev. Ind. Pharm., 16(8):1325.

Al-Achi, A. and Greenwood, R. (1993a) Drug Dev. Ind. Pharm., 19(6):673.

Al-Achi, A. and Greenwood, R. (1993b) Drug Dev. Ind. Pharm., 19(11):1303.

Bangham, A. D.; Standish, M. M. and Watkins, J. C. (1965) J. Mol. Biol., 13:238.

Connor, J. and Huang, L. (1986) Cancer Res., 461:3431.

DeLoach, J.; Peters, S.; Pinkard, O.; Glew, R. and Ihler, G. (1977) Biochim. Biophysics Acta, 496:507.

DeLoach, D. R. and Ihler, G. (1979) Biochimica et Biophysica Acta, 446:136

DeLoach, J. R. (1986) Med. Res. Rev., 6:487.

DeLoach, J. R.; Wagner, C. G. and Corrier, D. E. (1989) J. Contr. Rel., 9:243.

DeLoach, J. R. and Way, J. L. (1994) Am. J. Vet. Sci., 76:67.

Desnick, R. J.; Fiddler, M. B.; Donglas, S. D. and Hudson, L. D. S. (1978) Adv. Expt. Med. Biol., 101:753.

Diagnocure.com/eryl/prod/tech.htm

Eylar, C.K. (1962) J. Mem. Biol., 11:76.

Fiddler, M..; Hudson, L.D.S. and Desnick, N. (1977) Biochem. J., 168:141.

Frei, E. H. (1970) Crit. Re. Solid State Sci., 1:381.

Garret, N.M. (1965), J. Pharm. Sci., 54:1557.

Gregoriadis, G. (1972) TIBTECH, 13:527.

Gregoriadis, G. (1983) Pharm. International, 33:112.

Gupta, P. K. and Hung, C.T. (1989), Int. J. Pharm., 56:217.

Ihler, G. M.; Glew, R. H. and Schnure, F. W. (1973) Proc. Natl. Acad. Sci., 70, 2663.

Ihler, G.M.; Glew, R.H. and Schnure, F. W. (1983) Pharm. Ther., 20:151.

Jain, S. (1994) M. Pharm. Thesis, Dr. H. S. Gour University, Sagar, India.

Jain, S. and Jain, N. K. (1994) Proc. of 46th Pharmaceutical Association, Chandigarh, India, p. 76

Jain, S.; Jain, S. K. and Dixit, V. K. (1995a) Indian Drugs, 32(10):471.

Jain, S. and Jain, N. K. (1995b) Workshop on New drug delivery sytems, Manipal, India, p.4.

Jain, S. and Jain, N. K. (1995c) Proc. of 47th Indian Pharmaceutical Congress, Visakhapatanam, India, p.

Jain, S. and Jain, N. K. (1996a) Third International Symposium on Pharmaceutical Technology and Innovations, Ahmedabad, India, p.74

Jain, S. and Jain, N. K. (1996 b,c,d) 6th International Conference of ISURE, Germany, India, p. 11.

Jain, S. and Jain, N. K. (1996e) Proc. Indian Pharmaceutical Congress, Madras, India, p.94.

Jain, S. and Jain, N. K. (1997a) 24th International Conference of Controlled Release Society, Sweden, p. 108

Jain, S. and Jain, N. K. (1997b) Proc. of 3rd International conference on Cellular Engineering, Itlay, p.12.

Jain, S.; Jain, S. K. and Dixit, V. K. (1997c) Drug Dev. and Ind. Pharm., 23:999.

Jain, S. and Jain, N. K. (1997d) In : Controlled and Novel Drug Delivery [N.K.Jain (ed.)] CBS Publishers, N.Delhi, India, 1997, p.256

Jain, S. and Jain, N. K. (1997e) Proc. of 49th Indian Pharmaceutical Congress, Trivandrum, India, p.72

Jain, S. and Jain, N. K. (1997f) 24th International Conference of Controlled Release Society, Sweden, p. 113.

Jain, S. (1997g) Proc. of 12th M. P. Young Science Congress, Bilaspur, India, p.17

Jain, S. and Jain, N. K. (1997h) Indian J. Pharm. Sci., 59(6):275.

Jain, S. (1998) Proc. of 13th M. P. Young Science Congress, Gwalior, India, p.74

Jain, S. and Jain, N. K. (1998a) Die Pharmazie, 53(1):5.

Jain, S. and Jain, N. K. (1998b) National Seminar on Current Trends & Future Challenges in Pharmaceutics, Chandigarh, India, p.14.

Jain, S. and Jain, N. K. (1998c) Proc. of 25th International Conference of CRS, Las Vegas, USA, p.114.

Jain, S. and Jain, N. K. (1998d) Proc. of MPCOST, Bhopal, India, p.37.

Jain, S. (1999) Ph.D. Thesis, Dr. H. S. Gour University, Sagar, India.

Jain, S. and Jain, N.K. (1999a) Proc. Of 26th International Conference of Controlled Release Society, Swden, p.472.

Jain, S. and Jain, N.K. (1999b) Proc. Of 51st Indian Pharmaceutical Congress, Indore, India, p.76.

Jain, S. (2000) Proceedings of National Science Day, Sagar, India, p.6

Jain, S.K. and Vyas, S. P. (1994a) J. Microencap., 11:29.

Jain, S.K. and Vyas, S.P. (1994b) J. Microencap., 11:75.

Khopade, A. J.; Jain, S. and Jain, N. K. (1997) 24th International Conference of Controlled Release Society, Las Vegas, USA, p.458.

Kim, Y. W.; Fung, M. S. C.; Sun,, C. R. Y.; Chang, N. T. and Chang, T. W. (1996) J. Immunol., 144:1257.

King, J. and King, J. (1954) J. Pharm. Sci., 49:203.

Lejeune, A.; Moorjani, M.; Gicquard, C.; Lacroix, J.; Poyet, P. and Gauderault, R. (1994) Anticancer Research, 14:915.

Liautard, J. P.; Vidal, M. and Philpott, J. R. (1985) Biochemistry, 19:5376.

Lowery, O. H.; Rosebrough, N. J.; Farr, A.L. and Randall, R.I. (1951), J. of Biochem., 12:112.

Magnani, M.; Rossi, L.; Bianchi, M.; Serafini, S. and Stocchi, V. (1989) Acta Haematology, 82:27

Moorjani, M.; Lejune, A.; Gicquadid, C.; Lacroir, J.; Poyet, B. and Gaudreault, R. C. (1997) Anticancer Res., 16:2831

Mishra, P. R. and Jain, N. K. (2000) Drug Delivery, 7 : 1.

Reitman, S. and Frankel, A. S. (1957) Am. J. Clin. Pathol., 28:56.

Robinson, H. J. and Swintosky, J. V. (1959) J. Am. Pharm. Assoc., 48:473.

Sparndel, U. (1987) In:Advances in Biosciences (Ropers, C.; Chassaigne, M.; Nicolau, C.; eds.), Pergamon Press, New York., 67:243.

Steck, T. L.; Weinstein, R. S.; Straus, J. H. and Wallach, D.F.H. (1970) Science, 10:255.

Talwar, N. and Jain, N. K. (1992) Drug Dev. & Ind. Pharm., 8:199.

Tonetti, M.; Barotini, A.; Sobrero, A.; Guglielmi, A.; Felletti, R.; Gasparini, A.; Benatti, U. and DeFiora, A. (1994) In:Advances in Biosciences (DeLoach, J.R.; Way, J.L., eds.) Pergamon Press, New York.,92:169.

Thoppil, S. O. and Gandhi, A. K. (1999) Express Pharma Pulse, October 28, 1999, Vol.5 (49), p.14

Udupa, N. (1995) (ed.) Novel Drug Delivery Systems : Manipal Experience, p. 171.

Ulavel.ca./urr/rech/proj 62237.html

Vonderhoff, J.H. and Et-Assar, M. (1988) Theory of colloids in Pharmaceutical Dosage Forms: Disperse systems, Liberman, H. A.; Rieger, M.M.; Banker, G.S. (eds), Vol. A., Marcel Dekkar Inc, New York, p.93.

Voet, G. and Voet, J. (eds.) (1990) Biochemistry, John Wiley and Sons, New York, p.241.

Widder, K. J.; Senyei, A. E. and Scarpelli, D. G. (1978) Proceedings of the Society for Experimental Biology and Medicine, 58:141.

Widder, K. J.; Senyei, A. E. and Ranney, D. F. (1979) Advances in Pharmacology and Chemotherapy, 16:216.

Widder, K. J.; Senyei, A. E. and Ranney, D. F. (1980) Cancer Res., 40:3512

Wheeler, J.; Wong, K. M.; Ansell, S.M.; Masin, D. and Bally, M.B. (1994) J. Pharm. Sci., 83(11): 1558

Woolley, B. H. (1997), Therapeutic letter, 3(8): 2.

Zimmerman, U. (1992) Dentsche Apothekar Zefung, 12:1170.

Zimmermann, U. (1973) KFA-Report, p. 58.

Zimmermann, U. (1975) Chem. Eng. News. , 24:71.

Zimmermann, U.; Pilwat, U. (1976) Z. Naturforsch., 316:732.

Zocchi, E.; Tonetii, M.; Polvani, C.; Guida, L.; Benatti, U. and DeFlora, A. (1988), Biotechnol. Appl. Biochem., 10: 555.

Chapter 15

Dendrimers as Potential Delivery Systems for Bioactives

N. K. Jain, A.J. Khopade

In the search of novel biomaterials for controlled and targeted delivery of bioactives, starburst "dendrimers" is the latest star that bears promising properties for the delivery of bioactives ranging from drugs, vaccines, metals or genes to the desired site. They are highly branched structure obtained by iterative synthesis possessing unique properties. Inspite being polymer, they differ from conventional polymers but bear similarity to vesicles such as micelles, liposomes and globular proteins. The intriguing feature of dendrimer is their surface topology, shape and size, which open wide scope for their use as biomorphic/biomimetic moieties. Their hollow interior provides space to incorporate drugs and other bioactives physically or by various interactions to act as drug delivery vehicles. The present review highlights some of their distinguishing properties, brief account of synthesis and their potential applications in the field of novel drug delivery.

15.1 INTRODUCTION

Last one decade in particular has witnessed sea changes in the drug delivery concepts and the latest star on the horizon is visible, named "dendrimers". During this period several types of functional polymers with highly unusual architectures have appeared in the literature. These include sheet like two dimensional polymers (Stuff et al., 1993) as well as three dimensional structure dendrimers, hyperbranched polymers (Hawker et al., 1991) and the threaded linear polymers: polyrotoxanes (Gibson & Marand, 1993). In the late 1970's an interesting polymeric material began to appear in literature synthesized through various pathways. These materials share the features of defined composition, high molecular mass and highly branched architecture. This structure is accounted for by various names for these molecules such as 'cascade molecules', 'arborols', 'dendritic molecules' or 'dendrimers' (Tomalia et al., 1985; Newkome et al., 1985) and because of their minute size and monodispersity they are often referred to as nanoscopic compounds (Tomalia & Durst, 1993). The synthesis of functional polymers and copolymers with highly controlled architecture and precisely placed functional groups open new events for the preparation of well-defined molecular objects and devices.

The term dendrimer is derived from the word 'dendron', a Greek word for tree/branches, due to its resemblance with a tree and 'meros' meaning part. Dendrimers posses three distinguishing architectural components: (a) an initiator core, (b) interior layers (generations) composed of repeating units radially attached to the initiator core, and (c) exterior (terminal functionality) attached to the outermost interior generation. Due to high degree of branching large dendrimers adopt a globular shape in which all bonds converge to a focal point or central core unit. Of particular interest, in context of functional polymers, is the fact that dendrimers posses a very large number of chain ends. e.g. polyether dendrimers (Hawker & Frechet 1990). Dendrimers can be made from virtually any material. They start from a core molecule with at least three chemically reactive arms. To these arms, chemists attach multiple branches. Because these new branches end with same reactive groups as the original three arms, the process can be repeated many times. As the density of branches increases, the outermost branches arrange themselves in the form of sphere surrounding a lower density core. Drug deliverers are starting to control things outside and inside the dendrimers to make them functional e.g. mass, surface valency and surface directionality in dendrimer system. Dendrimer shapes have very unusual physical as well as chemical properties and other parameters that control solubility and miscibility. Dendrimers with hydrophilic surface groups are water-soluble while those with hydrophobic surfaces are hydrocarbon-soluble. The steric considerations that dictate the globular shape of dendrimers effect their ability to interact with neighbouring molecules.

Chemically bridging of fundamental building blocks "dendrimers" leads to a new class of topological macromolecules hence, referred to as "starburst polymers". This involves chemical reaction between nucleophilic dendrimers and dendrimers possessing electrophilic surfaces resulting in products with dramatically enhanced dimensions, about 100 nm, which are also referred to as nanoscopic compounds, clusters and polymers. These nanoscopic supramolecular compounds, clusters and assemblies can be observed directly by electron microscopy. They may be represented as:

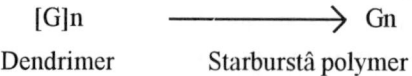

A number of different styles and designs of dendrimers have been reported with structural diversity in the repeat units ranging from pure hydrocarbons to peptides to co-ordination compounds. Especially in 1990's it has attracted drug deliverers in some parts of the world to explore the scope based on this concept and yearly the publications on this topic are increasing. A typical dendrimer structure is shown in Fig. 15.1.

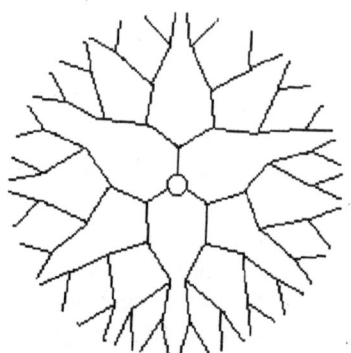

Fig 15.1: A typical dendrimer structure

15.2 MOLECULAR MODELLING OF DENDRIMERS

The conformation of dendrimer molecules in the solid state and in solution is still controversial. In particular, conflicting predictions on the shape of dendritic molecules have been made on the basis of theory and molecular modelling. The model of Gennes & Hervet (1983) suggests a density minimum at the center of dendrimer and predicts that ideal dendritic growth will only occur until a certain generation is reached, at which point steric congestion will prevent further growth. This was later called as "starburst effect" by Tomalia, (1994). Computer assisted molecular modelling experiments by Naylor et al.(1989) suggested that as size increases, the shapes of the starburst dendrimers progress from open structures to closed spheroids with well developed internal hollows and dense surfaces. This view is not shared by Lescanec & Muthukumar (1990) whose simplified kinetic model of dendritic growth predicts maximum density at the core of dendrimer and a distribution of end groups throughout the structures. The ends of the branches, the model suggests, are not positioned at the surface but are severely folded. This model has some valuable features but it fails to account for some properties of well-known dendrimers. Mansfield & Klushin (1993) reports similar results based on Monte Carlo simulations. The backfolding of chains hence radius of gyration of dendrimer depend upon polarity of solvent and increases with the generation (Murat & Grest, 1996). Using self consistent mean field model (SCMF) Boris & Rubinstein (1996) showed the maximum density at the core due to uniform distribution of end groups throughout the volume of dendrimer (Fig 15.2). There is also a different view of some scientists. Milkis et al (1997) and Cavallo & Fraternali (1998) have investigated through molecular dynamics study that some folding of terminal group does occur but not to the extent that core is completely filled. Monte Carlo simulations on dendrimers showed a dramatic change in dendrimer conformation upon addition of electrolyte. At high ionic strength, backfolding of the end groups takes place and a dense core dendritic structure is formed. At low ionic strengths, the molecule is stretched out to form a dense shell (Welch & Muthukumar, 1998).

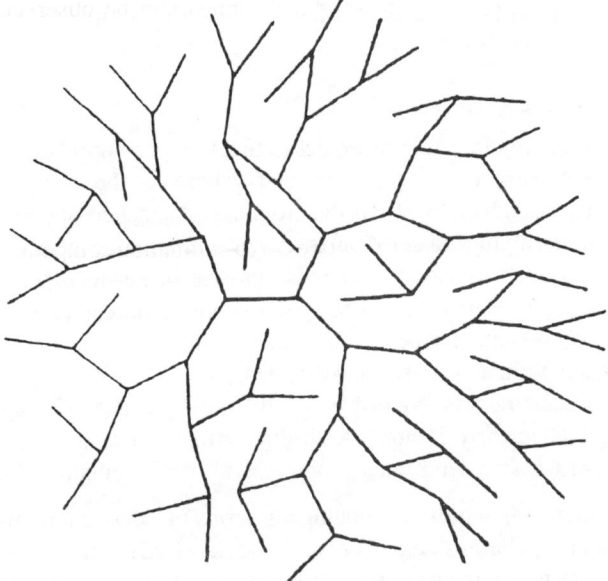

Fig15.2 : Schematic representation of backfolded dendrimer (Boris & Rubinstein, 1996)

Low Salt   High Salt

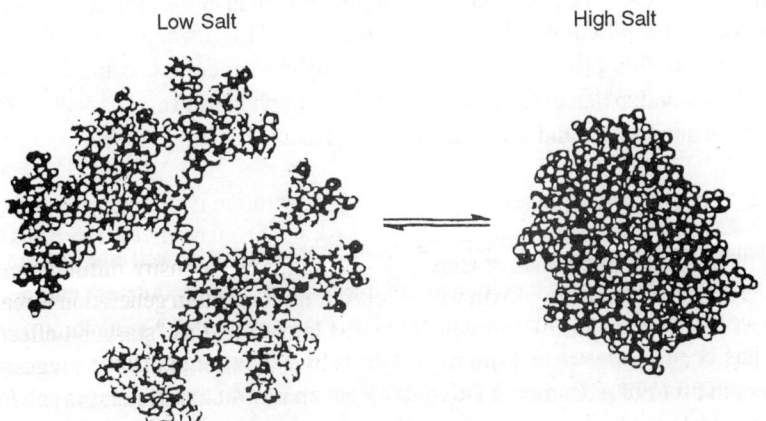

Fig15.3: Dense shell *vs* dense core: Effect of salt concentration (Welch & Muthukumar, 1998).

Table 15. 1: Difference between lower vs higher generation dendrimers

S.No.	Lower generation	Higher generation
1.	Polarity is high (Zimmerman et al., 1998)	Polarity decreases as generation increases.
2.	Open structure, size of encapsulation cavity is small.	Close and compact structure; size of cavity is large.
3.	Lower generation allows interaction with protein e.g. myoglobulin (Collman et al., 1997)	Higher generations do not allow interaction with protein due to closed structure.
4.	*In vivo* toxicity is not reported for 3rd and 5th generation PAMAM dendrimers.	*In vivo* toxicity is reported for 7th generation PAMAM dendrimer.
5.	*In-vitro* toxicity of (PAMAM) dendrimer for 3rd and 5th generation is less.	*In vitro* toxicity of PAMAM dendrimer for 7th generation is more.

15.3. DENDRIMERS VS. CONVENTIONAL POLYMERS

Dendrimers differ from classical random coil molecules in that they are highly branched, three-dimensional macromolecules with a branch point at each monomer unit. Therefore they are potentially the most highly branched structures that exist. Dendrimers also differ from hyperbranched polymers (Hawker et al, 1991). Hyperbranched polymers are also highly branched but their structure is neither regular nor highly symmetrical. Secondly, dendrimers are obtained by careful, stepwise growth of successive layers or generations but hyperbranched polymers are obtained in a single step by polycondensation of an X_2Y monomer that contains two reactive groups of type X and one of type Y. Functional groups X and Y are selected in such a way that they can react with each other to form a covalent bond (Frechet, 1996). A macroscopic illustration for comparison of linear polymers and dendrimers is "cooked spaghetti" and "green peas" respectively. The former is heavily entangled but the later clearly is not. A similar situation prevails for Tomalia's well known poly(amidoamine), (PAMAM) starburst dendrimers (Tomalia et al, 1985; Tomalia & Durst, 1993).

As molecular weight increases within a homologous series of dendrimers, the molecules undergo a transition from an extended to a globular shape. In case of classical linear polymers such as poly(styrene) the viscosity increases sharply with molecular weight according to the Mark-Houwink-Sakurada equation : $[\eta] = K.M^a$, where $[\eta]$ is the intrinsic viscosity of polymer, M is molecular weight , K and a are constants for a given polymer. Unlike almost all other macromolecules including branched and star polymers, dendrimers do not obey this relation once a threshold molecular weight is reached. This deviation is easily understood, if one considers that during generation growth, the volume of dendrimers increases cubically whereas their mass increases exponentially, a relation that does not hold true for other polymers (Tomalia et al., 1985; Moorey et al., 1992). Analogy between dendrimers and linear polymers is presented in Table 15.2.

15.4. DENDRIMER - MICELLE ANALOGY

It has been stated that aqueous micelles are "stable, disjoint, co-operative, closed equilibrium colloidal aggregates" (Frances et al, 1980) that posses topological order (an inside and an outside) and may be more accurately thought of as dimensionally discordant fractals (Butcher & Lamb, 1984; Mandelbrot, 1983). A variety of ingenious models has been proposed to explain certain of these aggregate structures and include those proposed by Menger & Dill (1984), Cantor & Dill (1984), Hartley (1948), Wennerstrom & Lindman (1979), Mitschell & Ninham (1981) etc. Unfortunately, there is no direct method available to date for equivocal determination of micellar structures (Fendler, 1984). Currently, there is some controversy over micellar structure (Dill & Flory, 1981) and possible perturbation effect caused by introduction of probe (guest) molecules into these aggregates. For this reason it would be of interest to mimic the fundamentals (i.e., size, shape, topology and chemical functionality) associated with these microenviroments in a "covalently fixed model". In the quest for

Table 15.2 : Difference between dendrimer vs. linear polymer molecules

S. N.	Parameter	Dendrimer	Linear polymer molecules
1.	Glass transition temperature (Tg) (Hawker et al., 1995)	Levels off at higher molecular weight dendrimer due to more end groups and less entanglements.	Levels off due to declining influence of the end group and more entanglement.
2.	Intrinsic viscosity	Does not obey Mark-Houwink-Sakurda equation i.e. intrinsic viscosity does not increase with molecular mass but reaches a maximum at certain dendrimer generation.	Obey Mark-Houwink- Sakurda equation, intrinsic viscosity increase with molecular mass.
3.	Solubility (Miller et al., 1992; Wooley et al., 1994)	More solubility in organic solvent in comparison to the analogous linear polymer e.g. 1,3,5 phenylene based dendrimer.	Less soluble than analogous dendrimer in organic solvent e.g. phenylene linear analogue.
4.	Reactivity (de Brabander et al., 1996)	The debenzylation of the polyesters via catalytic hydrogenation on $^{Pd}/_{c}$ is only possible e.g. Poly (propyleneimine) dendrimers with nitrile group.	Not possible. e.g. poly (acrylonitrile)
5.	Hydrodynamic volume	Hydrodynamic volume of fifth generation polyther dendrimer is approximately 30% smaller than that of its linear analogue	30% more
6.	Physical behaviour/ Crystallinity	More compact back folded - globular structure. The fifth generation dendrimer is completely amorphous and soluble in varieties of organic solvent.	Analogue of dendrimer is not compact. It is highly crystalline and poorly soluble in THF, acetone and chloroform.
7.	Architecture (Hawker et al., 1997)	Dendritic architecture has been shown as elegant, uniform, spherical and as "green peas". e.g. polyether dendrimer	Linear architecture has not been shown as elegant and can be visualised as "cooked spaghetti" e.g. polyether linear
8.	Size/polydispersity	Have certain size, monodisperse which shows significantly different physical behaviour.	Does not have certain size. Usually polydisperse.

such models, molecular architecture possessing regular dendritic branching and radial symmetry i.e. starburst dendrimers, were examined (Tomalia et al, 1984). Controlled branching reactions from an initiator core allow for the synthesis of particles with various types of surface groups that might be successfully compared to micellar structures without these dynamic structures. For example, an increase in the strength of the medium will change the aggregation number and size of micelles but not of the starburst particles (Maria et al, 1990). Dendrimers demonstrate controlled occupation of microspace in three dimensions as a function af size, shape and disposition of desired organic functionality. Dendrimers Vs micelles analogy has been given in Table 15.3.

Examples of covalently fixing (stabilizing) aqueous micelles into non-equilibrating unimolecular assemblies remain rare (Elias et al, 1972; Paleos et al, 1984). Unlike micelles, related assemblages such as liposomes (vesicles) have been successfully stabilized by polymerization (Fendler, 1985) of unsaturated amphiphiles to produce a wide variety of "membrane mimetic" systems (Fendler, 1984).

Inspection of unimolecular dendrimer structures reveals that they mimic the topology and discrete aggregation numbers noted for multimolecular micellar assemblies in that the number of dendrimer head groups (Z) is quantized as function of generation 1-5. Accumulation of Z groups per generation is equal to NcNrG-1, where Nc is the multiplicity of initiator core, Nr is the repeating unit multiplicity and G is the generation (Tomalia et al, 1987). With intrinsic viscosity measurements, hydrodynamic diameters and dendrimer surface area studies suggest that the dendrimers expand as a function of generation to a constant terminal group surface area in each series. Although this unique property is more characteristic for liposomes (vesicles) or "swollen micelles", it should be noted that these hydrodynamic diameters are much smaller and fall well within the traditional dimension (30-60 Å) reported for classical aqueous micelles (Fendler, 1984).

In recent years, the studies of photoinduced electron transfer quenching of ruthenium (II) polypyridyls to provide information about the structure of different microenvironments, such as micelles (Turro & Yekta, 1978), anionic polyelectrolytes (Duveneck et al, 1988), polynucleotides (Barton et al, 1986) and clay (Turro et a l, 1987) have been reported. The carboxylate-terminated sturburst dendrimers are very suitable candidates for the employment of this type of cationic probes, and systematic relationship between the external features of the former and quenching constant of the later is expected.

Table 15.3: Dendrimer vs. Micelles

Dendrimer	**Micelles**
Covalently fixed model	Fluid model with hydrophobic interactions
Possessing internal micro environment of similar or opposite nature than external	Internal microenvironment of opposite nature than external environment.
Dendrimers explain controlled occupation of micro-space in three dimension as a function of size, shape and disposition of organic functionality	Micelles explain change of strength of the medium by changing aggregation number and size. But unable to explain shape, topology, chemical functionality.

Dendrimers explain controlled occupation of micro-space in three dimension as a function of size, shape and disposition of organic functionality   Micelles explain change of strength of the medium by changing aggregation number and size. But unable to explain shape, topology, chemical functionality.

Dimension and shape corroboration of dendrimer-micelle analogy can be obtained by direct observation of individual dendrimer molecules via several electron microscopic techniques. Furthermore, one can readily alter the hydrophobic character of the interior by utilizing more hydrophobic amines such as 1-6, diamino hexane, 1-3 diamino propane or 1-2 diamio propane in place of 1,2 diamino ethane to more closely mimic an aqueous micelle. Likewise, the terminal surface groups (Z) can be converted to a wide variety of polar moieties (e.g. - hydroxyl, quarternary amine, carboxylic etc). Thus, these dendrimers should offer unique micelles/ liposomes like microenvironmental effects. Examination of parameters such as compartmentalization, preorientation, cage, localization, solubilization, polarity and surface group/counterion-ion effects should be of considerable interest to organic chemistry in their quest for novel catalysis and specificity media (Fendler, 1985).

15.5. DENDRIMERS-GLOBULAR PROTEIN ANALOGY

As stated earlier, dendrimers of lower generation exist in open forms while on increasing the number of generations they tend to adopt spherical three-dimensional structure, which bears similarity to globular protein. This suggests that they may function in the same way and might be used as models for various globular proteins. This is further supported by the fact that host-guest chemistry can take place in the hollow interior or on the dense periphery of the dendrimer in a manner similar to proteins where molecular recognition exhibited by them may occur deep within the biopolymer or at its surface. Binding groups on the interior of the dendrimer have been termed as 'endoreceptors' whereas peripheral or end groups involved in complexation are termed 'exoreceptors'. Mattei et al (1995) recently described dendrophanes containing a diphenylmethane-based cyclophane linked with four water-soluble dendrons. They were designated as models of globular protein based on their complexation chemistry in aqueous solution with aromatic guest molecules. A similar conclusion was made with another dendrimer containing larger cyclophanic core capable of binding steroids (Wallimann et al, 1996). Several dendrimers with metallo-porphyrin cores are synthesized to study the effect of dendrimer skeleton on the electrochemical or photochemical properties of the metalloporphyrins and designated as models for electron transfer proteins like cytochrome C in which the globular polypeptide is known to affect the metalloporphyrin redox potential (Dandliker et al, 1994). The effect on metal redox potential was determined by cyclic voltametry. Similarly, cytochrome C heme model was prepared using dendritic iron (II) porphyrin complexes (Dandliker et al, 1996) and zinc (II) porphyrin complexes (Tomoyose et al, 1996). The UV spectra of dendritic porphyrin in various solvents gave a clue to the microenvironment of the zinc porphyrin.

15.6 NON-COVALENT INTERACTIONS IN DENDRIMERS

The structural versatility of dendrimers makes them prone to participate in supramolecular chemistry i.e. non-covalent interactions. These interactions may be broadly classified as complexation and self-assembly.

15.6.1 Complexation

The complexation involves binding of molecules to dendritic host either at the interior core or at the periphery. The binding in the interior involves dendrimers of generation > 4 as the dendrimers have relatively open structures below this generation. The interaction is of "host-guest" type involving hydrophobic binding, hydrogen binding, co-ordination bonds and simple physical encapsulation. The hydrophobic binding involving $\pi-\pi$ interactions was suggested on the basis of upfield chemical shift of p-toluidine protons, indicating ability of polymer to bind the guest (Kim & Webster, 1990). The donor-acceptor-donor hydrogen bonding motif has been used to bind barbituric acids to dendrimers in which multiple hydrogen binding sites were incorporated (Newkome et al, 1996). These interactions are important as they are strong and directional however they are highly sensitive to the polarity of the solvent. Co-ordination bonding obviously involve metal : ligand interaction where the ligand is placed at the interior core of the dendrimer or at the surface. The complex is then formed using metal ion or the dendrons may be linked to preformed metal complex (Tzalis & Tor, 1996). The physical encapsulation of guest may be obtained by including guest by sonication or heating in higher generation dendrimers with very dense surface. Another method is by permanently capping host-guest complex using Boc or Fmoc protected amino acids (Jansen et al, 1994). The interactions at dendrimer surfaces are mainly of electrostatic type when their surfaces are charged. Thus they behave as polyelectrolyte and are likely to attract oppositely charged molecules e.g. aggregation of methylene blue at dendrimer surfaces (Jockush et al., 1995). The dendrimers with co-ordination centres at the periphery may interact with metal ions by co-ordination bonds e.g. dendrimers with phosphine groups on the periphery complexes with Au(I) ions at the surface (Slany et al, 1995).

15.6.2 Self-assembly

Self-assembly includes organization of monomeric dendrimers into aggregates, layers or different phases mainly involving hydrophobic effect as seen in the formation of lipidic assemblies. The dendrimeric amphiphiles, named bolaamphiphiles containing two dendritic polyols separated by a hydrophobic spacer are reported in literature. They form gel after a heating and cooling cycle at 80°C to 25°C. Various analytical studies have proved presence of rod-shaped aggregates (Newkome et al., 1990). Other types for application potential as molecular wires are prepared by Jorgenson et al. (1994). A polyethyleneglycol-polyether dendrimer hybrid capable of forming micellar aggregates at lower generation is also reported presumably driven by n-n interactions (Gitsov et al, 1992). The self-organization of hyperbranched polymers are reported by several research workers (Kim, 1992). The reports highlight organization dependent on intermolecular interactions and not discrete aggregation. The dendrimer in anti conformation adopt rod-like compact structure (nematic phase) while in gauche it remains monodisperse spherical (Li et al, 1996). The self-assembling dendrimers involving hydrogen bonding were synthesized based on the knowledge that isophthalic acid form hexamers by dicarboxylic acid dimer formation. Thus, tetraacids in which two isophthalic acid units were held in syn-orientation by rigid spacer were designed. Various instrumental analytical studies revealed formation of aggregates (Zimmerman et al, 1996). The self-assembly involving metal co-ordination has also been reported (Newkome et al, 1995) as photoactive dendrimer. PAMAM dendrimers and their various modifications have been described which can self-assemble on surfaces to form monolayers or multilayers. These surfaces have potential uses as sensors, in chromatographic separations and catalysts (Castagnola et al, 1995).

15.7 DENDRIMERS FOR MOLECULAR RECOGNITION

The dendrimer surfaces are modified using substrates/ligands that recognize receptors at the biological sites or on biologically important molecules. Since the dendrimer surface contains multiple copies of a particular functional group it is an ideal platform for amplification of substrate binding. They may display an increased affinity with a receptor. The presence of ligands in close proximity on dendrimer surface may help in increasing local concentration of particular ligand wherein the diffusion is a problem. Based on the interactions between monosaccharides and lectins, to study important biological processes like cell adhesion, recognition and infection, Sharon & Lis (1993) synthesized a number of branched glycosides. The binding to rabbit hepatic lectin was improved with increased affinity (Lee & Lee, 1995) due to 'cluster effect'. Later, Roy prepared glyco-polymers with lysine dendritic core capped with sialic acids (Roy, 1996). The fourth generation dendrimer was able to inhibit hemaglutination of human erythrocytes 158 times more effectively than analogous sialic acid or 10 times per sugar molecule. They prepared other types of glyco-dendrimers and established that the number of sugar valency required for maximum binding capacity is not necessarily correlated to the number of binding sites in lectin (Page et al., 1996). PAMAM dendrimer based glyco-dendrimers using glucose and galactose at the surface were able to bind concanavalin A with high affinity that 16 fold glucose was required to disrupt the binding (Aoi et al, 1995). The interesting finding from the studies is that the higher generation dendrimers are not useful as surface steric crowding leads to weaker carbohydrate-protein interactions. A spherical glyco-dendrimer may fail to interact because of poor complementarity.

15.8 CLASSIFICATION OF DENDRIMERS

We propose the following classification for the commonly reported dendrimer types although few dendrimer types may fit in one or more type of classes.

15.8.1 Simple dendrimers

They have simple monomer units e.g. poly(amidoamine) dendrimers composed of poly(amidoamine) segments named as "starburst" (trademark of Dendritech Inc., U.S.A.) dendrimers. Tomalia first reported the synthesis of starburst dendrimers in 1985. Few other examples of simple dendrimers are: poly(propyleneimine) dendrimers synthesized by divergent route starting from diaminobutane by a repetition of addition-reduction reactions (Jansen et al, 1995). The synthesis of polyamino- phosphine dendrimers-2$[G_0]$-2$[G_3]$ and 3$[G_0"]$-3$[G"_1]$ is achieved from the hexapodant N_3P_3 $(OC_6H_4CHO)_{6\text{-}2}[G_0]$ used as a core (Galliot et al, 1995). The convergent synthesis of a series of monodisperse arylester dendrimers related to 1,3,5-benzenetricarboxylic acid, based upon symmetrically substituted benzene tricarboxylic acid ester is described. These materials consist of 4, 10, 22 and 46 benzene rings connected symmetrically and have molecular diameters of upto 45A° (Miller et al, 1992).

15.8.2 Liquid crystalline dendrimers

They consist of mesogenic (liquid crystalline) monomers e.g. mesogen functionalized carbosilane dendrimers. Functionalization of end group of carbosilane dendrimers with 36 mesogenic units, attached through a C-5 spacer, leads to liquid crystalline dendrimers that form broad smectic A phase in the temperature range of 17°C to 130°C (Klaus et al 1996). In cholesterol containing polyorganosiloxane dendrimers, polyorganosiloxane dendrimer terminal groups are linked to cholesterol mesogenic groups through methylene spacers (Ponomarenko et al, 1994).

15.8.3 Chiral dendrimers

In chiral dendrimers the chirality is based on the construction of 4 constitutionally different but chemically similar branches to an achiral core e.g. chiral dendrimers derived from pentaerythritol (Kremers & Meijer, 1995).

15.8.4 Micellar dendrimers

These are unimolecular micellar structure e.g. water-soluble hyperbranched polyphenylene dendrimers. Fully aromatic, water-soluble dendrimers forming an array of aromatic polymeric chain were able to generate an environment that resembles some micellar structures, which could complex with small organic molecules in water (Kim & Webster, 1990a&b).

15.8.5 Hybrid dendrimers

These are combination of dendritic and linear polymer in hybrid block or graft copolymer forms. The small dendrimer segment coupled to multiple reactive chain ends provides an opportunity to use them as surface active agents, compatibilizers or adhesives, e.g. hybrid dendritic linear polymers (Gitsov et al, 1992,1993).

15.8.6 Amphiphilic dendrimers

These are classes of globular dendrimers that have unsymmetrical but highly controlled distribution of chain end chemistry. They are built with two segregated sites of chain end, half electron donating and half electron withdrawing. They may be oriented at interface forming interfacial liquid membranes for stabilizing aqueous-organic emulsion. They can be oriented under the influence of external stimulus e.g. electric field (Saville et al., 1993; Hawker et al., 1993; Wooley et al., 1993). Various types of amphiphilic dendrimers like hydra-amphiphiles (Chapman et al., 1994) and bola-amphiphiles (Escamilla & Newkome, 1994) have been reported.

15.8.7 Metallodendrimers

Dendrimers attached to metal ion by complexation either in the interior or on the periphery may be regarded as metallodendrimers (Liao & Moss, 1995). The ruthenium bipyridine complex based dendrimers have characteristic electrochemical and luminescence properties. The porphyrin metal complex based dendrimers as oxidation catalyst are also reported (Jin et al., 1993).

15.9 SYNTHESIS OF DENDRIMERS

Two fundamentally different methods have been developed for stepwise synthesis of dendritic polymers: the divergent approach in which the synthesis begins at the center of dendrimer and the convergent approach in which synthesis begins outside of dendrimers. The key contribution to divergent method came from Denkewalter et al (1984), Newkome et al (1986) and Tomalia et al. (1987). The convergent method was reported independently by Wooley et al (1991) and by Kwock et al (1991). Overview of all known strategies to dendrimer synthesis is given in Fig. 15.4.

15.9.1 Divergent growth method

Dendrimer synthesis based on divergent growth method exhibits the unique feature of transferring molecular level information from the initiator core, generation to generation. For that reason these constructions are referred to as geneologically directed synthesis (GDS). In this method, the core is reacted with two or more moles of reagent containing atleast two protecting branching sites, followed by removal of the protecting groups. The subsequent liberated reactive sites lead to the first generation dendrimer. This process is repeated until the dendrimer of the desired size is obtained (Tomalia, 1994) e.g. poly (amidoamine) starburst dendrimer prepared by divergent method. The synthesis begins with an initiator core such as ammonia (N series) or ethylenediamine (E series). The core molecule is then reacted in sequence, first with methylmethacrylate and then with ethylene diamine. The product of these reaction steps contains one free primary amine for each

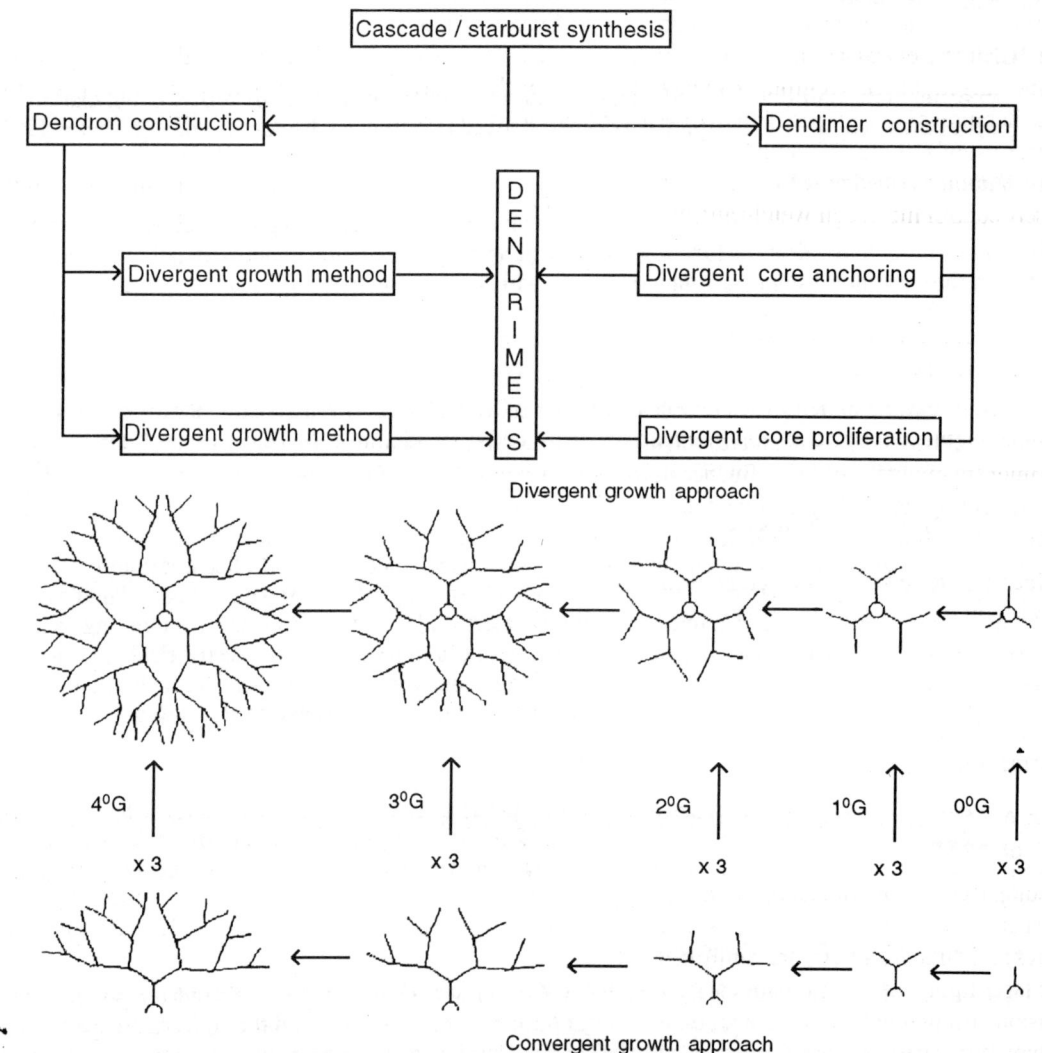

Fig 15.4: Overview of all known strategies to dendrimer synthesis

of the reactive hydrogen atoms originally present in the initiator core. This molecule is referred to as "generation zero" (G_0) of the dendrimer series. Each free amino group present in this branched molecule is then subsequently reacted with two additional molecules of methylmethacrylate monomer, followed by reaction with two more ethylenediamine molecules, to provide first generation (G_1) starburst dendrimers. This two step reaction sequence is repeated to provide subsequent generations of dendrimer (Singh et al, 1994). The disadvantage of this approach is that successive generations require a geometrically increasing number of reactions to be carried out on the growing dendrimer. Circumvention of this problem necessitates large excess of reactants and forcing conditions and causes difficulty in purification.

15.9.2 Convergent growth method

This is an alternative approach to dendrimer synthesis. The difficulty of many reactions that have to be performed on one molecule is overcome by starting the synthesis at the periphery and ending at the core. Convergent method involves two stages: namely, (i) a reiterative coupling of protected/deprotected branch to produce a focal point functionalized dendron, followed by (ii) a divergent core anchoring step to produce various multidendron dendrimers. In this method, progressively large dendrimer arms are prepared by the attachment of a small number (usually two) of smaller arms to a molecule having two functional groups X and Y. Each dendrimer arm has a functional group Z that reacts with only one of the two functional groups, e.g. X. The unchanged functional group Y in new larger arm is then converted to the functional group Z, permitting further iteration of this process. Finally, the completed dendrimer arms are coupled to a core containing a small number (usually three) of the functional group X. e.g. polyether dendrimers are prepared by convergent growth apporach (Hawker & Frechet, 1990). The advantages of the convergent approach include the ability to precisely control molecular weight and make material having functionalities in precise positions and numbers (Wallimann et al, 1996; Tomalia, 1994). The defective products are easier to separate hence the products are more homogeneous than those prepared by divergent strategy.

15.9.3 Factors affecting dendrimers synthesis

There are various factors which affect dendrimer synthesis (Tomalia et al, 1985). The nonideal dendrimer growth may be manifested in a variety of ways including (a) incomplete addition reaction, (b) intramolecular cyclization, (c) fragmentation, and (d) solvolysis of terminal functionalities. Some dendrimer defect events (eg. dendrimer fragmentation) can influence the degree of monodispersity during dendrimer growth. This is especially true if fragments posses amine functions which may participate with the propagation sequencing agents to produce new but 'regressed dendrimer' entities. They are usually due to following reasons:

1. Incomplete removal of reactant at each of generation sequences leads to polydispersity since residual reactant functions as an initiator core to produce 0.5 generation and subsequent lower generations.

2. Exposure of dendrimers to higher temperature causes cyclization of dendrimers by intramolecular reactions.

3. The incomplete amount of sequencing agent may cause bridging of dendrimer or nonideal dendrimer formation.

15.9.4 Analytical methods for structure validation of dendrimers (Pesak et al, 1997; Hummelen et al, 1997)

The complex structure of dendrimer moiety requires multiple methods for conclusive verification. The structural subtleties like elemental composition, molecular weight homogenity, interior and end group, topological features and dimensions etc. are confirmed by C, H, N analysis, mass spectroscopy, fragmentation pattern, low angle laser light scattering, chemical ionization and fast atom bombardment, vapour phase osmometry, size exclusion chromatography and electron microscopy, IR., ^{15}N, ^{13}C and ^{1}H NMR spectroscopy, titrimetry and stoichiometry with various reagents and rheological studies. Recent progress in electrospray ionization (ESI) and matrix-assisted laser desorption ionization (MALDI) mass spectrometry allow for an in-depth analysis and imperfections of dendrimers.

15.9.5 Dendrimers construction Vs atomic constructions (Aufbau Principle)

The systems that are constructed under well-defined rules follow various symmetries describing quantities of components involved in construction. The geometric or arithmetic pattern can be developed for the understanding of these systems, for example, Huckel's 4n+2 electron rule for aromaticity and electron orbital filling of elements. The mathematical predictability of monomer shell filling and the reactivity found in dendrimers can be compared with electron shell filling and reactivity of atomic entities. In order to develop this analogy the monomer units or branched shell in dendrimers are assumed as analogous to electrons in atoms. The monomers and electrons occupy space in predictable numbers around a core (nucleus) according to a defined but different mathematical rule in each case. They have defined upper and lower limits of proximity with respect to their core. In the case of dendrimers these relationships are Newtonian and determined by bonding connectivity to core and the space actually occupied by the atoms involved in dendrimeric organization whereas with atoms they are derived from charge neutralization and are quantum mechanically driven. In atoms, mass is located at the nucleus whereas in dendrimers it resides with the monomers in the functional shells surrounding the core. Just by defining the number of orthogonal orbitals for a given shell, maximum number of electrons residing in that shell can be obtained in a dendrimer. The core multiplicity and branch multiplicity determine the maximum number of monomer units residing in given dendrimer shell. Thus atomic orbitals fill electron in a sequence of 2, 8, 8, 18, 18, 32, etc., whereas the shells of dendrimers having the core multiplicity 3 (ammonia) and branched multiplicity 2 (ethylenediamine) fill with repeat units in sequence 3, 6, 12, 24, 48 etc.

In atoms, partially filled shells have unfilled orbitals, which impart chemical reactivity while a filled shell has a satisfied valency and requires extreme conditions for chemical reactions. Similarly, dendrimers possessing unfilled monomers are very reactive. They form nanoscopic compounds or produce macrocyclic sites by inter-dendrimer reaction and intramolecular combination respectively while dendrimers possessing saturated monomers shell are not reactive with each other.

Just as certain predictions about reactivity, morphological changes, dimensions, physical properties etc. can be made by vertical and horizontal inspection of atomic periodic table so can one make similar prediction about such properties within the molecular level dendrimeric periodic table. The atomic periodic table is limited to seven periods while dendrimeric periodic table is determined by number of different dendrimer families and the number of periods in each periodic table is determined by De-Gennes dense packing stages for each dendrimer family. The intriguing atomic feature is the directionality in bond formation, which is lacked in dendrimeric system. However, progress has been made in this regard by regioselective reactions to introduce surface groups protecting the dendron focal group. Deprotection of focal group followed by anchoring to various cores produces dendrimers with differentiated sectors whose interior electrons can be varied by changing branch shell composition. Applying the logic atomic chemistry set to dendrimers system, the mass, surface valency and surface directionality can be precisely controlled. Secondly, many classical issues of organic chemistry can be systematically examined. Besides, new issues such as nanoscopic steric effect, nanoscopic chirality, nanoscopic recognition can be understood.

15.10 ADVANTAGES OF DENDRIMERS

Dendrimers may offer following advantages over other systems:

1. Dendrimers show a structural uniformity and monodispersity.

2. Dendrimers have a better/greater targeting efficiency due to the presence of reactive functional groups on the surface of dendrimer. Terminal groups may also be modified to reorganise specific receptors.

3. The surface modification may allow to design dendrimers mimicking biological exo-receptors, substrates, inhibitors or cofactors.

4. The similarity of dendrimers structure with IgM antibodies (pentamers radially distributed) suggest that they may be used to function as antibodies e.g. activation of macrophages, recognition, and high affinity to antigen.

5. Dendrimers have the ability to deliver drug inside the cell or they may improve intracellular trafficking.

6. Dendrimers have a capability to entrap a variety of drugs having different types of functional groups in internal hollow core or by charge interactions.

7. Dendrimers can be made stimuli responsive.

8. Dendrimers have limited toxicity and immunogenicity but good biodegradability.

9. They have better colloidal, biological and shelf-stability.

10. They may be intrinsically anticancer agents in nature due to interferon, tumour necrosis factor inducing properties of acrylates.

15.11 DENDRIMERS APPLICATIONS

15.11.1 Solubilization

The dendrimer resembling micelles are formed when the surface of an apolar dendrimer contains charged functional groups. A unimolecular micelle of polyaryl ether dendrimers was prepared by Hawker et al (1993a&b) and used to investigate solubilization of nonpolar organic molecules. A linear relationship between amount of solubilized pyrene and the dendrimer concentration was observed. The solubilization efficiency was comparable to that of sodium lauryl sulfate (SLS) micelles. The dendrimer could solubilize as low as 5×10^{-7} mol/L concentration while SLS required its critical micelle concentration i.e. 8.1×10^{-3} mol/L. One dendrimer could solubilize approximately 0.45 molecules of pyrene, which was increased to 1.9 molecules by addition of NaCl probably due to quenching of water molecules from the interior of the dendrimer facilitating hydrophobic interior bonding. A series of inverted unimolecular micelles with hydrophobic shell and hydrophilic interior was prepared by Stevelmans et al (1996). The binding of Bengal rose in the interior was shown in hexane solution, which could be released by toluene but not water. Thus, polar molecules can be solubilized in apolar solvents using dendrimer. The dendritic 'box' prepared by Meijer and co-workers by capping dendrimer surfaces with aminoacids could irreversibly solubilize upto 4 molecules of Bengal rose and 8-10 molecules of 4-nitrobenzoic acid per molecule of dendrimer (Jansen et al, 1996). The use of crown ether dendrimers to solubilize peptides in organic solvents through peptide-NH^{+3}-crown ether interactions is also reported. The solubility of myoglobin in dimethyl formamide was dramatically increased with first generation dendrimer probably because of binding of lipophilic dendrimer at protein surface (Nagasaki et al, 1994). Chapman et al (1994) reported the synthesis of amphiphilic copolymers, named "hydraamphiphiles" derived from linear poly(ethyleneoxide) and Boc-terminated poly-α,ε-L-lysine dendrimers capable of forming micelles with critical micelle concentration of 8×10^{-5} M and compact aggregate surface. A dye, orange OT, was solubilized therein further supported their miceller behaviour. Other micelle forming copolymers were reported by Vanhest et al (1995) and Gitsov & Frechet (1993). Stimuli responsive unimolecular "wrappers" are reported which self-organize into different micellar structures as a function of environment (Gitsov & Frechet, 1996).

15.11.2 Controllable gene therapy / non-viral gene delivery

Gene therapy methods are designed to introduce genetic materials into patient's cells to cause these cells to produce therapeutic protein. For these approaches, there must be control over the location and functioning of an administered gene, that the gene should be administered by convenient and conventional route and that the product should be robust and have an acceptable cost/risk/benefit profile (Anderson, 1992; Ledley, 1993, 1994a&b).

Recently "starburst dendrimers" have been used for non-viral gene delivery. Gene expression system encoding reporter genes have been complexed with different generations of dendrimers through electrostatic interactions of their terminal amines with the phosphate group of DNA moleules and characteristics of such complex control the efficiency of delivery. The mean size of DNA dendrimer complexes is shown to be monodisperse and below 200 nm at various ratios of dendrimers to DNA. Increased transfection efficiency is observed for the 5th and 6th generation of dendrimers at ratios leading to a net positively charged complex (1:3,

1:6 -/+ ratio). As the ratio of dendrimers to DNA increased, the size of condensed particles decreased and transfection efficiency significantly increased (Tomlinson & Rolland, 1996).

Starburst (polyamidoamine) dendrimers have an ability to function as an effective delivery system for antisense oligonucleotides and "antisense expression plasmids" for the targeted modulation of gene expression. Cell line that permanently expresses luciferase gene was developed using dendrimers mediated transfection. Binding of the phosphodiester oligonucleotides to dendrimers also extended their intracellular survival. These results indicate that starburst dendrimers can be effective carriers to the introduction of regulatory nucleic acids and facilitate the suppression of the specific gene expression (Bielinska et al, 1996). The efficiency of plasmid DNA transfection using dendrimers was examined using two reporter gene system: firefly luciferase and bacterial β-galactosidase. The transfections were performed by using various dendrimers and levels of expression of the reporter protein were determined. Highly efficient transfections of a broad range of eukaryotic cells and cell lines were achieved with minimal cytotoxicity using the DNA /dendrimer complexes. The capability of the dendrimers to transfect cells appeared to depend on the size, shape and number of primary amino groups on the surface of the polymer. However, the specific dendrimers most efficient in achieving transfection varied between different types of cells (Kukowska et al, 1996). Haensler & Szoka (1993) showed using luciferase and b-galactosidase containing plasmids, that dendrimers mediate high efficiency transfection of a variety of suppression and adherent cultured mammalian cells and concluded that the precise control of structures, favourable pKa's and low toxicity make dendrimers suitable for gene transfer vehicle. Hughes et al (1996) found that fusogenic peptides GALA, dendrimers as well as the liposomal form of DIP (N-dodecyl 2- imidazole-propionate) could significantly enhance the effects of ODNS by using adjuvants that enhanced endosome to cytosol transfer of ODN.

15.11.3 Dendrimers based drug delivery

High charge density on dendrimers opens wide scope for making drug as well as metal-based complexes for targeted drug therapy. In our laboratory, we have prepared "methotrexate- dendrimer complex/conjugates" for improved cancer therapy. The "methotrexate-dendrimer complex" was found to be pH dependent and remains stable at physiological pH. The complex was found to be targeted substantially in the brain and bone marrow (Khopade & Jain, 1997). Malik et al (1997) prepared PAMAM dendrimer-platinate complex and extensively characterized it in-vitro. They reported improved antitumor activity of complex in all tumour models tested including platinum resistant tumour model. They have reported an increased potential for cancer chemo-therapy. Zhuo et al. (1999) prepared poly(amidoamine) dendrimers with a cyclic core, and attached 5-fluorouracil to G-4 and G-5 dendrimer to form conjugates. Subsequent hydrolysis of the conjugate in phosphate buffer pH 7.4 resulted in release of free 5-fluorouracil. Liu & Fretchet (1999) have recently reviewed the potential of designing dendrimer for drug delivery.

15.11.4 Dendrimer as magnetic resonance imaging contrast agents

Dendrimer based metal chelates act as a magnetic resonance imaging contrast agent. Wiener et al (1994) developed a new class of magnetic resonance (MR) imaging contrast agents with large proton relaxation enhancements and high molecular relaxivities by using polyamidoamine form of dendrimers in which free amines have been conjugated to chelator 2-(4-isothiocyanatobenzyl)-6-methyl-diethylene tri-amine pentaacetic acid and suggested that new and powerful class of contrast agents have the potentials for diverse and extensive application in MR imaging. This novel class compared to other polymeric or monovalent chelators exhibited greatly enhanced proton relaxation times indicating their superiority for MRI applications. Moreover, the sixth generation polygadolinium dendrimer displayed a prolonged enhancement with a half-life of 200 min compared to 24 min for monovalent gadolinium agent. This prolonged enhancement time is extremely useful for 3D time-of-flight MR angiography.

15.11.5 Boronated starburst dendrimers monoclonal antibody immunoconjugates

Boron neutron capture therapy is based on the nucleus capture reaction that occurs when boron-10, a stable isotope is irradiated with low energy or thermal neutrons to yield alpha particles and recoiling 7-Lithium nuclei. Approximately, 109-boron-10 atoms are delivered to each target cell in order to sustain a lethal reaction. If monoclonal antibodies are to be used for targeting boron-10, then it is essential that they recognize a surface membrane epitope that is highly expressed on tumor cells and that a large number of boron-10 atoms be attached to each antibody molecule. Barth et al (1994) utilized boronated starburst dendrimers to yield stable immunoconjugates for boron capture therapy of primary and metastatic brain tumours. Dendrimer surfaces have also been used as a platform to facilitate the conjugation of antibodies and small molecules. PAMAM dendrimers has been used to link porphyrin label to antibody by attaching porphyrin to dendrimer surface which was then conjugated to antibody followed by incorporation of copper-67 label into the porphyrin. This conjugate retained the immunoactivity of unmodified antibody (Roberts et al, 1990). Wu et al (1994) reported dendritic antibody metalchelate conjugate on similar lines and showed that dendrimer facilitated the conjugation.

15.11.6   Dendrimers as vaccines, artificial proteins and enzymes

Spetzler & Tam (1995) introduced two new site specific methods for preparing branched peptide dendrimers such as multiple antigen peptide (MAP). Both methods are based on general approach of exploiting the specific reaction between a weak base and an aldehyde under acidic conditions so that unprotected peptide can be used us building blocks. A weak base such as benzoyl hydrazine or 1,2- aminothiol of cysteine was attached to the N terminal of an unprotected peptide as nucleophilic to react with the alkyl aldehyde on the core matrix of a MAP to form a stable hydrazone linkage or a five membered thiazolidone ring respectively. Two synthetic peptides rich in basic amino acids such as lysine and arginine were used as models in the ligation reactions in solution to give peptide dendrimers containing four or eight copies of peptide immunogens. The phenyl hydrazone linkage and the five membered ring are found to be stable at physiological pH suitable for immunization. The antibodies induced by these peptide dendrimers in rabbits and mice were not only reactive but were specific to the corresponding peptide dendrimers, monovalent peptide and cognate native proteins. They extended this approach to the preparation of peptide dendrimer with multiple epitopes (Tam & Lu, 1989). The hepatitis B virus epitopes, S and pre S(2) peptide residues were incorporated in dendritic lysine core. These diepitope peptide dendrimers induced strong immunological response to both cognate native proteins. They have also designed an amphiphilic peptide dendrimer as a synthetic AIDS vaccine, capable of forming liposomes or micelles by attaching tripalmitoyl-s-glyceryl cysteine group to a tetravalent peptide antigen containing glycoprotein gp 120 of HIV-1 virus (Defoort et al, 1992).

15.11.7 Starburst dendrimers for enhanced performance and flexibility for immunoassays

Singh et al (1994) used dendrimers composed of polyamidoamine groups to which were coupled several specific antibodies, to investigate the potential formats based on radial partition immunoassay. The coupled antibodies retained their stability and immunological bonding after coupling, both in solution and when immobilized on to a solid support. On the basis of feasibility studies with model systems they concluded that immunoassays can be developed with performance equivalent to or better than that in many established systems and demonstrated enhanced sensitivity for creatinine kinase MB isoenzyme (CKBB), thyrotropin and myoglobin assays and reduced instrumental analysis time for the CKMB assay.

15.11.8 Biochemical analysis

The design of sugar binding receptor for detection of sugar levels in diabetic patients by introducing boronic acid base fluorescence sensor has been reported by James et al (1995). The anthracene units (chromophore) and boronic acid (sugar binding moiety) were attached to second generation PAMAM dendrimer through a tertiary amine. The enhanced binding was observed which was attributed to the high local concentration effect (James et al, 1996).

15.11.9 Isolation of biologicals

Dendrimers are isotropically soluble functional polymers with a great potential for precise arrangement or isolation of functional groups. Jin et al (1993) reported steric isolation of the metalloporphyrin, which is important to achieve certain biological functions.

15.12 Biocompatibility of dendrimers

It is clear that dendrimers have a great potential for drug delivery but, before proceeding to the third generation designs the biocompatibility and toxicity of dendrimers must be fully understood. There are few reports on biocompatibility of dendrimers. Roberts et al (1996) reported cytotoxicity of cationic PAMAM dendrimer is concentration and generation dependent. Duncan and co-workers recently systematically investigated in-vitro biocompatibility and cytotoxicity of broad range of dendritic structures including cationic and anionic PAMAM dendrimers, poly(propyleneimine) dendrimers, PEG-grafted carbo-silane dendrimers and other carboxyl terminated dendrimers. They found that hemolytic and toxic effects largely depend upon several parameters, such as type and number of surface groups, dendrimer size (generation) and its concentration. Unfortunately none of them exhibited great biocompatibility. In general, the anionic dendrimers were less toxic than the cationic counterparts. The PEG grafting greatly reduced the cytotoxicity (Malik et al, 1997). The biodistribution is another factor which deserves thorough consideration (Wilbur et al, 1998). The dendrimers should possess long circulation time to achieve therapeutic efficacy and to enable accumulation in targeted sites, such as tumour cells. They should be eliminated from the body to avoid unacceptable long-term accumulation. Some of the studies carried out in these directions instil optimism in pharmaceutical scientists.

15.13 Future prospects

Supramolecular/functional chemistry has gained much importance in recent years due to the focus of pharmaceutical industries on the drug design where understanding of structural and chemical interaction between host-guest system is essential for designing molecules. The pharmaceutical potential of the dendrimers application has hardly been realised. The future of dendrimeric drug delivery lies is fine tuning the carrier to incorporate variety of drugs and complex proteins to ensure the vectorization of dendrimer-complex/conjugates to desired cells/tissues. The major focus will be on development of dendrimers based on new concept of the biomimetism/biomorphism with increased plasma stability and capability to target cells in various body compartments. There are many issues that require further understanding. The detailed studies on these issues will undoubtedly involve the evolution of new concepts and characteristics of many biological nanostructures that are so intimately involved in sustaining life process. The application in the field of gene delivery holds promise. It is for the researchers in the field of pharmaceutical sciences to realise the broad spectrum of application of dendrimer based drug delivery systems. At the moment we can only predict that the dendrimer based drug delivery would be the most popular and dendrimers would be employed as golden carrier in twenty first century. Dendrimer based drug delivery is anticipated to be an answer for most of the problems related to drug targeting. Strategically dendrimer drug delivery should be most efficient, feasible both in terms of production and cost and system would perform reproducibly, reliably and safely, truly attaining the therapeutic objective.

REFERENCES

Anderson, W.F. (1992) Science, 256:808.

Aoi, K.; Itoh, K. and Okada, M. (1995) Macromolecules, 28:5391.

Barth, R.F.; Adams, D.M.; Soloway, A.H.; Alam, F. and Darby M.V. (1994) Bioconjug. Chem. 5:58.

Barton, J.K.; Kumar, C.V. and Turro, N.J. (1986) J. Am. Chem. Soc. 108:6391.

Bielinska A.; Kukowska-Latallo, J.F.; Johnson J.; Tomalia, D.A. and Baker, J.R.Jr. (1996) Nucleic Acids Res., 24:2176.

Boris, D. and Rubinstein, M. (1996) Macromolecules, 29:7251

Butcher, J.A.Jr. and Lamb, G.W. (1984) J. Am. Chem. Soc., 106:1217.

Cantor, R.S. and Dill, K.A. (1984) Macromolecules, 17:384.

Castagnola, M.; Cassiano, L.; Lupi, A.; Messana, I.; Patamia, M.; Rabino, R.; Rossetti, D.V. and Giardina, B. (1995) J. Chromatogr., 694:463.

Cavallo, L. and Fraternali, F. (1998) Chem. Eur. J. 4:927

Chapman, T.M.; Hillyer, G.L.; Mahan, E.J. and Shaffer, K.A. (1994) J. Am. Chem. Soc., 116:11195.

Collman, J.P.; Fu, L.; Zingg, A.; Diederich, F. (1997) Chem. Commun., 193.

Dandliker, P.J.; Diedrich, F.; Gisselbrecht, J.P.; Louati, A.; Gross, M. (1996) Angew Chem., Int. Ed. Engl., 34:2725.

Dandliker, P.J.; Diedrich, F.; Gross, M.; Knobler, C.B.; Louati, A. and Sanford, E.M. (1994) Angew Chem., Int. Ed. Engl., 33:1739.

de Brabander, E.M.M.; Brackman, J.; Mure.Mak, M.; de Man, H.;Hogeweg, M.; Keulen, J.; Scherrenberg, R.; Coussens, B.; Mengerink, Y. and van der Wal, S. (1996) Macromol. Symp., 102:9

Defoort, J.P.; Nardelli, B.; Huang, W.; Ho, D.D. and Tam, J.P. (1992) Proc. Natl. Acad. Sci., USA, 89:3879.

Denkewalter, R.G.; Kolc, J.F. and Lukasavage, M.J. (1984) Chem. Abstr., 100:103907.

Dill, K.A.; Flory, P.J. (1981) Proc. Natl. Acad. Sci., 78:676.

Duveneck, G.L.; Kumar, C.V.; Turro, N.J.; Barton, J.K. (1988) J. Phys. Chem., 92: 2028.

Elias, H.G.; Kammer, U.; Kolloid Z.Z. (1972) Polym., 250:344.

Escamilla, G.H. and Newkome, G.R. (1994) Angew. Chem. Int. Ed. Engl., 33:1937.

Fendler, J.H. (1984) Chem. Eng. News, 2:25.

Fendler, J.H. (1985) CHEMTECH, 686.

Franses, E.I.; David, H.T.; Miller, W.G. and Scriven, L. E. (1980) J. Phys. Chem., 84: 2413.

Frechet, J.M.J. (1996) Science, 263:1710.

Galliot, C.; Prevote, D.; Caninade, A.M. and Majoral, J.P. (1995) J. Am. Chem. Soc., 117:5470.

Gennes de, P.G.; Hervet, H.J. (1983) Phys. Lett. Pans., 44: 351.

Gibson, H.W.; Marand, H. (1993) Adv. Mater., 5:11.

Gitsov, I.; Wooley K.L. and Frechet, J.M.J. (1992) Angew. Chem., Int. Ed. Engl., 31:1200.

Gitsov, I. and Frechet, J.M.J. (1993) Macromolecules, 26: 6536.

Gitsov, I. and Frechet, J.M.J. (1996) J. Am. Chem. Soc., 118:3785.

Gitsov, I. and Frechet, J.M.J. (1993) Macromolecules, 26:6536.

Gitsov, I.; Wooley, K.L. and Frechet, J.M.J. (1992) Angew. Chem., 104:282.

Gitsov,I.; Wooley,K.L.; Hawker,C.J.; Ivanova, P.T. and Frechet, J.M.J. (1993) Macromolecules, 26:5621.

Haensler-J. and Szoka-FC. Jr. (1993) Bioconjug-Chem., 4: 372.

Hartley, G.S.Q. (1948) Rev. Chem. Soc., 2:152.

Hawker, C.J. and Frechet, J.M.J. (1990) J. Am. Chem. Soc., 112:7638.

Hawker, C.J.; Lee, R. and Frechet, J.M.J. (1991) J. Am. Chem. Soc., 113:4583.

Hawker, C.J.; Wooley, K.L. and Frechet, J.M.J. (1993) J. Chem. Soc., 1:1287.

Hawker, C.J.; Wooley, K.L. and Frechet, J.M.J. (1993) J. Chem. Soc. Perkin Transac., 21:1287.

Hawker, C.J.; Farrington, P.J.; Mackey, M.E.; Wooley, K.L. and Frechet, J.M.J. (1995) J. Am. Chem. Soc., 117: 4409

Hawker, C.J.; Malstrom, E.E.; Frank, C.W. and Kampf, J.P. (1997) J. Am. Chem. Soc., 119: 9903

Hughes, J.A.; Aronsohn, A.I.; Avrustskaya, A.V. and Juliano, R.L. (1996) Pharm. Res., 13:404.

Hummelen, J.C.; van Dongen, J.L.J. and Meijer, E.J. (1997) Chem. Eur. J., 3:1489

James, T.D.; Sandanayake, K.R.A.S.; Iguchi, R. and Shinkai, S. (1995) Nature, 374:345

James, T.D.; Shinmori, H.; Takeuchi, M. and Shinkai, S.A. (1996) Chem. Commun., 705.

Jansen, J.F.G.A.; Janseen, R.A.I.; Ellen, M.N.M. and Meijer, E.W. (1995) Adv. Mater., 7:561.

Jansen, J.F.G.A.; De Brabander van den Berg, E.M.M. and Meijer, E.W. (1994) Science, 266:1226.

Jansen, J.F.G.A.; Meijer, E.W. and De Brabender-van den Berg, E.M.M. (1996) Macromol Symp., 102:27.

Jin, R.H.; Aida, T. and Inoue, S. (1993) J. Chem. Soc. Chem. Commun., 1260.

Jockush, S.; Turro, N.J. and Tomalia, D.A. (1995) Macromolecules, 28:7416,

Jorgenson, M.; Bechgaard, K.; Bjornholm, T.; Sommer-Larson, P.; Hansen, L.G. and Schaumberg, K. (1994) J. Org. Chem., 59:5877.

Khopade, A.J. and Jain, N.K (1997).: Dendrimer delivery of methotrexate, Abstract book, Symposium on Particulate Systems, from Formulation to Production, Istanbul, 6-7 oct, 1997

Kim, Y.H. (1992) J. Am. Chem. Soc., 114:4947.

Kim, Y.H. and Webster, O.W. (1990) J. Am. Chem. Soc., 112:4592.

Kim, Y.H. and Webster, O.W. (1990) J. Am.Chem. Soc., 118:4592,

Kim, Y.W. and Webster, O.W. (1990) J. Am. Chem. Soc., 112:4592.

Klaus, L.; Dirk, H.; Bernd, S.; Rolf, M. and Holger, F. (1996) Adv. Mater., 8:414.

Kremers, J.A. and Meijer, E.W. (1995) Reactive and Functional Polymers, 26:13.

Kukowska, L.J.F.; Bielinsk A.V.; Johnson J.; Spindler R.; Tomalia, D.A.; Baker, J.R. Jr. (1996) Proc. Natl. Acad. Sci., 93:4897.

Kwock, E.W.; Neenan, T.X. and Miller, T.M. (1991) Chem. Mater., 3:775.

Ledley, F. D. (1993) Clin. Invest. Med., 16:78.

Ledley, F.D. (1994a) Exp. Op. Invest. Drugs, 3: 913.

Ledley, F.D. (1994b) Biotechnol., 5:626.

Lee, Y.C. and Lee, R.T. (1995) Acc. Chem. Res., 28:321.

Lescanec, R.L. and Muthulkumar, L. (1990) Macromolecules, 23:2280.

Li, J.F.; Crandall, K.A.; Chu, P.W.; Percec, V.; Petshek, R.G.; Rosenblatt, C. (1996) Macromolecules, 29:7813.

Liao, Y.H. and Moss, J.R. (1995) Organometallics, 14:2130

Liu, M. and Fretchet, J.M.J. (1999) Pharm. Sci. Tech. Today 2(10):393

Malik. N.; Evugorou, E. and Duncan, R. (1997) Proc. Int. Sym. Control. Release Bioact. Mater., 24:107

Mandelbrot, B.B. (1983) The Fractal Geometry of Nature.

Mansfield, M. and Klushin, L. (1993) Macromolecules 26:4262

Maria, C.M.; Orellana, G.; Turro, N.J. and Tomalia, D.A. (1990) Macromolecules, 23:910.

Mattei, S.; Seiler, P.; Diedrich, F. and Gramlich, V. (1995) Helv. Chim. Acta, 78:1904.

Menger, F.M. and Dill, D.W. (1984) J. Am. Chem. Soc., 106:1109.

Miller, T.M.; Kwock, E.W. and Neenan, T.X. (1992) J. Am. Chem. Soc., 25:3143.

Mitchell, D.J. and Ninham, B.W. (1981) J. Chem. Soc. Faraday Trans., 77:601.

Miklis, P.; Cagin, T. and Goddard, W.A. III (1997) J. Am. Chem. Soc., 119:7458

Moorey, T.H. et al. (1992) Macromolecules, 25:2401.

Murat, M. and Grest, G.S. (1996) Macromolecules, 29: 1278

Nagasaki, T.; Kimura, O.; Ukon, M.; Hamachi, I.; Shinkai, S. and Arimori, S. (1994) J. Chem. Soc. Perkin Transac., 1:75.

Naylor, A.M.; Goddard III, A.W.; Keifer, G. and Tomalia, D.A. (1989) J. Am. Chem Soc., 111:2339.

Newkome, G.R.; Baker, G.R.; Arai, S.; Saunders, M.J.; Russo, P.S.; Theriot, K.J.; Moorefield, C.N.; Rogers, L.E.; Miller, J.E.; Lieux,T.R.; Murray, M.E.; Phillips, B. and Pascal, L. (1990) J. Am. Chem. Soc., 112:8458.

Newkome, G.R.; Guther, R.; Moorefield, C.N.; Cardullo, F.; Echegoyen, L.; Perezcordero, E. and Luftman, H. (1995) Angew. Chem. Int Ed. Engl., 34:2023.

Newkome, G.R.; Yao, Z.; Baker, G.R. and Gupta, V. (1985) J. Org. Chem., 50:2003.

Newkome, G.R.; Yao, Z.Q.; Baker, G.R.; Gupta, V.K.; Russo, R.S. and Saunders, M.J. (1986) J. Am. Chem. Soc., 108:849.

Newkome,G.R.; Woosley,B.D.; He, E.; Moorefield, C.N.; Guther, R.; Baker, G.R.; Escamilla, G.H.; Merill, J. and Luftmann, H. (1996). Chem. Commun., 2737.

Page, D.; Zanini, D. and Roy, R. (1996) Bioorg. Med. Chem., 4.

Paleos, C.M.; Dais, P. and Malliaris, A. (1984) J. Polym. Sci. Polym. Chem. Ed., 22:3383.

Pesak, D.J.; Moore, J.S. and Wheat, D.E. (1997) Macromolecules, 30:6467

Ponomarenko,S.A.; Rebrov, E.A.; Bojko,N.I.; Vasilenko, N.G.; Muzafarov,A.M.N.; Frejdzon, Y.S. and Shibaev, V.P. (1994) Vysokomolekularnye Soedineniya, Seria A., 36:1086.

Roberts, J.C.; Adams, Y.E.; Tomalia, D.A.; Mercer-smith, J.A. and Lavallee, D.K. (1990) Bioconjug. Chem., 1:305.

Roy, R. (1996) Plym. News, 21:226.

Roberts, J.C.; Bhalgat, M.K. and Zera, R.T. (1996) J. Biomed. Mater. Res., 30:53

Saville, P.M.; White, J.W.; Hawker, C.J.; Wooley, K.L. and Frechet, J.M.J. (1993) J. Phys. Chem., 97:293.

Sharon, N. and Lis, H. (1993) Sci. Am., 82.

Singh, P.; Moll, III.F.; Lin, S.H.; Ferzli, C.; Kwok, S.Yu.; Koshi, R.K.; Saul, R.G. and Cronin, P. (1994) Clin. Chem., 40:1845

Slany, M.; Bardaji, M.; Casanov, M.J.; Caminade, A.M.; Majoral, J.P. and Chaudert, B. (1995) J.Am. Chem. Soc., 117:9764.

Spetzler J.C. and Tam, J.P. (1995) Int. J. Pept. Protein Res., 45:78.

Stevelmans, S.; Van Hest, J.C.M.; Jansen, J.F.G.A.; Van Boxte, D.A.F.J.; De Brabender-van den Berg, E.M.M. and Meijer, E.W. (1996) J. Am. Chem. Soc., 118:7398.

Stuff, S.I.; Son, S.; Lin, H.C.; Li S.L. (1993) Science 259:59.

Tam, J.P.; Lu, Y.A. (1989) Proc. Natl. Acad. Sci., 86:9084.

Tomalia D.A.; Berry, V.; Hall, M.; Hedstrand, D.M. (1987) Macromolecules, 20:1165.

Tomalia, D.A. (1994) Adv. Mater., 6:529.

Tomalia, D.A.; Baker, H.; Dewald, J.; Hall, M.; Kallos, G.; Martin, S.; Roeck, J.; Ryder, J. and Smith, P. (1985) Polymer J., 17 (1):117.

Tomalia, D.A.; Berry, V.; Hall, M. and Hedstrand, D.M. (1987) Macromolecules, 20:1164.

Tomalia, D.A. and Durst, H.D. (1993) Top. Curr. Chem., 165:193,

Tomalia, D.A. et. al. (1984) Presented at the 1st Society Polymer Science, Japan, International Polymer Conference, Kyoto Japan.

Tomlinson, E. and Rolland, A.P. (1996) J. Cont. Rel., 39:357.

Tomoyose, Y.; Jiang, D.L.; Jin, R.H.; Aida, T.; Yamashita, T.; Horie, K.; Yashima, E. and Okamoto, Y. (1996) Macromolecules, 29:5236.

Turro, N.J.; Kumar, C.V.; Grauer, Z. and Barton, J.K. (1987) Lamgmuir 3:1056.

Turro, N.J. and Yekta, A. (1978) J. Am. Chem. Soc., 100:5951.

Tzalis, D. and Tor, Y. (1996) Tetrahedron Lett., 37:8293.

Vanhest, J.C.M.; Delnoye, D.A.P.; Baars, M.W.P.L.; Vangenderen, M.H.P. and Meijer, E.W. (1995) Science 268:1592.

Wallimann, P.; Seiler, P. and Diedrich, F. (1996) Helv. Chim. Acta, 79:779.

Wennerstrom, H. and Lindman, B. (1979) Phys. Rep., 52:1.

Welch, P. and Muthukumar, M. (1998) Macromolecules 31:5892

Wiener, E. C.; Brechbiel M.W.; Brothers, H.; Magin, R.L.; Gansow D.A.; Tomalia D.A. and Lauterbur P.C. (1994) Magn. Reson Med., 31:1.

Wilbur et al. (1998) Bioconjugate Chem., 9:813

Wooley, K.L.; Hawker, C.J. and Frechet, J.M.J. (1991) J. Am. Chem. Soc., 113: 4252 .

Wooley, K.L.; Hawker, C.J. and Frechet, J.M.J. (1993) J. Am. Chem. Soc., 115:11496 .

Wooley, K.L.; Frechet, J.M.J. and Hawker, C.J. (1994) Polymer 35:4489

Wu, C.; Berchbiel, M.W.; Kozak, R.W. and Gansow, O.A. (1994) Bioorg. Med. Chem. Lett. 4:449.

Zhuo, R.X.; Du, B. and Lu, Z.R. (1999) J. Contrl. Rel. 57:249

Zimmerman, S.C.; Zeng, F.W.; Reichert, D.E.C. and Kolotuchin, S.V. (1996) Science 271:1095.

Chapter 16

Multiple Emulsions as Drug Delivery System

A. J. Khopade, N. K. Jain

16.1 INTRODUCTION

Although tremendous efforts have been devoted for designing carrier systems, their industrial and clinical applicability is limited by number of drawbacks. Some of the important concerns are: in-vitro and in-vivo stability, biocompatibility, toxicity and immunogenicity, economy, pilot-plant scaling and most importantly, any major improvement in therapeutic efficacy. Huge disappointments in developing carrier systems have led to the search for an ideal carrier system which considerably alleviate the limitations with the existing systems. A number of exciting and challenging carrier systems are reported in literature that include, bilayer vesicles and other supramolecular assemblies, polymeric micro- and nanoparticulates, cells, emulsions, functional polymers etc. It is almost two and a half decades that the concept of carrier assisted delivery of drug has evolved but only few carriers have the privilege to reach clinical trials and their claim to replace the existing conventional therapy is far away from reach. However, marketing of a couple of carrier based drug delivery systems retains an optimism in drug delivery scientist to search for new ideal carrier systems or to improve upon the limitations posed by the existing delivery systems. With this optimistic approach we have selected to work on multiple emulsions for controlled and targeted delivery of some bioactives. The following literature exhaustively reviews the system.

16.2 MULTIPLE EMULSIONS

Multiple emulsions are complex systems and may be called "emulsions of emulsions", "double or triple emulsions" since the internal phase itself contains dispersed globules which are miscible with the continuous phase. This leads to water-in-oil-in-water (w/o/w) or oil-in-water-in-oil (o/w/o) type, their two miscible phases are separated by an immiscible phase. This phase is sometimes called a "liquid membrane" which acts as semipermeable membrane through which a solute may diffuse from one phase to another, hence in some disciplines multiple emulsions are also called as 'liquid membrane systems' (Fig1). These systems are characterized by their low thermodynamic stability.

In most cases, the two aqueous phases are identical and therefore a w1/o/w1 emulsion is a second order two component system and an o1/w/o2 emulsion is a three component second order system. In this manner ternary, quaternary and even higher order emulsions can be envisioned. In principal, n order emulsion can be prepared by remicellization of an n-1 phase into another continuous phase. Recently, the ability to incorporate liquid crystals into emulsions lead to the development of new multiple phase system encompassing both liquid crystal and multiple emulsion technology (Bevacqua et al., 1991).

Although multiple emulsion is known for more than half a century when Seifriz, in 1925, first published a photograph of w/o/w type unique multiple emulsion. They have been patented more than three decades ago. But it is only the last twenty-five years that they have been extensively studied and investigated in the pharmaceutical and cosmetological field. The potential of multiple emulsions have been known for long period of time. Although there are some limitations in their manufacturing and application, focusing attention to the limitations and harnessing advantages numerous researches are currently being carried on multiple emulsion. As a result, today, a few commercial preparations of multiple emulsions are available in the market put in trade by Lancaster, Bioderma, Estee Lauder and Rubinstein laboratories (Yazan et al., 1993; Fox, 1986).

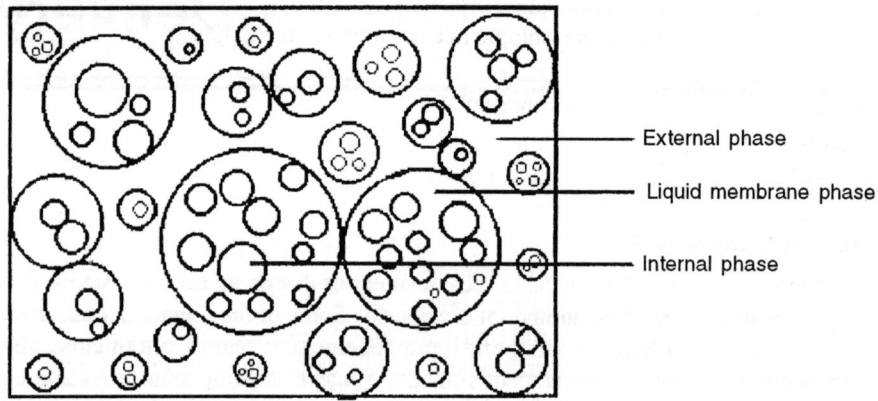

External phase

Liquid membrane phase

Internal phase

Fig 16.1: A typical multiple emulsion system

16.3 FORMULATION AND MANUFACTURE

The intent in preparing multiple emulsion systems is to introduce two different surfactants of opposite nature to the system. One surfactant stabilizes the w/o (lipophilic) emulsion while the other stabilizes the o/w (hydrophilic) emulsion. There are also some reports on accidental formation of multiple emulsion during normal emulsification processes especially during preparation of emulsion containing large volume of internal phase and inversion of emulsion. This is probably due to the partitioning of surfactant between the two phases. These systems have no reproducibility and stability and therefore are practically insignificant to the formulation chemist.

A multiple phase system can be obtained mainly by three methods:

i) Double emulsification

ii) One step emulsification/phase inversion

iii) Use of phase diagram of water-emulsifier-oil.

16.3.1 DOUBLE-EMULSIFICATION

In this method, the primary emulsion is prepared in an usual manner in the first step. Re-emulsification of primary emulsion in the second step leads to the formation of multiple emulsion. The w/o or o/w primary emulsion is prepared by employing lipophilic or hydrophilic surfactant respectively. For the production of w/o/w multiple emulsion, primary w/o emulsion is emulsified in aqueous phase containing hydrophilic surfactant with the aid of stirrer. In case of o/w/o emulsion, o/w primary emulsion is emulsified in second step using a hydrophobic surfactant in oily phase. The second emulsification step is crucial as it can lead to fracture of internal globules forming simple emulsion of either o/w or w/o type depending upon number of factors (Fukushima et al., 1983).

16. 3.2 PHASE INVERSION

The phase inversion of the emulsion occurs when the concentration of dispersed globules in the dispersion medium is quite high i.e. the globules are packed very closely in the suspending fluid. The concentrated o/w emulsion is thermally induced to produce w/o/w emulsion. When an aqueous solution of hydrophilic emulsifier is introduced into oil containing lipophilic surfactant, the w/o/w emulsion is obtained due to phase inversion of w/o emulsion. Phase inversion technique can be exploited to produce emulsions characterized by their fine droplet size (Matsumoto & Kanig, 1989). Improvement of the one-step emulsification by the addition of Fomblin HC (perfluoropolymethyl isopropyl ether) to conventional emulsion has been found to modify the physicochemical and the applicative properties. The most innovative feature is the formation of three phase systems since Fomblin HC is insoluble in both aqueous and oil phases (Brunetta & Pantini 1993).

16.3.3 USE OF PHASE DIAGRAMS OF WATER-EMULSIFIER-OIL

It has been shown that the multiple emulsion can be produced with the use of only one surfactant to stabilize both primary and secondary emulsion. But the incorporation of liquid crystalline mesophase in external phase of either primary or secondary emulsion is important. This is evident in the three phase region for such system where an aqueous micellar solution of the emulsifier and the oil rich solution of the emulsifier are in equilibrium with each other and with a mesomorphous phase. The presence of a liquid crystalline phase in the ternary system consisting of water- emulsifier-oil has been shown to greatly improve the stability of emulsions. The studies with ternary phase diagram consisting of nonylphenol diethyleneglycol ether (EMU 09), water and p-xylene shows an area where formation of multiple emulsion system with liquid crystalline phase is evident (Kavaliunas & Frank, 1978). Phase diagrams of four component systems containing light mineral oil, Span-80, Tween-20 and water at 25, 35 and 45°C were also studied. After gentle agitation of this component mixture for 48 hr various phases were observed including simple emulsions, mesophases and multiple emulsions. The regions of multiple emulsion decreased in area as the temperature was increased (Florence et al., 1989).

16.4. PARAMETERS AFFECTING MULTIPLE EMULSION PREPARATION

The critical, essential and non-essential parameters on manufacturing and formulation of w/o/w multiple emulsion preparations have been reported (Abd Elbary et al., 1990). In general, they are as follows:

16.4.1 COMPOSITION

16.4.1.1 Oils

Nature of oil is of great importance since it controls the permeability of the liquid membrane, which in turn controls the release of solute across it. The stability of oily layer against leakage of entrapped material depends upon the nature of oil (Omotosho et al., 1986). Besides the concentration of oil phase, the physicochemical characteristics of the oil used such as the density and viscosity influence the behaviour of the system. Depending on the conditions used for the manufacture, most of the oil -hydrocarbons, waxes, silicones, esters and triglycerides etc. form multiple emulsions. Refined hydrocarbon oils such as mineral oil and squalene have been used extensively. Esters of long chain fatty acids including isopropyl myristate or oleate and vegetable oils such as peanut oil, olive oil, sesame oil, maize/corn oil, jojoba oil and arachis oil have also been used to vary the physicochemical properties of multiple emulsions. A large number of non-polar lipophilic molecules (oil) have been investigated concerning their dielectric constant, size, shape and other properties (Lin & Wu, 1991). As the adsorption of emulsifier and emulsifier film formed at the oil-water interface will depend on the nature of oil phase, the multiple emulsion will be formed when there is a similarity between the hydrophobic part of the emulsifier and the oil phase.

16.4.1.2 Surfactants

As mentioned previously, the multiple emulsion formation requires at least two surfactants of different nature i.e. one hydrophilic and another lipophilic as primary and secondary surfactants depending upon the type of emulsion (o/w/o or w/o/w) required. The optimum concentration of surfactant required to emulsify given oil is determined by the use of hydrophile-lipophile balance (HLB) system. In a w/o/w emulsion, the optimal HLB value of the primary surfactant is usually in the range of 2-7 while 6-16 for the secondary surfactant. The concentration of secondary emulsifier is generally less than 1/5th of the primary emulsifier. If this value is high the primary surfactant will get incorporated in secondary surfactant micelles thus destabilizing primary emulsion. If the value of emulsifying mixture is less than 10, there is a risk of phase inversion and the formation of single emulsion. It is beneficial to use hydrophobic emulsifier in excess i.e. about 10-30% w/w of oil phase or primary emulsion whereas hydrophilic emulsifier is used in low concentration i.e. about 0.5 to 5% w/w of external phase. The addition of primary surfactant to the secondary surfactant during secondary emulsification improves stability due to avoidance of surfactant migration (Hameyer & Jenni, 1994; Abd Elbary et al., 1984).

Several investigators have tried various mixtures of surfactants mostly non-ionic at various concentrations to obtain stable systems. These emulsifiers are preferred because of their lower toxicity and also they are less likely to interact with other compounds. These surfactants are mannide monooleate, and polyoxyethylene (POE) sorbitan monooleate, polyoxyalkanol, sorbitan monooleate and POE sorbitan monolaurate, sorbitan sesquioleate and POE sorbitan monooleate, sorbitan monooleate and POE sorbitan monooleate, POE oleic alcohol and sorbitan monolaurate, sorbitan tristearate and POE sorbitan monooleate, cetearth 12 and POE octadecyl ethers, POE docosyl ethers (Adeyeye & Price, 1991).

A correlation between the oil-water interfacial tension and emulsifier has been reported. The concentration and type of emulsifier was optimized on the basis of concentration vs. interfacial tension relationship for various emulsifiers (Kover et al., 1997a,b). Two types of curves are generally obtained. The suitable surfactant is shown by a steep lowering curve with a sharp break at its optimum concentration. Other surfactants show relatively flat curve without a sharp break but with a slow change (Eros et al., 1990).

16.4.1.3 Phase volume

Over a range of low volume fractions, the secondary phase volume influences the yield of multiple drops. The multiple emulsions can be prepared using internal phase volume o:w/o in an optimal range of 25-50%. Later, the reports by Seiller and co-workers (1991) showed that the phase volume ratio of as large as 70-90% can produce a stable multiple emulsion. The order of addition of phases then becomes important for the required type of multiple emulsion. Usually slow addition of dispersed phase into continuous phase during emulsification is always advantageous. The rule that the continuous phase will be the one in which the surfactant is soluble (Bancroft's rule) is not always applicable to multiple emulsion because it is possible in some cases to prepare double emulsions (w/o first followed by its dispersion in water i.e. o/w) using a single surfactant. Internal phase volume influences the stability and release of solute from multiple emulsions.

16.4.2 Shear/Agitation

The choice of modes of emulsification is very important because the multiple emulsion systems are rather fragile systems. The shear rate and shear stress are two parameters specific of each system which again depends on type of phases and surfactants used to some extent. The high shear disrupts the large percentage of multiple drops and thus results in instability of the system. Therefore, the yield of the system falls rapidly as the homogenization time is increased. Many types of equipment are used for preparing multiple emulsions in laboratory which offer different shear rates and shear stresses ranging from simple magnetic stirrer, mechanical stirrer, homogenizer to ultrasonicator. For manufacturing purposes, pin mixers and micro-vortex stirrers are usually preferred to high shear producing Ultra-Turrax and ultrasonication. Ultra-Turrax causes incorporation of air hence excessive frothing resulting in loss of surfactant at air-water interface. Shear combined with air bubbles may lead to instability. Even if the formation of high yield emulsion is achieved the use of high energy like sonication leads to complete loss of multiple drops upon storage. However it is to be remembered that inspite of the best techniques used, a portion of multiple drops will always unavoidably be lost during preparation and storage. The rule of thumb is that high agitation speed for primary and lower speed for secondary emulsification are necessary for the manufacture of multiple emulsion. The minimum requirements seem to be 800rpm and 200rpm for primary and secondary emulsification, below which the multiple emulsion will tend to coalesce or cream. The maximum requirements vary depending upon the formulation composition (Yan et al., 1992).

16.4.3 Temperature

Temperature plays a significant role in the emulsion formation. It is advised to dissolve surfactant in respective phases completely, with the aid of heat, if required. The hydrophilic emulsifier becomes more lipophilic as it tends to precipitate upon increasing temperature from its solution (cloud point). The temperature must therefore be precisely controlled during the preparation of primary emulsion or multiple emulsion. The minimum temperatures are 70°C for primary emulsification and 10°C for multiple emulsion. The highest temperatures depend upon the composition e.g. the secondary emulsification temperature required to be maintained at 70°C if the additives like fatty acid, cetostearyl alcohol etc. causing gelling of oil phase are added (Khopade & Jain, 1997). The sudden cooling (quenching) to about 4°C is often suggested for such emulsions. When sonication is used for the preparation it is advised to cool the emulsion mixture to dissipate heat energy generated which otherwise causes rapid coalescence of droplets.

16.5. CHARACTERIZATION OF MULTIPLE EMULSIONS

Characterization of any drug delivery system is important both from the manufacturing and therapeutic points of view to obtain product reproducibility. Several methods allow determine the multiple character of the system while others determine the stability and efficacy. The important ones are discussed below:

16.5.1 Macroscopic examination

Colour, consistency and homogeneity are first investigated organoleptically in order to ensure formation of an emulsion. The control of type (o/w/o or w/o/w) is defined by dilution with the external phase.

16.5.2 Microscopic examination

The multiplicity of the multiple emulsion is verified by light microscopy and/or electron microscopic techniques. There are number of problems with this method. Firstly, the passage of small simple drops below large simple drops gives a false impression of multiple nature. Secondly, the internal droplets cannot be viewed if they are very small due to reflection of light from the surface of the oil droplets. Despite these problems, this method is simple and provides useful information on the character of multiple emulsion. The method also allows determination of droplet size. A suitable magnification may be used for the purpose. Using inverted phase contrast microscope and a high speed camera Florence & Whitehill (1982b) classified multiple emulsions into three types:

    (i) Type A composed of relatively small multiple drops of mean diameter 8.5 µm containing a few relatively large internal droplets of mean diameter 3.3 µm.

    (ii) Type B composed of larger multiple drops of mean diameter 19 µm containing smaller but more numerous multiple droplets of mean diameter 2.2 µm, and

    (iii) Type C with vast number of very small internal droplets entrapped.

A review of literature prompted the authors of this review to classify multiple emulsions based on their droplet size. We have proposed three types of multiple emulsions namely:

(i) Coarse multiple emulsions > 3 μm diameter,

(ii) Fine multiple emulsions of about 1-3 μm diameter, and

(iii) Micro-multiple emulsions < 1 μm diameter.

Very small multiple emulsion diameters are measured using Coulter-counter and their multiple nature is proved by calculating yield using suitable marker. A number of authors have used this method for determination of droplet size. The freeze fracture electron microscopy is yet another method to prove multiple nature of emulsion containing very fine internal droplets (nanometric range) or micellar droplets. The technique being time consuming and uneconomical, is not recommended for routine analysis.

A few scientists characterize multiple emulsions on the basis of internal droplet size for it was found to effect the release rate of entrapped drug and stability of multiple emulsion. A routine microscopic analysis is one method for larger internal droplets. Ohwaki et al. (1993b) reported a centrifugation-dilution method for nanometric internal droplets. The multiple emulsion was spun at 1000 rpm for 5 min. The w/o supernatant was removed and diluted with oil phase. It was stirred gently and the droplet size was determined on Coulter-counter operating on the principle of Brownian motion and photon correlation spectroscopy.

The multiple character of the emulsions and the location of fluorescent probes were observed by an optical microscope equipped with special optical filters adapted for fluorescent probe (Tokgoz et al., 1996).

16.5.3 Formation percentage of multiple emulsion, yield or entrapment efficiency

The yield or formation percentage of multiple emulsion is an indirect method for proving their multiple character. The use of an internal tracer is used to investigate the efficiency of entrapment of an impermeable marker molecule in the internal phase of the system. The method basically involves determination of unentrapped tracer or marker or drug. The entrapped drug is then obtained by subtracting untrapped amount from the amount added. There are four methods commonly used for determination of entrapment efficiency:

(i)   Dialysis,

(ii)   Centrifugation,

(iii) Filtration, and

(iv)   Conductivity measurements.

16.5.4 Nuclear magnetic resonance (NMR)

NMR is a new technique to verify the multiple character of the emulsion. It has been stated that the NMR signals of water protons are narrow and singlet in simple emulsions while the signals are widened or doubled in multiple emulsions.

16.5.5 Zeta potential

A relatively less number of studies are reported on the determination of zeta-potential of multiple emulsions but with the development of surface-modified multiple emulsion system the importance of determining zeta potential has increased. A study by Arai et al. (1994) was conducted to determine the effects of biologically important substances e.g. lipids and drugs, on modes of electric potential oscillation across liquid membrane of water-octanol-water system. The changes depended on the type and concentration of lipid and drug were correlated with drug's pharmacological activity. Wu et al. (1990b) formulated w/o/w emulsion by screening oils, emulsifiers and stabilizers by measuring critical properties including zeta potential.

16.5.6 Rheological analysis

Multiple emulsion systems exhibit viscoelastic properties hence rheological analysis is an important characterization parameter (Vasiljevic et al., 1994; Kovacic et al., 1992). The viscometer with cone and plate geometry is widely used, as it requires low sample volumes however spindle type viscometer may also be used. Rheological measurements are important from both stability and clinical point of view. Thus multiple emulsions are exposed to clinically relevant shear rates e.g. the maximum shear rate in human circulatory system in the capillary walls is about 1000 s-1.

Three different types of tests are performed (Terrisse et al., 1993):

(i) Oscillatory test,

(ii) Steady-state flow tests, and

(iii) Turbulence shock test.

16.5.7 Stability

The inherent instability of the multiple emulsions has lead researchers to study the factors causing it and to overcome this drawback as these systems find several potential applications. The mechanisms of instability are complex. Theoretical predictions and experimental results however show satisfactory relationship. The multiple emulsions of w/o/w type are widely studied for the mechanisms causing their instability. There are mainly four mechanisms which are identified (Baillet et al., 1994; Florence et al., 1989):

(i) Coalescence of the internal droplets,

(ii) Coalescence of the multiple emulsion drops,

(iii) Rupture of oil layer on the surface of internal drops i.e. expulsion of

internal droplet in external phase, and

(iv) Shrinkage and swelling of the internal drops due to osmotic gradient

across the oil membrane.

16.5.7.1 Approaches to improve stability

There have been a number of approaches to avoid the principal modes of instability described above to improve the stability of multiple emulsion. Fig 2 illustrates all the possible modes of stabilization. The methods available in literature and reviews summarise them mainly into three types (Florence et al., 1989) however, we have attempted to classify them into six types with subclassification therein:

(i) Gelation of phases

a. by gelating internal or external phase

b. by gelating oil phase

(ii) Formation of interfacial complex films

a. by in-situ polymerization at the interface (Law et al., 1983, 1986)

b. by interfacial interaction between a polymer and surfactants (Florence et al, 1982a)

(iii) Modulating surfactant concentration

a. by hydrophilic-lipophilic balance (HLB) approach

b. by liquid-crystal stabilization

(iv)   Additives in internal aqueous phase

   a. by addition of insoluble material (Oza & Frank, 1989a)

   b. by addition of soluble material (Kawashima et al., 1992)

(v)   Pro-multiple emulsion formation

   a. by solidification of multiple emulsions (Myers & Shively, 1992)

   b. by lyophilization of multiple emulsions

(vi)   Steric stabilization

16.5.7.2   Estimation of stability

Basic studies performed on multiple emulsion prepared freshly, and/or on storage for different time periods for the estimation of stability are:

(i)   Droplet size and polydispersity of internal and multiple droplets

(ii)   Phase separation

(iii)   Creaming

(iv)   Viscosity measurement

(v)   Drug leakage

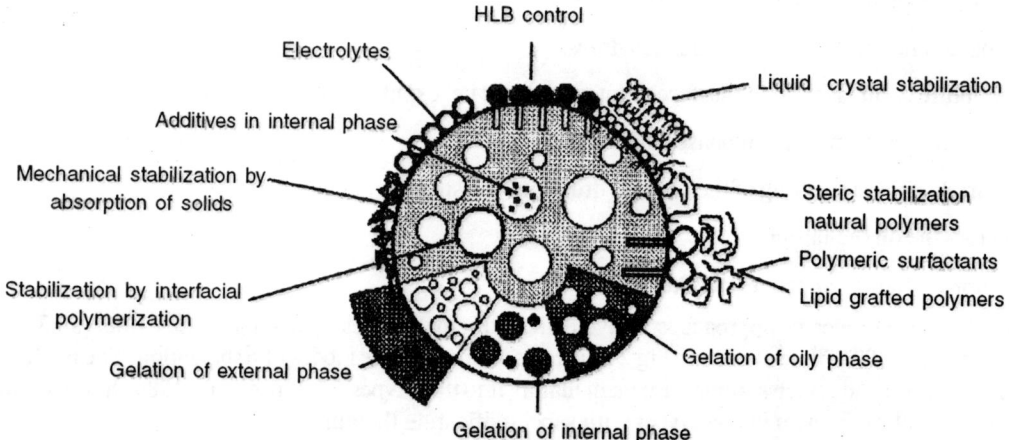

Fig 16.2 : Schematic illustration of modes of stabilization of multiple emulsion

For accelerated stability testing above basic tests are performed under following conditions:

(i)   Orthokinetic stress/ Turbulence shock

(ii)   Osmotic stress/ Dilution effect

(iii)   Centrifugal stress

(iv)   Electrokinetic stress

(v)   Thermal stress, determination of phase inversion temperature (Wu et al., 1990b)

16.5.8 Transport of solute from internal to external phase of multiple emulsion

A number of possible mechanisms by which materials may be transported across oily layer in w/o/w emulsion systems have been prepared and discussed (Fig 16.3). Some of them are (De-Luca et al., 1990):

16.5.9 Mathematical modelling

The complicated geometry of the multiple emulsion droplets makes it difficult to deal with drug release kinetics from them hence it is necessary to simplify the model of multiple emulsion droplets (Lin & Lui, 1992). The following discussion describes kinetic treatment of drug transport from internal to external phase as reported by various authors.

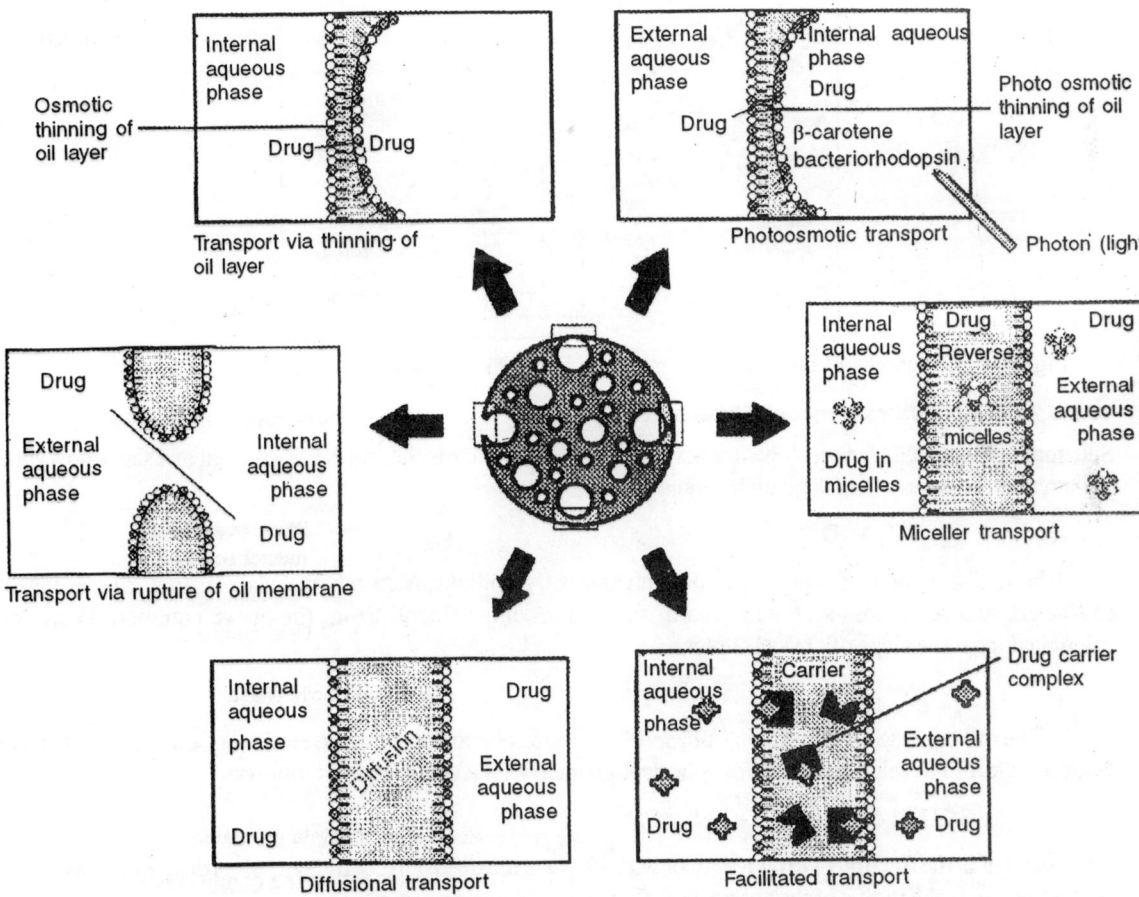

Fig 16.3: Schematic illustration of possible mechanisms of transport of solute across liquid membrane

    (i) Diffusion across oil membrane,

    (ii) Thinning of oil membrane,

    (iii) Rupture of oil membrane,

    (iv) Micellar transport,

    (v) Facilitated diffusion,

    (vi) Photo-osmotic transport (Madamwar & Jain, 1992,1993).

16.5.9.1 Diffusion model (Baker & Lonsdale, 1974)

The amount of drug released is given by the equation:

$$\text{Log } M_t = \frac{-A\,P_t}{2.303\,V_1} + \text{Log } M_o$$

where, M_o is initial amount of drug, M_t is the amount of drug remaining at time t, A is the area of mass transfer, V_1 is volume of internal aqueous phase and P is permeability coefficient. The model is illustrated in Fig 16.4.

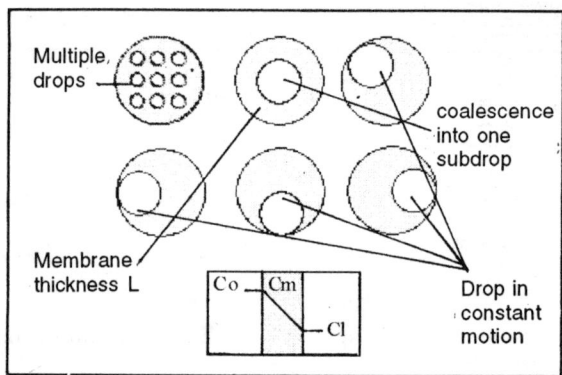

Fig 16.4 : Schematic illustration of diffusion model for the release of solute from multiple emulsion

16.5.9.2 Matrix diffusion model (Higuchi, 1962)

Schematic of matrix diffusion model is shown in Fig 16.5. From this theory of diffusion out of a slab into a sink, the amount of material lost is given by equation :

$$Q' = 2C_0\,A\,(Dt/p)^{1/2} \qquad\qquad (1)$$

where, Q' is amount of material lost per unit area, C0 is initial concentration of slab, t is time, D is diffusion coefficient and A is cross-sectional area of the donor compartment. From the above equation, D can be calculated from the slope of Q vs t1/2 plot.

$$D = \text{slope}/(2C_0\,A)\,p \qquad\qquad (2)$$

The full expression for release from spherical matrix is rather complex. However, some scientists have made an effort to develop equation for spherical geometry. The equation is as follows:

$$3/2[1-(1-F)^{2/3}] - F = 3DCst/r_0^2C_0 \qquad\qquad (3)$$

where, F is the fraction of drug released (M_t/M_0), D is the diffusion coefficient, Cs is drug solubility at the membrane, r0 is the radius of the sphere and C0 is initial drug concentration.

Magdassi & Garti (1995) developed this model for multiple emulsion where right hand term was denoted as B thus:

$$B = 3DCst/r_0^2\,C_0 \qquad\qquad (4)$$

or $\qquad B = 3De\,t/\cdot r_0^2\,C_0$

where, De is effective diffusion coefficient, De = D Cs

Plotting B against t gives straight line with a slope of $3De/r_0^2\,C_0$. A plot of B vs $_1/C_0$ was found to follow power law, and variable exponent n for the time (tn) ranged from 0.5 to 3.0 were calculated with correlation coefficient of 0.99 to 1. This indicates existence of mixed film at the interface and the presence of reverse micelles in oil phase. Thus this model is suitable for expressing micellar transport of drug (Sela et al., 1995).

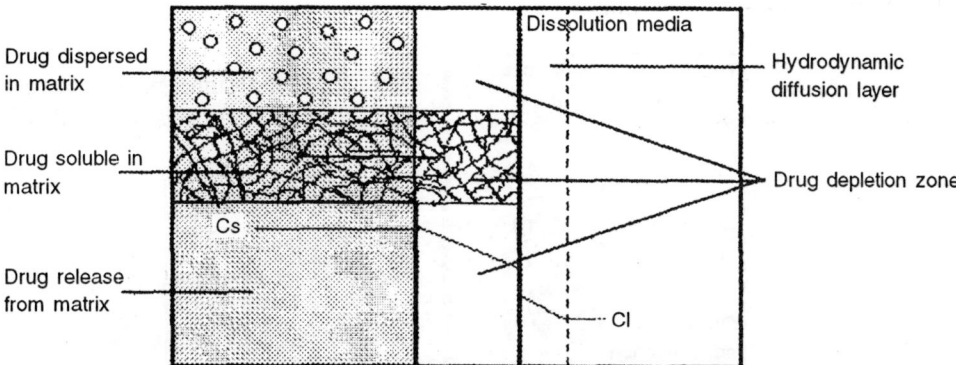

Fig 16.5 : Schematic illustration of matrix diffusion model for the release of solute from multiple emulsion

16.5.9.4 Rupture of oil membrane (Hino et al, 1995)

The release of solute by the rupture of oil membrane may be schematically shown as in Fig 6. The quantity of encapsulate released is given by:

$$\text{Log } V_0 - kt = \text{Log } Q \tag{5}$$

where,

$$Q = X \ \frac{Z(Y - C_3 V_3 - C_1 X)}{\{V_3 \, d \, C_3/dt - Z(C_1 - C_3)\}} \tag{6}$$

The parameters X, Y and Z are defined for simplification as under :

$$X = V_1 + V_2 = \frac{V_s(V_i + V_e)}{(V_i + V_o + V_e)} \tag{7}$$

$$Y = \frac{C_1 V_s V_i}{(V_i + V_o + V_e)} \tag{8}$$

$$Y = (C_1 V_1 + C_2 V_2 + C_3 V_3) \tag{9}$$

$$Z = D.S/h \tag{10}$$

The parameter Z is determined by :

$$P = Zt \tag{11}$$

where,

$$P = \{V_2 V_3/(V_2 + V_3)\} \times \text{Log}\{C_0 V_2 - C_3 V_2 - C_3 V_3\} \tag{12}$$

$$C_0 V_2 = C_2 V_2 + C_3 V_3 \tag{13}$$

Where V_1 and V_0 are volumes of inner aqueous phase at time t and zero (start of experiment) respectively, K is the rate constant (min^{-1}). D, S and h are diffusion coefficient of the drug in the pore of cellulose tube (cm^2.min^{-1}), the effective total cross sectional area (cm^2) of the pores and the thickness (cm) of the membrane of the tube, respectively. C_2, C_3 and V_3 are the concentration of drug in the outer aqueous phase in donor, outer aqueous phase in receptor and the volume of receptor phase respectively. V_2 is the volume of outer aqueous phase in donor, C_1 is the concentration of drug in the inner aqueous phase in receptor respectively. V_i, V_o, V_e are volumes of inner aqueous phase, oily phase and the outer aqueous phase respectively.

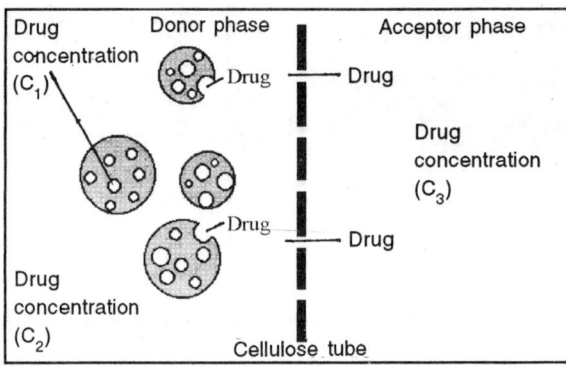

Fig 16.6 : Schematic illustration of model for the release of solute from multiple by the rupture of oil membrane

16.6. MARKERS USED IN MULTIPLE EMULSION STUDIES

Many types of markers have been used to study multiple emulsion characteristics, especially yield and release. The ideal requirement for a chemical to be used as marker seems to be its absolute insolubility in organic phase which is not possible. Hence, the materials with negligible solubility are used. Other requirements being easy detection and analysis, and inert nature i.e. should not effect formulation of the system. They may be divided into following categories:

(i)   Electrolytes e.g. NaCl, $MgSO_4.7H_2O$, $AgNO_3$, NaOH, HCl, H_2SO_4, $CuSO_4$, NaSCN.

(ii)   Dyes e.g. sulphane blue, polyporphyre, polytartarazine (Zatz & Cueman, 1988)

(iii)   Ionic drugs e.g. Ephedrine HCl

(iv)   Fluorescent markers e.g. Carboxyfluorescein and PMSA (Oba et al., 1992)

(v)   Radioactive tracer e.g. Tritiated water (Burbage & Davis, 1979)

(vi)   Organic solute e.g. new coccine (Ohwaki et al., 1993c).

16.7. BEHAVIOUR OF MULTIPLE EMULSION IN BIOLOGICAL SYSTEM

Multiple emulsions have been administered by oral, parenteral (i.v., i.p., s.c., i.m.) and topical (nasal, ocular, transdermal) routes. The fate of multiple emulsion after oral and parenteral administration requires insight from the stability, pharmacokinetic and pharmacodynamic point of view. After oral administration, emulsions are absorbed almost entirely through lymphatic pathway in association with intestinal lipoproteins namely chylomicrons, produced by enterocytes. They may directly be absorbed through the intestinal macrophage system and Payer's patches to gain access into mesenteric lymph from where they are drained into circulation through thoracic lymph duct. Thus, they are able to carry bioactives within them avoiding degradation in intestine as well as liver (first pass effect). After parenteral administration (i.v.), the emulsions are readily taken up by circulatory macrophage system to lymphatics as well as liver into fat metabolism pathway. Through other parenteral routes, the emulsion droplets gain access to nearby lymphatic node through interstitial spaces of lymphatic vessels which are relatively porous as compared to blood capillaries which have tight intracellular junctions. Thus, the system has an intrinsic lymphotropic characteristic hence is envisaged for the delivery of therapeutic agents for the treatment of cancer metastases and bacterial infections involving lymphatics.

16.8. APPLICATION OF MULTIPLE EMULSIONS AS DRUG DELIVERY VEHICLE: A LITERATURE REVIEW

16.8.1 Prolonged and controlled drug delivery

16.8.1.1 Analgesics and anti inflammatory drugs

The release of naltrexone from o/w/o emulsions and naltrexone HCl from w/o/w emulsions was studied in-vitro. The release was prolonged and found to depend on the additives that changed the property of the interface (Brodin et al., 1978).

Pandit et al. (1988) prepared o/w/o multiple emulsion system containing indomethacin. The prolonged action delivery system was confirmed by sustained plasma drug levels in mice following oral administration compared to plain drug. The brain homogenate levels of this formulation showed very strong prolonged effect, with a continuously rising level upto 6 hr and declining slowly thereafter.

Multiple emulsions, w/o/w and o/w/o type, containing pentazocine were prepared and tested in-vitro and in-vivo. Multiple emulsion gave higher extent of drug release than simple o/w emulsion. The in-vivo studies in mice showed prolonged tissue levels of pentazocine from multiple emulsion as compared to simple o/w, w/o or drug solution (Mishra & Pandit, 1989, 1990).

Adeyeye and Price (1991) prepared and evaluated sodium salicylate containing multiple emulsions.

Nakahare and Vyas (1994) showed prolonged release of diclofenac sodium from water-in-oil-in-water multiple emulsion.

Roy & Gupta (1993) prepared indomethacin loaded w/o/w emulsion and showed prolonged release of drug from the system. They also established positive correlation between in-vitro and in-vivo studies.

16.8.1.2 Antibacterials

A stable w/o/w emulsion encapsulating cefadroxil, cephradine, antipyrine and 4-aminoantipyrine was prepared using glyceryl tricaprylate as oil phase (Zhang et al., 1992). In-vivo release studies conducted by the same group of workers showed that the plasma levels of cefadroxil and cephradine were prolonged on i.v. administration of drugs in multiple emulsions compared to free drug solutions. The effect was attributed to long residence time and delayed release from w/o/w type multiple emulsions. The effect for antipyrine and 4-aminoantipyrine was decreased rapidly. These results correlated with in-vitro drug release observation (Miyakawa et al., 1993; Zhang et al., 1992; Goto et al., 1991)

Ferreira et al. (1994, 1995) studied the role of multiple emulsion on in-vitro absorption of water soluble drug, metronidazole, through rat skin. The absorption of drug was found to be similar to o/w emulsion but it was faster than from w/o emulsion.

The bioavailability of nitrofurantoin from multiple emulsions in healthy human volunteers was evaluated by urinary excretion studies of unchanged drug. The extent of absorption from soyabean oil emulsion was greater than that of arachis oil. The bioavailability from tablet dosage form with same dose (100 mg) was lower compared to both types of multiple emulsion. The results suggested improved therapeutic efficacy of the multiple emulsion. They also found increased gastrointestinal absorption of griseofulvin from w/o/w emulsion than o/w or tablet dosage form which lead to increased therapeutic efficacy of drug formulated in this system (Oyenji & Omotosho, 1993; Oyenji et al., 1992).

Nakahare and Vyas (1995) prepared and evaluated multiple emulsion containing rifampicin and studied release profile of drug. Results indicated that the pH of internal and external phase, nature of organic phase and partition coefficient of drug affected release profile of rifampicin. They also reported prolonged blood levels of drug in rats (Nakahare & Vyas, 1997)

Omotosho (1988) prepared stable multiple emulsion containing chloroquine phosphate. The rate of release was reduced and it was suggested that intramuscular injection of this formulation could reduce the frequency of administration, improve patient compliance and increase the therapeutic efficacy of chloroquine phosphate.

Khopade et al. (1996b) prepared and characterized multiple emulsion containing rifampicin for physical parameters and pharmacodynamic properties. The system showed high encapsulation efficiency and prolonged release in-vitro. The plasma and brain levels were prolonged when formulation was administered through both oral and nasal route compared to control plain drug solution. Substantial accumulation in brain, when administered through nasal route compared to oral, was attributed to prolonged release effect and presence of transport pathway from submucosal layer of nose to subarchanoid space in brain.

16.8.1.3 Cardiovascular/ANS/CNS acting drugs

The effect of polyhydric alcohols and polyvinylpyrrolidone, pH of the desorbing solution and viscosity of emulsion on the release characteristics of salbutamol sulphate from a w/o/w emulsion system was studied. The diffusion of drug was highly increased by each additive, the increase being in order: sorbitol > glycerol > mannitol > PVP (Pandit et al. 1987).

Kassem et al. (1995) prepared w/o/w emulsions containing prednisolone and studied the effect of external phase volume ratio on the percent mean change in intraocular pressure of the rabbit eye. The decrease in external phase-volume fraction ratio enhanced the bioavailability, maximum response, time of maximum response and half-value duration of drug. In a further study the effect of hydrophilic and lipophilic emulsifiers on drug bioavailability and duration of action was studied. The results showed that hydrophilic emulsifier reduced bioavailability while lipophilic emulsifier showed the reverse effect and decreasing hydrophilic-lipophilic balance favoured the bioavailability, intensity and duration of action (Kassem et al., 1994). The same group prepared and evaluated hydrocortisone multiple emulsion of both w/o/w and o/w/o types and measured their effect on intraocular pressure (Kassem et al., 1994).

Phenylephrine HCl containing ophthalmic o/w and w/o/w emulsions were prepared with hydrocolloid vehicles and evaluated in-vitro and in-vivo. The delayed release characteristics in-vitro and sustained effect was observed in-vivo (Mohammed et al., 1988b).

Diffusion coefficients of pilocarpine HCl in simple and multiple emulsion were determined and the effects of various systems on the miotic and intraocular pressure in rabbit eyes were assessed. Both types of multiple emulsion produced pronounced intraocular pressure decrease. Delays in time to peak response were 3.5 and 1.5 fold for intraocular pressure and miotic response (Attia & Habib , 1986).

Safwat et al. (1994a) studied effect of formulation variables on stability and antitremor and sedative activity of chlorphenoxamine HCl in mice and rats. They also studied formulation-performance relationship of multiple emulsions bearing cortisone and ocular activity (Safwat et al. 1994b).

Oza & Frank (1989b) prepared stable multiple emulsions containing lidocaine base and its HCl salt. They showed sustained release profile in-vitro.

Florence et al. (1976) studied duration of activity of intramuscular injections of phenothiazines in multiple emulsion system.

16.8.1.4 Anticancer drugs

The lipidiolized w/o and w/o/w multiple emulsions containing doxorubicin HCl with different emulsifiers were prepared to evaluate in-vitro sustained release behaviour, pharmacokinetic and tissue distribution function in Sprague Dawley rats. The results showed sustained release of drug in-vitro and prolongation of plasma drug levels in-vivo. The clearance was also decreased. The tissue retention of drug was dependent on the concentration of emulsifier and emulsion type. The results also indicated that lipidiol and HCO-60 (hydrogenated castor oil) play an important role in the prolongation and selective retention of w/o and w/o/w emulsion in-vivo (Lin et al., 1992).

The methotrexate loaded (s/o/w) multiple emulsion was prepared by using bovine serum albumin as stabilizer in internal phase. Using unique microwave technique, the albumin in internal aqueous phase was solidified to form microspheres-in-oil-in-water emulsion. The formulation and process variables were optimized to obtain methotrexate loaded (s/o/w) multiple emulsion. Its physicochemical characteristics such as microscopic structure, electrical charge, particle size distribution, rheological behaviour, yield, entrapment efficiency and release of drug and stability studies were performed. The emulsions were found to be stable and showed prolonged release in-vitro (Tao et al., 1992).

Release rate of methotrexate encapsulated in the internal phase of w/o/w emulsions stabilized by interfacial interaction between albumin and sorbitan monooleate was measured as function of two formulation variables-the oil phase and the secondary emulsifier composition. Release rate was significantly affected by the nature of oil phase and surfactants with high HLB value, used as secondary hydrophilic emulsifiers increased the release rates (Omotosho et al., 1989a).

Ma et al. (1993) prepared multiple emulsion containing etoposide and evaluated its physicochemical properties. The release was found to be biphasic, a fast phase releasing 50 % drug in 10 hr followed by slow phase in which upto 88 % drug was released in next 38 hr.

Fukushima et al. (1983) prepared multiple emulsions containing 5-fluorouracil and cytarabine by two step emulsification technique. They showed prolonged release of both drugs from the system and suggested its utility for sustained release preparations and the possibility to control the release. In a further study they used oily lymphographic agent as an oil phase to prepare w/o/w emulsion containing anticancer agent (Fukushima et al., 1987). Omotosho et al. (1989b) studied release of 5-fluorouracil from intramuscular w/o/w multiple emulsions.

Cytarabine loaded w/o/w multiple emulsions were prepared using non-ionic surfactants of Tween and Span types by emulsification-sonication technique and characterized by studying the osmotic behaviour. The system exhibited prolonged release pattern (Kim et al., 1995).

16.8.1.5 Peptide drugs

Ohwaki et al. (1993a,b) prepared water-in-oil-in-water emulsion containing secretin in internal phase for its application as nasal dosage form. The permeability tests were conducted in-vitro. The apparent permeation rate constants showed very slow release of secretin that was found to depend on the additives (NaCl and sodium octyl sulfonate) in internal phase.

Shively & Thompson (1995) with a view to study in-vivo characteristics, prepared solid-state emulsion of vancomycin, which is not normally absorbed from GI tract, with sesame oil and monoglycerol stearate as primary emulsifier. The findings show about 30 percent absorption of drug from oral route suggesting its potential for oral delivery of drugs that are incompatible with GI tract processes.

As early as 1968, Engel et al. showed intestinal absorption of insulin as w/o/w multiple emulsions.

Intraduodenal injection of a w/o/w emulsion containing insulin resulted in a significant hypoglycaemic activity in rats. In a further study, w/o/w emulsions when injected in jejunum of rabbits at doses of 100 IU/kg produced a fall in blood glucose. When administered orally, it produced fall in blood glucose in three out of seven rabbits. The same group studied the effect in alloxan induced diabetic rat model for absorption of insulin formulated in w/o/w emulsion. The urinary glucose levels were reduced in a dose equivalent to 25-50 IU/100gm body weight (Shichiri et al., 1974).

The insulin loaded multiple emulsion was prepared by two stage emulsification technique with 77.2 % yield and was orally administered to experimental diabetic mice at a dose level 70 IU/kg. It was compared with aqueous solution of drug administered similarly. The results showed that the former could reduce glucose levels from 154.7±36.1 to 40.1±25.3 mg/dl, while the latter failed completely (Wu et al., 1990a).

Nagai and co-workers showed enhanced absorption of insulin from enteral loops in rats using w/o/w multiple emulsion (Matsuzawa et al., 1995). They also studied effect of long-chain polyunsaturated fatty acids on colonic and rectal absorption of insulin (Suzuki et al., 1998). The results were promising for the use of multiple emulsion for the treatment of diabetes.

16.8.1.6 OXYGEN SUBSTITUTE

Zheng et al. (1991, 1992, 1993) performed feasibility studies to evaluate a prototype haemoglobin multiple emulsion containing haemoglobin solution-in-oil-in-water, as a stable oxygen carrying system. The studies using mineral oil demonstrated that Hb multiple emulsions have several important characteristics that are compatible with utility as blood substitute. These include satisfactory rheological properties and good hydro-dynamic stability compared to whole blood, high encapsulation efficiency with little meth-Hb generation and satisfactory oxygen affinity and cooperativity compared to whole blood. Isovolemic exchange with the developed emulsion could support life of rats with only 5 % hematocrit value with no visible acute toxicity.

16.8.2 Targeting of drugs

The successful application of carrier for the delivery of bioactive is its ability to accumulate in certain tissues or engineering to make them site specific. Multiple emulsions as a targetable delivery system was first reviewed by Davis & Walker (1987). The reports on targeting of multiple emulsions are rare, however those available in literature are reviewed below.

16.8.2.1 Lymphatic targeting

Multiple emulsions are intrinsically lymphotropic in nature, thus their use in the treatment of diseases involving lymphatics is suggested. Takahashi et al., (1973) studied the delivery of labeled 5-fluorouracil to regional lymph nodes following intratesticular administration. They found that the emulsion reached regional lymph nodes within 15 min and remained there for about 7 days. The influence of the nature of oil phase of w/o/w emulsions on the oral absorption of 5-fluorouracil in the rat was determined by measuring liver and lymphatic accumulation of drug. The multiple emulsion system showed potential as lymphotropic carrier to the mesenteric lymph nodes following oral administration (Omotosho et al., 1990). Multiple emulsion system containing 5-fluorouracil was evaluated through intramuscular route. The sustained blood levels were obtained as compared to free drug solution (Omotosho et al., 1989b). Hashida et al., (1977) have demonstrated that the sesame oil labeled with 14C tripalmitin and 131iodohippuric acid entrapped in gelled gelatin phase of w/o emulsion could be converted into a crude gel/o/w type emulsion which is then transported to regional lymph nodes. Subsequently, Yoshioka et al. (1982) prepared microsphere-in-oil-in-water multiple emulsion containing bleomycin and showed prolonged plasma concentration of drug after intramuscular injection of the formulation to rats. After administration in appendix of rabbits, the system was transported to lymphatics. Takahashi et al., (1973) used sesame oil based multiple emulsion system for local administration to tumours. The drug, bleomycin, was retained in the tumour tissue and was slowly delivered to the regional lymph node. They also reported complete absence of toxicity.

16.8.2.2 Lung targeting

Magnetic guidance of magnetic emulsion for site specific delivery was investigated both in-vitro and in-vivo. The magnetic emulsion was characterized in-vitro for its magnetic responsiveness using a constant flow apparatus, and its high retention by magnetic field was confirmed. After i.v. injection in rat, magnetic emulsions were localized to the lungs by application of an electromagnet to the lungs. The drug nitrosourea derivative (methyl CCNU) contained therein was also targeted to the site. Such preferential localization suggested use of magnetic emulsions for site specific delivery of chemotherapeutic agents (Akimoto & Morimoto, 1983).

The preferential accumulation of mannanylated multiple emulsion to the lungs is reported by Khopade et al. (1996a). The lipid grafted mannan was coated over the surface of the emulsion droplets whose droplet size was reduced by filtration to $< 5\mu m$ to avoid passive embolism. The tissue distribution studies showed higher accumulation into the lungs. The system was non-toxic to cultured cells.

16.8.2.3 Liver/spleen targeting

The oleic acid multiple emulsion was skinned with a polymer layer by localized pH induced interfacial polymerization of 4-vinyl pyridine. The drug, isoniazid, contained therein was highly accumulated in liver and to relatively greater extent in spleen compared to uncoated emulsion (Khopade & Jain 1998).

16.8.2.4 Inflammatory-site targeting

Khopade et al. (1995) prepared dextran coated w/o/w multiple emulsion by anchoring palmitoyl dextran by slow stirring. The encapsulant was diclofenac sodium. Sustained release of drug was obtained in-vitro and in-vivo studies demonstrated increase in plasma drug half-life. The antiinflammatory studies using carageenan induced rat paw oedema model showed significant activity with faster onset of action. This was attributed to improvement in circulation-life of the system and accumulation to inflammatory sites which became more permeable due to inflammatory reaction.

16.8.3 As adjuvant

An oil emulsion as an adjuvant was first used in 1916, when Le Moignic and Penoy found that a suspension of killed Salmonella typhimurium in mineral oil increased immune response. Later, Freund (1956) demonstrated adjuvant effect of mineral oil with killed mycobacterium. The Freund's complete adjuvant and Freund's incomplete adjuvant (FIA) were used for long time in experimental animals and veterinary vaccines. The mode of action was found to be the slow release and accumulation in regional lymph nodes. But the side effects were so severe that search for non-toxic adjuvant was continued with oils. Herbert (1965, 1967) first reported the use of multiple emulsions as adjuvants. Taylor et al., (1969) conducted experiments and studied comparative antibody responses and reactions to aqueous influenza vaccine, simple emulsion and multiple emulsion vaccine. They demonstrated satisfactory response greater than solution or emulsion vaccine. Non-specific antibody response in mice was studied by encapsulating endotoxin in multiple emulsion. The non-specific resistance to endotoxin in mice was enhanced but the toxicity of endotoxin was not reduced which was attributed to the presence of free endotoxin in external phase. Kimura et al. (1978a) employed sesame oil to make w/o/w emulsion for adjuvant activity. The activity in human was found to be less than FIA but better than plain influenza vaccine. This type of emulsion was almost equally potent to o/w type emulsion, less viscous and easy to administer, more stable and produced fewer nodules at the site of injection. Kimura et al. (1978b), developed w/o/w emulsion without the use of Arlacel A (which was found to be carcinogenic) that could be metabolized. This preparation showed good adjuvant effect on antibody response in mice. The mode of action suggested was slow release and targeting to lymph glands.

16.8.4 Cosmetology

Multiple emulsion systems have been designed to be applied cosmetically because of their ease in skin application and encapsulation character. In several formulation studies multiple emulsions have been claimed to be useful when applied as suncreams, moisturising, nutritive and protective hand creams, make-up cleansers, shaving creams, antiperspirants and perfume preparations by incorporating the active ingredients either in internal or external phases (Yazan, 1993).

The healthy look of the skin could be maintained by a multiple emulsion containing protein derivatives in the external phase and lanolin hydroxyethylene in the internal phase. For an antiperspirant-desodorisant preparation, aluminium derivatives have been incorporated in external phase and bacteriosides like trichlorocarbanilide in internal phase. Protective creams for hands have been suggested to include a hydrosoluble citron extract in external phase and a depigmentant like hydroquinones in internal phase (Seiller et al., 1991).

A makeup cleanser preparation was prepared by incorporating polyethylene particles in external phase and humectants like hyaluronic acid in internal phase while body care preparations were formulated with sodium lactate in external phase and glycerine in internal phase (Yazan, 1993).

Various cosmetic formulations based on multiple emulsion systems are commercially available; marketed by Bioderma, Estee Lauder and Rubinstein Laboratories.

16.8.5 Masking of taste

Encapsulating active ingredients in the internal phase of multiple emulsion have also been used to overcome the bad taste of drugs like chlorpromazine HCl and chloroquine (Garti et al., 1983; Florence et al., 1989).

16.8.6 Drug overdosage treatment

The excess drug can be removed by extraction into the internal aqueous phase of a w/o/w system because the diffusion of unionized lipid soluble material takes place. Acidic drugs such as aspirin or barbiturates, when administered orally, exist at low pH values as the unionized form and therefore would be readily soluble in unionized form. The internal aqueous phase is formulated in basic buffer so as to ionise the drugs and entrap the materials (Chiang et al., 1978).

Detoxication potential of multiple (w/o/w) emulsion for the treatment of drug overdose by drug extraction into the emulsion in the GI tract was studied using rabbit as model animal (Morimoto et al., 1979). The same group showed detoxification of quinine sulphate by coadministration of multiple emulsion in the GI tract of rabbits (Morimoto et al., 1982).

16.8.7 Immobilization of enzymes

The immobilization technique as substrate processing units was invented by May & Li (1972). They immobilized urease in liquid surfactant membranes. Later, they utilized the system for reduction and separation of nitrate and nitrite by liquid surfactant encapsulated enzymes and whole cells (Mohan & Li, 1974, 1975).

The conversion of a-ketoisocaproate to L-leucine by L-leucine dehydrogenase by reductive amidation has been carried out using multiple emulsion system. NADH is oxidized in this reaction and is reduced continuously via a second enzyme, formate dehydrogenase. The method is called co-factor recycling method. The liquid membrane system was prepared from liquid paraffin with 5% Span 80 and 1% Adogen 464. The system worked for one week (Makryaleas et al., 1985).

The conversion of alcohol to acetaldehyde was achieved by immobilising alcohol dehydrogenase and second enzyme, diaphorase, to reduce NADH produced during the reaction (May & Landgraff, 1976).

16.8.8 Extraction/separation of components

Lee & Lee (1992) determined optimum conditions for penicillin G extraction from a model media using an emulsion liquid membrane. They also proposed a theoretical model of product decomposition based on these studies.

It is demonstrated that proteins and nucleic acids can be transported through liquid membranes via non-specific complex formation with detergents. The rate of detergent facilitated transport of proteins is not a function of molecular weight but the hydrophobicity of the complex formed. Thus, albumin can be transported faster than insulin that is less than 1/10th of its size (Bromberg & Kibanov, 1994).

Transport of adenine mono- and dinucleoside monophosphates across liquid membranes and extraction of oligonucleotides with the use of synthetic carriers have been suggested by Andreu et al. (1994).

Scholler et al. (1993) reported extraction of lactic acid from the fermentation broth using emulsion liquid membrane system of Span-80/n-heptane/paraffin and Alamine 336 as selective carrier.

Extraction and recovery of heavy metals from waste water is suggested as superior method than precipitation where the sludges have to be disposed in landfills. Raghuraman et al. (1994) successfully carried out extraction of Cu, Ni and Zn using various extractants in liquid membrane system.

Menger & Lee (1993) showed extraction of Cu(II) using six long chain ligands through liquid membrane system. The transport was proton driven and capable of moving Cu(II) 'uphill'.

16.8.9 As a basic preparative step for microencapsulation

A double emulsion film dehydration/rehydration approach was developed for encapsulation of haemoglobin at high concentration in liposomes. A double emulsion containing haemoglobin in internal aqueous phase and lipids in organic phase was prepared. The organic phase was then evaporated and water was dehydrated to form haemoglobin-lipid film that upon rehydration gave liposome encapsulated haemoglobin (Zheng et al., 1994).

Shah et al. (1987) prepared and evaluated albumin microcapsules containing sulphadiazine by o/w/o emulsification technique. Heat was utilized to denature albumin to form rigid capsule shell. The effect of viscosity of inner oil phase of multiple emulsion on size of capsules and release of drug was investigated.

Wang et al. (1992) reported formulation and process variables for the preparation of biodegradable poly-DL-lactide microspheres by multiple emulsion polymer precipitation technique.

Iwata & McGinity (1992) prepared multiphase microspheres of poly D, L-lacticglycolic acid containing chlorphenaramine maleate by multiple emulsion solvent evaporation technique and studied their dissolution, stability and morphological properties.

Alonso et al. (1994) prepared biodegradable microspheres of poly L-lactic acid, poly D, L-lacticglycolic acid by solvent evaporation/extraction method carried out in a w/o/w multiple emulsion system. The results suggested their use in producing higher and more sustained antibody levels.

Microballoons with hollow structure were prepared as a novel multi-unit floating device for use in stomach by emulsion solvent diffusion method. An antiallergic drug, transilast, was embedded in the shell of microballoon. In-vivo studies showed that the microballoons were dispersed in upper part of intestine against peristaltic motion (Kawashima et al., 1991).

Bodmeier et al. (1992) studied formulation and process variables for the preparation of wax microparticles by w/o/w emulsion technique.

16.8.10 Food applications

The loss of flavour (volatile compound 1-butanol as model) into gas phase from protein stabilized w/o/w multiple emulsion have been investigated using a head space analysis technique. Incorporation of butanol in multiple emulsion droplets leads to a reduction in the rate of release by about a factor of two (Dickinson et al., 1994).

Stability and nutrient release from model w/o/w multiple emulsion based on kerosene, Span 80 and Tween 20 was studied. The release of L-tryptophan and vitamin B2 was found to follow first order release with the release increasing near isoelectric point (Owusu et al., 1992).

16.9. CONCLUSIONS AND FUTURE PROSPECTS

Multiple emulsions offer interesting advantages as drug delivery system in that:

(i) they protect bioactives from degradation,

(ii) they are easy to administer via oral, parenteral, nasal, ocular or any other route,

(iii) they offer encapsulating compartments for both hydrophilic and lipophilic compounds with very high efficiency, the drug may be encapsulated as solution or suspension,

(iv) the drug release pattern may be prolonged or controlled,

(v) they may be targeted by both passive and active means by surface-modification,

(vi) they utilize pharmaceutically acceptable components which are non-toxic, non-immunogenic and biocompatible/biodegradable,

(vii) the components of formulation are economical and manufacturing equipments are easily accessible, there is no special requirement,

(viii) easy to produce and scale up.

Some aspect of multiple emulsions are not yet fully explored and require further study, such as :

(i) Optimizing stability of oil membrane.

(ii) Reducing the size of multiple emulsion droplets.

(iii) Potential as single-unit, multiple-drug encapsulated system.

(iv) Targeting of the system through surface modification.

(v) Pro-multiple emulsion formulation.

REFERENCES

Abd Elbary, A.; Nour, S.A.; Ibrahim, I. (1990) "Physical stability and rheological properties of w/o/w emulsions as a function of electrolytes." Pharm. Ind., 52(3): 357-363.

Abd Elbary, A.; Nour, S.A.; Mansour, F.F. (1984) "Efficacy of different emulsifying agents in preparing o/w/o and w/o/w multiple emulsions." Pharm. Ind., 46(9): 964-969.

Adeyeye, C.M.; Price J.C. (1991) "Effect of non-ionic surfactant concentration and type on the formation and stability of w/o/w multiple emulsions: microscopic and conductimetric evaluation." Drug. Dev. Ind. Pharm., 17(5): 725-736.

Akimoto, M.; Morimoto, Y. (1983) "Use of magnetic emulsion as a novel drug carrier for chemotherapeutic agents." Biomaterials, 4(1): 49-51.

Alonso, M.J.; Gupta, R.K.; Min, C.; Siber, G.R.; Langer, R. (1994) "Biodegradable microspheres as controlled-release tetanus toxoid delivery systems." Vaccine, 12(4): 299-306.

Andreu, C.; Galan, A.; Kobiro, K.; De Mendoza, J.; Park, T.K.; Rebek, J. Jr.; Salmeron, A.; Usman, N. (1994) "Transport of adenine mono and di nucleoside monophosphates across liquid membranes and extraction of oligonucleotides with synthetic carriers." J. Am. Chem. Soc., 116(12): 5501-5502.

Arai, K.; Fukuyama, S.; Kusu, F.; Takamura, K. (1994) "Effects of biologically important substances on spontaneous electrical potential oscillation across a liquid membrane of a water octanol water system." Bioelectrochemistry and bioenergetics, 33(2): 159-166.

Attia, M.A.; Habib, F.S. (1986) "Pilocarpine delivery from multiple emulsions." S.T.P. Pharm. Pract. 2: 636-640.

Baillet, A.; Pirishi, E.; Vaution, C.; Grossiord, J.L.; Ferrier-Baylocq, D.; Seiller, M. (1994) "Multiple emulsion of water in oil in water type: preparation and breakdown mechanisms." Int. J. Cosmet. Sci., 16(1): 1-15.

Baker, R.W.; Lonsdale, H.K. (1974) In: Controlled Release: Mechanisms and Rates. Controlled Release of Biologically Active Agents, Tonquary, A.O. and Lacey, R.E. (Eds.), Plenum press, New York, p.15-40.

Bevacqua, A.J.; Lahanas, K.M.; Cohen, I.D.; Cioca, G. (1991) "Liquid crystals in multiple emulsions." Cosmet. Toilet., 106: 53-56.

Bodmeier, R.; Wang, J.; Bhagwatwar, H. (1992) "Process and formulation variables in the preparation of wax microparticles by a melt dispersion technique: II. W/O/W multiple emulsion technique for water-soluble drugs." J. Microencap, 9(1): 99-108.

Brodin, A.F. , Kavaliunas, D.R.; Frank, S.G. (1978) "Prolonged release from multiple emulsions." Acta. Pharm. Suec., 15(1): 1-12.

Bromberg, L.E.; Klibanov, A.M. (1994) "Detergent-enabled transport of proteins and nucleic acids through hydrophobic solvents." Proceed, Natl. Acad. Sci. USA, 91(1): 143-147.

Brunetta, F.; Pantini, G. (1993) "Multiple emulsion comprising a perfluoropolyether (Fomblin HC)." Seifen Oele Fette Wachse, 119: 625-630.

Burbage, A.S.; Davis, S.S. (1979) "The characterization of multiple (W/O/W) emulsion using a radio-tracer technique." J. Pharm. Pharmacol., Suppl. 31: 6P.

Chiang, C.W.; Fuller, G.C.; Frankenfeld, J.W.; Rhodes, C.T. (1978) "Potential use of liquid membranes for drug overdose treatment : in vitro studies." J. Pharm. Sci., 67: 63-66.

Davis, S.S.; Walker, I. (1987) "Multiple emulsions as targetable delivery systems." Methods Enzymol., 149: 51-64.

De-Luca, M.; Grossiord, J.L.; Vaution, C.; Seiller, M. (1990) "W-O-W multiple emulsions: release mechanisms." Anais de Academia Bracileria de Ciencias, 62(3): 283-290.

Dickinson, E.; Evison, J.; Gramshaw, J.W.; Schwope, D. (1994) "Flavour release from protein-stabilized water-in-oil-in-water emulsion." Food Hydrocolloids, 8(1): 63-67.

Engel, R.H.; Riggi, S.J.; Fahrenbach, M.J. (1968) "Insulin: intestinal absorption as water-in-oil-in-water multiple emulsions." Nature, 219: 856-857.

Eros, I.; Balazs, J.; Peter,I.; Tacsi, M. (1990) "Investigation of drug-containing multiple phase emulsions." Pharmazie, 45(6): 419-422.

Ferreira, L.A.M.; Seiller, M.; Grossiord, J.L.; Marty, J.P.; Wepierre, J. (1994) "Vehicle influence on in vitro release of metronidazole: Role of w/o/w multiple emulsion." Int. J. Pharm., 109(3): 251-259.

Ferreira, L.A.M.; Doucet, J.; Seiller, M.; Grossiord, J.L.; Marty, J.P.; Wepierre, J. (1995) "In vitro percutaneous absorption of metronidazole and glucose: comparison of o/w, w/o/w, w/o systems." Int. J. Pharm., 121: 169-179.

Florence, A.T.; Jenkins, A.W.; Loveless, A.H. (1976) "Effect of formulation of intramuscular injections of phenothiazines on duration of activity." J. Pharm. Sci., 65: 1665-1668.

Florence, A.T.; Whitehill, D. (1982a) "Stabilization of multiple emulsions by polymerization of aqueous phases." J. Pharm. Pharmacol., 34(11): 687-691.

Florence, A.T.; Whitehill, D. (1982b) "The formulation and stability of multiple emulsions." Int. J. Pharm., 11: 277-308.

Florence, A.T.; Omotosho, J.A.; Whateley, T.L. (1989) "Multiple w/o/w emulsions as drug vehicles." In: Morton,R.(Ed.) Controlled release of drugs: polymers and aggregated systems, VCH Publishers, pp.163-183.

Fox, C. (1986) "Introduction to multiple emulsions." Cosmet. Toilet., 101: 101-106.

Freund, J. (1956) "The mode of action of immunological adjuvants." Adv. Tuberc. Res., 7: 130.

Fukushima, S, Juni, K.; Nakano, M. (1983) "Preparation of and drug release from w/o/w type double emulsions containing anticancer agents." Chem Pharm. Bull., 31 (11): 4048-4056.

Fukushima, S.; Nishida, M.; Nakano, M. (1987) "Preparation of and drug release from w/o/w type double emulsions containing anticancer agents using an oily lymphographic agent as an oil phase." Chem Pharm. Bull., 35: 3375-3381.

Garti, N.; Frenkel, M.; Shwartz, R. (1983) "Multiple emulsions: Part-2. Proposed technique to overcome unpleasant taste of drugs." J. Disp. Sci. Tech., 4(3): 237-252.

Goto, S.; Nakata, K.; Miyakawa, T.; Zhang, W.; Uchida, T. (1991) "Releasing properties of water-soluble drug in internal water phase of W/O/W multiple emulsions." Yakugaku Zasshi, 111(11): 702-708.

Hameyer, P.; Jenni, K.R. (1994) "Emulsifiers for multiple emulsions- optimization of stability by constitution and molecular weight." Perfum. Kosmet., 75: 819-850.

Hashida, M.; Muranishi, S.; Sezaki, H. (1977) J. Pharmacokin. Biopharma., 5: 241-247.

Herbert, W.J. (1965) "Multiple emulsion as adjuvants." Lancet, 2: 771-772.

Herbert, W.J. (1967) "Multiple emulsion adjuvants." Symp. Series Immunobio., 6: 89-90.

Higuchi, W.I. (1962) "Analysis of data on the medicament release from ointments." J. Pharm. Sci., 51: 802-810.

Hino, T.; Takeuchi, H.T.; Niwa, T.; Kitagawa, M.; Kawashima, Y. (1995) "The analysis of drug release from diluted water/oil/water emulsion by a model of the rupture of oil membrane." J.Pharm. Pharmacol., 47: 1-7.

Iwata, M.; Mc Ginity, J.W. (1992) "Preparation of multiphase microspheres of poly(D,L-lactic acid) and poly(D,L-lactic-co-glycolic acid) containing a w/o emulsion by a multiple emulsion solvent evaporation technique." J. Microencap., 9(2): 202-214.

Kassem, M.A.; Safwat, S.M.; Attia, M.A.; El-Mahdy, M.M. (1995) "Influence of phase volume ration of multiple emulsions on the ocular activity of prednisolone." S.T.P. Pharm. Sci., 5(4): 309-315.

Kassem, M.A.; Safwat, S.M.; Attia, M.A.; El-Mahdy, M.M. (1994) "Preparation and evaluation of hydrocortisone multiple emulsions in rabbits eye." Pharm. Ind., 56(6): 584-588.

Kavaliunas, D.R.; Frank, S.G. (1978) "Liquid crystal stabilization of multiple emulsion." J. Colloid Inter. Sci., 66(3): 586-588.

Kawashima, Y.; Hino, T.; Takeuchi, H.; Niwa, T. (1992) "Stabilization of water/oil/water multiple emulsion with hypertonic inner aqueous phase." Chem. Pharm. Bull., 40(5): 1240-1246.

Kawashima, Y.; Niwa, T.; Takeuchi, H.; Hino, T. and Ito, Y. (1991) "Preparation of multiple unit hollow microspheres (microballoons) with acrylic resin containing tranilast and their drug release characteristics (in vitro) and floating behaviour (in vivo)." J. Contrl. Rel., 16(3): 279-290.

Khopade, A.J.; Mahadik, K.R. and Kadam, S.S. (1995) "Stealth multiple emulsions for passive targeting of an antiinflammatory drug", Abstracts Book, International Seminar on Recent Trends in Pharmaceutical Sciences, Ootacamund, Feb. 18-20, C-5.

Khopade, A.J.; Mahadik, K.R. and Jain, N.K. (1996a) "Targeting of multiple emulsions to the lungs." Pharmazie, 51(8): 558-562.

Khopade, A.J.; Mahadik, K.R.; and Jain, N.K. (1996b) "Enhanced brain uptake of rifampicin from multiple emulsion via nasal route." Ind. J. Pharm. Sci., 2: 83-85

Khopade, A.J. and Jain, N.K. (1997) "Stabilized multiple emulsions uni/oligo droplet internal phase." Pharmazie, 52: 562-563

Khopade, A.J. and Jain, N.K. (1998) "Surface-modified multiple emulsions containing isoniazid for liver targeting." (unpublished results)

Kim, C.K.; Kim, S.C.; Shin, S.J.; Kim, K.M.; Oh, K.H.; Lee, Y.B. and Oh, I.J. (1995) "Preparation and characterization of cytarabine-loaded w/o/w multiple emulsion." Int. J. Pharm., 124: 61-67.

Kimura, J.; Nariuchi, H.; Watanabe, T.; Matuhasi, T.; Okayasu, I. and Hatakeyama, S. (1978a) "Studies on the adjuvant effect of water-in-oil-in-water emulsion in sesame oil I. Enhanced and persistent antibody formation by antigen incorporated into the water-in-oil-in-water emulsion." Jpn. J. Exp. Med., 48: 149-156.

Kover, T.; Csoka, I. and Eros,I. (1997a) "Formation and stability of multiple phase (w/o/w) emulsions Part 1: Investigation of the primary interface." Pharmazie, 52: 166-167

Kover, T.; Csoka, I. and Eros,I. (1997b) "Formation and stability of multiple phase (w/o/w) emulsions Part 2: Relationship between primary interface saturation and formation." Pharmazie, 52: 328-328.

Kovacic, D.; Vuleta, G.; Primorac, M. (1992) "Rheological characteristics of w/o/w multiple emulsions." Pharmazie, 47: 233-234.

Law, T.K.; Florence, A.T.; Whateley, T.L. (1983) "Release from multiple emulsion (w/o/w) stabilized by interfacial complexation." J. Pharm. Pharmacol., 36: 50-55.

Law, T.K.; Whateley, T.L.; Florence, A.T. (1986) "Stabilization of w/o/w multiple emulsion by interfacial complexation of macromolecule and non-ionic surfactant." J. Contrl. Rel., 3: 279-290.

Lee, S.C.; Lee, W.K. (1992) "Extraction of penicillin G from simulated media by an emulsion liquid membrane process." J. Chem. Tech. Biotech., 55(3): 251-261.

Le Moignic ; Penoy (1916) "Application to man of vaccines consisting of emulsions in fatty substances (lipovaccines) Comp." Rend. Soc. Biol., 79: 352.

Lin, S.Y.; Wu, W.H.; Lui, W.Y. (1992) "In-vitro release, pharmacokinetic and tissue distribution studies of doxorubicin hydrochloride (Adriamycin HCl) encapsulated in lipiodolized w/o emulsion and w/o/w multiple emulsion." Pharmazie, 47(6): 439-443.

Lin, S.Y.; Wu, W.H. (1991) "Physical parameters and release behaviours of w/o/w multiple emulsions containing cosurfactants and different specific gravity of oils." Pharm. Acta. Helv., 66(12): 342-347.

Lin, S.Y; Lui, W.Y (1992) "Zero-order or first-order release kinetics of water- in-oil-in-water (W/O/W) multiple emulsions of lipiodol dependent on the types of surfactants." Chem. Pharm. Bull., 40(10): 2860-2863.

Ma, J.L.; Xiaong, Q.M.; Tao, T.; Chen, R.Z. (1993) "Physicochemical properties and its release in-vitro of multiple emulsion containing etoposide." Chinese J. Pharm., 24(8): 357-360.

Madamwar, D.; Jain, N. (1992) "Photoosmosis through liquid membrane bilayers generated by mixture of bacteriorhodopsin and cyanocobalamin." J. Colloid Inter. Sci., 153(1): 152-156.

Madamwar, D.; Jain, N. (1993) "Photoosmosis through liquid membrane bilayers generated by mixture of beta-carotene coupled with bacteriorhodopsin." Appl. Biochem. Biotechnol., 37(2): 191-199.

Magdassi, S.; Garti, N. (1995) "Release of markers from the inner water phase of w/o/w emulsions stabilized by silicon based polymeric surfactants." J. Controlled Release, 33: 1-12.

Makryaleas, K.; Scheper, T.; Schugerl, K.; Kula, M.R. (1985) "Enzymatic production of L-amino acid with continuous co-enzyme regeneration by liquid membrane technique." Germ. Chem. Eng., 6: 345-350.

Matsumoto, S.; Kanig, W.W. (1989) "Formation and applications of multiple emulsions." J. Disp. Sci. Tech., 10(4-5): 455-482.

Matsuzawa, A.; Morishita,M.; Takayama, K.; Nagai, T. (1995) "Absorption of insulin using water-in-oil-in-water emulsion from enteral loop in rats." Biol. Pharm. Bull, 18: 1718-1723.

May, S.W.; Li, N.N. (1972) "The immobilization of urease using liquid surfactant membranes." Biochim. Biophys. Res. Commun. 47(5): 1179-1185.

May. S.W.; Landgraff, L.M. (1976) "Cofactor cycling in liquid membrane surfactant systems." Biochim. Biophys. Res. Commun., 68(3): 786-792.

Menger, F.M.; Lee, J.J. (1993) "Lipid-catalyzed transport of copper(II) through liquid membranes." J. Org. Chem., 58(7): 1909-1916.

Mishra, B.; Pandit, J.K. (1989) "Prolonged release of pentazocine from multiple O/W/O emulsions." Drug Dev. Ind. Pharm., 15(8): 1217-1230.

Mishra, B.; Pandit, J.K. (1990) "Prolonged tissue levels of pentazocine from W/O/W emulsions in mice." Drug Dev. Ind. Pharm., 16(6): 1073-1078.

Miyakawa, T.; Zhang, W.; Uchida, T.; Kim, N.S.; Goto, S. (1993) "In-vivo release of water soluble drug from stabilized water-in-oil-in-water (w/o/w) type multiple emulsions following intravenous administration using rats." Biol. Pharm. Bull., 16(3): 268-272.

Mohan, R.R.; Li, N.N. (1974) "Reduction and separation of nitrate and nitrite by liquid membrane encapsulated enzyme." Biotechnol. Bioenerg., 16: 513-523.

Mohan, R.R.; Li, N.N. (1975) "Nitrate and nitrite reduction by liquid membrane encapsulated whole cells." Biotechnol. Bioenerg., 17: 1137-1156.

Mohammed, A.A.; Ismail, S.; Habib, F.S.; Attia, M.A. (1988) "Availability of phenylephrine hydrochloride from ophthalmic multiple emulsions." Bull. Pharm. Sci. (Assiut Univ.) 11(2): 248-260.

Morimoto, Y.; Sugibayashi, K.; Yamaguchi, Y.; Kato, Y. (1979) "Detoxication capacity of multiple (w/o/w) emulsion for the treatment of drug overdose: drug extraction into the emulsion in the gastrointestinal tract of rabbits." Chem. Pharm. Bull., 27(12):3188-3192.

Morimoto, Y.; Yamaguchi, Y.; Sugibayashi, K. (1982) "Detoxication capacity of multiple (w/o/w) emulsion for the treatment of drug overdosage Part 2. Detoxication of quinine sulfate with the emulsion in the gastrointestinal tract of rabbits." Chem. Pharm. Bull., 30: 2980-2985.

Myers, S.L.; Shively, M.L. (1992) "Preparation and characterization of emulsifiable glasses: oil-in water and water-in-oil-in-water emulsions." J. Colloid Inter. Sci., 149(1): 271-278.

Nakhare, S.; Vyas, S.P. (1997) "Multiple emulsion based system for prolonged delivery of rifampicin." Pharmazie, 52: 224-226.

Nakhare, S.; Vyas, S.P. (1995) "Prolonged release multiple emulsion based system bearing rifampicin: in-vitro characterization." Drug. Dev. Ind. Pharm., 21(7): 869-878.

Nakhare, S.; Vyas, S.P. (1994) "Prolonged release of diclofenac sodium from multiple W/O/W emulsion systems." Pharmazie, 49: 842-845.

Oba, N.; Sigimura, H.; Umehara, Y.; Yoshida, M.; Kimura, T.; Yamaguchi, T. (1992) "Evaluation of an oleic acid water-in-oil-in-water-type multiple emulsion as potential drug carrier via the enteral route." Lipids, 27(9): 701-705.

Ohwaki, T.; Machida, R.; Ozawa, H.; Kawashima, Y.; Niwa, T. (1993a) "Improvement in stability of water-in-oil-in-water multiple emulsion by addition of surfactants in the internal aqueous phase of the emulsions." Int. J. Pharm., 93: 61-74.

Ohwaki, T.; Nakamura, M.; Ozawa, H.; Kawashima, Y.; Hino, T.; Takeuchi, H.; Niwa, T. (1993b) "Drug release from water-in-oil-in-water multiple emulsion in-vitro: II. Effects of addition of hydrophilic surfactants to the internal aqueous compartment on the release rate of secretin." Chem. Pharm. Bull., 41(4): 741-746.

Ohwaki, T.; Nakamura, M.; Ozawa, H.; Kawashima, Y.; Hino, T.; Takeuchi, H.; Niwa, T. (1993c) "Drug release from water-in-oil-in-water multiple emulsion in-vitro: II. Effects of addition of hydrophilic surfactants to the internal aqueous compartment on the release rate of water soluble drug." Yakuziagaku, 53(1): 44-54.

Omotosho, J.A.; Whateley, T.L.; Law, T.K.; Florence, A.T. (1986) "Nature of oil phase and the release of solutes from multiple (w/o/w) emulsions." J. Pharm. Pharmacol., 38: 865-870.

Omotosho, J.A. (1988) "Effect of chloroquine on globule structure of certain water-in-oil-in-water multiple emulsions." Pharm. World J., 5: 312-316.

Omotosho, J.A.; Whateley, T.L.; Florence, A.T. (1989a) "Methotrexate transport from internal phase of w/o/w emulsion." J. Microencapsulation, 6(2): 183-192.

Omotosho, J.A.; Florence, A.T.; Whateley, T.L. (1989b) "Release of 5-fluorouracil from intramuscular w/o/w multiple emulsions." Biopharm. Drug Dispo., 10: 257-268.

Omotosho, J.A.; Florence, A.T.; Whateley, T.L. (1990) "Absorption and lymphatic uptake of 5-fluorouracil in the rat following oral administration of multiple emulsion." Int. J. Pharm., 61: 51-56.

Owusu, R.K.; Zhu, Q.; Dickinson, E. (1992) "Controlled release of L-tryptophan and vitamin B-2 from model water/oil/water multiple emulsions." Food Hydrocolloids, 6(5): 443-453.

Oyenji, C.O.; Omotosho, J.A.; Ogunbona, F.A. (1992) "Increased gastrointestinal absorption from w/o/w emulsions." Ind. J. Pharm. Sci., 53(6): 256-258.

Oyenji, C.O.; Omotosho, J.A. (1993) "Bioavailability of nitrofurantoin from multiple w/o/w emulsions in man and the influence of the oil phase of the emulsion." Ind. J. Pharm. Sci., 55(1): 14-18.

Oza, K.P.; Frank, S.G. (1989a) "Multiple emulsion stabilized by colloidal microcrystalline cellulose." J. Disp. Sci. Tech., 10(2): 163-185.

Oza, K.P.; Frank, S.G. (1989b) "Drug release from emulsions stabilized by colloidal microcrystalline cellulose." J. Disp. Sci. Tech., 10(2): 187-210.

Pandit, J.K.; Misra, B.; Chand, B. (1987) "Drug release from multiple w/o/w emulsion." Ind. J. Pharm. Sci., 3: 103-105.

Pandit, J.K.; Misra, B.; Krishnaswamy, Y.; Mishra, D.N. (1988) "Prolonged plasma and brain levels of indomethacin from o/w/o emulsions." Ind. J. Pharm. Sci., 5: 274-275.

Raghuraman, B.; Termizi, N.; Weincek, J. (1994) "Emulsion liquid membranes for waste water treatment: Equilibrium models for some typical metal-extractant systems." Environ. Sci. Tech., 28(6): 1090-1098.

Roy, S.; Gupta, B.K. (1993) "In vitro- in vivo correlation of indomethacin release from prolonged release w/o/w multiple emulsion system." Drug. Dev. Ind. Pharm., 19(15): 1965-1980.

Safwat, S.M.; Samy, I.M.; Abdel-Rahman, M. (1994a) "Effect of formulation variables of multiple emulsion on the stability and antitremor activity of chlorphenoxamine hydrochloride." Bull. Pharm. Sci. (Assiut University), 17(2): 165-176.

Safwat, S.M.; Kassem, M.A.; Attia, M.A.; El-Mahdy, M.M. (1994b) "Formulation-performance relationship of multiple emulsions and ocular activity." J. Contrl. Rel., 32: 259-268.

Scholler, C.; Chauduri, J.B.; Pyle, D.L. (1993) "Emulsion liquid membrane extraction of lactic acid from aqueous solutions and fermentation broth." Biotechnol. Bioeng., 42(1): 50-58.

Sela, Y.; Magdassi, S.; Garti, N. (1995) "Release of markers from inner water phase of w/o/w emulsions stabilized by silicone based polymeric surfactants." J. Contrl. Rel. 33: 1-12.

Seifriz, W. (1925) "Studies in emulsions." J. Phy. Chem., 29: 738-749.

Seiller, M.; Vaution, C.; Grossiord, J.L.; Rabaron, A. (1991) "Multiple emulsion for skin care preparations." Actualities Pharmaceutiques, 41: 55-68.

Shah, M.V.; De Gennaro, M.D.; Suryakasuma, H. (1987) "An evaluation of albumin microcapsules prepared using a multiple emulsion technique." J. Microencap., 4(3): 223-238

Shichiri, M.; Shimizu, Y.; Yoshida, Y.; Kawamori, R.; Fukuchi, M.; Shigeta, Y.; Abe, H. (1974) "Enteral absorption of water-in-oil-in-water insulin emulsions in rabbits." Diabetalogia, 10: 317-324.

Shively, M.L.; Thompson, D.C. (1995) "Oral bioavailability of vancomycin solid-state emulsion." Int. J. Pharm. 117: 119-122.

Suzuki, A.; Morishita, M.; Kajita, M.; Takayama, K.; Isowa,K.; Chiba, Y.; Tokiwa, S.; Nagai,T (1998) "Enhanced colonic and rectal absorption of insulin using a multiple emulsion containing eicosapentaenoic acid and docosahexaenoic acid." J. Pharm. Sci., 87(10): 1196-1202.

Takahashi, T.; Mizuno, M.; Fujita, Y.; Ueda, S.; Nishioka, B.; Mazima, S. (1973) Gann., 64: 345-350.

Tao, T.; Ma, J.L.; Xiong, Q..M.; Chen, R.Z (1992) "Study on preparation of methotrexate-loaded multiple emulsion." Chinese J. Pharm., 23(9): 393-396.

Taylor, P.J.; Miller, C.L.; Pollock, T.M.; Perkins, F.T.; Westwood, M.A. (1969) "Antibody response and reaction to aqueous influenza vaccine, simple emulsion vaccine and multiple emulsion vaccine." J. hyg. (Camb.), 67:485-490.

Terrisse, I.; Seiller, M.; Rabaron, A.; Grossiord, J.L. (1993) "Rheology: how to characterize and to predict the evolution of w/o/w multiple emulsions." Int. J. Cosmet. Sci., 15(2): 53-62.

Tokgoz, N.S.; Grossiord, J.L.; Fructus, A.; Seiller, M.; Prognon, P. (1996) "Evaluation of two fluorescent probes for the characterization of W/O/W emulsions." Int. J. Pharm., 141: 27-37.

Vasiljevic, D.; Vuleta, G.; Dakovic L.J.; Primorac, M. (1994) "Influence of emulsifier concentration on rheological behaviour of w/o/w multiple emulsions." Pharmazie, 49: 933-934.

Wang, C.J.; Kuo, P.C.; Tien, J.H. (1992) "Process and formulation variables in the preparation of biodegradable microspheres by sovent evaporation method: I. W/O/W technique for water soluble drugs." Chinese Pharm. J., 44(3): 199-210.

Wu, Q.Z.; Ping, Q.N.; Liu, G.H. (1990a) "Blood glucose-reduced efficiency of insulin multiple emulsion for experimental diabetic mice by oral administration." Chinese J. Pharm., 21(10): 445-448.

Wu, Q.Z.; Ping, Q.N.; Liu, G.H. (1990b) "Formulation and physical stability of W/O/W multiple emulsion." Chinese J. Pharm., 21(6): 252-255.

Yan, N.; Zhang, M.; Ni, P. (1992) "A study of stability of W/O/W multiple emulsions." J. Microencap., 9(2): 143-151.

Yazan, Y.; Seiller, M.; Puisieux, F. (1993) "Multiple emulsions." Boll. Chim. Farmaceutico., 132: 187-196.

Yoshioka, T.; Ikeuchi, K.; Hashida, M.; Muranishi, S.; Sezaki, H. (1982) "Prolonged release of Bleomycin from parenteral gelatin-sphere-in-oil-in-water multiple emulsion." Chem. Pharm. Bull., 30(4): 1408-1415.

Zatz, J.L.; Cueman, G.H. (1988) "Assesment of stability in water-in-oil-in-water multiple emulsions." J. Soc. Cosmet. Chem., 39: 211-222.

Zheng, S.; Beissenger, R.L.; Wasan, D.T. (1991) "The stabilization of hemoglobin multiple emulsion for use as a red cell substitute." J. Colloid Inter. Sci., 144(1): 72-85.

Zheng, S.; Beissenger, R.L.; Wasan, D.T. (1992) "Measurement of yield of hemoglobin (HB)-in oil-in water multiple emulsion based on HB encapsulation efficiency." J. Disp. Sci. Tech., 13(1): 33-44.

Zheng, S.; Zheng, Y.; Beissenger, R.L.; Wasan, D.T.; McCormick, D.L. (1993) "Hemoglobin multiple emulsion as an oxygen delivery system." Biochim. Biophys. Acta, 1158: 65-74.

Zheng, S.; Zheng, Y.; Beissenger, R.L.; Fresco, R. (1994) "Microencapsulation of hemoglobin in liposome using a double emulsion film dehydration/rehydration approach." Biochim. Biophys. Acta, 1196(2): 123-130.

Chapter 17 _____

Solid Lipid Nanoparticles

Shelly Utreja , N.K.Jain

17.1 INTRODUCTION

Solid lipid nanoparticle (SLN) dispersions have been proposed as a new type of colloidal drug carrier system suitable for intravenous administration. The system consists of spherical solid lipid particles in the nanometer range, which are dispersed in water or in aqueous surfactant solution. Generally, they are made of solid hydrophobic core having a monolayer of phospholipid coating .The solid core contains the drug dissolved or dispersed in the solid high melting fat matrix. The hydrophobic chains of phospholipid are embedded in the fat matrix. They have potential to carry lipophilic or hydrophilic drugs or diagnostics. (Domb, 1993).

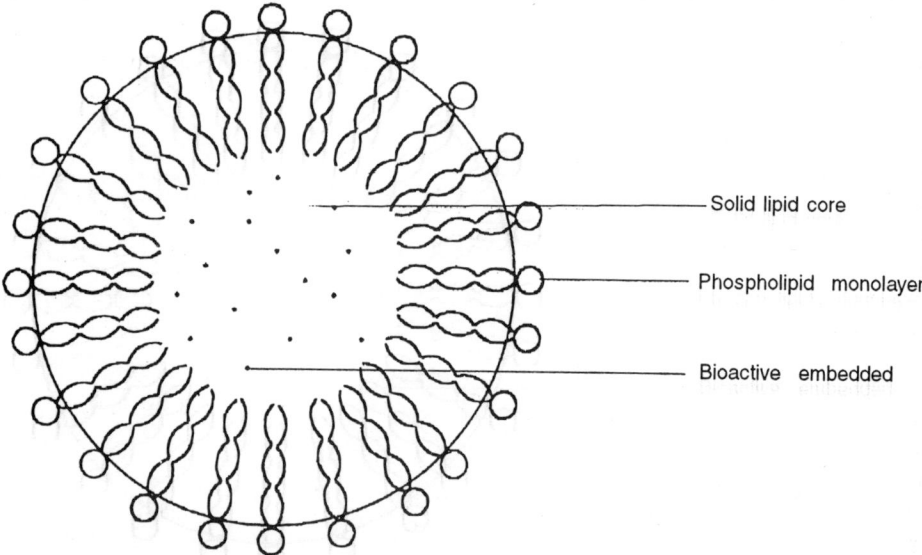

        — Solid lipid core

        — Phospholipid monolayer

        — Bioactive embedded

Fig 17.1 Schematic illustration of proposed structure of SLN

   Various colloidal drug carrier systems such as liposomes, fat emulsions, nanoparticles for the controlled delivery of drugs by intravenous route are well known. Each of these particulate carriers possesses specific advantages and disadvantages (Table17.1) (Schwarz et al., 1994).

   There are major differences between lipid emulsions and liposomes. The basic structure of a lipid emulsion is a neutral lipophilic oil core surrounded by a monolayer of amphiphilic lipid (phospholipid). In contrast, liposomes contain an outer bilayer of amphipathic molecule such as phospholipid with an aqueous compartment inside. The amount of poorly water-soluble drug that is possible to incorporate is, however, limited due to the relatively small volume (0.7ml /mmol of lipid) of the hydrophobic region of the lipid bilayer in comparison to

Table 1: Comparative Properties of Solid Lipid Nanoparticles, Polymer nanoparticles, Liposomes, Lipid emulsions

S. No.	Property	SLN	Polymer nanoparticles	Liposomes	Lipid emulsions
1.	Systemic toxicity	Low	>or=to SLN	Low	Low
2.	Cytotoxicity	Low	>=to SLN	Low	Low
3.	Residues from organic solvents	No	Yes	May or may not	No
4.	Large scale production	Yes	No	Yes	Yes
5.	Sterilization by autoclaving	Yes	No	No	Yes
6.	Sustained Release	Yes	Yes	< or =to SLN	No
7.	Avoidance of RES	?	No	Yes	Yes

the aqueous interior (2-3 ml/mmol of lipid). Emulsifier/ drug ratio is high in case of liposomes. Moreover, incorporation of a lipophilic drug into bilayer membrane changes the properties of the particles and results in loss of control of delivery. A satisfactory long-term physical and chemical stability for liposomes is hard to achieve (Shaw et al., 1976). They tend to fuse and are therefore relatively unstable on storage. They often display instability in the vascular system due to lipid exchange with lipoproteins (Allen, 1981). Liposomes have been sterilized by g radiations. However, this treatment causes the loss of integrity of bilayer component (Sculier et al., 1986).

Commercially available phospholipid-triglyceride emulsions such as Intralipid 10% and 20% (Kabivitrum), LipofundinS (Braun), Travemulsion (Travenol) and Liposyn (Abbott) widely used in clinical medicine for parenteral nutrition over long periods of time, have been investigated as a parenteral drug delivery system especially for lipophilic drugs (Garti, 1996; Me Niff, 1977; Davis et al., 1987; Lundberg, 1991; Paborji et al., 1988 ; Prankered et al., 1988).They are non toxic and are sufficiently stable to be stored at room temperature for long periods. They are autoclavable (Mizushima, 1985). However, they are hardly suited for sustained release in any case because of rapid immobilization of incorporated drug molecule due to fluid core.

The solid nanoparticulate supports, which are generally made with suitable biodegradable polymers, such as polyalkylcyanoacrylate, polymethylmethacrylate have been shown to prolong the release of the incorporated drugs (Couvreur, 1996; Fessi et al., 1988; Puisieux et al., 1994). The major disadvantages of polymeric nanoparticles are their relatively slow biodegradability (upto 3-4weeks), which might cause systemic toxicity by impairment of reticuloendothelial system as well as cytotoxicity towards macrophages, presence of residual toxic agents (organic solvents) employed during preparation and lack of reproducibility (Kante et al.,1982). Polymeric nanoparticles cannot be sterilized by autoclaving. They have been sterilized by γ radiation. However, this treatment causes the formation of unacceptable toxic reaction products.

Solid lipid nanoparticles (SLNs) combine advantages of polymeric nanoparticles, fat emulsions and liposomes but simultaneously avoid some of their disadvantages. They are biodegradable and non-toxic; stable against coalescence, drug leakage, hydrolysis, particle growth oftenly observed in lipid emulsions and liposomes. Unlike lipid emulsions, which have a fluid core, they possess a solid matrix, which has the potential for allowing drug release over a prolonged period. Other advantages include low cost of ingredients, ease of preparation and scale up, high dispersibility in an aqueous medium, high entrapment of hydrophobic drug, controlled particle size and extended release of entrapped drug after single injection from few hours to several days. The perspectives for the use of SLN for controlled drug delivery were discussed by Muller & Mehnert, (1995) in detail. They reported a prolonged in vitro release of upto 6 weeks for prednisolone.

17.2 METHODS OF PREPARATIONS

Various methods have been developed for the preparation of aqueous dispersions of lipid nanoparticles. The different production methods use biocompatible lipids or lipid molecules with a history of safe use in medicine. The essential excipients of SLNs are solid lipids as matrix material and amphipathic lipids as surface stabilizer. Solid lipids such as saturated monoacid triglycerides (tristearin, tripalmitin, trilaurin etc), hard fat, cetyl palmitate, fatty acids (stearic acid, behenic acid etc) and cholesteryl acetate are recommended to be used as matrix for solid lipid nanoparticles. Physiologically compatible emulsifiers such as phospholipids, bile salts and Poloxamers are preferred as stabilizers.

17.2.1 Melt-homogenization technique

SLNs can be produced by homogenization of the molten lipids in an aqueous phase (Siekmann & Westesen, 1992; Muller et al., 1993). The preparation of solid lipid nanoparticles by this technique involves two steps. First, the lipids are heated at least 10°C above their melting point. The melted lipids are then dispersed in hot aqueous medium using a suitable dispersing agent. Dispersion is accomplished using mechanical stirring or by ultrasonication. The pre-mix formed is then passed through a thermostatized high-pressure homogenizer under optimum homogenization conditions. The second step involves the solidification of oil droplets by cooling the hot dispersion to room temperature. For drug loaded SLNs, the drug is dissolved either in melted lipid or in hot aqueous phase prior to emulsification.

This technique uses high-pressure homogenizer, which reduces efficiently the number of large particles and produces particle dispersions suitable for I.V. injections. A combination of shear, turbulence, collision, cavitation forces and intense mixing are among the factors responsible for the production of fine droplets with a narrow size distribution. There are a number of production parameters (matrix constituents, type and amount of emulsifying agent, volume fraction of the dispersed phase, pressure and the number of homogenization cycles) inherent in this process which may have profound effects on physical stability of the product. As far as homogenization parameters (pressure, number of cycles) are concerned, it has been found that a moderate increase in homogenization pressure and number of cycles reduce the number of large particles due to progressing dispersion of the oil phase. But this effect reaches a plateau value at some point, which must be determined during process development. The constant particle number indicates the plateau value or the dispersion limit. Once the dispersion limit is reached, further increase in homogenization pressure or cycle number can cause breaking of emulsion due to droplet coalescence. The droplets coalesce due to their high kinetic energy, which overcome the stabilizing energy barrier of electrostatic repulsion. It should be kept in mind that optimum homogenization conditions differ for each nanoparticle system and cannot be generalized. The difference may be due to the difference in the diffusion velocity of the surfactant monomers from the bulk phase into the interface. The limiting factor is the substitution of monomers removed from the bulk phase by monomers from micelles or undissolved surfactant. Diameter of SLNs has been found to decrease as the molar ratio of core/coating material increases, until a plateau is reached. After this point the diameter of SLNs is unaffected by further increase in the molar ratio. Increase in surfactant concentration reduces the diameter of bulk population.

17.2.2 Microemulsification -solidification

SLNs can be produced by microemulsification of molten lipids, as the internal phase, and subsequent dispersion of the microemulsion in aqueous medium under mechanical stirring (Cavalli et al., 1995; Gasco & Morel, 1990; Gasco et al, 1992a,b). Microemulsions are clear, thermodynamically stable, microheterogeneous dispersions usually obtained by mixing oil, water, surfactant and co-surfactant. The diameter of the disperse phase droplet is always below 100nm (Shah, 1985). Moreover, their preparation doesnot require energy. Rapid crystallization of oil droplet on dispersion in cold aqueous medium produces lipid nanoparticles with solid matrix. Cavalli et al, (1993) prepared solid lipid nanoparticles incorporating doxorubicin and idarubicin from o/w microemulsion prepared at 65-70°C. The microemulsion was prepared using stearic acid as internal phase, purified egg lecithin as surfactant, taurodeoxycholate sodium as co-surfactant and distilled water as continuous phase. Drug loaded SLNs were prepared by adding drug to melted stearic acid at about 65-70° C. Surfactant, warm water, and the co-surfactant were successively added to the melted mixture. A clear microemulsion was easily obtained under stirring at about 65-70°C. SLNs were then obtained by dispersing the warm microemulsion in distilled cold water (2-3°C) under mechanical stirring; the dispersion were washed twice with distilled water by ultrafiltration. After washing, the suspension was freeze-dried.

The microemulsions require presence of a co-surfactant for their production. When lecithin alone is used as a single surfactant it will not produce balanced microemulsion. It favors the formation of reverse microemulsion over a very limited range of concentration. This is because the lecithin molecule is too lipophilic; it has a critical packing parameter, Cpp, of approx. 0.8 favoring the formation of lamellar phase or bilayers. The Cpp is further increased in a microemulsion if the oil phase of a microemulsion penetrates into the long alkyl chains of the lecithin. In order to produce a balanced lecithin microemulsion, it is necessary to reduce its effective Cpp. This can be achieved by the use of co-surfactants. They can alter the effective Cpp in one of two ways, either by making the aqueous phase less hydrophilic and/or by their incorporation into the interfacial film. The co-surfactant can also have a third effect, in that it can reduce the tendency of lecithin to form highly rigid films thus allowing the interfacial film sufficient flexibility to take up the different curvatures required to form balanced microemulsion. So we can say that the co-surfactant acts in bulk aqueous phase (to decrease the effective Cpp) and in the interfacial layer (to decrease the effective Cpp and rigidity of the lecithin monolayer) to produce balanced lecithin microemulsion. However, the ideal co-surfactant would exert an effect on the interfacial surfactant layer, which would allow the infinite dilution of the microemulsion without destruction due to the dilution of the co-surfactant below effective levels (Aboofazeli et al, 1994).

Utreja et al, (1999) prepared lipid nanoparticles for the delivery of MTX by instantaneous cooling of the microemulsion. Gasco et al, (1992a) prepared lipospheres containing timolol maleate as ion pairs. The amount of drug incorporated varied from 2.7 to 4.8% due to the difference in the lipophilicity of the ion pairs of the drug.

17.2.3 Multiple microemulsification solidification

Multiple emulsions are complex systems, often called emulsions of emulsions, in which drops of dispersed phases contain smaller droplets that have the same composition as the external phase. Like simple emulsions, multiple emulsions are also considered to be of two types: oil-in-water-in-oil (o/w/o) and water-in-oil-in-water (w/o/w). Multiple emulsions have shown potential applications in controlled release for drug delivery (Mishra et al., 1988; Khopade & Jain, 1996). Multiple microemulsions (w/o/w) can be used to prepare SLNs with potential to vectorize hydrophilic drug.

Warm w/o/w multiple microemulsion can be prepared in two steps. Firstly, w/o microemulsion is prepared by adding an aqueous solution containing drug to a mixture of melted lipid, surfactant and co-surfactant at a temperature slightly above the melting point of lipid to obtain a clear system. In second step, the formed w/o microemulsion is added to a mixture of water, surfactant and co-surfactant to obtain a clear w/o/w system. SLNs can be obtained by dispersing the warm micromultiple emulsion in cold aqueous medium in a fixed ratio, under mechanical stirring. The suspension of lipid particles is then washed with dispersion medium by ultrafiltration system.

Multiple emulsions have inherent instabilities due to coalescence of the internal aqueous droplets within the oil phase, coalescence of the oil droplets, and rupture of the oil layer on the surface of the internal droplets (Florence & Whitehill, 1982). In case of SLNs production, they have to be stable for few minutes, the time between the preparation of the clear multiple microemulsion and its quenching in cold aqueous medium, which is possible to achieve. This method of SLNs production needs to be investigated. Only few reports based on this methodology are available. Morel et al., (1994) exploited this method to prepare solid lipospheres containing hydrophilic drug- the peptide [D-Trp-6] LHRH. A system with following composition was used to incorporate the drug (Table 17.2).

Table 17.2

S.NO.	Component	Composition %	
		W/O Microemulsion	W/O/W Microemulsion
1	Stearic acid	55 %	-
2	Egg lecithin	14%	7%
3	Butyric acid	20%	7%
4	Aqueous solution of peptide	11%	-
5	Taurodeoxycholate	-	7%
6	W/o(internal phase)	-	7%
7	Water	-	72%

17.3 CHARACTERIZATION OF SLNs

In order to develop a drug product of high quality, a precise physico-chemical characterization of solid lipid nanoparticles is necessary. The parameters generally used to ensure that a standard product is made by the process in use include the particle size and its distribution, morphology, and surface charge, the drug loading capacity, the drug release profile, and the physical state of the lipid particles.

17.3.1 Particle size, morphology, and zeta potential

Particle size characteristics are of great importance for dispersions suitable for parenteral administration. The limiting factor for i.v. administration is the number of large particles (greater than 5 μm) which can potentially block blood capillaries. The USP XXIII limits the particulate matter in small volume injections (100 ml or less) to 6000 particles per container equal or greater than 10 μm For i.v. use of SLN dispersions the presence of particles of average diameter above 5 μm should in any case be avoided. To assess i.v. injectability, the SLN dispersions are compared with emulsions for parenteral nutrition, with regard to the particles in the micrometer range (Muller et al., 1995). The required maximum injection volume of SLN dispersions can be estimated by considering the necessary single dose of the drug, the typical loading capacity of the lipid matrix and the maximum lipid content of the SLN dispersion.

Modification of the size significantly affects the physical stability and the biofate of the nanoparticles. The average size and size distribution of solid lipid nanoparticles is also important with respect to the release rate of the loaded drug. So the size of SLNs will have to be controlled within reasonable limits.

The particle size depends on the matrix constituents as well as on the type and amount of emulsifying agent. The choice of the lipid has been found to affect SLNs diameter. Systems containing the suppository mass Witepsol W35 as the lipid component have been found to form the finest dispersions compared to tripalmitate containing systems, which may be attributed to the presence of surface-active mono- and diglycerides, which probably facilitate emulsification. It has been reported that the increase in the amount of emulsifier generally decreases the mean diameter of the bulk population but not significantly effecting the Polydispersity Index (PI) (Westesen et al., 1993). Particle size depends on the molar ratio of the total amount of oil and emulsifier. Heiati et al., (1996) observed the decrease in the mean diameter of the SLN comprised of a high melting triglyceride (TG) core with a phospholipid (PL) coating as the molar ratio of PL to TG was increased. The diameter decreased as the molar ratio was increased until a plateau was reached at a molar ratio of 0.15. After this point the diameter of the SLNs was unaffected by further increase in the molar ratio. They demonstrated that high molar ratio of PL to TG causes the formation of multiple bilayer structure around the solid lipid core of SLNs. The size and the structure of the incorporated drug is also a factor affecting SLNs size and tends to increase the average diameter and PI of SLNs (Cavalli et al., 1998).

The size of particles obtained from saturated monoacid triglycerides tends to increase with triglyceride chain length, which may be due to the increasing viscosity of the triglyceride melts (Bunjes et al., 1996). The choice of the emulsifying agent has been found to affect SLNs diameter. The phospholipid/ tyloxapol (P/T) blend yields smaller particles than the phospholipid /bile salt (P/Bs) blend. The smaller particle sizes observed in P/T stabilized dispersions may partially be attributed to the higher surfactant/triglyceride (S/T) ratio. Preparation of P/T stabilized lipid nanoparticles requires larger amounts of emulsifier to obtain dispersions with homogeneous size distribution than preparation with P/Bs blends (Westesen et al.,1993; Siekmann & Westesen, 1994; Westesen et al.,1997). The choice of the dispersion method is also found to affect the size of SLNs. Production of SLNs by high-pressure homogenization (HPH) proved to be most effective in reducing the number of large particles.

There are a number of methods used to determine this physical attributes, but photon correlation spectroscopy and electron microscopy techniques are the most commonly used tools.

Photon Correlation Spectroscopy (PCS): It is an established technique based on dynamic laser light scattering due to Brownian motion of particles in solution/ suspension, suitable for the measurement of particles in the range of 3nm to 3mm. The PCS device consists of a laser source, a temperature-controlled sample cell, and a photomultiplier for detection of the scattered light. The PCS diameter is based on the intensity of the light scattering from the particles. Nanoparticles are generally polydisperse in size, and the polydispersity index (PI) give a measure of the size distribution of the nanoparticle population (Koppel, 1972). Theoretically, PI is zero for a monodisperse colloidal suspension, however, standard latex particles with a polydispersity index of about 0.05 are practically 'monodisperse'. Polydispersity index (PI) greater than 0.5 indicate a very broad size distribution. From the PCS data, the mean particle diameter of the bulk population and the PI of the SLN dispersions can be calculated. The popularity of this method depends on its ease of operation and the speed by which one can obtain data. To be analyzed, the samples only need to be diluted to an appropriate concentration in a solvent, which is usually filtered water.

Atomic Force Microscopy (AFM) Advanced microscopic technique, such as atomic force microscopy is applied as a new tool to image the original unaltered shape and surface properties of the particles. In AFM, a small probe is brought into close proximity to the object and this technique utilizes the force acting between the surface and the probing tip resulting in a spatial resolution of upto 0.01nm for imaging. A striking advantage of AFM is the simple sample preparation as no vacuum is needed during operation and the sample need not be conductive. Hence, it allows the analysis of hydrated, solvent containing samples. The speed at which AFM obtains images is fast enough to permit the observation of in situ processes occurring at interface.

For AFM investigations, the particles are fixed on an appropriate smooth substrate surface to allow an unambiguous distinction between the particles and the surface. For non-contact mode imaging standard polished silicon water surface with a roughness below 1nm can be used to place the nanoparticles. In case of contact mode operation the tip touches the sample surface and may result in alterations of the sample surface, such as the removal of particles from the area under investigation. This can be avoided by fixing the nanoparticles on silicon water surface roughened to values of up to 10nm by etching the wafers in hydrofluoric acid and ammonium fluoride. The measurements are performed under ambient air conditions. In addition to topography imaging, AFM allows the study of mechanical properties of the system. Monitoring the force acting between the tip and the sample while the tip is approaching the sample surface can reveal the hardness of the sample. Muhlen, (1996) demonstrated that the results of particle size measurements by PCS and AFM are in the same magnitude of size.

Electron Microscopy: Electron microscopy techniques such as SEM and TEM are very useful in ascertaining the overall shape and morphology of lipid nanoparticles. It allows the determination of particle size and distribution. SEM uses electrons transmitted from the specimen surface while TEM uses electrons transmitted through their specimen. SEM has high resolution and the sample preparation is relatively easy. However, to be analyzed the nanoparticles must be able to withstand a strong vacuum and they have to be conductive. Therefore, the surface of the sample is coated with conductive metal (gold), but this can modify the original aspect of the particles.

Zeta potential is a measure of charge on the particles. It imparts colloidal stability due to particle-particle repulsion. A zeta potential measurement also helps in designing particles with reduced reticuloendothelial (RES) uptake. In order to divert SLNs away from the RES or lymphatic system, the surface of the particles should be hydrophilic and non-charged (Muller,1991). Siekmann, (1995) incubated freshly prepared lecithin-stabilized tripalmitate lipospheres with Poloxamer 407 and Poloxamine 908 solution and confirmed polymer adsorption by measurements of the zeta-potential employing Laser Doppler Anemometry. The zeta potential was considerably reduced i.e. from -29.6 mV to -1.9 & -2.9 mV for fresh liposphere and Poloxamer 407 & Poloxamine 908 coated lipospheres.

Structure of SLNs   The structure of SLNs can be determined by 31P nuclear magnetic resonance (NMR) technique after Mn2+ or Pr3+ ion complexation . The other methods include labeling of SLNs formulation containing phosphatidylethanolamine with trinitro benzene sulphonic acid (TNBS). The agent reacts specifically with surface polar phosphate heads on SLNs. There is a optimum ratio of core lipid: phospholipid when surface phosphate groups are maximum. When phospholipid is further increased there is a decrease in surface phosphate groups resulting into decrease in 31P nuclear magnetic resonance peak area. It has been seen that other phospholipid structures such as liposomes are formed inside where many polar phosphate groups are concealed inside concentric bilayers (Heiati et al., 1996).

17.3.2 Crystallization Tendency and Polymorphic Behavior of SLN

Solid lipid nanoparticles are based on physiologically tolerable lipids, predominantly saturated monoacid triglycerides or hard fats that are solid at room temperature as matrix constituents. The rationale behind the use of lipids that are solid at room temperature as a carrier matrix is that emulsified molten lipids resolidify on cooling producing solid particles. The solid state of the particles is of prime importance, as it reduces the mobility of incorporated drug and thus prevents drug leakage from the carrier. Moreover, the rigid solid particles are less prone to stability problems (coalescence). As the potential advantages of these novel drug carrier systems essentially rely on the solid state of the lipid particles, the solidification of the particles after the homogenization process must be ensured. It has to be taken into consideration that some lipid particles may not recrystallize in the colloidally dispersed state and can remain in the supercooled state for a long period of time.

The melting and crystallization behavior or the kinetics of polymorphic transitions of lipids in the dispersed state can differ significantly from that of their bulk material. The presence of emulsifiers, the preparative method and the high dispersity as well as the small particle size of the colloidal drug carrier systems may account for changes in the crystallization behavior, the degree of crystallinity, and the crystal modifications of the matrix constituents compared to the bulk materials. Before going into details, it is necessary to understand the polymorphic behavior of triglycerides (matrix constituents). Triglyceride molecules have the ability to reveal different unit cell structures in crystal, originating from a variety of molecular conformations and molecular packing or we can say that they have the ability to crystallize as more than one distinct crystalline species and are said to be polymorphic. The main polymorphic forms are the a, b', and b forms. These different polymorphs have different melting points, X-ray diffraction patterns, and solubilities, even though they are chemically identical. a is the least stable form and can be obtained on cooling from melt. The progression of polymorphic transitions occurs in this direction:

| Liquid | → | alpha (α) | → beta prime (β') | → | beta form (β) |
| (melt) | | (low melting meta stable) | | | (high melting stable form) |

This transition is the pathway for triglycerides to the optimum form of the molecule i.e. more stable crystalline structure and cannot occur in the opposite direction. Dispersed triglyceride particles recrystallize on rapid cooling in the metastable a form and transform rapidly via the b' form into the thermodynamically stable b form upon heating or storage. These transitions are slow in bulk triglycerides. The recrystallization of the colloidally dispersed triglycerides occurs at lower temperature than that of the bulk material. Emulsions of supercooled melts rather than dispersions of solid particles are formed when the particles do not recrystallize even on enforced cooling below a critical recrystallization temperature.

The nanoemulsions of supercooled melts deviate substantially from solid lipid nanoparticles in their properties. Severe stability problems related to recrystallization of the lipids, such as the formation of gel-like system, considerable particle growth and expulsion of incorporated drug do not occur in nanoemulsions of supercooled melts. Although their drug incorporation capacity is higher than that of crystallized nanoparticles, yet they are thermodynamically unstable. The physical state of the matrix influences the in-vitro and in-vivo release characteristics of dispersions. Drug release from solid matrix is expected to be degradation controlled and slower than diffusion controlled release from emulsions.

Basic techniques to determine the physico-chemical state of particles include thermal analysis and X-ray diffraction.

Thermal Analysis It covers a group of techniques in which a physical property of a substance is monitored as a function of controlled temperature. The techniques most commonly used in pharmacy include differential thermal analysis (DTA) and differential scanning calorimetery (DSC). DTA measures the temperature differences between a reference material and the sample, whereas DSC quantifies the enthalpic changes during endothermic or exothermic thermodynamic phase transitions. Among these methods, differential scanning calorimetery is quite diverse a technique in measuring enthalpic changes during endothermic or exothermic thermodynamic phase transitions accurately. Melting and crystallization generally produce endothermic and exothermic effects respectively. Fig 17.2 illustrates a schematic of a typical DSC thermogram.

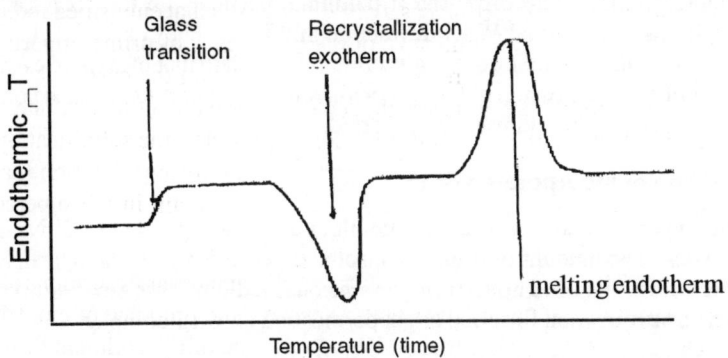

Fig 17.2 : Schematic of typical DSC thermogram

The maxima and minima in the DSC thermogram indicate the melting and recrystallization temperature of the lipid respectively. Supercooling is given as the difference between these two temperatures. The different polymorphic forms can be assigned by correlation with the X-ray data. There are very few reports on the DSC curves and X-ray diffraction pattern of triglyceride nanoparticles in the literature.

Tristearin and tripalmitin nanoparticles are crystalline when stored at room temperature, while trimyristin and trilaurin nanoparticles show no sign of crystallinity and remain in the liquid state for at least several months of storage. Supercooled trilaurin nanoparticles can be forced to recrystallize at subzero temperature, while in contrast, supercooled trimyristate particles crystallize immediately when stored below their critical recrystallization temperature of around 10^0C. The tendency of colloidally dispersed triglycerides towards the formation of supercooled melts increases with decreasing triglycerides chain length.

X-Ray Diffraction When a monochromatic x-ray beam is focused on a crystal, the regularly placed atoms scatter the x-ray beam in a specific diffracting pattern, producing a finger-print for each atomic crystal or molecule. The wavelength of x-rays, λ, is related to the angle of incidence, q, and the interatomic distance, d, by Bragg's equation

$$n\lambda = 2d \, Sin\theta$$

Where n is the order of the distance, 1,2,3 etc. The direction of the diffracted beam and its intensity are characteristic for a given polymorph of a substance. This technique is able to discriminate between amorphous and crystalline substances. Since amorphous materials have no orderly arranged crystal lattice, they display a more or less regular baseline, crystalline materials on the other hand are reflected in many diffraction bands.

Synchrotron radiation X-ray (SAX) is a diffraction technique, which provides an efficient way to compare the recrystallization of the lipid nanosuspension with that of the bulk material. It allows one to identify the crystal modification even in dilute suspensions of submicron particles. Its ability to perform simultaneously time resolved small and wide-angle diffraction measurements allow a very comprehensive study on physical state and on the polymorphism of the glyceride dispersions.

Westesen et al., (1993) investigated lipid dispersions containing approximately 10% lipid (w/w) by Synchrotron radiation small angle and wide angle X-ray diffraction. SAX diffraction studies confirmed the crystalline state of particles but failed to permit a clear distinction between the crystal modification. WAX diffraction measurements revealed that all investigated carrier systems were in the β crystalline modification at room temperature. At body temperature the carriers were either β -crystalline or amorphous liquids depending on the matrix constituents. Time resolved X-ray diffraction measurements during temperature scans demonstrated that the dispersed lipids recrystallize in the a-form whereas the bulk lipids recrystallize in the b' modification and transform rapidly into the β-form. Bunjes et.al., (1994) studied the effect of incorporation of lipophilic drug ubidecarenone into dispersed tripalmitate particles on the recrystallization tendency and polymorphic transitions by SAX and WAX diffraction and DSC. They observed that incorporation of drug had no effect on the crystalline structure of the glyceride compared to that of an pure carrier, high concentration of drug caused a significant depression of the recrystallization temperature. An accelerating effect of the drug on the formation of the b polymorph was also reported.

17.3.3 Determination of incorporated drug

It is of prime importance to measure the amount of drug incorporated in SLNs, since it influences the release characteristics. The amount of drug encapsulated per unit wt. of nanoparticles is determined after separation of the free drug and solid lipids from the aqueous medium. This separation can be carried out using ultracentrifugation, centrifugation filtration or gel permeation chromatography.

In centrifugation filtration the filters such as Ultrafree →-MC (Millipore) or Ultrasart→ 10 (Sartorius) are used along with classical centrifugation techniques. The degree of encapsulation can be assessed indirectly by determining the amount of drug remaining in the supernatant after centrifugation filtration /ultracentrifugation of SLN suspension or alternatively by dissolution of the sediment in an appropriate solvent and subsequent analysis. Standard analytical techniques such as spectrophotometry, spectrofluorophotometry, high-performance liquid chromatography, or liquid scintillation counting can be used to assay the drug (Magenheim & Benita, 1991). In gel permeation chromatography Sephadex® and Sepharose® gels are used for removal of free drug from SLN preparations. First, preliminary calibration of column is carried out using SLNs and free drug. SLN preparations are applied to the column and eluted with suitable buffer. Fractions containing SLNs can be collected and analyzed for the actual drug content after dissolution/extraction with appropriate solvent.

Drug content can also be determined directly in SLNs by extracting the drug with suitable solvent under optimum conditions and subsequent analysis of aqueous extract.

17.3.4 In-vitro drug release studies

In vitro drug release studies are mainly useful for quality control as well as for the prediction of in-vivo kinetics. Unfortunately, due to the very small size of the particles, the release rate observed in vivo can differ greatly from the release obtained in a buffer solution. However, in vitro release studies remain very useful for quality control as well as for evaluation of the influence of process parameters on the release rate of active compounds.

In vitro drug release profile from SLNs can be evaluated by various experimental methods. Release profile of drug can be conducted in dialysis tubing or without tubing. In dialysis, the SLN dispersion is introduced into prewashed dialysis tubing, which is then hermetically sealed. The dialysis sac is dialyzed against dissolution medium at constant temperature with constant stirring. The released drug diffuses through the dialysis membrane. Samples from dissolution medium are taken at discrete times, centrifuged, and assayed for drug content. The sink conditions must be maintained during release studies (Fig 17.3). Washington, (1989) criticized this method and claimed that perfect sink conditions are not maintained during release studies, since SLN dispersions are not directly diluted in the dissolution medium. As a result, the rate of drug appearance in the dissolution medium does not reflect its real release rate, but rather the concentration gradient between the continuous phase of the SLN dispersion and the dissolution medium. Levy & Benita, (1990) reported a technique, which avoids the enclosure of the colloidal drug carrier in a dialysis sac. This technique is based on reverse dialysis. In this technique, the SLN dispersion is directly diluted in the release medium so that perfect sink conditions can be maintained. A number of small dialysis sacs containing 1ml of buffer are then suspended in the release medium for the monitoring of amount of drug released. The potential drawback of this method is that it is not 'sensitive' enough to characterize rapid release rate of drug from colloidal carrier. However, it can be assumed that if the drug is released over much more than one hour, then this method can be used for in vitro release profile investigation from colloidal carriers.

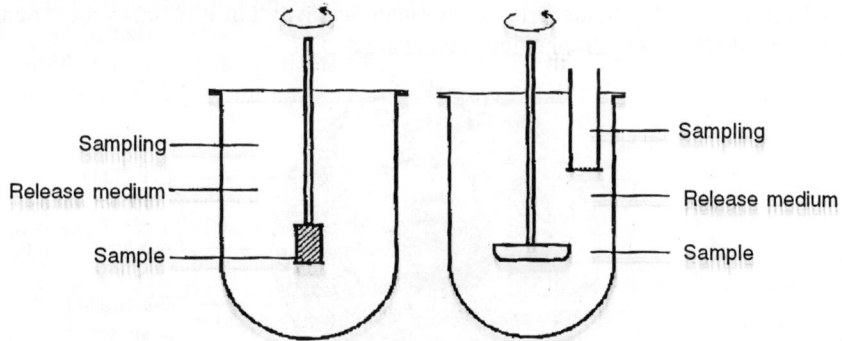

Fig 17.3 : Diagrammatic representation of the appratus used for drug release studies

The in vitro kinetic methods based on dilution and separation (Tsai et al., 1986; Farah et al., 1987) employ direct dispersion of lipid nanoparticles in the release medium. At specified time intervals, samples of the diluted dispersion solution are withdrawn. After separation of solution from the SLNs the amount of drug released in the solution can be assessed. This method is efficient only if successful and rapid separation of the SLNs from the aqueous phase is achieved to prevent further drug release in release medium after sampling. Because of small size of the SLNs this is likely to be difficult.

17.3.5 Rheology

Rheological measurements of formulations can be conducted in a Brookefield Viscometer, using an appropriate spindle number. The viscosity depends upon the dispersed lipid content. Usually flow is newtonian but becomes non-newtonian for high lipid content.

17.3.6 Storage stability

The physical stability of the SLNs during prolonged storage can be determined by monitoring changes in particle size, drug content, appearance, viscosity as a function of time. Since with the passage of time the PC components can be hydrolyzed to lyso-PCs, the chemical changes also need to be monitored. This can be accomplished by thin -layer chromatography.

17.4 STEALTH SLNs

One of the main obstacle in systemic use of colloidal carriers designed to deliver active principles to targeted tissues is the presence of reticuloendothelial system (RES) which recognizes them as foreign products and quickly removes them from blood circulation. The rate of RES mediated clearance of colloidal carriers is so fast that the half-life of the carrier reduces significantly. It is therefore very much necessary to overcome such recognition and capture occurring. The clearance of particles from blood stream is believed to be related to the process of their interaction with blood plasma proteins (opsonins), resulting in attachment of the particles to the membrane of macrophages (opsonization). The capacity of the carriers to avoid opsonization and, consequently, macrophage uptake mainly depends on their size, surface hydrophobicity, surface mobility (Muller, 1991; Illum & Davis, 1984). Many strategies have been proposed to prolong the circulation lifetime of SLNs by avoiding RES recognition. The hydrophilic and flexible polymer coating on SLNs is thought to mask the surface from opsonins marking the particle for uptake by RES. Bocca et al., (1998) obtained sterically stabilized SLNs, using two lipid derivatives of monomethyl poly (ethylene) glycol 2000 (PEG 2000) as stealthing agents: dipalmitoyl phosphatidylethanolamine-PEG 2000 and stearic acid-PEG 2000. The molecules of these two stealthing agents consist of a hydrophilic and lipophilic moiety; PEG 2000 represents hydrophilic part in both cases. The hydrophilic PEG chains form a conformational hydrophilic cloud over the nanoparticles that protect the SLNs and affect their hydrophobicity and charge.

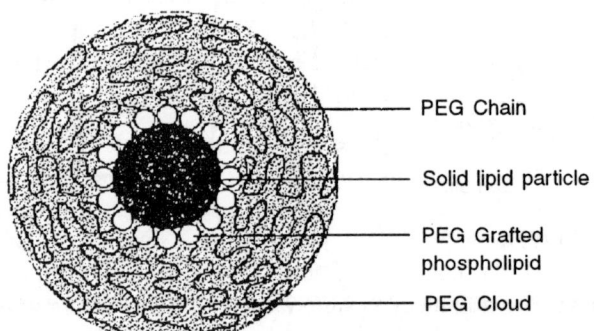

PEG Chain

Solid lipid particle

PEG Grafted phospholipid

PEG Cloud

Fig 17.4 : Stealth solid lipid nanoparticles

A decrease in zeta potential of stealth SLNs results consequently. The hydrophilic nanoparicles escape from recognition by RES and can remain in circulation for prolonged periods; on the contrary, hydrophobic nanoparticles are phagocytized actively. The amount of stealthing agent to be used is critical. Too high amount of stealthing agent may not be able to decrease SLNs uptake by macrophages. Jeon et al., (1991) proposed that the high surface density and long chain lengths of PEG are necessary for low protein adsorption and that surface density has a greater effect than chain length on steric repulsion and Van der Waals attraction.

Stabilization of SLNs with Poloxamer also leads to a distinct reduction in phagocytosis, consequently, resulting in prolonged blood circulation. The Poloxamer is added during the production process of the SLNs. It adsorbs partially on particle and partially grafts into the particle surface during homogenization. The adsorption layer increases the surface hydrophilicity, minimizing adherence to cell membranes by hydrophobic interaction, the first required step for phagocytosis (Muller, 1991). In general, the surface hydrophilicity of the Poloxamer adsorption layer increases with increasing adsorption layer thickness and ultimately leads to a decrease in phagocytic uptake (Muller & Blunk, 1989).

17.5 EX-VIVO STUDIES

17.5.1 Phagocytosis assay of SLN

The in vitro phagocytosis of SLNs can be assessed by chemiluminescence (CL) and fluorimetry. Chemiluminescence allows continuous measurements of the phagocytic uptake regardless of the nanoparticle type and does not require labeling of the particles. The main drawback of CL is that it gives no information on the adsorption process (Rudt & Muller, 1992). A fluorimetric method allows the simultaneous analysis of mixed cell populations by cell-by-cell fluorescence measurement (Leroux et al., 1994). In this technique the choice of fluorescent marker is of prime importance. Whatever the assay chosen, a careful selection of the incubation medium and cell model is necessary to study the effect of modifying the nanoparticle surface on their uptake by cells. Macrophages and blood cells such as granulocytes can be used as a model to study phagocytosis.

Culture of macrophages

Bocca et al., (1998) in a study used Murine macrophages cell line J 744 A12 to assess the phagocytic uptake of SLNs. The cells were grown in monolayers in RPMI 1664 medium supplemented with 10% fetal bovine serum at 37^0C and 5% CO_2. After incubating the cells for 24 hrs at 37^0C in a 24 well culture plate they were washed to remove non-adherent cells. The adherent cells were further incubated in DME F12 medium (Gibco) with 10% fetal bovine serum. Cell numbers were adjusted so that each well contained about $5x10^5$ cells. After 24h incubation, 24ml of aqueous dispersion of fluorescent SLNs were added. Following incubation periods of 2.5,5,10,40,60,90 min., the cells were washed and rinsed twice with the culture medium to remove the non phagocytosed SLNs. The extent of phagocytosis was assessed by measuring the concentration of the phagocytosed SLNs in the resuspended cells as a function of intensity of fluorescence. The results are expressed as percentage of the dose/$1x10^6$ cells.

Muller et al., (1997) studied the in vitro phagocytosis of SLNs in suspension of human granulocytes. Human granulocytes were obtained by density centrifugation. Briefly, three ml of blood were added to 3ml of M-PRM medium and centrifuged at 400g for 30 min. The granulocytes suspension was adjusted with Dulbecco's phosphate buffer (PBC) to 5x106 cells per ml, 50ml of this suspension were given per well of microtitre plates (250000 cells/well). The uptake of particles by human granulocytes was determined by chemiluminescence. For the CL assay the granulocytes were incubated with 100ml luminol solution per well for 30 min. One hundred ml of SLN were added to each well and the CL intensity (arbitrary unit) recorded for 120 min. The uptake was quantified by calculating the area under the curve (AUC) of the intensity/time profiles (integration of CL in arbitrary units, time in minutes, yielding arbitrary AUC units). The AUC was found to be correlated with total particle mass internalized at the analytical parameters applied in the assay. As an alternate to the AUC the maximum CL intensity can be used as a measure for phagocytic uptake. In order to define adequate in vitro models, the choice of the incubation conditions should be reevaluated continuously depending on the in vivo results. These in vitro models represent promising in vitro tools for predicting the in vivo fate of the particles.

17.5.2 Cytotoxicity assessment

To assess the injectability of SLNs with regard to toxicological acceptance, the in vitro cytotoxicity of the SLNs needs to be investigated. The viability can be chosen as cytotoxicity parameter and can be determined using the MTT (3-(4,5-dimethylthiazol-2yl)-2,5-diphenyltetrazolium bromide) test on microtitre plates (Mosmann, 1983). Muller et al., (1997) observed the cytotoxicity of the glyceride SLNs -10 fold below the one of polylactide/glycolide nanoparticles. For cytotoxicity assessment, the granulocytes (50ml) are incubated with SLN (50ml) for 120 min., MTT solution (100ml) is added and further incubated for 4h. Living cells take up the MTT, which is reduced in the mitochondria to the blue tetrazolium, salt. The formed blue crystals can be dissolved in isopropanol (100 ml) and the absorbance is then measured at 550 nm.

17.6 STERILIZATION OF SOLID LIPID NANOPARTICLES

For parenteral administration, the sterility of the solid lipid nanoparticles is of utmost importance. Aseptic production, filtration, g-irradiation and autoclaving are commonly used to achieve sterilization. Filtrative sterilization of the dispersed system needs high pressure and is not applicable to nanoparticles (Weinstein & Leserman, 1984). However, the filtration method using nylon 66 Ultipor® 0.45mm membrane with CWST (critical water surface tension) value >80 dynes/cm may be used if mean particle size is less than 0.45 mm. Such membrane can be obtained by treating nylon 66 membrane with acrylates possessing -OH groups in their side chains. Aseptic procedures can be applied in order to produce sterile SLN but are very complex and expensive. Gamma sterilization can be chosen, but this treatment has been reported to cause unacceptable chemical breakdown of bilayer components in phospholipid based drug carriers such as liposomes (Sculier et al., 1986). The most popular and convenient method is sterilization by autoclaving at 121°C for at least 15 min.

With SLN dispersions, the high temperature reached during sterilization by autoclaving presumably causes a hot o/w microemulsion to form in the autoclave, and probably induces change in the size of the hot particles. On subsequent slow cooling, the SLNs reform, but nanodroplets may coalesce, producing larger SLNs than the initial ones. During heat sterilization, chemical composition of the carrier and incorporated drug may also undergo changes. Drug may also leak out of the carrier. Therefore, it is highly desirable to study the stability of SLNs following sterilization. Heiati et al., (1988) reported insignificant changes in SLNs mean diameter, zeta potential and incorporated drug content after autoclaving (Table 17.3).

Table17.3 : Mean diameter, zeta potential and drug content of SLN's constituted of trilaurin (core) and phospholipid coating.

SLN	Before autoclaving			After autoclaving		
	Diameter (nm)	Zeta Potential (mV)	Incorporated AZT–P (%)	Diameter (nm)	Zeta Potential (mV)	Incorporated AZT–P (%)
Neutral	200 $\pm$ 30	-5 $\pm$ 3	72 $\pm$ 5	219 $\pm$ 29	-5 $\pm$ 2	62 $\pm$ 6
Negative	294 $\pm$ 27	-15 $\pm$ 3	92 $\pm$ 4	311 $\pm$ 28	-13 $\pm$ 2	80 $\pm$ 5

Mean ± SD of three experiment; Neutral SLN's contains DPPC as the PL & negative SLNs contains DPPC : DMPG (95:5 molar ratios) as the PL.

They subjected SLN preparations to temperature stability testing as the thermal stress is reported to have an effect on the characteristics of dispersed submicron particles (Klang et al., 1994). For thermal stability testing, the SLNs were incubated for 10 weeks at 4, 20, 37°C. The SLNs mean diameter, zeta potential and incorporated drug content were determined during the incubation period. It was observed that autoclaved SLNs were stable for a period of 10 weeks at 20°C but an increase in particle size and loss of drug occurred at 4 and 37°C (Fig 17.5).

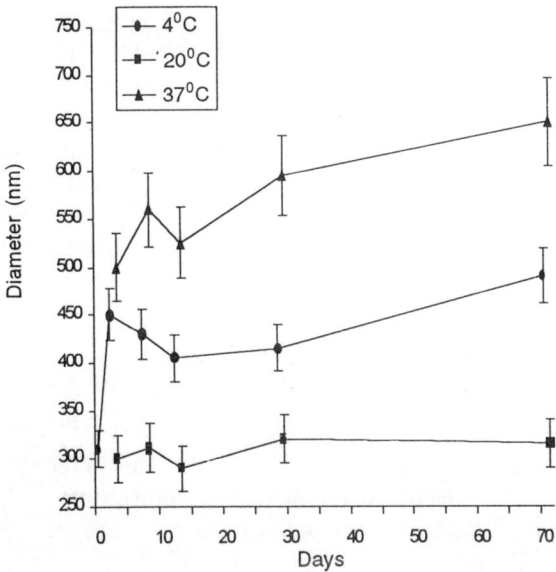

Fig 17.5 : Effect of thermal stress on the stability of negatively charged SLNs. (The stability profile of neutral SLNs was identical to that of negatively charged SLNs.)

Cavalli et al., (1997) reported the physical stability of SLNs during sterilization. They confirmed by TEM analysis that SLN maintained a spherical shape and narrow size distribution after sterilization (Fig 17.6).

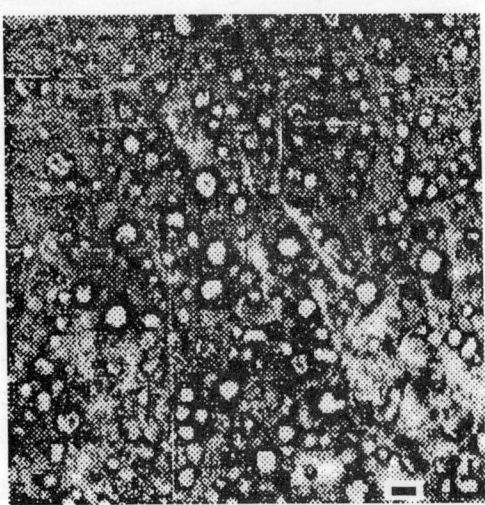

Fig 17.6 : Sterilized SLN consititued of behenic acid after 15 months at 40°C Bar =100μm

It was observed that all dispersions presented nanoparticles in the colloidal range after sterilization (Table 17. 4).

Table 17.4 : Average diameter and polydispersity index of SLNs containing diazepam, before and after sterlization.

Lipid Used	Average Diameter(nm)		Polydispersity Index	
	Drug Free SLN	**Drug Loaded SLN**	**Drug Free SLN**	**Drug Loaded SLN**
Stearic acid				
Before	78.5	55.0	0.16	0.20
After	120.0	110.0	0.20	0.25
Behenic acid				
Before	86.0	70.0	0.15	0.21
After	116.0	135.0	0.18	0.22
Acidan NI$_2$				
Before	70.0	60.0	0.18	0.23
After	75.5	65.0	0.16	0.22

To verify the effect of storage conditions on SLNs size they monitored the stability of sterilized SLNs over time by measuring the size of nanoparticles after fixed storage times (1day, 2,4,6,8,10,12 months at 40^0C). It was observed that all dispersions were uniform, with no separation between aqueous phase and nanoparticles after more than 1year.

17.7 LYOPHILIZATION

It involves the removal of water from products in the frozen state at extremely low pressure and has great potential to extend the shelf- life of drugs and drug carriers. Dry products with sufficient long-term stability and reconstitution properties can be obtained by lyophilization.

Because of limited stability of SLNs as aqueous dispersions, it is highly desirable to have a freeze-dried SLNs formulation available. A prerequisite is a good reconstitution performance. The freeze-drying process may change the size and shape of the SLNs. As the size of SLNs is a limiting factor for parenteral administration, it is very much necessary to control the size and avoid nanoparticle growth during freeze-drying. The use of cryoprotectants can protect SLNs against the formation of aggregates during freeze- thaw or freeze drying process. Lyophilization can induce structural and functional damage to phospholipid membrane. Cryoprotective sugars have been reported to minimize the damage to PL membranes due to their ability to form hydrogen-bond to phospholipid head groups, thus supplanting water as the membrane stabilizer (Crowe et al., 1988; Ma et al., 1994). According to Crowe et al., (1985) it is desirable to have carbohydrate on both sides of PL membrane to ensure its stabilization during freeze-drying. The choice of the appropriate type and concentration of cryoprotectant for a maximum of protection can be made by freeze-thaw cycles. The cryoprotectants which proved most effective in the freeze-thaw pre-test are then employed in a standard lyophilization process. Usually, for freeze-drying the SLN dispersions are diluted with the cryoprotectant solution and are rapidly frozen at temperatures ranging from -40^0C to -60^0C in an acetone/dry ice bath or in liquid nitrogen. Lyophilization is then carried out under vacuum for periods ranging from 24 to 90h. Changes in particle size distribution during lyophilization can be minimized by optimizing the parameters of lyophilization process like freezing velocity, pressure, and temperature and redispersion method. Schwarz & Mehnert, (1997) studied the effect of freezing velocity by adding SLNs dispersion dropwise to liquid nitrogen (Method A) or by dipping the whole vial of SLNs into liquid nitrogen (Method B). They observed fast freezing by method B to be most efficient for trehalose and glucose protected Dynasan-SLNs (Fig 17.7)

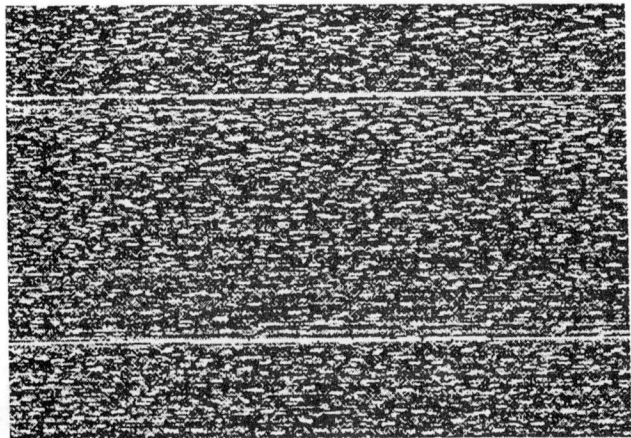

Fig 17.7 : Diameters 10, 50, 90, 95 and 99% of reconstituted lyophilised Dynasan-SLNs

Cryoprotectants were trehalose 15% (left) and glucose 15% (right).

Freezing methods: slow freezing on the shelves (-25^{0}C), rapid freezing by addition of SLNs dropwise to liquid nitrogen (-196^{0}C (A)) or by dipping the whole vial into liquid nitrogen

(-196^{0}C (B)). Redispersion by manual shaking.

They also investigated the influence of redispersion method and reported that manual shaking and dispergator were slightly less effective for Dynasan-SLNs than sonication. Lyophilised SLNs can be reconstituted in a quality considered suitable for I.V. injection with regard to the size distribution. Heiati et al (1998) observed 100% drug retention in SLNs after reconstitution and concluded that drug loaded SLNs can be lyophilized and reconstituted without significant changes in size and zeta potential.

17.8 CONCLUSION

Solid lipid nanoparticles represent a particulate system which can be produced with an established technique. They present an interesting approach to the parenteral administration of poorly water-soluble drugs. The advantages of SLNs as a potential carrier for hydrophobic drugs are their safety and biocompatibility. The possibility of preparing multiple, warm microemulsions means that SLNs carrying hydrophilic drugs can be obtained, realizing a prolonged release. Due to their solid physical state they can circumvent or reduce the pitfalls of conventional drug delivery system. Depending on the matrix constituent the lipid carriers display differences in their physical state at body temperature which may influence their biopharmaceutical behaviour. The behavior of SLNs is generally constrained by phagocytic cells of the RE system. However, stealth SLNs with their size in nanometer range, might provide a way to circumvent this problem and allow the escape from the RES while ensuring efficient targeting. Although, no marketed product has yet emerged, it is surely a matter of time as extensive research work give cause for optimism. We are confident that SLNs will prove its place in enhancing the effectiveness, convenience, and general utility of new and existing drugs.

REFERENCES

Aboofazeli, R.; Lawrence, C.B.; Wicks, S.R.; Lawrence, M.J. (1994) Int. J. Pharm., 111:63.

Allen, T.M. (1981) Biochim. Biophys. Acta, 640:385

Bocca, C.; Caputo, O.; Cavalli, R.; Gabriel. L.; Miglietta, A.; Gasco, M.R. (1998) Int. J. Pharm., 175:185.

Bunjes, H.; Westesen, K.; Koch, M.H.J. (1996) Int. J. Pharm., 129:159.

Bunjes, H.; Westesen, K.; Koch, M.H.J. (1994) Eur. J. Pharm. Sci., 2:177

Cavalli, R.; Caputo, O.; Marengo, E.; Pattarino, F.; Gasco, M.R. (1998) Pharmazie, 53:392

Cavalli, R.; Caputo, O.; Carlotti, M.R.; Trotta, M.; Scarnecchia, C.; Gasco, M.R. (1997) Int. J. Pharm., 148:47

Cavalli, R.; Caputo, O.; Gasco, M.R. (1993) Int. J. Pharm., 89:R9.

Cavalli, R.; Morel, S.; Gasco, M.R.; Chetoni, P.; Saettone, M.F. (1995) Int. J. Pharm., 117:243.

Couvreur, P.; Couarraze, G.; Devissaguet, J.P.; Puisieux, F. (1996) In : Microencapsulation Methods & Industrial application, Marcel Dekker Inc., New York, Basel & Hongkong, pp 183

Crowe, J.H.; Crowe, L.M.; Carpenter, J.F.; Rudolph, A.S.; Wistrom, C.A.; Spargo, B.J.; Anchordoguy, T. (1988) Biochim. Biophys. Acta, 947:367

Crowe, L.M.; Crowe, J.H.; Rudolph, A.S.; Womersley, C.; Appel, L. (1985) Arch. Biochem. Biophys., 242:240

Davis, S.S.; Washington, C.; West, P.; Illum, L.; Liversidge, G.; Sternson, L.; Kirsh, R. (1987) Ann. N.Y. Acad. Sci., 507:75

Domb, A.J. (1993) U. S. Patent, 5, 188:837

Farah, N.; Bouzon, J.; Rollet, M.; Taverdet, J.L.; Vergnaud, J.M. (1987) Int. J. Pharm., 36:81

Fessi, H.; Puisieux, F.; Devissaguet, J.P. (1998) U.S. Patent No. 5118528

Florence, A.T.; Whitehill, D. (1982) Int. J. Pharm., 11:277.

Garti, N.; Aserin, A. (1996) In : Microencapsulation Methods & Industrial Application, Benita, S. (Ed), Marcel Dekker Inc., New York, Basel & Hongkong, pp 45.

Gasco, M.R.; Cavalli, R.; Carlotti; M.E. (1992a) Pharmazie, 47:119.

Gasco, M.R.; Morel, S.; Carpignano, R. (1992b) Eur. J. Pharm. Biopharm., 38:7.

Gasco, M.R.; Morel, S. (1990) Farmaco, 45(Oct) : 1127.

Heiati, H.; Phillips, N.C.; Tawashi, R. (1996) Pharm. Res., 13(9) : 1406.

Heiati, H.; Tawashi, R.; Phillips, N.C. (1998) J. Microencap., 15(2):173.

Illum, L.; Davis, S.S. (1984) FEBS Lett., 767:79.

Jeon, S.I.; Lee, J.H.; Audrade, J.D.; deGennes, P.G. (1991) J. Coll. Int. Sci., 142:149.

Kante, B.; Couvreur, P.; Dubois-Krack, G.; De Meester, C.; Guiot, P.; Roland, M.; Speiser, P. (1982) J. Pharm. Sci., 71:786

Khopade, A.J.; Jain, N.K. (1996) Pharmazie, 51:558.

Klang, S.H.; Frucht-Pery, J.; Hoffman, A.; Benita, S. (1994) J. Pharm. Pharmacol., 46:986.

Koppel, D.E. (1972) J. Chem. Phys., 57:4814.

Leroux, J.C.; Gravel, P.; Balant, L.; Volet, B.; Anner, B.M.; Allemann, E.; Doelker, E.; Gurny, R. (1994) J. Biomed. Mater. Res., 28:471.

Levy, M.Y.; Benita, S. (1990) Int. J. Pharm., 66:29.

Lundberg, B. (1991) : In Lipoproteins as Carriers of Pharmacological Agents, Shaw, J.M. (Ed), Marcel Dekker Inc., New York , pp 97

Ma, X.; Santiago, N.; Chen, Y.S.; Chaudhary, K.; Milstein, S.J.; Baughman, R.A. (1994) J. Drug. Targeting, 2:9.

Magenheim, B.; Benita, S. (1991) S.T.P. Pharma. Sci., 1:221.

MeNiff, B.L. (1977) Am. J. Hosp. Pharm., 34:1080

Mishra, B.; Pandit, J.K.; Tiwari, P. (1988) Eastern Pharmacist, XXXI:77

Mizushima, S. (1985) Drugs Exp. Clin. Res., 11:595.

Morel,S.; Gasco, M.R.; Cavalli, R. (1994) Int. J. Pharm., 105:R1

Mosmann,T. (1983) J. Immunol. Meth., 65:55.

Muhlen, A.Z.; Muhlen, E.Z.; Niehus,H.; Mehnert, W. (1996) Pharm. Res., 13(9) :1411.

Muller, R.H. (1991) In : Colloidal Carriers for Controlled Drug Delivery & Targeting, Wissenschaftliche Verlagsgesellschaft, Stuttgartuller, CRC Press Bola Raton.

Muller, R.H.; Schwarz, C.; Mehnert, W.; Lucks, J.S. (1993) Proc. Int. Symp. Controlled Release Bioactive Mater., 20:480.

Muller, R.H.; Maassen,S.; Schwarz, C.; Mehnert, W. (1997) J. Control. Rel., 47:261

Muller, R.H.; Blunk, T. (1989) Arch. Pharm., 322:699.

Muller, R.H.; Mehnert, W.; Lucks, J.S.; Schwarz, C.; Zur Muhlen, A.; Weyhers, H.; Freitas, C.; Ruhl,D. (1995) Eur. J. Pharm. Biopharm., 41 (1) :62

Muller, R.H.; Mehnert, W. (1995) Dtech. Apoth. Ztq., 135(Jul.13): 35-36, 39-41.

Paborji, M.; Riley, C.; Stella, V. (1988) Int. J. Pharm., 42:243.

Prankered, R.; Frank, S.; Stella, V. (1988) J. Parenter. Sci. Technol., 42:76.

Puisieux, F.; Barratt, G.; Couarraze, G.; Couvreur, P.; Devissaguet, J.P.; Dubernet, C.; Fattal, E.; Fessi, H.; Vauthier, C.; Benita, S. (1994) In : Polymeric Biomaterials, Dumitriu (Ed), Marcel Dekker Inc., New York, pp 749

Rudt, S.; Muller, R.H. (1992) J. Control. Rel., 22:263.

Schwarz, C.; Mehnert, W. (1997) Int. J. Pharm., 157:171.

Schwarz, C.; Mehnert, W.; Lucks, J.S.; Muller, R.H. (1994) J. Control. Rel., 30:83.

Sculier, J.P.; Coune, A.; Brassine, C.; Laduron, C.; Atassi, G.; Ruysschert, G.M.; Fruhling, J. (1986) J. Clin. Oncol., 4:789.

Shah, D.S. (1985) In : Macro and Microemulsions, Theories and Applications, A.C.S. Symposium Series.

Shaw, I.H.; Knight, C.G.; Dingle, J.T. (1976) Biochem. J., 158:473

Siekmann, B ; Westesen, K. (1992) Pharm. Pharmacol. Lett., 1:123

Siekmann, B. (1995) Ph. D. Thesis, University of Braunschweig.

Siekmann, B.; Westesen, K. (1994) Pharm. Pharmacol. Lett., 3:194

Tsai, D.C.; Howard,S. A.; Hogan, T.F.; Malanga, C.J.; Kandzari, S.J.; Ma, J.K.H. (1986) J. Microencap., 3:181

Utreja ,S.; Khopade, A.J.; Jain, N.K. (1999) Pharm. Acta Helv.,73:275

Washington, C. (1989) Int. J. Pharm., 56:71.

Weinstein,J.N.; Leserman, L.D. (1984) Pharmacology & Therapeutics, 24:207.

Westesen, K.; Bunjes, H.; Koch, M. H.J. (1997) J. Control. Rel., 48:223.

Westesen, K; Siekmann, B.; Koch, M.H.J. (1993) Int. J. Pharm., 93:189

Chapter 18

Transfersomes - A Novel Carrier for Effective Transdermal Drug Delivery

Subheet Jain, Sanjay Jain, Dipankar Bhadra, N.K.Jain

18.1 INTRODUCTION

Poor patient compliance is a frequent problem in daily clinical practice. The unfavorable pharmacokinetic of the drug, the inconveniences of the standard form of such drug application and the side effects due to the administration route often are the reasons for this. Consequently much effort has been put into the development of strategies that could improve the patient compliance with new modes of drug application. Delivery via the transdermal route is an interesting option in this respect because transdermal route is convenient and safe. This offers several potential advantages over conventional routes (Shaw & Chandrasekaran, 1989) like avoidance of first pass metabolism, predictable and extended duration of activity, minimizing undesirable side effects, utility of short half-life drugs, improving physiological and pharmacological response, avoiding the fluctuation in drug levels, inter- and intra-patient variations, and most importantly, it provides patient convenience. But one of the major problem in transdermal drug delivery is the low penetration rate through the outermost layer of the skin, the stratum corneum (Schatzlein & Cevc, 1995; Cevc, 1997). To date many chemical and physical approaches have been applied to increase the efficacy of the material transfer across the intact skin, by use of the penetration enhancers, iontophoresis, sonophoresis and the use of colloidal carriers such as lipid vesicles (liposomes and proliposomes) and nonionic surfactant vesicles (niosomes and proniosomes). Initially various chemical additives (such as alcohols, azones, surfactants etc.) (Cooper, 1987) were used to increase the lipid fluidity in the outer skin layers and thus improve the skin permeability to various agents. Use of penetration enhancers has some limitations like applicable only for low molecular weight drugs (smaller than 500 to 1000 Da), skin irritation, immunogenicity etc. (Walters, 1989). Physical methods like electrophoresis, iontophoresis (Burnette & Ongpipattanakul, 1987), moreover can transfer some intermediate size charged molecules, but the resulting overall material transfer efficiency is rather low (less than 10%), and applicable only for charged drugs (Cevc et al, 1993).

Vesicular carrier systems like liposomes and niosomes have both received lot of attention over the last decade as a means for the transdermal drug delivery (Schreier & Bouwastra, 1994). Initially the use of liposomes on the skin was reported (Mezei & Gulasekharam, 1980), since then a wide range of agents loaded in liposomes have been tested on the skin, with different rationalities in mind. In most cases transdermal drug penetration has not been achieved. To overcome all the problems mentioned above a new type of carrier system called a "transfersomes" was introduced recently for the effective transdermal delivery of number of low and high molecular weight drugs (Schatzlein & Cevc, 1995). A transfersomes, in the widest sense of the word, is any supramacromolecular entity that can pass spontaneously through a permeability barrier and thereby transport material from the application to the destination site. In order to meet the goal, however, a tranfersomes must adjust its properties, most notably its deformability to the shape and the size of the pores in the barrier. A tranfersomes, in functional terms, may be described as lipid droplets of such deformability that permit its easy penetration through the pores much smaller than the droplets' size. In thermodynamic terms this typically corresponds to an aggregate in the quasi-metastable state, which facilitates the formation of highly curved bilayers. From the composition point of view, a transfersomes is a self-adaptable and optimized mixed lipid aggregate (Cevc, 1996).

18.2 THE PENETRATION BARRIER OF THE INTACT SKIN

In the field of the dermal or transdermal drug delivery the skin represents the application site and sometimes also the target, but it is the main obstacle for efficient drug and/or carrier penetration. The main barrier is the so-called horny layer, or stratum corneum, which is illustrated in Fig. 18.1

The skin (cutis) consists of two histologically and functionally different parts: the inner part, the dermis, is 10 to 20 times thicker than the outer part, the epidermis that is usually approximately 4 mm thick .The dermis encompasses a variety of specialized cells, tissues, blood vessels, lymph ducts, glands, hair follicles, and sensory and immunocompetent cells. Each of these fulfills a range of important tasks. One of the important functions of the dermis is to nourish the cells of the epidermis. The main function of the epidermis is to render the skin mechanically stable and chemically and environmentally resistant, the low permeability is part of this.

The predominant cell type in the epidermis is the keratinocyte. Other cells, such as melanocytes (for UV protection), Langerhans cells (for immune response), and Merkel cells (part of sensory system) etc., play an important role in the function of the skin as well. The keratinocytes at the basal membrane of the epidermis continuously produce new cells. These then gradually move toward the skin surface and thus replace the shedding cells of the stratum corneum. The stratum corneum consists of several layers of dead, flattened cells (corneocytes) embedded into a quasi-lamellar lipid matrix (Christophers et al, 1974). Cells originating from the same keratinocyte stem cell remain organized in a columnar stack during the terminal differentiation. Corneocytes of neighboring stacks interdigitate at their edges (Christophers, 1988). This structure is often referred to as the "brick and mortar" model of stratum corneum; the corneocytes represent the bricks, and the mortar consists of the intercellular lipid lamellae. The latter are believed to be crucial for the skin permeability barrier (Swartzendraber et al, 1989).

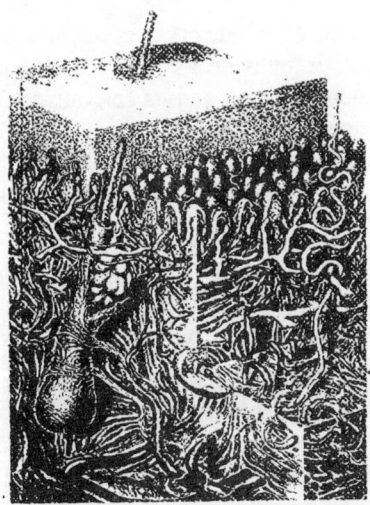

Fig. 18.1: Schematic representation of human skin

18.3 NOVEL METHODS IN TRANSDERMAL DRUG DELIVERY

New dosage forms and drug delivery systems providing excellent improvement in drug therapy are termed as novel drug delivery systems. These are termed 'novel' due to recent development with satisfactory results in the field of drug delivery (Juliano, 1980).

Some of these novel advanced transdermal technologies include (Prausnitz & Allen, 1998):

1. Penetration enhancers

2. Iontophoresis

3. Electroporation and sonophoresis

4. Microfabricated microneedles and microchips

5. Vesicular approaches

18.3.1 Penetration enhancers

Transdermal drug delivery has been a subject of research interest since the first introduction of transdermal patch of scopolamine for motion sickness in 1981 (Chowdary & Naidu, 1995). The most recent developments center around methodologies to increase molecular transport across the skin. Much effort has been directed towards the search for specific chemicals or combination of chemicals that act as penetration enhancers. The diffusional resistance of the stratum corneum is a challenge accepted by the research scientists and considerable progress has been made towards percutaneous enhancement technologies.

An ideal enhancer should be pharmacologically inactive, non-irritant and should not damage the skin irreversibly. The effects of an enhancer on the permeation of a drug usually depend upon the physico-chemical characteristics of the permeant as well as the enhancer molecule. The penetration of the enhancers into the stratum corneum is a basic requirement for their efficacy. It is possible to facilitate the penetration of the drug by appropriate pretreatment of the skin with penetration enhancer. The lipid-protein-partitioning theory of Barry offers the most acceptable explanation for the possible interaction between penetration enhancers and the stratum corneum (Barry, 1991). Accordingly, the main reasons for enhancements include:

• Interactions with the intercellular lipids and intracellular keratin

• Increased penetration of high amounts of enhancers or cosolvents into the stratum corneum due to the improved dissolving capacity of the barrier to the drugs. Many of the chemical enhancers such as dimethyl sulfoxide (Barry, 1991), surfactants, alcohols, urea and its derivatives (Wong & Tsuzuki, 1988) have been screened for their penetration enhancement. The adverse effects caused by some of these enhancers restrict their use widely. Currently, there has been an upsurge in the use of naturally occurring chemicals like terpenes as enhancers. Terpenes isolated from natural essential oils are currently under investigation as safe and non-irritating penetration enhancers (Williams et al, 1990).

Terpene enhancers such as L-menthol, D-limonene, menthone, carvone and 1-8 cineole have been used to enhance the transdermal delivery of drugs including 5-fluorouracil (William & Barry, 1991), indomethacin, zidovudine and diclofenac sodium. These chemicals have exhibited low cutaneous irritation potential and reversible alterations of skin barrier function.

18.3.2 Iontophoresis

The drawbacks associated with chemical enhancers include the unsuitability for delivery of new biotechnological products like peptides, small proteins, and oligonucleotides. Hence a renaissance of interest was shown towards iontophoresis developed over the last decade (Sage et al, 1995).

Iontophoresis is a process or technique involving the transport of ionic or charged molecules into a tissue by the passage of direct or periodic electric current through an electrolyte solution containing the ionic molecules to be delivered using an appropriate electrode polarity (Bellantone et al, 1986). The process involves the transfer of ions into the body by an electromotive force. Ions with positive charge are driven into the skin at the anode and those with the negative charge at the cathode (Stillwell, 1971). In the conventional topical treatment by iontophoresis, the drug is administrated through an electrode having the same charge as the drug and a return electrode opposite in charge to the drug is placed at a neutral site on the body surface. The operator then selects a current intensity below the pain threshold level of the patient and allows the current to flow for an appropriate period of time (Banga & Chien, 1988). The current intensity should be increased slowly, maintained for the length of the treatment and decreased slowly at the end of the treatment. The current must be within comfortable toleration of the patient with a current density less than 0.5 ma/cm^2 of the electrode surface has been found to be tolerable by the patient. Interposition of a moist pad between the electrode plate and the skin is necessary for making a perfect contact, preventing any skin burns, overcoming skin resistance and protecting the skin from absorbing any caustic metallic compound formed on the metal plate surface (Banga & Chien, 1988). It is critically important that the drug be applied through the electrode with correct polarity, since any reversal of the polarity may result in no penetration of the drug. The electrode must not come in any direct contact with skin as it may cause burns (Stillwell, 1971; Sounderson et al, 1987).

Inspite of its extensive application, the drawbacks associated with the technology include the possibility of electric shock, skin irritation, burns and cost of treatment. Recent efforts in this technology have resulted in the design of iontophoretic electrodes, which avoids burns (Masada et al, 1985). The technique has gained acceptance for local therapy. Its application for systemic medication will require further research to elucidate simple means of drug delivery. The development of iontophoresis can broaden the scope of transdermal delivery to the absorption of poorly absorbed ionic drugs. User acceptance will probably depend on success in miniaturization of the assembly.

18.3.3 Electroporation

The drawbacks associated with chemical enhancers and iontophoresis can be overcome to a certain extent by electroporation technology developed in recent years. In a more futuristic way, the technology has been developed to overcome the most daunting challenges of transdermal drug delivery. The process involves the application of transient high voltage electrical pulse to cause rapid dissociation of the stratum corneum through which large and small peptides, oligonucleotides and other drugs can pass in significant amounts (Kiro et al, 1987). The degree of enhancement achieved in vitro is related to the applied voltage, number and duration of the pulses offering the possibility of a controllable phenomenon.

Electroporation is a technique in which the drug encapsulated in vesicles or particles is delivered into the skin by applying a pulse causing a breakdown of the stratum corneum (Weaver et al, 1996). Pressure mediated electroincorporation has been used to deliver leuprolide acetate microspheres into hairless mouse skin and human skin xenografted on immunodeficient nude mice. It has been shown that application of continuous low voltage resulted in a calcein flux with three orders of magnitude (Prausnitz, 1997).

Beside the model compound calcein, other drugs investigated for transdermal delivery by electroporation include metaprolol, flurbiprofen, cyclosporin, heparin, fentanyl and oligonucleotides (Prausnitz et al., 1995).

The studies with model compounds have given excellent mechanistic insights into the magnitude of flux enhancement. These reports may not be applicable for all drugs. Hence each drug needs to be studied as a separate entity. More human clinical data is however required before the technology can be commercialized.

18.3.4 Sonophoresis

Another technique besides electroporation attempting to overcome the challenges of transdermal drug delivery involves the usage of high frequency ultrasound waves. The application of low frequency ultrasound was shown to increase the permeability of human skin to many drugs including high molecular weight proteins by several orders of magnitude, thus making transdermal administration of these molecules potentially feasible. Low- frequency ultrasound is thus a potential, non-invasive technology for transdermal drug delivery.

Despite the excitement these findings have provoked, it is necessary to maintain an appropriate perspective until several basic questions are answered with respect to mechanism of action, toxicity, economical and technological feasibility. Furthermore, optimal parameters such as frequency, pulse length and intensity should be observed carefully to ensure a safe and efficacious application (Levy et al, 1989).

18.3.5 Microfabricated microneedles

Recently a novel method has been developed for enhancing transport of molecules across the skin. The microfabricated microneedles technology employs micron-sized needles made from silicon (Kenry et al, 1998). These microneedle arrays after insertion into the skin create conduits for transport of drug across the stratum corneum. The drug after crossing the stratum corneum diffuses rapidly through deeper tissue and taken up by capillaries for systemic administration. Microneedles penetrate the skin about 10-15 mm deep inside the skin but do not reach the nerves found in deeper tissue, so are painless. The microneedles were made using the microfabrication technology similar to that of making integrated circuits (Runyan & Bean,1990). The microfabrication technology is simple for cheap and mass production of micron sized structures. For the drug delivery, a three-dimensional array of sharp-tipped microneedles with approximately 150 mm in lengths were fabricated. A deep reactive ion etching process was used to microfabricate the needles for drug delivery. The reactive ion etching technique is based on the black silicon method (Jansen et al,1995). Each microneedle is about 1 mm in diameter or one hundredth of the diameter of a human hair and can be seen only under a microscope. A microprocessor is attached to a tiny pump for delivering tiny amounts of the drug. The microprocessor and pump automatically inject the right dosage of the drug. The microneedles have extremely sharp tips with radius of curvature less than 1mm facilitating easy piercing into the skin. The microfabrication technique can be easily modified to make longer or shorter needles according to the requirement. Microneedles after insertion into skin, are found to be mechanically strong, can be removed without difficulty as well as reinserted into skin multiple times. The experiments were also conducted on human volunteers by inserting microneedles into the skin of the forearm or hand. As reported, the volunteer never felt pain, but mild wearing or a weak pressure with the feeling of a piece of tape affixed to the skin. Inspection of the site after insertion showed no erythema, edema or other reaction to microneedles over the hours and days. Microneedles are still a long way from being marketed. It may take some years to perfect and test the technology for safety and clinical studies before gaining approval from Food and Drug Administration (Kulkarni et al, 2000).

18.3.6 Vesicular approaches

The encapsulation of drug in lipid vesicles prepared from phospholipids and nonionic surfactant is used for transport of drug into and across the skin. The rationale for use of lipid vesicles as a topical drug carrier is as follows (Schreier & Bouwstra, 1994; Cevc, 1992a):

- Vesicles may serve as rate-limiting membrane barrier for systemic absorption of drug.

- Because of the amphiphilic nature of the vesicles, these vesicles may serve as non-toxic penetration enhancer for drugs.

- They may serve as "organic solvent" for the solubilization of poorly soluble drugs.

- Vesicles can incorporate both hydrophilic and lipophilic drugs.

The vesicular approach e.g. liposomes in transdermal drug delivery systems have been studied for many purposes, but their unstable nature limits their use at clinical and industrial levels. In order to increase the stability of liposomes concept of proliposomes has been proposed. This approach has been extended to niosomes which exhibit superior stability compared to liposomes and attempts have been made to further stabilize them and overcome their limitation by proniosomal approach. But all approaches because of their poor skin permeability, breaking of vesicles, leakage of drug, aggregation and fusion of vesicles are not much successful for effective transdermal delivery (Cevc et al, 1997; Lasch et al, 1991).

Specially optimized, ultradeformable lipid supramolecular aggregates known as transfersomes, are able to penetrate the mammalian skin intact. Each transfersomes consists of at least one inner aqueous compartment, this is surrounded by a lipid bilayer with specially tailored properties (Planas et al, 1992; Cevc, 1991a). These novel carrier are applied in the form of semi-dilute suspension, without occlusion and offer the efficient dermal and transcutaneous drug delivery of high and low molecular weight substances. If properly made and optimally applied, these drug carrier can regularly bring more than 85-90% of the applied agent across the intact skin (Cevc, 1992a).

18.4 TRANSFERSOMES

Transfersomes were developed in order to take the advantage of phospholipid vesicles as transdermal drug carrier. These self-optimized aggregates, with the ultraflexible membrane, are able to deliver the drug reproducibly either into or through the skin, depending on the choice of administration or application, with high efficiency. These vesicular transfersomes are several orders of magnitudes more elastic than the standard liposomes and thus well suited for the skin penetration. Transfersomes overcome the skin penetration difficulty by squeezing themselves along the intracellular sealing lipids of the stratum corneum. There is provision for this, because of the high vesicle deformability, which permits the entry due to the mechanical stress of surrounding, in a self-adapting manner. Flexibility of transfersomes membrane is achieved by mixing suitable surface-active components in the proper ratios (Cevc, 1992b). The resulting flexibility of transfersome membrane minimizes the risk of complete vesicle rupture in the skin and allows transfersomes to follow the natural water gradient across the epidermis, when applied under nonocclusive condition. Transfersomes can penetrate the intact stratum corneum spontaneously along two routes in the intracellular lipid that differ in their bilayer properties (Schatzlein & Cevc, 1995). The following figure (Fig.18.2) shows possible microroutes for drug penetration across human skin intracellular and transcellular (Panchagnula, 1997)

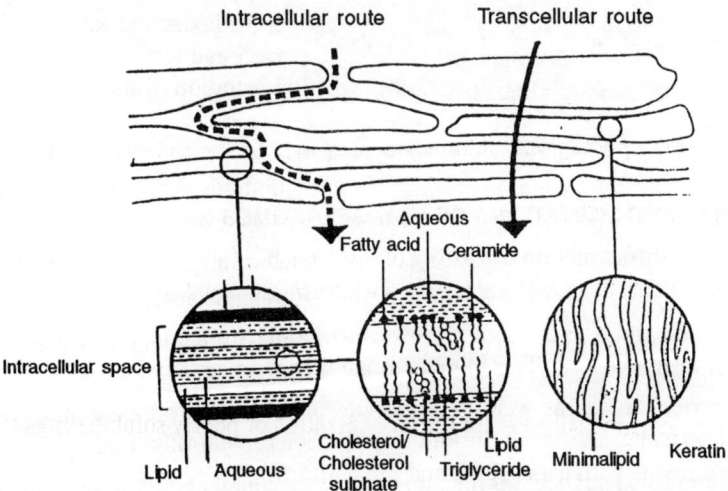

Fig. 18.2 : Possible micro-routes for drug penetration across human skin

The high and self-optimizing deformability of typical composite transfersomes membrane, which are adaptable to ambient stress allow the ultradeformable transfersomes to change its membrane composition locally and reversibly, when it is pressed against or attracted into a narrow pore. The transfersomes components that sustain strong membrane deformation preferentially accumulate, while the less adaptable molecules are diluted at sites of great stress. This dramatically lowers the energetic cost of membrane deformation and permits the resulting, highly flexible particles, first to enter and then to pass through the pores rapidly and efficiently. This behavior is not limited to one type of pore and has been observed in natural barriers such as in intact skin (Cevc, 1993a; Paul et al, 1995).

Natural transdermal water concentration gradients consequently drive high number of the specially designed lipid vesicles across the hydrophobic outer skin layers. This does not pertain to all lipid vesicles, for example, the available transdermal osmotic pressure difference is too low to push the standard lipid vesicles (liposomes) through an intact mammalian stratum corneum. Dermally applied lipid vesicles can only penetrate into rather than across this region. The reason for this is the prohibitively high cost of the standard liposome deformation. In order to increase the efficacy of vesicle penetration through the skin it is therefore necessary to minimize this cost for each given vesicles type. It had been by adjusting the lipid bilayer composition until the maximum of the tolerable vesicles surface flexibility was achieved. Such an optimization yields transfersomes. Owing to their hyperflexibility the latter can transfer as much as 0.1 mg of lipid per hour and cm^2 across the intact skin, if applied under suitable conditions. Furthermore, transfersomes can mediate an efficient transepidermal transport of the water soluble substances, such as proteins or polypeptides (Cevc, 1991b; Cevc et al, 1993).

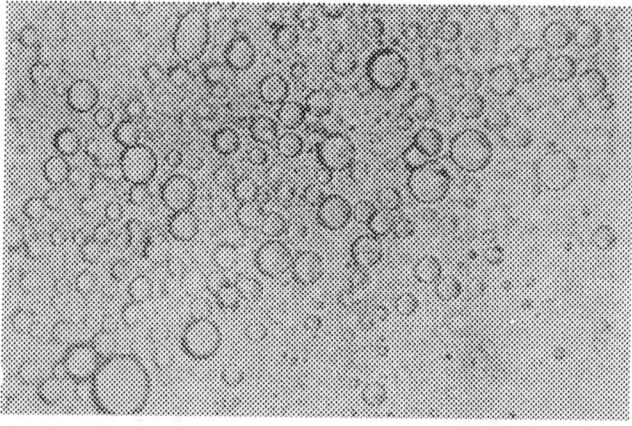

Fig 18.3 : Microphotograph of transfersomes without sonication (at 1000X)

18.5 SALIENT FEATURES AND LIMITATIONS OF TRANSFERSOMES

1. Transfersomes possess an infrastructure consisting of hydrophobic and hydrophilic moieties together and as a result can accommodate drug molecules with a wide range of solubility.

2. Transfersomes can deform and pass through narrow constriction (from 5 to 10 times less than their own diameter) without measurable loss. This high deformability gives better penetration of intact vesicles.

3. They can act as a carrier for low as well as high molecular weight drugs e.g. analgesic, anesthetic, corticosteroids, sex hormone, anticancer, insulin, gap junction protein, albumin.

4. They are biocompatible and biodegradable as they are made from natural phospholipids similar to liposomes.

5. They have high entrapment efficiency, in case of lipophilic drug near to 90%.

6. They protect the encapsulated drug from metabolic degradation.

7. They act as depot, releasing their contents slowly and gradually.

8. They can be used for both systemic as well as topical delivery of drug.

9. Easy to scale up, as procedure is simple, do not involve lengthy procedure and unnecessary use of pharmaceutically unacceptable additives.

18.5.1 Limitations of transfersomes

1. Transfersomes are chemically unstable because of their predisposition to oxidative degradation.

2. Purity of natural phospholipids is another criteria militating against adoption of transfersomes as drug delivery vehicles.

3. Transfersome formulations are expensive.

18.6 TRANSFERSOMES Vs OTHER CARRIER SYSTEMS

At first glance, transfersomes appear to be remotely related to lipid bilayer vesicle, liposomes. However in functional terms, transfersomes differ vastly from commonly used liposomes in that they are much more flexible and adaptable. The extremely high flexibility of their membrane permits transfersomes to squeeze themselves even through pores much smaller than their own diameter. This is due to high flexibility of the transfersomes membrane and is achieved by judiciously combining at least two lipophilic/amphiphilic components (phospholipid plus biosurfactant) with sufficiently different packing characteristics into a single bilayer. The high resulting aggregate deformability permits transfersomes to penetrate the skin spontaneously. This tendency is supported by the high transfersomes surface hydrophilicity that enforce the search for surrounding of high water activity. It is almost certain that the high penetration potential of the transfersomes is not primarily a consequence of stratum corneum fluidization by the surfactant because micellar suspension contains much more surfactant than transfersomes (PC/Sodium cholate 65/35 w/w %, respectively). Thus, if the penetration enhancement via the solubilization of the skin lipids was the reason for the superior penetration capability of transfersomes, one would expect an even better penetration performance of the micelles. In contrast to this postulate, the higher surfactant concentration in the mixed micelles does not improve the efficacy of material transport into the skin. On the contrary, mixed micelles stay confined to the topmost part of the stratum corneum even they are applied non occlusively (Cevc et al, 1993). The reason for this is that mixed micelles are much less sensitive to the transepidermal water activity gradient than transfersomes. Transfersomes differ in at least two basic features from the mixed micelles, first a transfersomes is normally by one to two order of magnitude (in size) greater than a standard lipid micelles. Secondly and more importantly, each vesicular transfersomes contains a water filled core whereas a micelle is just a simple fatty droplet. Transfersomes thus carry water as well as fat-soluble agent in comparision to micelles that can only incorporate lipoidal substances (Schatzlein & Cevc, 1995; Planas et al, 1992).

To differentiate the penetration ability of all these carrier systems Cevc et al., (1996) proposed the distribution profiles of fluorescently labelled mixed lipid micelles, liposomes and transfersomes as measured by the Confocal Scanning Laser Microscopy (CSLM) in the intact murine skin. In all these vesicles the highly deformable transfersomes transverse the stratum corneum and enter into the viable epidermis in significant quantity (Fig 18.4)

Chapman & Walsh, (1990) also showed that the former two types of aggregates are confined to the outer half of the horny layer, where the cellular packing and intercellular seals are already compromised by the desquamation process. Pure lipid vesicles or micelles seem to have access to the low-resistance pathway only and thus very seldom reach the lower stratum corneum or even get into the viable parts of the skin in significant quantities.

Table18. 1: Comparison of different approaches for transdermal drug delivery

Method	Advantage	Disadvantage
Penetration enhancers (Walters, 1989)	Increase penetration through skin and give both local and systemic effect	Skin irritation, Immunogenicity, only for low molecular weight drugs
Physical methods e.g. Iontophoresis (Cevc et al, 1995)	Increase penetration of intermediate size charged molecule	Only for charged drugs, transfer efficiency is low (less than 10%)
Liposomes (Hadgraft & Guy, 1989)	Phospholipid vesicle, biocompatible, biodegradable	Less skin penetration, less stable
Proliposome	Phospholipid vesicle, more stable than liposomes	Less penetration, cause aggregation and fusion of vesicles
Niosomes (Schreier & Bouwstra,1994) (Holland et al, 1995)	Non-ionic surfactants vesicles, greater stability,	Less skin penetration easy handling
Proniosomes	Will convert into niosome in situ, stable	But will not reach upto deeper skin layer
Transfersomes and Protransfersomes (Cevc et al, 1996)	More stable, high penetration due to high deformability, biocompatible and biodegradable, suitable for both low and high molecular weight and also for lipophilic as well as hydrophilic drugs and reach upto the deeper skin layers.	None, but for some limitations.

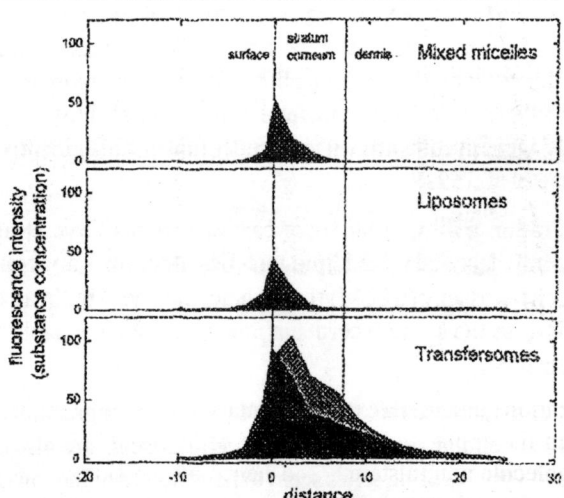

Fig 18.4 : Distribution profiles of fluorescently labelled mixed lipid micelles, liposomes, transfersomes as measured with the confocal scanning laser microscopy in the intact murine skin.

In contrast to this, the much more deformable vesicles can use intra- as well as inter-cluster pathway by virtue of their capability to squeeze themselves into the smallest pores. Such lipid aggregates, consequently, are found in the stratum corneum as well as in the viable skin and even bring their associated material deep into the body (Cevc, 1996).

18.7 MECHANISM OF PENETRATION OF TRANSFERSOMES

Transfersomes when applied under suitable condition can transfer 0.1 mg to 0.5 mg of lipid per hour and cm^2 area across the intact skin. This value is substantially higher than that which is typically driven by the transdermal concentration gradients. The reason for this high flux rate is naturally occurring "transdermal osmotic gradients" i.e. another much more prominent gradient is available across the skin (Gompper & Kroll, 1995). This osmotic gradient is developed due to the skin penetration barrier, prevents water loss through the skin and maintains a water activity difference in the viable part of the epidermis (75% water content) and nearly completely dry stratum corneum, near to the skin surface (15% water content) (Warner et al, 1988). This gradient is very stable because ambient air is a perfect sink for the water molecule even when the transdermal water loss is unphysiologically high. All polar lipids attract some water, this is due to the energetically favourable interaction between the hydrophilic lipid residues and their proximal water. Most lipid bilayers thus spontaneously resist an induced dehydration (Rand & Porsegian, 1990; Cevc & Marsh, 1987). Consequently all lipid vesicles made from the polar lipid vesicles move from the rather dry location to the sites with a sufficiently high water concentration (Cevc, 1985,1987,1990). So when a lipid suspension (transfersomes) is placed on the skin surface, that is partly dehydrated by the water evaporation loss and then the lipid vesicles feel this "osmotic gradient" and try to escape complete drying by moving along this gradient (Schatziein & Cevc, 1995). They can only achieve this if they are sufficiently deformable to pass through the narrow pores in the skin, because transfersomes composed of surfactant have more suitable rheologic and hydration properties than that responsible for their greater deformability (Cevc, 1990). Less deformable vesicles including standard liposomes are confined to the skin surface, where they dehydrate completely and fuse, so they have less penetration power than transfersomes. Transfersomes are optimized in this respect and thus attain maximum flexibility, so they can take full advantages of the transepidermal osmotic gradient (water concentration gradient) (Cevc & Blume, 1992).

The transfersomes vesicle penetration through skin and their deformability was represented in different stages by Cevc et al (1996). They showed that vesicle larger than the narrow pore segment is first pressed against the pore entry, where it fluctuates until it deforms enough to fit in to the constriction. Upon complete elongation it feels further resistance and than through the pore easily (Fig.18. 5)

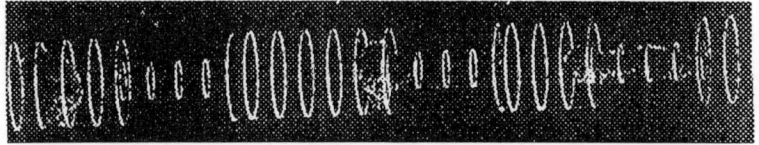

Fig.18. 5 : Mechanism of penetration of transfersomes

18.7.1 Propensity of penetration

Any epicutaneous lipid application generates a transepidermal concentration gradient and thus should result in the transport of lipids from the application site into the body, if only possible. The likelihood for this dependson the mobility of molecule administered, and hence on the skin as well as subcutaneous tissue permeabilities. The magnitude of the transport driving force, of course, also plays an important role:

Flow = Area x (Barrier) Permeability x (Trans-barrier) Force

Therefore, the chemically driven lipid flow across the skin always decreases dramatically when lipid solution is replaced by the some amount of lipids in a suspension. The reason for this is that lipid aggregation always decreases the effective transcutaneous concentration gradient by at least 4 order of magnitude, owing to the inverse dependence of vesicle concentration on the number of molecules in each vesicle:

$$\Delta c_{agg} = \frac{\Delta c_{\,monomer}}{Aggreg.\ number}$$

This then suggests that : Flow α $\Delta c_{\,monomer}$ / Aggreg. number

In contrast to this, the aggregate sensitivity to an external potential that can act on all lipid molecules increases with the aggregation number:

$$n_{w.\ aggregate} = n_{m.monomer} \cdot Aggreg.\ number$$

Aggregation thus promotes the flow of lipids under the influence of any fixed or naturally occurring gradient, such as the trans-epidermal water concentration gradient, Δaw : flow α $nm_{\,monomer} \cdot$ aggreg. number Δaw. Increasing the monomer hydrophilicity, which is roughly proportional to the $nm_{\,monomer}$, also enhance the transport of hydrophilic material or hydrophilic aggregate in the water activity gradient, for example, across the stratum corneum region. This positive size dependence of the transport-driving hydrotaxis suggests that large and more polar lipid aggregates will have a higher propensity to enforce their passage through the skin than the small or moderately polar entities (Cevc, 1996)

18.8 MATERIALS AND METHODS OF PREPARATION

Materials commonly used for the preparation of transfersomes are summarized in Table 18.2. The method of preparation of transfersomes has been shown schematically in Fig 18.6

Table18.2 : Different additives used in formulation of transfersomes.

Class	Example	Uses	References
Phospholipids	Soya phosphatidyl choline	Vesicles forming	Cevc et al, 1997
	Egg phosphatidyl choline	component	Cevc, 1992$_b$
	Dipalmitoyl phosphatidyl choline		
	Distearoyl phosphatidyl choline		
Surfactant	Sod. cholate	For providing flexibility	Schubert et al, 1986
	Sod. deoxycholate		Schubert et al, 1988
	Tween-80		Cevc et al, 1995
	Span-80		Gamal et al, 1999
Alcohol	Ethanol	As a solvent	Planas et al, 1992
	Methanol		Gamal et al, 1999
Dye	Rhodamine-123	For CSLM study	Cevc et al, 1995
	Rhodamine-DHPE		Schatzlein & Cevc, 1998
	Fluorescein-DHPE		
	Nile-red		
Buffering agent	Saline phosphate buffer (pH 6.4)	As a hydrating medium	Cevc, 1993

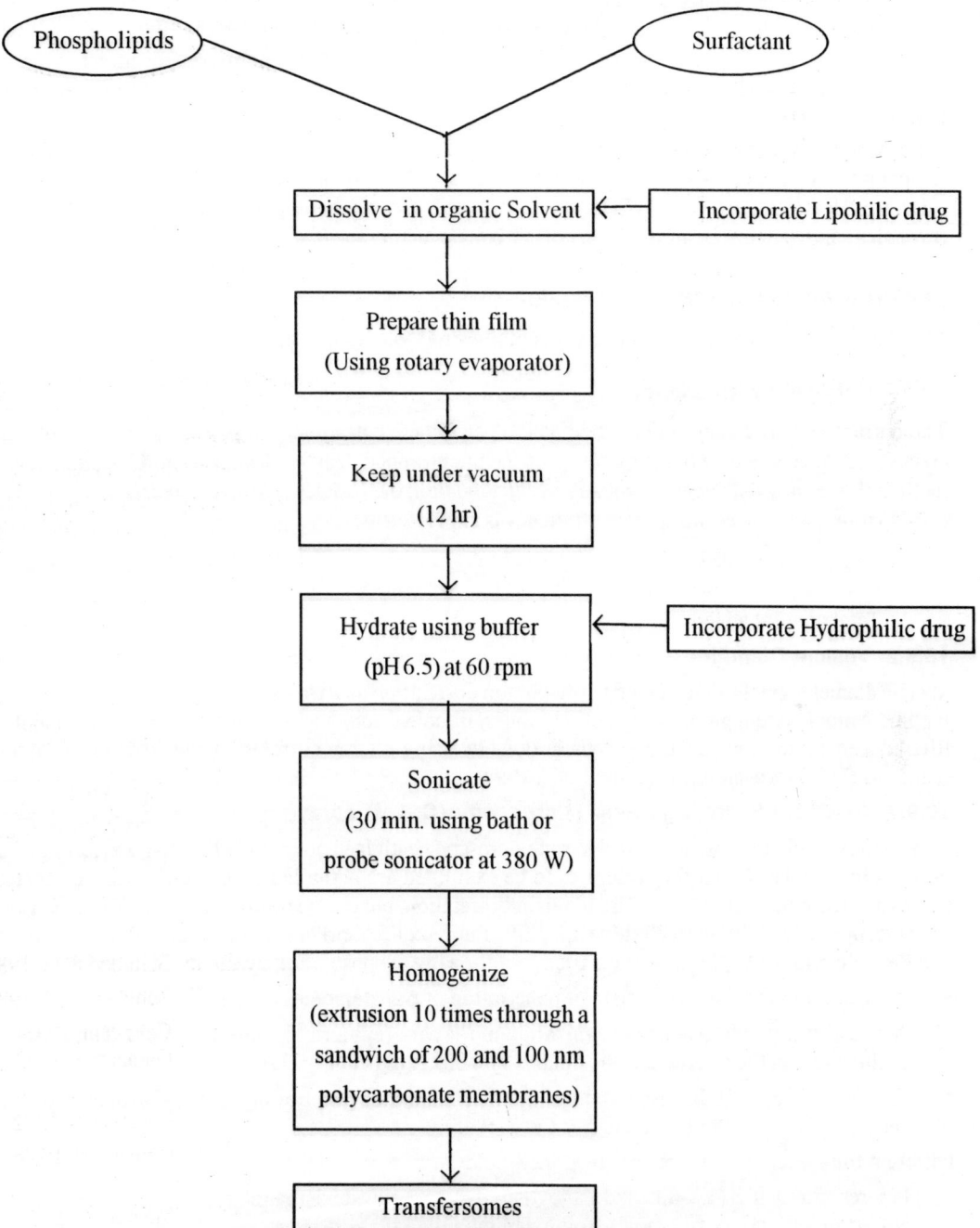

Fig18. 6 : Method of preparation of transfersomes

All the methods of preparation of transfersomes are comprised of two steps. First, a thin film is prepared, hydrated and then brought to the desired size by sonication; and secondly, sonicated vesicles are homogenized by extrusion through a polycarbonate membrane.

The mixture of vesicles forming ingredients, that is phospholipid and surfactant were dissolved in volatile organic solvent (chloroform-methanol), organic solvent evaporated above the lipid transition temperature (room temp. for pure PC vesicles, or 50°C for dipalmitoyl phosphatidyl choline) using a rotary evaporator. Final traces of solvent were removed under vacuum for overnight. The deposited lipid films were hydrated with buffer (pH 6.5) by rotation at 60 rpm min^{-1} for 1 hr at the corresponding temperature. The resulting vesicles were swollen for 2 hr at room temperature. To prepare small vesicles, resulting LMVs were sonicated at room temperature or 50°C for 30 min. using a B-12 FTZ bath sonicator or probe sonicated at 4°C for 30 min (titanium microtip, Heat Systems W 380). The sonicated vesicles were homogenized by manual extrusion 10 times through a sandwich of 200 and 100 nm polycarbonate membrane (Cevc et al, 1998).

18.9 CHARACTERIZATION OF TRANSFERSOMES

The characterization of transfersomes is generally similar to liposomes, niosomes and micelles.

18.9.1 Entrapment Efficiency

The entrapment efficiency is expressed as the percentage entrapment of the drug added. Entrapment efficiency was determined by first separation of the unentrapped drug by the use of mini-column centrifugation method (Fry et al, 1978; New, 1990). After centrifugation, the vesicles were disrupted using 0.1% Triton X-100 or 50% n-propanol. The entrapment efficiency is expressed as:

$$\frac{\text{Amount entrapped}}{\text{Total amount added}} \times 100$$

18.9.2 Vesicle Diameter

Vesicle diameter can be determined using photon correlation spectroscopy or dynamic light scattering (DLS) method. Samples were prepared in distilled water, filtered through a 0.2 mm membrane filter and diluted with filtered saline and than size measurement done by using photon correlation spectroscopy or dynamic light scattering (DLS) measurements (Gamal et al, 1999).

18.9.3 Confocal Scanning Laser Microscopy (CSLM) study

Conventional light microscopy and electron microscopy both face problem of fixation, sectioning and staining of the skin samples. Often the structures to be examined are actually incompatible with the corresponding processing techniques, these give rise to misinterpretation, but can be minimized by Confocal Scanning Laser Microscopy (CSLM). In this technique lipophilic fluorescence markers are incorporated into the transfersomes and the light emitted by these markers used for following purpose (Schatzlein & Cevc, 1998):

*   for investigating the mechanism of penetration of transfersomes across the skin,

*   for determining histological organization of the skin (epidermal columns, interdigitation), shapes and architecture of the skin penetration pathways (Simonetti et al, 1995),

*   for comparison and differentiation of the mechanism of penetration of transfersomes with liposomes, niosomes and micelles (Schatzlein & Cevc, 1995).

Different fluorescence markers used in CSLM study are

   I. Fluorescein-DHPE (1,2-dihexadecanoyl-sn-glycero-3-phosphoethanolamine-N-(5- fluoresdenthiocarbamoyl), triethylammonium salt)

   II. Rhodamine-DHPE (1,2-dihexadecanoyl-sn-glycero-3-phosphoethanolamine-N -Lissamine^{Tm} rhodamine B sulfonyl), triethanolamine salt)

   III. NBD-PE (1,2-dihexadecanoyl-sn-glycero-3-phosphoethanolamine-N-(7-nitro- Benz-2-oxa- 1,3-diazol-4-yl) triethanolamine salt)

   IV. Nile red.

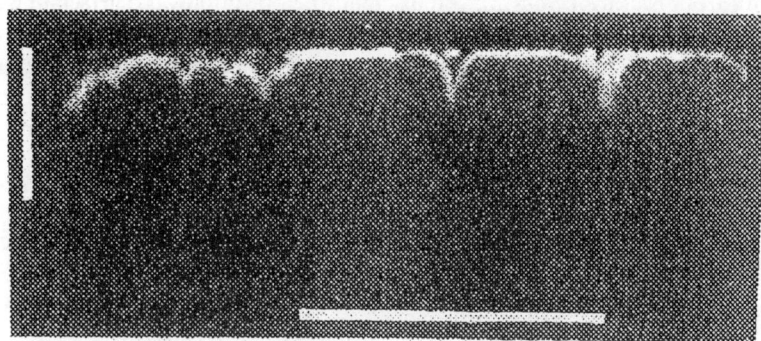

Fig. 18.7: Tranfersomes penetration with the intact murine skin visualized by CSLM

18.9.4 Degree of Deformability or Permeability Measurement

In the case of transfersomes, the permeability study is one of the important and unique parameter for characterization. The deformability study is done against the pure water as standard. Transfersomal preparation is passed through a large number of pores of known size (through a sandwich of different microporous filters, with pore diameter between 50 nm and 400 nm, depending on the starting transfersomes suspension). Particle size and size distributions are noted after each pass by dynamic light scattering (DLS) measurements (Cevc et al, 1998).

18.9.5 In Vitro Drug Release

In vitro drug release study is performed for determining the permeation rate. Time needed to attain steady state permeation and the permeation flux at steady state and the information from in-vitro studies are used to optimize the formulation before more expensive in vivo studies are performed. For determining drug release, transfersomes suspension is incubated at 32^0C and samples are taken at different times and the free drug is separated by minicolumn centrifugation (Fry et al., 1978). The amount of drug released is then calculated indirectly from the amount of drug entrapped at zero times as the initial amount (100% entrapped and 0% released) (Gamal et al, 1999)

18.10 IN VIVO FATE OF TRANSFERSOMES AND KINETICS OF TRANSFERSOMES PENETRATION

After having penetrated through the outermost skin layers, transfersomes reach the deeper skin layer, the dermis. From this latter skin region they are normally washed out, via the lymph, into the blood circulation and through the latter throughout the body, if applied under suitable conditions. Transfersomes can thus reach all such body tissues that are accessible to the subcutaneously injected liposomes (Cevc et al, 1995).

The kinetics of action of an epicutaneously-applied agent depends on the velocity of carrier penetration as well as on the speed of drug (re)distribution and the action after this passage. The most important single factors in this process are:

· Carrier in-flow

· Carrier accumulation at the target site

· Carrier elimination

The onset of penetration-driving force depends on the volume of the suspension medium that must evaporate from the skin surface before the sufficiently strong trans-cutaneous chemical potential or water activity gradient is established. Using less solvent is favorable in this respect.

The rate of carrier passage across the skin is chiefly determined by the activation energy for the carrier deformation. The magnitude of the penetration driving force also plays a big role. This explains, for example, why the occlusion of an application site or the use of too strongly diluted suspension hampers the penetration process (Cevc & Blume, 1992)

Carrier elimination from the subcutis is primarily affected by the lymphatic flow; general anesthesia or any other factor that affects this flow, consequently, is prone to modify the rate of transcutaneous carrier transport. While it has been estimated that approximately 10% of the cardiac blood flow pass through each gram of living skin tissue, no comparable quotation is available for the lymph. Further, drug distribution is also sensitive to the number of carrier used, as this may affect the rate of vehicle degradation and/or filtration in the lymph nodes.

The lag between the time of application and the time of drug appearance in the body, therefore, is always quite long, complex, and strongly sensitive to the type of drug and formulation administration.

In the best case, the skin penetration lag amounts to approximately 15 min. if rapidly exchanging agents such as local analgesics are detected right under the skin permeability barrier (Planas et al., 1992). Less rapidly exchanging molecules or molecules measured in the blood compartment are typically detected with a lag time between 2 and 6 hr. depending on the details of drug formulation. Molecules that do not diffuse readily from the carriers or agents delivered with the suboptimal carriers normally fall in this category. The kinetics of vesicle penetration into and across the skin can be controlled to a large extent by fixing the physicochemical characteristics of the drug carrier suspension. This is shown in fig.18.8 for several agent molecules of different kind, size, and type of labelling.

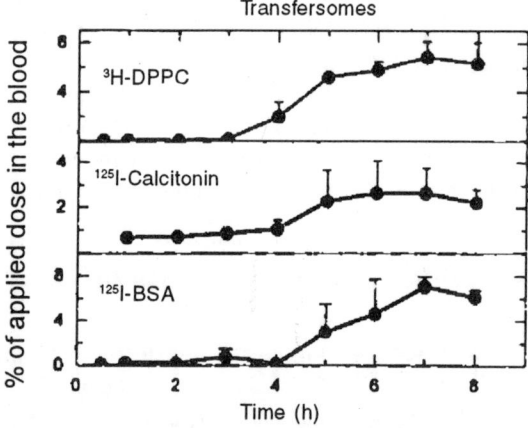

Fig.18.8: The kinetics of penetration through the intact murine skin of several epicutaneously administered transfersome preparations containing radioactiviely phospholipids (3H-dipalmitoyl phosphatidylcholine; top), polypeptides (125-calcitonin; middle) or proteins (125-bovine serum albumin). In all cases, the radioactivity appears in the blood compartment after comparable lag time of approx. 6 hr.

Kinetics of the transfersomes penetration through the intact skin is best studied in the direct biological assays in which vesicle associated drugs exert their action directly under the skin surface. Local analgesics are useful for this purpose (Planas et al, 1992). For determining the kinetics of penetration, various lidocaine-loaded vesicles were left to dry out on the intact skin. Corresponding subcutaneous injection is used as control. The animal's sensitivity to pain at the treated site after each application was then measured as a function of time. Dermally applied standard drug carrying liposomes or simple lidocaine solution have never caused any analgesic effect. It was necessary to inject such agent preparations to achieve significant pain suppression. In contrast to this, the lidocaine-loaded transfersomes were analgesically active even when applied dermally. Maximum analgesic effect with the latter type of drug application was typically observed 15 minutes after the drug application. A marked analgesic effect was still noticeable after very long time. The precise reach as well as kinetics of transfersomes penetration through the skin are affected by:

- drug carrier interaction,
- carrier characteristics,
- application condition or form,
- skin characteristics,
- applied dose.

18.10.1 Drug carrier interaction

Agents must have a high carrier affinity because agents with a low carrier affinity are more difficult to target into selected tissue. Such agents are also burdened with a lower efficiency of transfer across the intact skin (Cevc et al, 1995).

18.10.2 Carrier characteristics

For a rapid and efficient delivery of drug in dermis region or in blood circulation, the carrier must have a high flexibility, hence for this purpose transfersomes are optimized in terms of the type of surfactant and their concentration. If transfersomes is highly or sufficiently flexible then very rapid and efficient delivery of drug occurred (Cevc et al, 1996).

18.10.3 Application condition or form

Transfersomes associated drug applied in an open patch or as an open droplets (nonocclusively) can get very efficiently into and across the intact skin. If applied occlusively then transfersomes do not penetrate deep into the skin. Owing to the permanent lipid overhydration (W-local > 85%), that is caused by the water-tight skin wrapping, so "osmotic gradient" across the skin is lost that is the most important gradient for penetration of transfersomes. Wet skin surface thus normally retains at least 90% of the total dose on the top or in the outermost stratum corneum layers (Cevc & Blume, 1992).

18.10.4 Skin characteristics

The energetic cost of drug carrier penetration through the intact skin depends on the carrier as well as skin characteristics. Partly damaged or very thin skin is probably more permeable to the superficially applied vesicles. Wet or strongly macerated skin, on the other hand, is expected to interfere with the transdermal transport of such vesicles. It should be possible to compensate for this latter difficulty by choosing sufficiently polar and flexible lipid bilayers.

The enhanced water flow toward the skin surface that results from the lipid excess at the application site may change the kinetics of the lipid vesicles penetration through the intact skin. Such water "counterflow" however seems not to affect overall efficacy of the inwards directed lipid transport. The reason for this is rather simple. As long as enough water is lost at the skin surface to keep the superficial water concentration lower than the vesicle, driving force will persist and vesicles flow into the skin will continue (Cevc et al, 1993).

18.10.5 Applied dose

The efficacy and the depth of the transfersomes penetration in the intact skin are strongly affected by the applied carrier dose. Transfersomes applied at small doses permeate across the skin rather inefficiently. When ultraflexible vesicles with an optimal composition are applied in sufficiently high but not in excessive quantities, they can transport upto 90% of their associated lipid mass into and through the intact horny layers (Cevc et al, 1996).

18.11 TRANSFERSOMES AS DRUG CARRIER

Drug carrier must fulfill two basic criteria for a successful transdermal drug delivery effect if they are to bring an appreciable amount of their payload from the skin strata: (a) drug carrier should respond to or create a gradient that drives the drug carrier complex from the skin surface into the skin interior, and (b) drug vesicles should be able to pass the skin barrier without uncontrollably loosing too much of the enclosed therapeutic material (Planas et al, 1992). Transfersomes also fulfill the other basic properties of the carrier system.

Transfersomes have been proposed for a variety of applications in humans. Various applications can be summarized as under.

1. Transfersomes as a carrier for proteins

2. Transfersomes as a carrier for insulin.

3. Transfersomes as a carrier for interferon.

4. Transfersomes as a means of transdermal immunization.

5. Transfersome as a carrier for corticosteroids.

6. Transfersomes as a carrier for topical analgesic and anesthetic agents.

7. Transfersomes as a carrier for non steroidal anti-inflammatory drugs.

8. Transfersomes as a carrier for anticancer drugs.

18.11.1 Transfersomes as a carrier for proteins

The delivery of large biogenic molecules such as peptides or proteins into the body is difficult. When given orally, they are completely degraded in the GI tract; when used in a degradation preventing formulation, their uptake in the gut becomes problematic and extremely insufficient, even with the best currently available formulation. These are the reasons why nearly all therapeutic peptides still have to be introduced into the body through an injection needle, in spite of the inconvenience of this method. To overcome above problems numerous attempts have therefore been made for the delivery of peptides and proteins across the skin (Hadgraft & Guy, 1989). All recent approaches, either chemical (penetration enhancers, lipid vesicles) or physical (iontophoresis, sonophoresis) have some limitations and improve this situation somewhat. However even the most efficient established methods for transdermal peptide delivery to date only achieve a transport efficiency of a few percent (Wearley, 1991).

Proteins and other molecules normally do not cross the intact mammalian skin. Despite this it elicits antibodies against the transcutaneously applied proteins, such as fluorescein-isothiocyanate-labelled bovine serum albumin (FITC-BSA), if these macromolecules are associated with the specially optimized and ultradeformable agent carriers (Paul & Cevc, 1995)

The transfersomes-mediated bioavailability of serum albumin (at t = 24 hr., > 50%), for example, is very similar to that resulting from a subcutaneous injection of the same protein suspension. Fig.18.9 documents this. The transfersomal preparations of this protein also induce a strong immune response after the repeated epicutaneous applications: the adjuvant immunogenic bovine serum albumin in transfersomes, for example, after several dermal challenges is as active immunologically as is the corresponding injected proteo-tranfersomes preparations. The measured titer reaches ~70% of that of the commercial anti-BSA solution. The less immunogenic FITC-moiety attached to the BSA molecules and delivered epicutaneously or subcutaneously by means of transfersomes gives maximum reading of around 40% (35 to 65%) of the value characterizing a commercial anti-FITC ascites. The dermally applied liposomal or mixed micellar immunogens are biologically inactive, as are simple protein solutions.

Judicious combination of the integral membrane proteins and ultradeformable membrane also provides a solution to the problem of the noninvasive delivery of such molecules. Incorporation of gap junction protein (GJP) into transfersomes, for example, results in a maximum immune response to this type of macromolecules. GJP-transfersomes give rise to the specific antibody titers that are marginally higher than those elicited by the subcutaneous GJP injections. The use of transfersomes may even increase the relative immunoglobulin-A (IgA) levels (Paul et al., 1995)

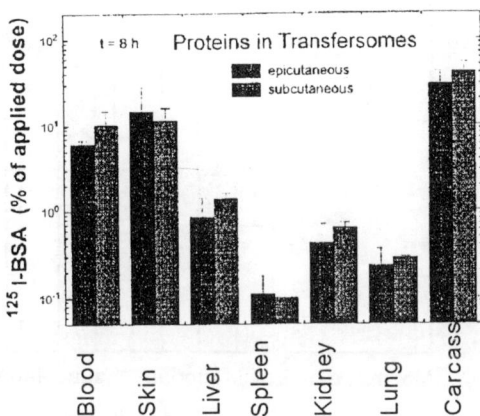

Fig.18.9 : Biodistribution of the ^{125}I-BSA derived radioactivity 8 hr. after the protein application on (black columns) or after the protein injection under (gray columns) the skin of the NMRI-mice by means of transfersomes. The radioactivity biodistribution is in both cases nearly the same and also comparable reproducible (adapted from Cevc, 1996)

18.11.2 Transfersomes as a carrier for insulin

Delivery of peptides by transfersomes provides a very successful means for the noninvasive therapeutic use of such large molecular weight drugs on the skin (Cevc et al, 1990). For example, insulin is a most commonly and regularly used drug. It is generally administered by subcutaneous route that is inconvenient. Encapsulation of insulin into transfersomes (Transfersulin) overcomes these entire problems. Cevc et al, (1998) studied insulin-loaded transfersomes and concluded that transfersomes-associated insulin is carried across the skin with an efficacy of >50% (and often >80%, if properly optimized).

Insulin associated with the ultradeformable vesicles (Transfersulin^{Tm}) was used to lower the blood glucose level in animals and in humans noninvasively (Cevc, 1993$_b$). After each transfersulin application on the intact skin, the first signs of systemic hypoglycemia are observed after 90 to 180 min, depending on the specific carrier composition. This result, which is nearly the same in mice, pigs, or humans, implies a delay of 45 to 145 min. relative to the onset of the subcutaneous insulin action. Maximum transfersomes-mediated decrease in the blood glucose concentration is estimated to be approximately ($35 \pm 10\%$) of the effect of similar subcutaneously injected insulin dose, but the cumulative effect is much higher (> 70%) and often approaches 100%. The results of epicutaneously applied mixed micelles or liposomes are negative in the investigated time period (Cevc et al., 1996)

18.11.3 Transfersomes as a carrier for interferon

Leukocytic derived interferon-a (INF-α) is a naturally occurring protein, having antiviral, antiproliferative and some immunomodulatry effects. Because of these properties, INF-α has found its place in therapy of several viral diseases and exhibits encouraging anticancer activities. Interferon-α is chemically protein so its delivery is very difficult. Transferesomes as drug delivery systems have the potential for providing controlled release of the administered drug and increasing the stability of labile drugs. Hafer et. al. studied the formulation of interleukin-2 and interferon-α containing transfersomes for potential transdermal application. They reported delivery of IL-2 and INF-α trapped by transfersomes in sufficient concentration for immunotherapy (Hafer et al, 1999).

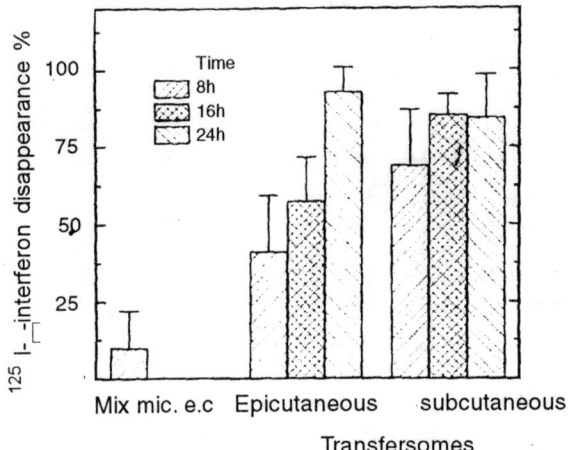

Fig. 18.10 : The trasport of ^{125}I-γ-interferon by means of transfersomes across the intact murine skin, as deduced from the disappearance of the agent-derived radioactivity from the body, measured by the whole body camera as a function of time (adapted from Cevc, 1996)

18.11.4 Transfersomes as a means of transdermal immunization

Many environmental pathogens attempt to enter the body through the skin. Skin, therefore, has evolved into an excellent protective barrier, which is also immunologically active. On the basis of above fact another most important application of transfersomes is transdermal immunization using transfersomes loaded with soluble protein like integral membrane protein, human serum albumin, gap junction protein. This approach offers at least two advantages, first they are applicable without injection and second, they give rise to rather high titers and possibly, to relatively high IgA levels (Paul et al, 1995, 1998).

18.11.5 Transfersomes as a carrier for corticosteroids

Corticosteroids are used topically for a large variety of dermatological conditions. They benefit by virtue of their anti-inflammatory, immunosuppressive, vasoconstrictor and antiproliferative action, which is used in atopic eczema, allergic contact dermatitis, arthritis, rash, sunburn, neurodermatitis, and psoriasis. The generally available corticosteroid formulations for topical use fulfill only a few of the therapeutics goals. The dermally administered corticosteroids typically fail to deliver a sufficiently large drug amount into the body for the successful therapy of the tissue deep under the application site. General problems in topical corticosteroids therapy of the present generation are :

1. local irritation, dermal atrophy on application of steroid topically in the form of cream and ointment,

2. systemic absorption of steroid occurs, which leads to systemic toxicity,

3. higher amounts of drugs are required when given in the form of cream and ointment because of the barrier function of skin, which results in poor permeability of drug,

4. occlusive dressing markedly enhances absorption of steroid, retains moisture and results in maceration of the horny layer, but continuous occlusion promotes bacterial and fungal growth,

5. use of penetration enhancer increases the permeability of drug across the skin in various commercial products, causes skin irritation and immunogenicity due to the local and systemic toxicity of chemical used (Schatzlein & cevc. 1995),

6. use of the highly concentrated or even supersaturated drug solution on the skin leads to the problem of drug precipitation and higher chances of the adverse effects (Cevc at el., 1995; Davis & Hadgraft, 1991)

To overcome all these problems complex lipid vesicles, transfersomes were used, which adapt their shape and properties to the surrounding stress and thus penetrate through the skin barrier . The advantages of transfersomes as a carrier for corticosteroid are :

1. transfersomes improve the site specificity and overall drug safety of corticosteroids delivery into skin by optimizing the epicutaneously administered drug dose (Cevc et al, 1997),

2. transfersome based corticosteroids are biologically active at doses several times lower than the currently used formulation for the treatment of skin diseases (Cevc et al, 1997),

3. by choosing a sufficiently high applied drug amount, epicutaneously administered transfersomes are made to transport enough agent into the blood circulation to bring the systemic corticosteroid concentration close to the value achieved by a subcutaneous injection of similar drug formulation in somewhat lower quantity (Cevc et al, 1997).

18.11.6 Transfersomes as a Carrier for Topical Analgesics and Anaesthetic Agents

The most popular route for the introduction of analgesics into the body is per OS. The effects of oral pain treatment are often relatively diffuse and weak, however in the case of strong peripheral pain subcutaneous drug injection are therefore therapy of choice. Analgesic drugs are hardly ever applied percutaneously owing to the poor therapeutic efficiency of such application resulting from the inadequate penetration of most analgesics through the intact skin. Owing to their low molecular weight and high water solubility, most of the standard monomolecular analgesics do not respond to a strong transdermal gradient, nor do they adequately permeate the skin. Thus analgesics in an aqueous solution, applied topically do not cross the skin permeability barrier and thus do not significantly suppress local pain. This is the case before, during and after evaporation of superficially applied water from the site of application.

Lipophilic analgesics have a somewhat higher chance of achieving the desired therapeutic effect, provided that they are applied under appropriate conditions. However, even with sufficiently lipophilic drugs used in combination with skin fluidizers, the analgesia after a dermal drug application is, as a rule, rather low

A new type of drug carrier, transfersomes, can circumvent this problem and provide formulations of unprecedented quality for the induction of local anesthesia and newly developed analgesics transfersomes for the management of local pain in rats and humans. These analgesics transfersomes can penetrate rapidly through the intact dermis and can also bring appreciable amounts of analgesic drugs into the skin. Depending on their composition, size and concentration, the transfersomal drug carrier can reach the cutis as well as the subcutis and consequently, may effect strongly the physiological functions of nociceptors and other nerve endings. With the use of analgesics transfersomes, peripheral transfersomes, peripheral pains can thus be suppressed at their very roots (Planas et al, 1992).

Application of anesthetics in the suspension of highly deformable vesicles, transfersomes, induces a topical anesthesia, under appropriate conditions, within less than 10 min. Maximum resulting pain insensitivity is nearly as strong (80%) as that of a comparable subcutaneous bolus injection, but the effect of tranfersomal anesthetics lasts longer. For example, the pain insensitivity mediated by the anesthetic transferesomes persists for at least 30 min. after a single drug application. Repeated use of transfersomal analgesics (e.g. 3 x every 2 to 3 min) extends the duration of drug action to 3 hr. and more; simultaneously, the maximum depth of the local anesthesia is increased. Injection induced anesthesia only lasts for less than 30 min (Planas et al., 1992)

18.11.7 Transfersomes as carrier for non-steroidal antiinflammatory agents

Nonsteroidal antiinflammatory agents have also been applied on the skin many times by means of lipid suspensions. The results obtained with the transfersomal formulations of diclofenac are elucidating and encouraging in this respect: 12 hr. after a single application of diclofenac in the ultradeformable vesicles, up to one order of magnitude higher drug concentration are measured in the soft tissue under the application site in comparison with the conventional hydrogel preparations.

The main advantages of transfersomal formulation of diclofenac are lowering the drug dose because the gel formulation only permits this drug to penetrate to a depth of 3 to 4 mm. In contrast to this, the transfersomal formulation of diclofenac always makes sure that the drug concentration in the soft tissues under the application site is by at least a factor of 4- and often by a factor of more than 10- higher than in the former case. In all species investigated so far (mice, rats, pigs) diclofenac was also found to penetrate deep into the soft tissues under the drug application site from the transfersomes. Similar observation was also made for ibuprofen delivery by means of tranfersomes. Thus, transfersomes not only dramatically improve the efficacy of diclofenac penetration through the intact skin permeability barrier, they also carry most of their associated agents directly into the depth of the soft tissues under the application site. The probable reason for this is the (transient) drug confinement to the carrier that prevents rapid agent elimination after the passage through the skin, being too big to disappear in the blood capillaries (Cevc, 1996)

18.11.8 Transfersomes as a carrier for anticancer drugs

Tamoxifen is the most common agent for the treatment of all stages of breast cancer. Despite the widespread use of this anti-oestrogen, it would be very desirable to develop a regio-selective and convenient-to-use formulation of the drug to lower the incident of side effects, such as depressions or thrombosis.

Cevc et al., (1996) developed tamoxifen formulation based on ultradeformable vesicles and applied on the shaved murine back, then most of the epidermally applied transfersomes penetrated the skin, leaving less than 5% of the drug-derived radioactivity on the body surface. Simultaneously, the integrated dose of tamoxifen (AUC) in the uterus, an organ with targatable estrogens receptors, is by the factor of 2 higher than that achieved by an oral application of the same amount of drug.

Experiments with the radioactively labelled tamoxifen in transfersomes in mice reveal significantly higher drug concentration in the body and better site-specificity after epicutaneous applications when compared with the orally administered tamoxifen. The biological activity of tamoxifen administrations on the skin by means of transfersomes is equally impressive. Such treatment accelerates the growth of murine uteri even at doses as low as 0.1 to 0.2 mg/kg/d. Ten-fold higher amounts of tamoxifen in soy oil must be injected subcutaneously in mice to achieve comparable biological effects by the nontrasfersomal formulations. Tamoxifen in soy oil given orally is also significantly less efficient than the epicutaneously used transfersomal drug formulation (Cevc, 1996)

18.12 CONCLUSION

Transfersomes are specially optimized particles or vesicles, which can respond to an external stress by rapid and energetically inexpensive, shape transformations. Such highly deformable particles can thus be used to bring drugs across the biological permeability barriers, such as skin. When tested in artificial systems. transfersomes can pass through even tiny pores (100 nm) nearly as efficiently as water, which is 1500 times smaller.

Drug laden transfersomes can carry unprecedented amounts of drug per unit time across the skin (up to 100mg cm^2 h^{-1}). The systemic drug availability thus mediated is frequently higher than, or at least approaches 80-90%. The biodistribution of radioactively labelled phospholipids applied in the form of transfersomes after

Table. 18. 3 : Different drugs used and results obtained of different studies of transfersomes for transdermal application.

Drug	Results	References
Insulin	High encapsulation efficacy	Cevc et al, 1998
	Transfer across the skin with an efficacy of >50%	
	Provide noninvasive means of therapeutic use	
Interferon-α	Efficient delivery means (because delivery by other	Hafer et al, 1999
Interleukin-2	route is difficult)	
	Controlled release	
	Overcome stability problem	
Soluble proteins	Permits non-invasive immunization through normal	Paul et al, 1995
Gap junction protein	skin	
Human serum albumin	Antibody titer is similar or even slightly higher than	Paul et al, 1998
Integral membrane protein	subcutaneous injection	Paul & Cevc 1995
Corticosteroids	Improve site specificity and overall drug safety	Cevc et al, 1997
Hydrocortisone	Biologically active at dose several times lower	
Triamcinolone acetonide	than the currently used formulation	
	Used both for local and systemic delivery	
Topical analgesic and	Suitable means for the noninvasive treatment of	Planas et al, 1992
anesthetic agent	local pain on direct topical drug application.	
Tetracaine		
Lidocaine		
Oestradiol	Improved transdermal flux	Maghraby et al, 1998
		Gamal et al, 1999
Tamoxifen	Improved transdermal flux	
Norgesterel	Improved transdermal permeation	Jain et al, 1998.

24 hr is essentially the same after an epicutaneous application or subcutaneous injection of the preparations. When used under different application conditions, transfersomes can also be positioned nearly exclusively and essentially quantitatively into the viable skin region.

Such a high efficacy of skin passage by transfersomes is quite reproducible even when carrier are loaded with the peptide molecules with a molecular weight of several KDa. Increasing the carrier deformability, however does speed up the skin penetration by transfersomes.

Transfersomes thus offer a singularly good opportunity for the non-invasive delivery of small, medium and large sized drugs. The results of the first human trials with the epicutaneously applied transfersomal insulin support this conclusion. The Transfersulin-induced systemic hypoglycemia in these experiments is found to reach approximately 30% of that induced by subcutaneous insulin injections, the cumulative efficiency over a period of 12 hr being comparable (>75-100%) in both cases. The former has a much slower action, however several unrelated transfersulin formulations were proven to be active hypoglycemically when applied on the intact skin.

Multiliter quantities of sterile, well defined transfersomes containing agent can be and have been prepared relatively easily. It therefore should be not before long that the corresponding drug formulation will find their way into clinics to be tested for the widespread usages.

This it can be a logical conclusion that transfersomes hold a promising future in effective transdermal delivery.

REFERENCES

Banga, A.K.; Chien, Y.W. (1988) "Iontophoretic delivery of drugs, fundamentals, developments and biomedical applications", J. Control. Rel., 7: 1-24

Barry, B.W. (1991) "LPP theory of skin penetration enhancement", J. Control. Rel., 15: 237-248

Bellantone, N.H.; Francoeur, M.L.; Rasadi, B. (1986) "Enhanced percutaneous absorption via iontophoresis. I. Evaluation of an in vitro system and transport of model compounds", Int. J. Pharm., 30: 72-80

Burnette, R.R.; Ongpipattanakul, B. (1987) "Characterization of the permselective properties of excised human skin during iontophoresis", J. Pharm. Sci., 76: 765-773

Cevc, G. (1985) "Molecular force theory of solvation of the polar solutes. The mean field solvation model, its implication and examples from lipid/water mixtures", Chem. Scripta, 25: 97-110

Cevc, G. (1987) "How membrane chain melting properties are controlled by the polar surface of the lipid bilayers", Biochemistry, 26: 6305-6318

Cevc, G. (1990) "Membrane electrostatics", Biochem. Biophys. Acta., 1031: 311-325

Cevc, G. (1991a) "How membrane chain-melting phase transition temperature is affected by the lipid chain-asymmetry and degree of unsaturation: analysis and prediction based on the effective chain length model", Biochemistry, 30/29: 7186-7202

Cevc, G. (1991b) "Isothermal lipid phase transition", Chem. Phys. Lipids, 57: 293-299

Cevc, G. (1992a) " Rationale for production and dermal application of lipid vesicles", In: Broun, O.; Korting, H. C.; Malbach, H. I. (Eds)., Liposome dermatics, Springer Verlag Berlin, Germany, 82-90

Cevc, G. (1992b) "Lipid properties as a basis for the modeling and design of liposome membrane", In: Liposome technology, 2nd ed., Gregoriadis G., (Ed.), CRC Press, Boca Raton, FL, 1-43

Cevc, G. (Ed.), (1993a) "Phospholipids Handbook", Marcel Dekker, New York, Basel, Hong Kong, 215-240

Cevc, G. (1993b) "Lipid hydration, In: Hydration of biological macromolecules", Westhof, E. (Ed.), Macmillan Press, New York, 338-351

Cevc, G. (1994), "Material transport across permeability barriers by means of lipid vesicles", In: Hand book of physics of biological systems", Lipowsky, R. (Ed.), Vol. I, Elsevier Sciences, Amsterdam, 441-466

Cevc, G. (1996) "Transferomes, liposomes and other lipid suspensions on the skin, permeation enhancement, vesicles penetratuion and transdermal drug delivery", Crit. Rev. Ther. Drug Carrier Syst., 13: 257-388

Cevc, G. (1997) "Drug delivery across the skin", Exp. Opinion. Invest. Drugs, 6: 1887-1937

Cevc, G.; Blume, G. (1992) "Lipid vesicles penetrate into intact skin owing to the transdermal osmotic gradients and hydration force", Biochem. Biophys Acta., 1104: 226-232

Cevc, G.; Blume, G.; Schatzlein, A. (1997) "Transfersomes-mediated transepidermal delivery improves the regiospecificity and biological activity of corticosteroids in vivo", J. Control. Rel., 45: 211-226

Cevc, G.; Blume, G.; Schatzlein, A.; Gebauer, D.; Paul, A. (1996) "The skin : a pathway for the systemic treatment with patches and lipid based agent carriers", Adv. Drug. Deliv. Rev. 18: 349-378

Cevc, G.; Grbauer, D.; Schatzlein, A.; Blume, G. (1993) "Ultra high efficiency of drug and peptide transfer through the intact skin by means of novel drug carriers, Transfersomes", *In*: Bain, K.R.; Hadgkraft, A J.; James, W.J.; Water, K.A. (Eds.), Prediction of percutaneous penetration, Vol. 3b, STS Publishing, Cardiff, 226-234

Cevc, G.; Grbauer, D.; Schatzlein, A.; Blume, G. (1998) "Ultraflexible vesicles transfersomes have an extremely therapeutic amount of insulin across the intact mammalian skin", Biochem. Biophys. Acta., 1368: 201-215

Cevc G.; Marsh D. (1995) "Phospholipid Bilayers Physical Principals and Models". Wiley Intersciences, New York, 235-250

Cevc, G.; Schatzlein, A.; Blume G. (1995) "Transdermal drug carrier basic properties , optimization and transfer efficiency in the case of epicutaneously applied peptides", J. Control. Rel. 36: 3-16

Cevc, G.; Strahmaier, L.; Berkhalz, J.; Blume G. (1990) "Molecular mechanism of protein interaction with the lipid bilayer membrane", Stud. Biophys., 138: 57-70

Chapman, S.J.; Walsh, A. (1990) "Desmosomes, corneosomes and desquamation. An ultrastructural study of adult pig epidermis", Arch. Dermatol. Res. 282: 304-320

Chowdary, K.P.R.; Naidu, R.A.S. (1995) "Transdermal drug delivery; a review of current status", Indian drugs, 32(9): 414-422.

Christophers, E. (1988) *In* : The skin of vertebrates, Spearman, R.I.C.; Riley, P.A.; (Eds.), Academic Press, London, 137-139

Christophers, E.; Walff, H.H.; Laurence, E.B. (1974) "The formation of epidermal cell columns", J. Invest. Dermatol., 62: 556-564

Cooper, E.R. (1987) "Alteration in skin permeability", *In*: Transdermal controlled systemic medication ,Chien, Y.W. (Ed.), Mercel Dekker, New York, 83-92

Davis, A.F.; Hadgraft, J. (1991) "Effects of supersaturation on membrane transport: I. Hydrocortisone acetate", Int. J. Pharm., 76: 1-8

Fry, D. W.; White, J.C.; Goldman, I. D. (1978) "Rapid seperation of low molecular weight solutes from liposome without dilution", J. Anal. Biochem., 90: 809-815

Gamal, M.; El Maghraby, M.; Williams, A.C.; Barry B.W. (1999) "Skin delivery of oestradiol from deformable and traditional liposomes : Mechanistic studies", J. Pharm. Pharmacol., 51: 1123-1134

Gompper, G.; Kroll, D. M. (1995) "Driven transport of fluid vesicles through narrow pores", Phys. Rev., E.52: 4198-4211

Hadgraft, J.; Guy, R.H. (Eds.), (1989) "Transdermal drug delivery: Development issues and Research initiative", Marcel Dekker, New York, 1-22

Hafer, C.; Goble, R.; Deering P.; Lehmer, A.; Breut, J. (1999), "Formulation of interleukin-2 and interferon-a containing ultradeformable carriers for potential transdermal application", Anticancer Res., 19(2c): 1505-1512

Holland, H.E.J.; Bouwstra, JA.; Spies, A. (1995) "Interactions between nonionic surfactant vesicles and human stratum corneum in vitro", J. Liposome Res., 5: 241-64.

Jain, S.; Sapre,R. and Jain, N.K. (1998) "Pro-ultraflexible lipid vesicles for effective transdermal delivery of Norgestrel." Proceeding of 25th Conferance of CRS, U.S.A.,32.

Jansen H.; Deboer, M.; Elwenspoet B. (1995) "The back silicon method IV, micro electro. Mechanical systems", Institute of electrical and electronics Engineers, Piscataway, NJ. 88-93.

Juliano, R.L. (1980) "Drug delivery systems". Oxford University Press, New York, 15.

Kenry, S.; Devom, V.; Mark, G.A.; Prausnitz, M.R. (1998) "Micro fabricated micro needles; A novel approach to transdermal drug delivery", J. Pharm. Sci., 87 (8): 922-925.

Kiro, P.C.; Kiu, J. C.; Change, S.F.; Chien, Y.W. (1987) "Transdermal delivery of oxycodone enhancement mechanism with iontophoresis", Pharm. Res., 4: 62-78

Kulkarni, R.G.; Jain S.; Agrawal G.P.; Chourasia M.; Jain S.; Jain N.K. (2000) "Advances in transdermal drug delivery systems", Pharma Times, 32(5): 21-24

Lasch, J.; Laub, P.; Wohlrab, W. (1991) "How deep intact liposome penetrate the human skin", J. Control. Rel. 18: 55-58

Levy, D.; Kost, J.; Meshulam, Y.; Langer, R. (1989) "Effect of ultrasound on transdermal drug delivery to rats and guinea pigs", J. Clni. Invest., 83: 2074-2078

Maghraby, E.l.; Willams, M.; Barry, B.W. (1998) "Optimization of deformable vesicles for epidermal delivery of oestradiol", J. Pharm. Pharnacol. 50(Suppl.), 146

Masada, J.; Rous, U.; Higuchi, W.; Behl, C.; Malick W.; Goldberg, A. K.; Pous S. (1985) "Examination of iontophoretic transport of ionic drugs across skin Baseline studies with four electrode systems", Abstrats of 39th National Meting of the Academy of Pharmaceutical Sciences, Minneapolis, MN, 15, 73.

Mezei, M.; Gulasekharam, V. (1980) "Liposomes: a selective drug delivery system for the topical route of administration. I. Lotion dosage form", Life Sci., 26: 1473-1477

New, R.R.C. (1990) "Liposomes: A practical approach", Oxford University Press, Oxford, 1-15

Panchagnula, R. (1997) "Transdermal delivery of drugs", Ind J. Pharmacol., 29: 140-156

Paul, A.; Cevc G.; Bachhawat, B.K. (1995) "Transdermal immunization with large proteins by means of ultradeformable drug carriers", Eur. J. Immunol., 25: 3521-3524

Paul, A.; Cevc, G.; Bachhawat, B.K. (1998) "Transdermal immunisation with an integral membrane component, gap junction protein, by means of ultradefromable drug carriers, transfersomes", Vaccine, 16: 188-195

Paul, A.; Cevc, G., (1995) "Non-invasive administration of protein antigens. Epicutaneous with the bovine serum albumin", Vaccine Research, 4: 145-164

Planas, M.E.; Gonzalez, P.; Rodriguez, S.; Sanchez, G.; Cevc. G. (1992) "Noninvasive percutaneous induction of topical analgesia by a new type drug carrier and prolongation of the local pain intensity by liposomes", Anesth. Analg., 95: 615-621

Praousnitz, M.R.; Edelman, E.R.; Gimm, J.A.; Langer, R.; Weaver, J.C. (1995) "Transdermal delivery of heparin by skin electroporation", Biotechnology, 12: 1205-1209.

Prausnitz, M.R.; Allen, M.G. (1998) J. Pharm. Sci., 87(8): 925

Prousnitz, M.R. (1997) "Reversible skin permeabilization for transdermal delivery of macromolecules", Crit. Rev. Ther. Drug. Carrier Syst., 14(4): 455-483

Rand, R.P.; Parsegian, V.A. (1989) "Hydrophilic force between phospholipid bilayers", Biochem. Biophys. Acta, 988: 351-377

Runyan, W.R.; Bean, K.E. (1990) "Semiconductor integrated circuit processing technology", Addison-Wesley, New York,.

Sage, B.H. (1995) Iontophoresis. *In* : Smith, E.W.; Maibach, H.I. (Eds.), Percutanous Penetration Enhancers, CRC Press, Boca Raton, 351-368.

Schatzlein, A.; Cevc, G. (1995) "Skin penetration by phospholipid vesicles, Transfersomes as visualized by means of the Confocal Scanning Laser Microscopy, *In*: Phospholipids characterization, metabolisim, and novel biological applications" (Cevc, G.; Paltauf, E., Eds.), Champaign, AOCS Press, 191-209

Schatzlein, A.; Cevc, G. (1998) "Non-uniform cellular packing of the stratum corneum and permeability barrier function of intact skin : a high resolution Confocal Scanning Laser Microscopy study using highly deformable vesicles (Transfersomes)", Brit. J. Dermatol., 138: 583-598

Schreier, H.; Bouwstra, J. (1994) "Liposome and niosomes as topical drug carriers : dermal and transdermal drug delivery", J. Control. Rel., 30: 1-15

Schubert, R.; Beyer, K.; Wolburg, H.; Schmidt, K.H. (1986) "Structural changes in vesicles membranes of large unilamellar vesicles after binding of sodium cholate", Biochemistry, 25, 5263-5271

Schubert, R.; Beyer, K.; Wolburg, H.; Schmidt, K. H. (1988) "Structural change in vesicles membrane and mixed micelles of various lipid compositions after binding of different bile salts", Biochemistry, 27, 8787-8796

Shaw, J.E.; Chandrasekaran, S.K. (1989) *In*: pharmacology of the skin", Greaves, M.W.; Shuster S. (Eds.), Springer- Verlag, Berlin, 115-122

Simonetti, O.; Hoogstraate, J.; Bodde, H.E. (1995) "Visualization of diffusion pathways across the stratum corneum of native and in-vitro-reconstructed epidermis by confocal laser scanning microscopy", Arch. Dermatol. Res., 287: 465-473

Sounderson, J.E.; Coldwell, R.W.; Hsio, J.; Dixon, R. (1987) "Noninvasive delivery of a novel inotsopic catecholamine iontophoretic. Versus intravenous infusion in dogs". J. Pharm. Sci, 76: 215-218

Stillwell, G.K. "Electrical stimulation and iontophoresis" *In*: Krussen, F.H., (Ed.), Handbook of physical medicine and rehabilitation, W.B. Saunders company, St. Louis, Mo, 1971, chap. 14

Swartzendruber, D.C.; Wertz, P.D.; Kitko, D.J. (1989), "Molecular models of intercellular lipid lamellae in mammalian stratum corneum", J. Invest. Dermatol., 92: 251-258

Walters, K.A. (1989) *In*:Transdermal drug delivery", Development issues and research initiatives, Hadgraft, J.; Guy, R.H. (Ed.) Marcel Dekker, New York, , 197-246

Wang, S.; Kara, M.; Rjishnan, T.R. (1997) "Topical delivery of cyclosporin A coevaporate using electroporation technique". Drug Dev. Ind. Pharm., 23: 657-663.

Warner, R.R.; Myers, M.C.; Taylar, D.A. (1988) "Electron probe analysis of human skin determination of the water concentration profiles", J. Inves. Dermatol., 90: 218-224

Wearley, L.L.; (1991) "Recent progress in protein and peptide delivery by noninvasive routes", Crit. Rev. Drug Carr. Sys., 8, 331-394

Weaver, J.C.; Chizmadzhev Y., (1996), "Electroporation", *In* : Polte, C.; Postow, E. (Eds.), "Biological effects of electromagnetic fields", CRC, press, Boca Raton, NY, 247-274.

Willams, A.C.; Barry, B.W. (1992) " Skin absorption enhencers", Crit. Rev. Drug Carr. Sys., 9, 305-353

Williams, A.C.; Barry, B.W. (1990), *In*: Scott, R.C.; Guy, R.H.; Hadgraft, J. (Eds.) "Prediction of percutaneous penetration", I.B.C, Technical services, London, 2, 224-230

Chapter 19 _____

Targeted Delivery of Drugs

Roop K. Khar, Manish Diwan

19.1 INTRODUCTION

Drug targeting is the delivery of drugs to receptors or organs or any other specific part of the body to which one wishes to deliver the drug exclusively. The drug's therapeutic index (TI), as measured by its pharmacological response and safety, relies in the access and specific interaction of the drug with its candidate receptor, whilst minimizing its interaction with non-target tissue. The desired differential distribution of drug by its targeted delivery would spare the rest of the body and thus significantly reduce the overall toxicity while maintaining its therapeutic benefits. The targeted or site-specific delivery of drugs is indeed a very attractive goal because this provides one of the most potential ways to improve the therapeutic index of the drugs. The need for targeted delivery of drugs is best illustrated with peptide drugs where failure in the clinic may not be due to a poor intrinsic activity, but rather due to transport factors including widespread disposition, rapid catabolism and excretion, variable or inefficient extravasation, and the subsequent high dosing levels required to obtain a therapeutic effect (Tomlinson et al, 1986). Earlier work done between late 1960s and the mid 1980s stressed the need for drug-carrier systems primarily to alter the pharmacokinetics of the already proven drugs whose efficacy might be improved by altering the rates of metabolism in liver or clearance by the kidneys (Pozansky & Juliano,1984). These approaches generally were not focussed to achieve site-specific or targeted delivery such as getting a cytotoxic drug to cancerous tissue while sparing other normal, though equally sensitive tissue (Papahadjopoulos, 1978). With the advancement in the 'carrier technology' the issue of delivering either individual drug molecule or the entire carrier to the desired site has been addressed during the last few years.

The targeted delivery of drugs may be achieved by different approaches that may be classified broadly into three categories. These are as follows:

1. Physical or mechanical approach

2. Biological approach

3. Chemical approach

19.2 PHYSICAL OR MECHANICAL APPROACH

It requires formulation of the drug using a particulate delivery device, which by virtue of its physical localization will allow differential release of the drug. The site specificity is due to the exclusive generation of higher drug concentrations at the site of localization of the device, while the drug concentration in the rest of the body is very much diminished due to the simple dilution factor. This type of targeting is referred as 'passive targeting' which exploits the natural fate of the particles given intravenously or orally.

The carrier systems employed are either solid particulates such as microspheres, nanoparticles, or liquid colloids such as liposomes. The microparticulate carriers can be monolithic or capsular in construction. These may range from 20nm to 20mm in diameter. Colloidal particles in the nanometre size range (less than 1µm) can be engineered to provide site-specific delivery of encapsulated drugs after injection into the general circulation or lymphatic systems. The particulate carriers may target liver (Kupffer cells and hepatocytes), endothelial cells, sites of inflammation and lymph nodes. The size and surface of the particles are crucial factors in targeting. Several anatomical compartments exist where particulates are retained due to either the physical properties of the environment or the biophysical interactions of particles with the cellular components of the target tissue. The delivery of drug in this manner yields a persistent and sustained supply of the drug at the target site.

19.2.1 Localization of particulate carriers

Fate of intravenously injected microparticulate carriers largely depends on their sizes. Particles small enough to escape capillary filtration, are generally taken up by cells of the mononuclear phagocytic system. The blood carries the 'particle-loaded' macrophages through the liver, spleen and bone marrow. About 90% of these macrophages are removed by the Kupffer cells, 5% by the spleen and the few remaining percent by the bone marrow (Bradfield, 1980). The dominance of the liver as the prominent site for clearance reflects the accessibility and capacity of the uptake of the drug carrying particles. The extent of particle clearance by the mononuclear phagocytic system is further influenced by the surface characteristics, hydrophilicity and hydrophobicity and the net charge on the particles (Davis, 1997; Gregoriadis et al, 1985).

Orally administered microspheres are taken up from the intestine by Peyer's patches which are present in the GI tract (Eldridge et al, 1989). This passive localization of the carriers facilitates selective delivery of carrier-associated materials to the gut associated or systemic lymphoid organs. In addition, encapsulation of the biologically labile drugs such as proteins or nucleotides, protect them from inactivation or degradation by enzymes, acids or hydrolysis in vivo. These particulate carriers therefore, can be designed to carry the therapeutic or diagnostic agents in intact particles for the manifestation of the desired action both by parenteral and mucosal applications.

19.2.1.1 Targeting to the mononuclear phagocytic system

Passive localization of intravenously administered liposomes within the macrophages of the mononuclear phagocytic system (MPS) can be exploited to deliver bioactive agents selectively to these cells for enhanced therapeutic activity. This system is a connective tissue of cells mesenchymal in origin. The main functions of the MPS include the clearance of a large variety of potentially harmful substances from the plasma, catabolism of macromolecules, participation in the immune response and the synthesis and secretion of various effector molecules. Targeting of gamma-interferon, or other immunomodulators, to macrophages transforms these cells into more competent host defence cells with the capacity to kill tumor cells (Bugelsky et al, 1985).

Specific targeting of antivirals such as azidothymidine (AZT) to macrophages has been described by using nanoparticles as colloidal drug carrier. The routes of administration employed were intravenous and oral. The drug concentrations in organs belonging to the reticuloendothelial system were 18 folds higher when the drug was administered as bound to nanoparticles, than the drug levels achieved after intravenous injection of aqueous AZT solution. Administration of drug-nanoparticles conjugate by oral route also gave better results than the free drug in solution. The increase in the drug concentrations at sites containing higher number of macrophages may also be of utility in reduction of dosage to avoid or reduce the systemic toxicity (Lobenberg & Kreuter, 1996).

An immunostimulator, muryl dipeptide (MDP) loaded in liposomes when injected in mice by intravenous route showed significant higher macrophage-mediated tumoricidal activity as compared to the animal group to which it was delivered in saline (Fidler & Raz, 1981).

Intravenous injection of a liposomal preparation carrying MDP and human C-reactive protein showed significant reduction in established metastases produced by several murine tumors (Fidler et al, 1980). Multiple metastatic lesions containing several thousand tumor cells were present in the mice footpad at the onset of therapy. After 3-4 days of therapy with liposomes-encapsulated macrophage activating agents the 'primary lesions' at the tumor site disappeared. At the end of the therapy period of 3 weeks no macro- or microscopic tumor were noticed in 70% of the treated animals. In the control group, receiving no therapy, these metastatic 'primary lesions' progressed to form large colonies exceeding 2-3 μm in diameter at the time of death (Deodhar et al, 1982). Furthermore, liposomal delivery of compounds such as MDP may provide extended retention which otherwise shows rapid blood clearance when administered in saline (90% of MDP injected intravenously can be detected in the urine within 2 hr) (Parant et al, 1979).

Intracellular infections caused by a number of bacteria, fungi, viruses and pathogenic protozoa are usually difficult to manage clinically with conventional chemotherapy due to limited permeation of drugs into the cells. Administration of antimicrobial drugs in liposomes offers a possible solution to this problem. The phagocytic uptake of the systemically delivered drug-loaded liposome provides an efficient method for delivery of drug directly to the site of infection. The encapsulation of various chemotherapeutic agents in liposomes has been described to achieve enhanced intracellular concentration of these agents. It has resulted not only in the reduction of drug toxicity, at the same time there was no adverse effect on the efficacy of drug as seen in the treatment of systemic fungal infections such as candidosis, histoplasmosis and cryptococcosis. Some of the drugs delivered in liposomes include, cephalothin for murine salmonellosis (Desiderio & Campbell, 1983), amikacin, gentamicin, kanamycin and tobramycin against S.aureus (Fountain et al, 1981), pentostam for leishmaniasis (New et al, 1981), amphotericin B for histoplasmosis and cryptococosis (Taylor et al, 1982; Lopez-Berstein et al, 1983), ribavirin against Rift Valley viral fever (Kende et al, 1985), and idoxuridine for herpes simplex keratitis (Smolin et al, 1981).

19.2.1.2 Targeting to the pulmonary region

The microparticulate drug carriers have also been employed for pulmonary drug targeting. It has been observed that instilled microspheres larger than 7μm are effectively lodged in the pulmonary region. Particles of 3 to 7μm in diameter, instilled into the lungs of the beagle dogs can translocate to the tracheobroncheal lymph nodes (Snipes et al, 1984) and appear to be extracellularly accumulated (Lehnert et al, 1968). Small liposomes of 50nm are retained for many hours, though those depositing in the tracheal bronchial regions are physically cleared within 6 hrs by the mucocilliary escalator (Juliano & McCullough, 1980). Liposomes and microspheres have been used effectively to provide a sustained input of the encapsulated drugs to the lung tissue leading to an increase in drug efficacy and a decrease in drug toxicity (Mufson & Szoka, 1985).

Intravenous administration of radiolabeled microspheres leads to localization in the lungs, which has applications in diagnostics (Al-Janabi et al, 1984). Particles larger than 7μm get entrapped in the capillaries of the lung. This phenomenon has been employed for the scintigraphic examination of tumor masses within the lung (Widder et al, 1983).

Similarly, the approach can also be utilized in the treatment of emphysema. Martodam et al (1979) have demonstrated the feasibility of passive targeting to the lungs in case of a peptide-linked inhibitor of human leukocyte elastase covalently coupled to the surface of human serum albumin microspheres.

19.2.1.3 Extravascular delivery

The ability to leave the blood pool or 'extravasation' in a reproducible, efficient manner is critical to the drug's action delivered using carriers. The potential for particulate extravasation being limited, it is argued that the use of these carriers will probably be restricted to targets within discrete anatomical compartments, to intravascular targets, or to extravascular targets at highly specialized areas of endothelia, or where the pathology at the site permits particulate extravasation.

Solid lipid nanoparticles have been shown to be preferentially accumulated in the brain upon intravenous administration (Yang et al, 1999). An anticancer drug, camptothecin, loaded in these nanoparticles of 196.8nm mean diameter was given as 0.1% suspension alongwith 2% stearic acid, 1.5% soybean lecithin and 0.5% Poloxamer 188. The average mean residence time after intravenous administration of the encapsulated camptothecin was much higher than the soluble drug, especially in brain, heart and reticuloendothelial cells containing organs.

The dalargin does not normally penetrate the blood brain barrier when given intravenously. Poly(butyl cyanoacrylate) nanoparticles coated with polysorbate 80 were investigated as drug carriers for delivery across the BBB. The dalargin loaded nanoparticles coated with polysorbate 80 induced an analgesic effect at a minimum dose of 5mg/Kg. On the other hand, neither the intravenous injection of dalargin alone at various dose levels nor the mixture of dalargin loaded nanoparticles without the polysorbate 80 were able to induce an analgesic activity (Schroder & Sabel, 1996).

The application of a drug in solution to the eye, suffers from the limitations of dilution or wash out effects with lachrymal fluid resulting in a short span of availability for manifestation of drug's pharmacological action. A pH sensitive nanoparticle suspension, which gels in neutral pH environment of the cul-de-sac of the eye, has been described by Gurny et al (1985). The drug was delivered as adsorbed on the particles. The changes in the visco-elastic properties of the particle suspension from fluid (at the acid pH of lachrymal fluid) to gel resulted in ocular retention of the dosage form and enhanced therapeutic profile of the drug compared to a solution of the free drug applied topically.

The inraarticular administration of liposomes containing the sterol cortisol palmitate has been shown to persist within the joint (Ratcliffe et al, 1984). These were used successfully in the treatment of experimental rabbits' arthritis of the knee joints at relatively lower than the recommended normal dose of the drug when delivered conventionally (Dingle et al, 1978). The larger microparticles (7-15 μm in diameter) are retained for longer periods with evidence of uptake by the macrophages within the synovium (Noble et al, 1983).

19.2.1.4 Mucosal delivery of antigens

The mucosal surfaces, including lining of gastro-intestinal (GI) tract, lungs, nose and vagina, are the sites of entry of most pathogens into the body. For this reason, the ability to induce high titers of secretory immunoglobulin fraction A (IgA) may be important for mucosal immunity to protect against challenge by many infectious agents. Parenteral injections of antigen are usually the least effective at stimulating production of IgA, which is most effectively elicited by immunization of mucosal surfaces for example, oral and intratracheal administration. Oral immunization offers the advantages of convenience, reduced cost of administration and greater patient acceptance. Bacterial vaccines, recombinant proteins or DNA vaccines none can be administered orally as these antigens undergo enzymatic or hydrolytic degradation under the influence of gastric juices and acidic pH conditions.

Orally administered microspheres are taken up from the intestine by Peyer's patches, hence these have considerable potential as carriers for oral immunization (Eldridge et al, 1989; O'Hagan, 1990; Ermak et al, 1995). The polymer wall of microspheres protects encapsulated vaccine from degradation by the low pH of the gastric juice and from proteolysis in the gut. Administration of vaccines loaded in microspheres, orally often leads to the induction of IgA antibody production not only in the mucosa of the gut, but also in the other mucosal surfaces of the body, including the genitourinary and respiratory tracts (Challacombe et al, 1997). Eldridge et al (1990) have shown that orally administered microspheres containing Staphylococcal enterotoxin B (SEB) toxoid targeted to Peyer's patches induced not only circulating immunoglobulin fraction M (IgM), immunoglobulin fraction G (IgG) and IgA antitoxin antibody, but also a disseminated mucosal IgA response in mice. In contrast, oral immunization with the same amount of fluid antigen resulted in minimal to no antibody titers of all classes.

Size of the microspheres employed for targeting plays a significant role in determining the type and quality of the immune response to oral immunization. Eldridge and colleagues (1990) also showed that orally administered microspheres less than 10 μm in diameter are preferentially absorbed by the Peyer's patches in the GI tract and passed to the immune inductive environment of both Peyer's patches and systemic lymphoid organs. Time course studies performed to know the fate of the microspheres within the gut-associated lymphoid tissue showed that the majority of microspheres less than 5μm in diameter were transported through the efferent lymphatics within macrophages, while the majority of those more than 5μm in diameter remained in the Peyer's patches for upto 35 days. This pattern of absorption and redistribution suggests that particle size may be determinant in the type of immune response i.e. systemic or mucosal, elicited by oral vaccination with antigen-containing microspheres.

Microencapsulated oral vaccines designed to protect against diarrhoea induced by enterotoxigenic E. coli are currently in the early stages of development (Edelman, 1993). Encapsulation of a pilus protein (colonization factor antigen) in microspheres has been shown to preserve its immunogenicity on oral administration and, subsequently uptake of antigen loaded microspheres by the Peyer's patches (McQueen, 1993). This resulted in the induction of high systemic (IgG) and mucosal (IgA) antibody response and protection of rabbits when challenged with the pathogen (Reid et al, 1993).

Mucosal immunization with encapsulated antigen has shown a great deal of potential as a means of boosting the immune response to achieve a high level of local mucosal IgA antibody. For example, oral or intratracheal (i.t.) boosting of mice that received intraperitoneal (i.p.) primary immunizations with microencapsulated SEB toxoid was as effective at inducing disseminated mucosal IgA antitoxin antibodies as three oral doses in microspheres. On the other hand, soluble toxoid was ineffective for boosting (Eldridge et al, 1991). In a subsequent study, rhesus macaques that received two intramuscular (i.m.) primary immunizations, followed by i.t. boosting, were protected against aerosol challenge with lethal doses of SEB (Staas et al, 1993).

19.2.1.5 Magnetic drug targeting

Anticancer drugs reversibly bound to magnetic fluids called ferrofluids, could be concentrated in locally advanced tumors by magnetic fields that are arranged at the tumor surface outside of the subject. A magnetic fluid has been reported to which the drugs, cytokines and other molecules can be chemically bound to enable those agents to be directed within the subject under influence of high-energy magnetic fields. In one such example, epidoxorubicin was chemically conjugated with the ferrofluid which act as a vehicle to concentrate the drug locally in tumours. The magnetic fluid mediated treatment was found safe in an experimental human kidney and in a xenotransplanted colon carcinoma model (Lubbe et al, 1996a). Phase I clinical trials using this approach in 14 patients with advanced and unsuccessfully pretreated cancers or sarcomas have been conducted. Nine such patients received two treatment courses, 3 patients received one course of magnetic drug targeting consisting of the infusion of epirubicin in increasing doses (from 5 to 10mg/m^2) that had been chemically bound to a magnetic fluid and the application of magnetic fields to the tumors for 60-120min. Based on magnetic resonance tomographic techniques, pharmacokinetics, and the histological detection of magnetites, it was shown that the ferrofluid was successfully directed to the tumors in about one-half of the patients (Lubbe et al, 1996b).

19.3 BIOLOGICAL APPROACH

Of particular importance and most viable among the three approaches explored for the targeted delivery, is biological. It involves delivery of the drug using a carrier system with targeting moiety either in-built (by virtue of the structure of the carrier) or is chemically coupled. The concept of "magic bullets" for drug targeting was given by the great cell biologist, Paul Ehrlich (Ehrlich, 1906). His statement "...bodies which possess a particular affinity for a certain organ? a carrier to bring therapeutically active groups to the organ in question" was made in 1898 at a time when antibodies had not yet been discovered.

A wide variety of macromolecular, particulate and cellular matrices have been proposed for use as carriers for drug targeting. These include microspheres, nanoparticles, liposomes, erythrocytes, antibodies, dextrans, plasma proteins, polynucleotides, polymorphonuclear leukocytes, etc. Four targeting strategies seem to have dominated this approach which are:

(1) antibodies directed against specific cell surface antigens,

(2) endogenous carbohydrate-binding proteins (lectins),

(3) glycoconjugates functioning as specific ligands for receptors on specific cells that recognize particular sugar residues, and

(4) hormones functioning as specific ligands for receptors on specific targets.

19.3.1 Antibodies for antigen targeting

It has been postulated that the need for non-specific immunostimulators for eliciting strong responses to weak antigens is related to the poor antigen processing efficacy or their poor recognition by receptors of T-cells and/or B-cells. It may be possible to achieve much higher immune responses to antigens without the use of potent adjuvants if antigens are directed to antigen presenting cells (APCs) and lymphocytes by coupling them with a ligand of strong binding affinity for molecules of the Major Histocompatibility Complex (MHC). This approach is particularly attractive for the delivery of synthetic peptides or small recombinant antigens where the attraction of large number of mononuclear cells to the site of injection is normally needed in order to affect adequate processing and presentation of small molecules.

Studies in mice have demonstrated that the coupling of viral antigens to monoclonal antibodies against a mouse Class II MHC molecule has elicited antibody response with much less antigen than needed without the use of the targeting molecule (Carayanniotis & Barber, 1987). These responses were obtained without any adjuvant and suggested a promising approach to safer vaccines. This study indicated that the targeted antigen may be needed only in the first injection to prime the response and that unconjugated antigen could be used to stimulate secondary responses.

It is noteworthy that in vitro studies of antigen presentation to T-cells have indicated that the efficiency of presentation can be enhanced as much as 1,000 fold by coupling antigen with antibodies specific for determinants on the APCs (Snider and Segal, 1987).

Studies have also been reported using cell targets other than MHC molecules which have successfully used immunotargeting for T-cells (Staerz & Bevan, 1986), follicular dendritic cells (Inaba & Steinman, 1985) and B-cells (Casten et al, 1988). In the studies involving B-cells the targeting of cell surface antigens specific for this cell type, markedly facilitated the processing and presentation of antigens by B-cells. Thus, it may be possible to use more than one target by coupling antigens with multiple cell-specific ligands in appropriate proportions for optimal responses. The means for targeting antigens have been the use of mouse monoclonal antibodies (mAbs) directed to cellular molecules. These mAbs are unlikely to be suitable for immunizing non-rodents but humanized mAbs or other specific ligands may render this approach practical for vaccine development.

It is possible to coat drug loaded erythrocytes with biotinylated antibodies in the presence of avidin or streptavidin. These immunoerythrocytes bind specifically to the immobilized antigens and are susceptible to complement mediated lysis. This helps in achieving high local concentration of the encapsulated drug which gets released after the lysis of RBCs. The in-vitro model described in the report describes the possibilty of coating with specific antibody that leads to site-specific/targeted delivery of drug (Muzykantov et al, 1996).

Conjugation of drugs with antibodies to surface endothelial antigens is a potential strategy for drug delivery to endothelium. The antibodies to platelet-endothelial adhesion molecule 1 (PECAM-1), however are poorly internalized by the endothelial cells and accumulated poorly after intravenous administration in mice and rats. It was shown that conjugation of biotinylated anti-PECAM antibodies with streptavidin markedly stimulated uptake and internalization of anti-PECAM by endothelial cells and by cells expressing PECAM after either intravenous or intraarterial injection (Muzykantov et al, 1999).

Cholera toxin is well adapted to the GI tract. It is acid-stable, is not bound by mucins, and uses a receptor glycolipid (ganglioside GM1) present in high concentrations on intestinal epithelial cell surfaces. Cholera toxin subunit B (CTB) is a unique adjuvant for mucosal vaccines by virtue of its uptake by M cells. These M cells deliver foreign material by transepithelial transport from lumen to the organized lymphoid tissue, within the mucosa (Peyer's patches) that are the sites of T-cell helper responses and for production of secretory (IgA) antibodies by B-cells (Nedrud & Lamm, 1991). CTB is the non-toxic pentameric portion of the cholera toxin responsible for binding to GM1 can enhance the mucosal immune response when coupled directly to antigen (Dertzbaugh & Elson, 1991). This suggested that the presence of CTB on the surface of particulate carriers such as microspheres encapsulating vaccines, would enhance M-cell uptake of the particles and hence immune response. In our laboratory, microspheres were prepared using biodegradable poly-lactide-co-glycolide (50:50 PLGA) copolymers encapsulating tetanus toxoid as a model protein. During microspheres preparation, dextran-oleates linked to SPDP were employed as 'phase stabilizers', which made it possible to covalently couple CTB (via SPDP) at the exposed conjugation sites on the surface of the microspheres. The presence of immunoreactive CTB on the surface of microspheres was confirmed by immunofluorescence using primary antibodies (raised against CTB in rats) and FITC-labeled secondary antibodies (Fig 19.1). The size of the microspheres was maintained below 5 μm (range 0.5 - 5μm). Microspheres equivalent to 5Lf tetanus toxoid suspended in saline were administered to animals by oral route followed by an oral booster after 8 days. It was observed that systemic antibody response could be elicited by CTB conjugated microspheres (Fig 19.2; Diwan M, Khar RK and Talwar GP; unpublished data).

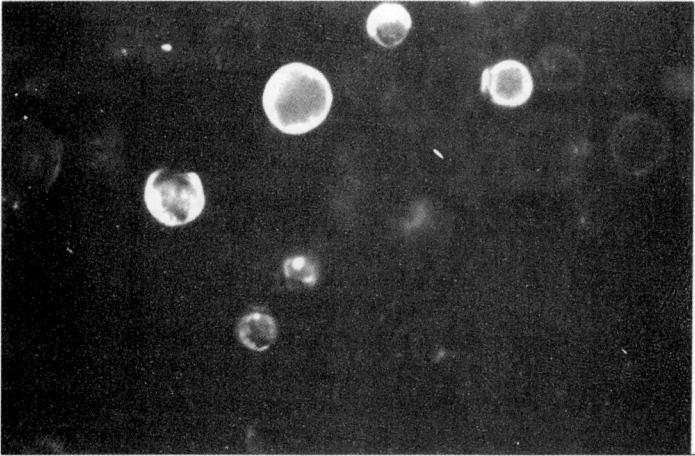

Fig 19.1: Photomicrograph shows fluorescent TT microspheres carrying CTB on their surface as homing agent for Peyer's patches. Primary antibodies were rat anti-CTB while the secondary were anti-rat IgG labelled with FITC. The fluorescence on the surface of microshperes shows the presence of CTB.

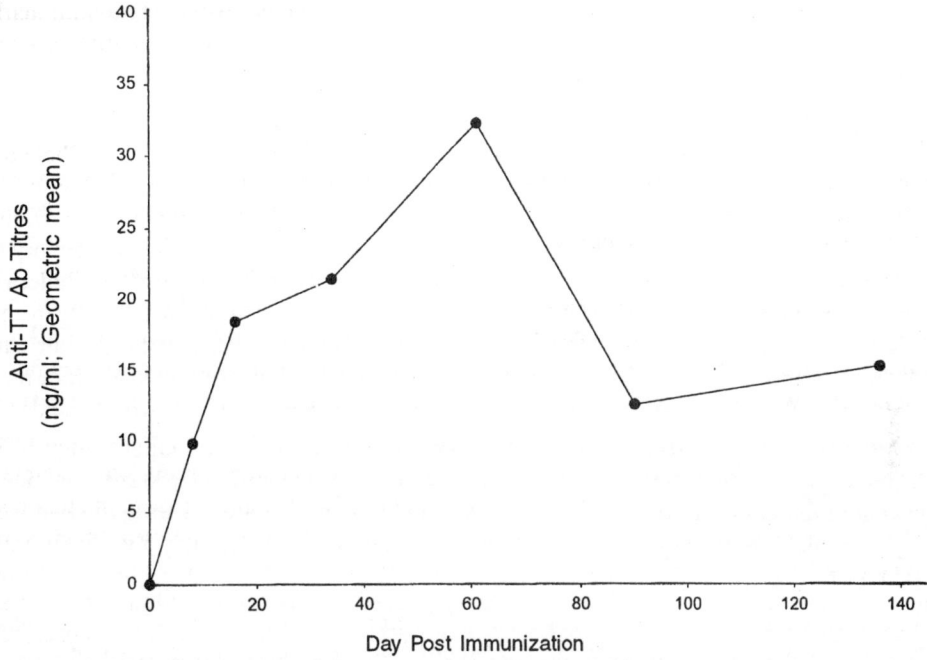

Fig 19. 2: The graph shows kinetics of immune response generated against tetanus toxoid in Wistar rats. Animals were immunized with TT encapsulated microspheres with a homing agent, CTB, present on the surface. Microspheres equivalent to 5Lf TT were orally administered on day 0 followed by a booster dose of 5Lf on day 8 in saline.

19.3.2 Lectins as targeting agents

Endogenous carbohydrate-binding proteins of tumors are commonly known as lectins. These act in recognitive and growth processes relevant to tumor growth and spread (Gabius et al, 1986). As lectins have been detected in a variety of human tumor cells, these may be utilized for better clinical management of tumors with a selective lectin-mediated uptake of therapeutically active glycoproteins by the infected cells (Wirth et al, 1998a). The carrier potential of glycoproteins or synthetic neoglycoproteins in this system of specific carbohydrate-protein interaction can thus be exploited to direct drugs to certain cell types. Whereas carbohydrates on the carrier render it accessible to the lectin-mediated uptake, the co-transported drugs will be released after intracellular proteolysis of the carrier. For human embryonic carcinoma cell lines, the use of fluorosceinated neoglycoproteins chemically coupled to etoposide, cis-Pt, or methotrexate, revealed that neoglycoproteins serve as significantly better carriers as compared to nonglycosylated carrier. Glycosylation of the carrier (serum albumin) with lactose, melibiose or maltose confered upto 10-fold increase in cytotoxicity to the drug-carrier conjugate as compared to the conjugate of nonglycosylated albumin (Gabius et al, 1987). In the case of melanoma cell lines, lactose and mannose proved to be effective for glycosylation (Gabius & Vehmeyer, 1987).

Wirth and colleagues (1998b) explored the potential of the wheat germ agglutinin (WGA) as a targeting agent for an acid-labile chemotherapeutic prodrug of doxorubicin, for the colon carcinoma cells in vitro. The lectin-prodrug conjugate's binding capacity and anti-proliferative activity on Caco-2 cells was measured. The lectin conjugated prodrug yielded 160% of the cytostatic activity as compared with that of free doxorubicin.

Lectins for different tissues and tumors show restricted expression. With the preparation of more refined carbohydrate structures on glycoproteins, matching the specificity of the target lectin, neoglycoproteins can thus become alternatives to monoclonal antibodies as carriers. They have the further advantage over monoclonal antibodies for high drug loading by chemical conjugation without loss of activity. This is of paramount importance for drugs that are poorly taken up by cells and for drug-resistant cells that get low local concentrations of drug (Pozansky & Juliano, 1984).

19.3.3 Low molecular weight proteins for renal drug targeting

Low molecular-weight proteins accumulate in the proximal tubular cells of the kidney, which makes these proteins interesting tools for renal drug targeting. A renal-specific controlled release of an active drug may enable a reduction in the required dose and may provide a reduction in the extra-renal toxicity. Haas et al (1997) studied the targeting of the NSAID naproxen to the kidney using the low molecular weight protein, lysozyme, as carrier since it is mainly taken up and catabolized in the proximal tubules of the kidney. It was observed that, as native lysozyme, the conjugate was predominantly and rapidly (within 20 min) taken up by the kidney. No detectable amounts of free naproxen were present in the plasma after administration of the conjugate. The conjugation of the drug with lysozyme resulted in a 70-fold increase of naproxen accumulation in the kidney.

Lysozyme was studied as a carrier for the angiotensin-converting enzyme inhibitor captopril that was conjugated to lysozyme and administered in rats. The total amount of captopril in the kidney was detected as six times higher after the administration of the conjugate than the administration of an equivalent amount of free captopril. It was also observed that the circulating concentration of the free drug was also reduced after conjugation (Kok et al, 1999).

When the tubular reabsorption of a low molecular weight protein such as lysozyme, can be prevented, the protein will be excreted in the urine. The lysozyme (LZM) drug conjugates may then also be used as carriers for targeting to the urinary tract. A positively charged protein carrier was synthesized with FITC conjugated to lysozyme (FITC-LZM). The positive charge of the conjugate was neutralized by succinylation of the conjugate (Suc-FITC-LZM) at the free amino acids sites. By decreasing the positive charge on the carrier surface, the excretion of the drug-lysozyme conjugate was increased in the urine from 29% to 45% (Kok et al, 1998).

Human serum albumin has also been described as a carrier for targeting naproxen to non-parenchymal liver cells to protect against endotoxin induced liver damage (Lebbe et al, 1997).

In normal rat livers, cell-sensitive delivery of drugs to hepatocytes, endothelial cells and Kupffer cells can be achieved by coupling drugs to lactosaminated human serum albumin (HSA), succinylated HSA and lactosaminated HSA, respectively (Beljaars et al, 1998). It was reported that cell-specific delivery of sugar and charge-modified albumins in fibrotic livers is possible. Despite the increased matrix deposition during fibrosis, the accessibility of different liver cell types for the carriers was not significantly altered as compared to normal livers. These sugar- and charge-modified albumins provide opportunities for development of effective therapeutic strategies based on targeting the drug to the specific cell types of liver.

Dextran has been investigated for its intestinal absorption behaviour in view of its receptor-mediated transportation. The results suggested high potential of the polysaccharide as an oral drug carrier (Koyama et al, 1992; Hovgaard & Brondsted, 1995).

Receptor-mediated targeting of cytosine b-D arabinoside, a model drug, to liver has been described using glycosylated dextran as macromolecular carrier. Dextran (T70) was selected because of its high water-solubility, many hydroxyl groups (which are easily modified chemically) and low immunogenicity (Koyama et al, 1996; Nishikawa et al, 1992).

In another study, a polymeric prodrug of streptomycin was coupled via a spacer, glycine hydrazide, onto derivatized dextran for the treatment of intracellular infections. For targeting to macrophages, 6-aminohexyl-a-D-mannopyranoside groups were introduced on the carrier. It was observed that streptomycin in vitro release from the carrier was faster in the lysosomal pH of 5.2 (Coessens et al, 1996).

Inulin hydrogels as carrier for colonic drug targeting have also been reported (Vervoort et al, 1997).

19.3.4 Hormones functioning as specific ligands for receptors on the specific targets

Insulin has been examined as enzyme carrier in vitro with a possibility of correcting an enzyme deficiency disease in fibroblasts from a patient with a cholesterol storage disease. The approach was to use insulin as a targeting agent with a view that following binding to the insulin receptor on the cell surface, the complex would undergo internalization by a process resembling receptor-mediated endocytosis with the eventual deposition of the complex in the lysosome. Incubating fibroblast cells with enzyme that was conjugated with excess of insulin resulted in a highly significant reduction in the cholesterol ester and a concomitant increase in free cholesterol levels (Pozansky et al, 1984).

19.4 CHEMICAL APPROACH

Chemical approach incorporates targeting considerations into the drug design process and represents a novel, systematic methodology for the design of a safe, localized delivery of compounds. The chemical delivery systems allow targeting of active biological molecules to specific target sites or organs, based on predictable enzymatic activation. Also, incorporation of some groups in the structure of the active molecule is done so as to deactivate and detoxify the drug subsequent to exerting its biological effects (Bodor & Buchwald, 1997).

The site-specific chemical delivery system (CDS) is produced by chemical reactions with the target drug, which is then covalently coupled with one or more carrier moieties and if necessary one or more protective moieties. By design, after delivery the CDS will undergo a variety of enzymatic conversions, which produce intermediates such as CDS1 CDS2 ... CDSn, all having different physical properties and varying rates of formation and elimination, thus ultimately allowing a preferential and favourable distribution of the precursor drug [PD] at the site of action where ultimately the drug is released. The complex design process thus involves knowledge and use of the various enzymatic reactions and the rate differences between these reactions and eliminations. One important concern is that the various forms of CDS, including the direct precursor are inactive and non-toxic, thus allowing that the distributional processes will lead to the release of the active drug only at the site. This is summarized as follows:

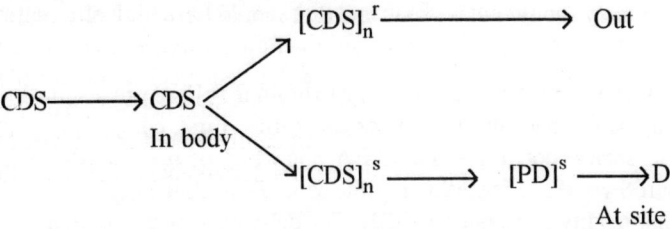

('s' superscript indicates the site and superscript 'r' the rest of the body)

Thus the concentration of the important precursors and intermediates will be significantly higher at the site of action than the rest of the body.

This approach can allow not only the site-enhanced specific delivery, but also the sustained release of pharmacologically active concentrations at the active sites as desired. The drug released at the site will then produce the desired pharmacological activity, after which it will undergo the usual metabolism-elimination. By design, the ultimate and the intermediate moieties produced by the various enzymatic reactions should also be nontoxic and easily eliminated from the body.

In another case, where the intermediate or final enzymatic reactions occur only at the site of action, the drug can directly be released specifically at the site of action. Here, the drug is released only at the site of action as enzymatic reactions responsible for producing the drug do not take place at or, if they do, at a much lower rate in the rest of the body, than at the site. For example, enzymes present in the iris-ciliary body are used to produce the active drugs only at that site, which is the site of action, while CDS distributed throughout the rest of body will not produce the active drug.

19.4.1 Drug targeting to lungs

A novel approach using chemical delivery system to a delivery mechanism for drug targeting to lung tissue was reported by Saah et al (1996). The 1,2-dithiolane-3-pentyl moiety of lipoic acid was used as the 'targeting moiety'. The in vitro kinetic and in vivo pharmacokinetic studies showed that the chemical delivery systems comprising of ester derivatives of the two drugs, chlorambucil and cromolyn, were sufficiently stable in buffer and biological media. In the lung tissue these hydrolyzed rapidly into the respective active parent drugs, and significantly enhanced delivery and retention of the active compounds to lung tissue in comparison with the underivatized parent compounds used in conventional therapy.

19.4.2 Drug targeting to brain

The blood-brain barrier (BBB) is a unique protective barrier that provides a very efficient exclusion of a variety of blood-borne compounds from the brain by obstructing the free flow of blood between brain and the rest of the body (Pardridge et al, 1975; Rapoport, 1976). This also prevents the penetration of hydrophilic compounds such as various neurotransmitters, amino acids etc. unless these are transported into the brain by an active transport system. The amount of a drug that reaches the brain depends on molecular size, lipophilicity and largely on its affinity for various blood proteins, specific enzymes in the blood or BBB. The impermeability of BBB for hydrophilic substances such as the neurotransmitters prevents their loss to blood plasma after synthesis in the brain which confines the neurotransmitters to near site of release and action. This recognition that the BBB should act as a barrier against the efflux of hydrophilic molecules formed in situ has lead to the development of brain targeting of drugs by 'chemical approach' or 'redox chemical delivery system' (Bodor et al, 1981). The basic principle being if by using an enzymatic process, ubiquitous in nature, a lipophilic molecule that can penetrate the BBB is converted into a hydrophilic compound, then its efflux from the brain will be restricted while at the same time its elimination from the rest of the body is accelerated. Importantly, the enzymatic modifications of the properties of the whole molecule should not affect the pharmacologically active compound. Also, the separated carrier moiety should not be toxic and that should have high elimination rate from the brain.

The use of the 'redox chemical delivery system' for drug targeting to brain may be of great significance to many substrate drugs. These drugs may be divided into two major categories. First, compounds that have difficulty in penetrating the BBB defense, such as dopamine and GABA; and which do not cross the BBB at all, such as antiviral compounds like trifluorothymidine, or antibiotics like penicillins, cephalosporins, etc. In the second category, fall the compounds that readily penetrate the BBB. The delivery of these compounds to the brain by this approach will result in substantial and effective separation of the brain and the rest of the body to reduce the peripheral effects and toxicity. For example, drugs such as steroid hormones like estradiol, or various antiepileptic drugs like phenytoin, valproic acid, etc.

In one such study, dopamine was delivered using the N1-substituted dihydropyridine-pyridinium salt-type redox system. This drug-carrier complex was sufficiently lipophilic for distribution throughout the body after intravenous administration to rats. The lipophilic drug-carrier complex had to undergo steps of sequential hydrolytic and oxidative conversions at the redox carrier part to generate ultimately the precursor drug which on further cleavage lead to the release of dopamine in the brain. A 15-fold difference in the brain and blood concentration for the drug was measured after 40 minutes of delivery (Bodor & Farag, 1983). A 1mg/Kg dose of dopamine as drug-carrier complex resulted in about 80% decrease in the serum prolactin levels which sustained for over 12 hours in the experimental rats (Bodor & Simpkins, 1983).

Similarly, GABA was delivered in rats using the redox chemical system. The delivery system showed significant CNS activity both as an anticonvulsant and anxiolytic (Anderson et al ,1987).

Radiolabeled Abetal-40 images brain amyloid in tissue sections of Alzhemier's disease autopsy of brain, but this peptide radiopharmaceutical can not be used for imaging brain amyloid in vivo owing to negligible transport through the BBB. Wu and colleagues (1997) studied the possibility of brain targeting of I125-Abetal-40. Monobiotinylated radioactive-Abetal was conjugated to a BBB delivery system comprising of a complex of the monoclonal antibody to the human insulin receptor, which was coupled to streptavidin. A marked uptake of the peptide was noticed within 3 hours of intravenous administration. The radioactive peptide was degraded in brain with export of the iodide radioactivity, and by 48 hours 90% of the radioactivity was cleared from the brain. Other peptide-radiopharmaceuticals may also be targeted using this methodology for imaging brain disorders.

19.4.3 Osteotropic drug delivery

A bisphosphonic (BP) prodrug for 17 beta-estradiol (E2) was developed for the estrogen replacement therapy in the patients of post menopausal oesteoporosis. Intravenous administration of E2-BP in ovariectomized rats resulted in rapid uptake of E2, which showed a half-life of 13.5 days. The bone concentration of regenerated estradiol was maintained for 28 days after a single application, which was significantly higher than free E2 administered either by intravenous or oral routes. The drug delivered by such a delivery system is expected to result in lower adverse effects and less frequent medication in the long-term E2 replacement therapy (Fujisaki et al, 1997).

19.5 CONCLUDING REMARKS

It is very difficult for a drug molecule to reach its destination (site of action) in the complex cellular network of an organism. Targeted delivery of drugs, as the name suggests, is to assist the drug molecule to reach preferably to the desired site. The inherent advantage of this technique has been the reduction in the dose and side effects of the drug.

By virtue of their size smaller than that of blood capillaries, intravenously administered particulate drug carriers get accumulated in the liver cells. Among the particulate drug carriers liposomes are a potential mode of delivery for the treatment of intracellular infections as the cells of mononuclear phagocytic system easily take these up.

Microparticles may serve as future mode of delivery for oral route especially for the drugs of protein nature. Orally delivered microparticles (<5 μm in size) are taken up by the Peyer's patches. This leads to induction of immune response against the antigen released from the microparticles. Also, the antigen is protected from the loss of activity in the GI tract. A major limitation is the effective uptake of these particles from the GI tract, which is even less than 1%. However, a combination of biological approach such as incorporation of specific ligands on the surface of these particles enhances their uptake.

Magnetic drug targeting, even though is effective but can not be employed in routine clinical applications. The use of strong magnetic fields and the unknown long term toxicity status of the ferrofluids are factors associated with its limited implementation.

Of course, biological approach is more specific but at the same time the biology is notoriously known for variations and mutations. The highly specific monoclonal antibodies may also show cross-reactivity. The common source of the mAbs employed in the targeting studies is rodents, which can not be used for humans. Interestingly, technologies are now available to 'humanize' such antibodies. The biological approach may find ultimately great clinical applications.

Neoglycoproteins (lectins) are also useful targeting agents. These offer certain advantages over mAbs such as higher drug loading and retention of the activity after chemical conjugation with the drug moieties.

The chemical approach looks impressive especially for the drug delivery to the brain which may not be possible using the conventional modes of delivery. It is however very difficult to design and control the pharmacokinetics of chemical delivery system involving several prodrugs and intermediates. The acute and chronic toxicity of every component other than the whole moiety needs to be established.

Overall it may be concluded that with the vast database of the in vitro and animal studies, the science of site specific or targeted delivery has become wiser. Manifestation of these strategies in clinics now seems possible in near future.

REFERENCES

Al-Janabi, M.A.A.; Heyam, A.Y. and Al-Salem, A.M. (1984) Int J Appl Radiat Iso, 35 : 209-214.

Anderson, W.; Simpkins, J.; Woodard, P.; Winwood Stern W. and Bodor, N. (1987) Psychopharmacology, 92 :157-163.

Beljaars, L.; Poelstra, K.; Molema G and Meijer DK (1998) J Hepatol, 29: 579-588.

Bodor, N. and Buchwald, P. (1997) Pharmacol ther, 76: 1-27.

Bodor, N. and Farag, H. (1983) J Med Chem, 26: 528-534.

Bodor, N. and Simpkins. J. (1983) Science, 221: 65-67.

Bodor. N.; Farag, H. and Brewster, M. (1981) Science, 214 : 1370-1372.

Bradfield, J.W.B. (1980) Br J Exp Path, 61: 617-623.

Bugelsky, P; Kirsch, R.; Sowinski, J.M. and Poste, G. (1985) Am J Pathol, 118 : 419-424.

Carayanniotis, G. and Barber, B.H. (1987) Nature, 327 : 59-61.

Casten, L.A.; Kaumaya, P. and Pierce, S.K. (1988) J Exp Med, 168 : 171-180.

Challacombe, S.J.; Rahman, D. and O'Hagan, D.T. (1997) Vaccine, 15 : 169-175.

Coessens, V.; Schacht, E. and Domurado, D. (1996) J Control Rel, 38 : 141-150.

Davis, S.S. (1997) Trends Biotechnol, 15 : 217-224

Deodhar, S.D.; Barna, B.P.; Edinger, M. and Chiang, T. (1982) J Biol Resp Modifiers, 1 : 27-34.

Dertzbaugh, M.T. and Elson, C.O. (1991) In: Topics in vaccine adjuvant research. Spriggs, D.R. and Koff, W.C. (Eds) CBC Press, Boca Raton, Florida, 119-132.

Desiderio, J.V. and Campbell, S.G. (1983) J Reticuloendothelial Soc, 34: 279-287.

Dingle, J.T.; Gordon, J.C.; Hazelman, B.L.; Knight, C.G.; Thomas, D.P.P.; Phillips, N.C.; Shaw, I.H.; Fildes, F.J.T.; Oliver, J.E.; Jones, G.; Turner, E.A. and Lowe, J.S. (1978) Nature, 271 : 372-373.

Edelman, R.; Russell, R.G., Losonsky, G.; Tall, B.D.; Tacket, C.O.; Levine, M.M. and Lewis, D.H. (1993) Vaccine, 11: 155-158.

Ehrlich, P. (1906) In: Collected Studies on Immunity.2: 442-447.

Eldridge, J.H.; Hammond, C.J.; Meulbroek, J.A.; Staas, .J.K.; Gilley, R.M. and Tice, T.R. (1990) J Control Rel, 11 : 205-214.

Eldridge, J.H.; Meulbroek, J.A.; Staas, J.K.; Tice, T.R. and Gilley, R.M. (1989) Adv Exp Med Biol, 251: 192-202.

Eldridge, J.H.; Stass, J.K.; Meulbroek, J.A.; Tice, T.R. and Gilley, R.M. (1991) Infect Immun, 9 : 2978-2986.

Ermak, T.H.; Dougherty, E.P.; Bhagat, H.R.; Kabok, Z. and Pappo, J. (1995) Cell Tissue Res, 279 : 433-436.

Fidler, I.J, and Raz, A. (1981) In: Lymphokines. Pick, E. (Ed): 345-364. Academic Press, New York.

Fidler, I.J.; Hart, I.R.; Raz, A.; Fogler, W.E.; Kirsh, R. and Poste, G. (1980) In: Liposome and Immunobiology. Tom BH and Six H (Eds): 109-118. Elsevier, New York.

Fountain, M.W.; Dees, C. and Schultz, R.D. (1981) Curr Microbiol, 6 : 373-376.

Fujisaki, J.; Tokunga, Y.; Takahashi, T.; Kimura, S.; Shimojo, F. and Hata, T. (1997) Biol Pharm Bull, 20 : 1183-1187.

Gabius, H.J. and Vehmeyer, K. (1987) Naturwissenschaften, 74: 37-38.

Gabius, H.J.; Bokemeyer, C.; Hellmann, T. and Schmoll, H.J. (1987) J Cancer Res Clin Oncol, 113 :126-130.

Gabius, HJ.; Vehmeyer, K.; Engelhardt, R.; Nagel, G.A. and Cramer, F. (1986) Cell Tissue Res, 246 : 515-521.

Gregoriadis, G.; Senior, J.; Wolfe, B. and Kirby, C. (1985) Ann NY Aced Sci, 446 : 319-340.

Gurny, R.; Boye, T. and Ibrahim, H. (1985) J Control Rel, 2 : 353-361.

Haas, M.; Kluppel, A.C.; Wartna, E.S.; Moolenaar, F.; Meijer, D.K. de Jong, P.E. and de Zeeuw, D. (1997) Kidney Int, 52 : 1693-1699.

Hovgaard, L. and Brondsted, H. (1995) J Control Rel, 36 : 159-166.

Inaba, K. and Steinman, R.M. (1985) Science, 229 : 475-479.

Juliano, R.L. and McCullough, H.N. (1980) J Pharmacol Exp Ther, 214 : 381-387.

Kende, M.; Alving, C.R.; Rill, W.L.; Swatz, G.M. and Cononico, P.G. (1985) Antimicrob Agents Chemother, 27: 903-907.

Kok, R.J.; Haas, M.; Moolenaar, F.; de Zeeuw, D. and Meijer, D.K. (1998) Ren Fail, 20 : 211-217.

Kok, R.J.; Grijpstra, F. Walthuis, R.B.; Moolenaar, F. de Zeeuw, D. and Meijer, D.K. (1999) J Pharmacol Exp Ther, 288 : 281-285.

Koyama, Y.; Kawaide, A. and Katoake, K. (1992) Procee Intern Sym Control Rel Bioact Mater, 19 : 38-39.

Koyama, Y.; Miya gawa, T.; Kawaide, A. and Kataoka, K. (1996) J Control Rel, 41: 171-176.

Lebbe, C.; Reichen, J.; Wartna, E.; Sagessar, H.; Poelstra, K. and Meijer, D.K. (1997) J Drug Target, 4 : 303-310.

Lehnert, B.E.; Valdez, Y.E. and Stewart, C.C. (1968) Exp Lung Res, 10: 245-266.

Lobenberg, R. and Kreuter, J. (1996) AIDS Res Human Retroviruses, 12: 1709-1715.

Lopez-Berstein, G.; Mehta, R.; Hopfer, R.L.; Mills, K.; Kasi, L.; Mehta, K,.; Fainstein, V.; Luna, M.; Hersh, E.M. and Juliano, R. (1983) J. Infect. Dis. 5 : 939-945.

Lubbe, A.S.; Bergemann, C.;Huhnt, W.; Fricke. T,; Riess, H.; Brock, J.W. and Huhn, D. (1996a) Cancer Res., 56 : 4694-4701.

Lubbe, A.S.; Bergemann,C.; Riess, H.; Schriever, F.; Reichardt, P.; Possinger, K.; Matthias, M.; Dorken, B.;, Herrmann, F.; Gurtler, R.; Hohenberger, P.; Haas, N.; Sohr, R.; Sander, B.; Lemke, A.J.; Ohlendorff, D.; Huhnt, W. and Huhn, D. (1996b) Cancer Res, 56 : 4686-4693.

Martodam, R.R.; Twumasi, D.Y.; Liener, I.E.; Powers, J.C.;, Nishino, N. and Krejcarek, G. (1979) Proc. Natl. Acad Sci. USA, 76 : 2128-2132.

McQueen, C.E.; Boedeker, E.C.; Reid, R.; Jarboe, D.; Wolf, M.; Le, M. and Brown, W.R. (1993) Vaccine, 11 : 201-206.

Mufson D and Szoka FC (1985) Pharm Technol, 1 : 16-21.

Muzykantov V.R.; Zaltsman A.B.; Smirnov M.D.; Samokhin G.P and Morgan B.P (1996) Biochim Biophys Acta, 1279 :137-143.

Muzykantov, V.R.; Christofidou-Solomidou, M.; Balyasnikova, I.; Harshaw D.W.; Schultz L.; Fisher A.B and Albelda S.M (1999) Proc Natl Acad Sci, USA, 96 : 2379-2384.

Nedrud, J.G. and Lamm, M.E. (1991) In: Topics in vaccine adjuvant research. Spriggs DR and Koff WC (Eds) CBC Press, Boca Raton, Florida, 54-67.

New, R.R.C.; Chance M.L. and Heath, S. (1981) Parasitol, 83 : 519-527.

Nishikawa, M.; Yamashita F, Takakura Y, Hashida M and Sezaki H (1992) Procee Intern Sym Control Rel Bioact Mater, 19 : 133-134.

Noble J, Jones A.G, Davis M.A, Sledge C.B, Kramer R.I and Levini E (1983) J Bone Joint Surg, 65A : 381-389.

O'Hagan D.T (1990) Adv Drug Del Rev, 5 : 265-285.

Papahadjopoulos, D. (Ed) 1978. Liposomes and their Use in Biology and Medicine. Ann NY Acad Sci, 398.

Parant, M.; Parant, F.; Chedid, L.; Yapo, A.; Petit, J.F and Lederer, L (1979) Int J Immunopharmacol, 1: 35-41.

Pardridge, W.; Connor, J.D and Crawford, LL (1975) CRC Crit Rev Toxic, 3 : 159-199.

Poznansky, M.J and Juliano, R.J (1984) Pharmacol Rev, 36 : 278-336.

Poznansky, M.J.; Singh, R.; Singh, B. and Fantus, G. (1984) Science, 223 : 1304-1306.

Rapoport S.I. (1976) Raven Press, New York.

Ratcliffe, J.H.; Hunneyball, I.M.; Wilson, C.G.; Smith, A. and Davis, S.S. (1984) In: Microspheres and Drug Therapy. Pharmaceutical, Immunological and Medicinal Aspects. Davis SS, Illum L, McVie JG and Tomlinson, E. (Eds) 345-346, Elsevier, Amsterdam.

Reid, R.H.; Boedeker, E.C.; McQueen, C.E.; Davis, D.; Tseng L.Y.; Kodak, J.; Sau, K.; Wilhelmsen, C.L.; Nellore, R.; Dalal, P. and Bhagat, H.R. (1993) Vaccine, 11: 159-167.

Saah, M.; Wu, W.M.; Eberst, K.; Marvanyos, E. and Bodor, N. (1996) J Pharm Sci, 85 : 496-504.

Schroder, U. and Sabel B.A. (1996) Brain Res, 710 : 121-124.

Smolin, G.; Okumoto, M.; Feiler, S. and Condon, D. (1981) Am J Opthalmol, 91: 220-225.

Snider, D.P. and Segal, D.M. (1987) J Immunol, 139 : 1609-1616.

Snipes M.B, Chavez G.T and Muggenburg B.A. (1984) Environ Res, 33 : 333-342.

Staas, J.K.; Hunt, R.E.; Marx, P.A.; Compans, R.W.; Smith, J.F.; Eldridge, J.H.; Gibson, J.W.; Tice, T.R. and Gilley, R.M. (1993) Proceed Intern Symp Control Rel Bioact Mater, 20 : 63-64.

Staerz, U.D. and Bevan, M.J. (1986) Immunol Today, 7, 241.

Taylor, R.L.; Williams, D.M.; Craven, P.C.; Graybill, J.R.; Drytz, J. and Magee, W.E. (1982) Am Rev Respir Dis, 125, 610-611.

Tomlinson, E.; Davis, S.S. and Illum, L. (1986) In Delivery Systems for peptide drugs. In: Davis, S.S.; Illum, L. and Tomlinson, E. (Eds) Plenum Press, New York, 351-355.

Vervoort, L.; Van de Mooter, G.; Augustijns, P.; Busson, R.; Toppet, S. and Kinget, R. (1997) Pharm Res, 14: 1730-1737.

Widder KJ, Marino PA, Morriss RM, Howard DP, Poor GA and Senyei AE (1983) Eur J Cancer Clin Oncol, 19: 141-147.

Wirth, M.; Hamilton, G. and Gabor, F. (1998a) J Drug Target, 6: 95-104.

Wirth, M.; Fuchs, A.; Wolf, M.; Ertl. B. and Gabor, F. (1998b) Pharm Res, 15: 1031-1037.

Wu, D.; Yang, J. and Pradridge, W.M. (1997) J Clin Invest, 100: 1804-1812.

Yang, S.C.; Lu, Lf.; Cai, Y.; Zhu, J.B.; Liang, B.W. and Yang, C.Z. (1999) J Control Rel, 59: 299-307.

Index